Case Management in Healthcare

Case Management in Healthcare

A PRACTICAL GUIDE

Peggy Rossi, RN, MPA, CCM

President, Case Management Society of America
  Northern California
Director of Medical Management
Western Health Advantage
Sacramento, California

W.B. SAUNDERS COMPANY
A Division of Harcourt Brace & Company
Philadelphia   London   Toronto   Montreal   Sydney   Tokyo

W.B. SAUNDERS COMPANY
A Division of Harcourt Brace & Company

The Curtis Center
Independence Square West
Philadelphia, Pennsylvania 19106

Library of Congress Cataloging-in-Publication Data

Rossi, Peggy Gray.

Case management in healthcare: a practical guide / Peggy Gray Rossi.—1st ed.

p.   cm.

Includes bibliographical references and index.

ISBN 0–7216–7175–6

1. Community health services—Case studies.   2. Medical care—Case
   studies.   I. Title. [DNLM: 1. Case Management.   2. Delivery of
   Health Care. W 84.7 R833c 1999]

RA427.R67   1999   362.1—dc21

DNLM/DLC   98-9757

CASE MANAGEMENT IN HEALTHCARE: A PRACTICAL GUIDE   ISBN 0-7216-7175-6

Printed in the United States of America.

Last digit is the print number: 9   8   7   6   5   4   3   2   1

IN MEMORY

This book is dedicated to the memory of my dad who, because of two horrific back injuries and then the prior stigma associated with mental health, the lack of mental health benefits, and more importantly, a lack of understanding of pain management, died a premature death—all from the ravages of pain. As a result of these events, I always strive to educate patients and families about the alternatives available, making every attempt to link them to the appropriate resources. With this education, hopefully the patients and families can have some quality and normalcy to their lives.

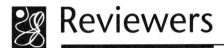

Reviewers

Kathleen M. Andolina, RN, MS, CS

Clinical Nurse Specialist, Adult Psychiatric
  Nursing
Bournewood Health Systems
Brookline, Massachusetts
Adjunct Assistant Professor
Department of Nursing
Massachusetts College of Pharmacy and Allied
  Health Sciences
Boston, Massachusetts

Vicky A. Mahn, RN, MS

Senior Consultant, Outcome Management
MIDS, Inc.
Tucson, Arizona

Carol Y. Phillips, PhD, RN

Chair and Professor, Department of Nursing
Millersville University
Millersville, Pennsylvania

Janet M. Stallmeyer, MSN, MBA

Principal Health Care of Kansas City
Kansas City, Missouri

Preface

The writing of *Case Management in Healthcare: A Practical Guide* has been an exciting endeavor that started several years ago at the prodding of newly hired case managers. These nurses were struggling with their cases and seeking "basic" solutions. As I would give them information, they kept expressing a desire for "more" in the form of a concrete reference manual. Thus, now their wish is fulfilled.

Certainly, *Case Management in Healthcare: A Practical Guide* is by no means a cookbook for case management. Such a task would be impossible because the accuracy of such a book could never be maintained to its final completion. This is true not only because of our ever-changing healthcare environment but also because of the multiplicity of case variables encountered with each patient. Another reason is that agency names and the services they render vary drastically not only from state to state but also often from county to county within a state. Budgetary constraints of many organizations may lead to programs that are here today and gone tomorrow. As we in healthcare know, when this occurs patients and healthcare workers are left scrambling for alternative sources for payment or provisions for the care and services. Thus, with the many name and service changes, the book would be out of date before printing.

As a result, I have made every attempt to write *Case Management in Healthcare: A Practical Guide* in such a way that it gives the basics required to complete a case manager's tasks. From these basics the case manager can further research the community to determine which agency or resources are available to provide the care.

I am a strong believer that the key to establishing services for patients is a keen awareness of the services and resources and their availability whether it be in the immediate service area, regionally, or nationally. This key is further expanded by a basic knowledge of alternate funding programs, as well as the types of patients served by the major agencies or programs, the services or benefits they provide, their referral processes, and in some cases, the appeal processes.

What is the best way to keep abreast of resources and changes? Networking with your peers in the industry. This can be done in person, by telephone, or by joining the various professional organizations. Also, as I tell new case managers—"learn to let our fingers do the walking, make extensive notes of the services provided by the various agencies and providers, and always get personal names and phone numbers for future use."

We in the case management industry know that case management is a labor intensive process. In most cases the rewards of success can be the most exhilarating of experiences. Case management challenges us to constantly keep our clinical, business, management, and other skills (e.g., thinking, analytic, and research abilities) attuned and sharp. It also challenges us to be diverse, creative, and innovative if we are to be effective and assist patients and families in accessing and using the healthcare delivery system appropriately. More importantly, case management challenges us to be effective communicators, interacting and collaborating with all levels of case management (i.e., facility-based, community-based, home health, healthcare payor) and the healthcare team.

Case management comes in many types; it is provided by various levels of expertise; and it is influenced by differing organizational goals. No one type of case management is more important or "professional" than the other. We all have our place if, as a team, we are to move the patient through the continuum of care.

With this in mind, *Case Management in Healthcare: A Practical Guide* is written to offer a comprehensive reference of the basics for establishing care, services, and alternate funding for patients. The book draws from my background as a discharge planner, utilization reviewer, and healthcare payor case manager. I have attempted to focus on the importance of all case managers working closely with each other for joint planning. I have included the healthcare payor case management perspective, as it can offer valuable input into overall planning. Far too often case managers are left out of the picture, as their role is often confused with that of the healthcare payor's utilization review nurses.

The focus of the healthcare payor's case manager is included largely because the healthcare industry has shifted its operating model to managed care. Sharing knowledge among all case managers is especially important because of shorter lengths of stay and a more technology-dependent post-acute care population. The payor's perspective is also included because linkage with the appropriate provider is important. A client's care needs not only must be met, but

the client's resources, healthcare benefits, and payor conditions must be wisely managed to ensure they have been applied to effective and appropriate care. Thus, we must all work collaboratively in this new "business": cost-conscious healthcare delivery.

My purpose in writing this book is to foster a basic awareness of the various resources available in any given community or region and the impact the healthcare payor and the patient's healthcare coverage has on the overall process. I also wish to encourage my colleagues to make use of their clinical expertise, skills, and creativity in navigating the existing managed care enviroment.

My thanks and gratitude to all who made this book possible. Thank you, Thank you!

PEGGY ROSSI

Acknowledgments

A special acknowledgment goes to my friend, Eleanor Soltau, RN, BA, BSN, Director of Case Management, First Care Healthcare, Austin, Texas. Eleanor was my driving force to complete this project. Without her prodding and nagging, it might never have materialized. Eleanor served as my main editor, editing this text more than once. To her I will be eternally grateful.

My husband, Nick, who was virtually an author's widower, spending hours alone as I read, researched, or wrote.

My daughter, Debbie, who spent thousands of hours typing and retyping all that I wrote. My daughter, Michele, who helped in the final hours of typing and assembly.

My friend, Glenda Evans-Shaw, BSN, RN, PHN, CIRS, CCM, who also assisted in editing this massive undertaking. Glenda is an experienced case manager who owns her own business, Nursing Concepts Incorporated in Amador City, California.

My friend, Lt. Col. Susan Repp, BSN, MPH, COHN, who edited the manuscript from a point of view of wanting to become a case manager when she retires from active military service and military public health nursing.

I would like to thank and acknowledge the following organizations or professionals who had an active role either in contributing information or reviewing what I had written. Sherill Gray, RN, Independent Case Manager, Sacramento, CA; Ann McAfee, RN, BSN, HIV/AIDS Case Manager, Davies Medical Center, San Francisco, CA; Debbie Glynn, RN, Aetna Government Health Plans, Mental Health, Fairfield, CA; Dr. Cheryl Harris, Director of Gerontology, Sutter Health Systems, Sacramento, CA; Pat Harra, Physical Therapist/Pulmonary Rehabilitation, Sutter Community Hospitals, Sacramento, CA; Greg Barlow, Physical Therapist/Cardiac Rehabilitation, Anberry Rehabilitation Hospital, Merced, CA; Donna Hope Wegener, Child Institute for Health Policy, University of Florida, Gainsville, FL; State of California Department of Rehabilitation; State of California Department of Education; Social Security Administration; State Department of Health Services/California Children's Services; The staff of Mercy American River Rehabilitation Hospital, Sacramento, CA; State of California Department of Veterans Affairs; Sally Kimball, RN, Director of Operations, OPTIONCARE Home Intravenous and Nutritional Services, Sacramento, CA; State of California Department of Developmental Services, especially John Moise; Patricia Pearson, RN, Respiratory Care Specialist, John Davis Durable Medical Equipment Company, Sacramento, CA; Sacramento County Department of Social Services.

To the nurses at University of California, Davis Medical Center, Sacramento, CA, who edited and commented on the medical technical sections of the manual—a big thank you! They were Carol Williams, RN, BS, Certified Enterostomal Therapy and Ostomy Nurse Specialist (CETN); Barbara Lord, RN, MSN, Certified Nurse Specialist Rehabilitation Nursing (CNRN); Karen Smith, RN, MSN, Certified Nurse Specialist Neurological Nursing (CNRN); Margaret Friend, RN, BSN, Certified Clinical Transplant Coordinator (CCTC); Michelle Sturges, RN, BSN, Certified Clinical Transplant Coordinator (CCTC); JoAnn Booth, RN, MA, Behavioral Sciences, Pulmonary Nurse Specialist; Joan Worblin, RN, Clinical Nurse Specialist Diabetes; Ann E. F. Sievers, RN, MACORLN, Clinical Nurse Specialist Otolaryngology UCD, and Adjunct Clinical Professor UCSF, Physiologic Nursing; Pamela Cronwell, RN, CM, Clinical Nurse III, Burn Unit.

PEGGY ROSSI

Contents

1 OVERVIEW OF CASE MANAGEMENT **1**

Origins of Case Management 2

Case Managers as Health Arena Guides 2

Definition of Case Management 4

Case Management Versus Utilization Review 4

Expertise of the Case Manager 5

Demographics Affecting Case Management 8

Case Variables and Most Common Diagnoses 8

Determination of Caseloads 9

Case Management Process 12

Case Planners 12

Communication 13

Healthcare Payor Types 14

Legislative Forces Affecting Case Management and the Continuum of Care 15

Alternate Payors 16

Common Problems in Obtaining Access to Care 17

Caregiver Burnout 18

Case Management Tools 19

Intent of Manual 20

2 CASE MANAGEMENT PROCESS **23**

Referrals 25

Verification of Eligibility 29

Preliminary Screening or Assessment 29

Clinical Assessments 30

Interviews 35

Case Management Plan 37

Implementation 40

Monitoring and Reassessments 41

Case Closure 43

Case Management Reports 43

3 FINANCIAL CONSIDERATIONS IN CASE MANAGEMENT **47**

Providers 48

Steps in Negotiating Reduced Rates 51

Cost Savings, Cost Avoidance, or Cost Benefit Analysis Reporting 53

Other Case Managers 55

Extra Contractual Process 55

Case Closure 57

4 FUNDING **59**

Financial Resources 60

Potential Financial Resources for Families 62

Title V of The Social Security Act of 1953: Children's Medical Services 64

Medicaid 69

Special Education 73

Veterans Benefits 81

Civilian Health and Medical Programs of the Uniformed Services 86

TRICARE 86

Social Security Programs 93

State Department of Rehabilitation 102

State Agency for Developmental Disabilities 104

5 BARRIERS TO EFFECTIVE CASE MANAGEMENT **111**

Questions to be Addressed Prior to Discharge of Case-Managed Patients 112

Common Barriers to Discharge 115

Overcoming Barriers to Case Management 116

6 UTILIZATION REVIEW **127**

Purpose 128

Case Management as Intensive Care Unit ... 128

Case Management Involving
Two Companies 128

Types and Categories of
Utilization Review 129

Overutilization Versus Underutilization 129

Techniques and Criteria Used in
Utilization Review 129

Levels of Review 130

Second Opinions 131

Referral Flags 131

**7 LEGAL ASPECTS OF CASE
MANAGEMENT** **133**

Confidentiality 134

Patient Rights 135

Conservatorship Versus Power of Attorney
and Durable Power of Attorney 135

Antitrust Law 137

Patient Abuse 137

Wickline Case 138

Abandonment 138

Standards of Care and Negligent
Referral 138

Provider and Patient Fraud and Abuse of
the System 139

8 GENERAL SERVICES **143**

Care of the Caregiver 144

Hiring Help for Home Care 145

Recreational Activities 148

Transportation and Travel 149

9 ANCILLARY SERVICES **155**

Durable Medical Equipment and Supplies ... 156

Self-Help Devices or Adaptive Equipment,
Other Tips for Use of Durable Medical
Equipment, and Home Modifications 162

Pharmaceuticals and Enteral Therapy 168

**10 CASE MANAGEMENT IN SPECIFIC
CLINICAL SITUATIONS** **175**

Common High-Risk Catastrophic Cases 176

Case Management of the Patient
With AIDS 198

Case Management of Cancer and
Hospice Patients 205

Case Management of the End-Stage Renal
Disease Patient 214

Case Management of the Chronically Ill or
Disabled Child or the Child With
Special Needs 219

Case Management of the
Diabetic Patient 230

Case Management of the
Geriatric Patient 234

Case Management of the Mentally
Ill Patient 241

Case Management of the Neurologically
Impaired Patient 248

Case Management of the
Transplant Patient 264

Case Management of Respiratory
Disease Patients 277

Case Management of the Cardiac Patient ... 285

Case Management of Patients Requiring
Technologically Complex
Antibiotic Therapy 289

Case Management of the Burn Patient 291

Case Management of the Patient Receiving
Total Parenteral Nutrition 294

Case Management of Patients Needing
Complex Wound Care 296

11 POST-ACUTE CARE **305**

Principles for Determining Skilled Versus
Custodial Service 306

Home Placement Versus Out-of-Home
Placement 310

Rehabilitation 316

Skilled Nursing Facility 329

Home Health Agency Care 333

**APPENDIX: COMMUNITY
RESOURCES** **341**

GLOSSARY **355**

INDEX **381**

Chapter 1

Overview of Case Management

ORIGINS OF CASE MANAGEMENT

Historically, case management as a profession has been around for years.[1] It was used formerly by administrators in many public and social programs to coordinate individual methods of locating resources, primarily for children who had benefit coverage under the Children's Medical Services program (Title V of the 1935 Social Security Act), military servicemen returning from World War II, the elderly or persons with a mental illness who were at risk of placement in long-term care facilities.

However, when case management became the newest buzz word and specialty in the medical arena in the 1980s and 1990s, it acquired a new focus. Medical and nursing case management evolved during the late 1980s, when some healthcare payors patterned their "medical case management programs" after workers' compensation management programs, offering similar services to their clients who had "catastrophic" or highly expensive medical illnesses. It was soon found that, as in workers' compensation case management, the nurses working with these patients could control costs while maintaining quality. These benefits resulted when someone remained involved with the case to ensure that the necessary resources were available and then coordinated, implemented, and monitored the case as necessary; and as problems were identified or encountered or as the patient's condition progressed, regressed, or stayed the same, this person initiated new linkages to other services. By the mid-1980s, hospitals were likewise finding that nursing case management provided assistance with the education and discharge of their more difficult patients and ultimately improved the hospital's productivity and fiscal viability.[2] Thus, these experiences provided further impetus for professional case management.

CASE MANAGERS AS HEALTH ARENA GUIDES

Many factors have contributed to the complexity of our healthcare system. Our system is now more scientific and more dependent on technology than it was formerly. These improvements have increased the average lifespan, which means that because people live longer, they also require more long-term care. The increased lifespan in turn has led to increased demands on services and resources and strained budgets to meet the demand. Ultimately, when needs cannot be met, fragmentation occurs. In addition, our healthcare system must operate under increased ethical and legal pressures, increased restraints on provider usage by healthcare payors, increased government regulations, tighter market competition, organizational mergers, and further economic constraints. Although many of these pressures are focused on containing costs, the result has been to shift care to alternative sites and create changes in healthcare payor reimbursement mechanisms.[3-6]

Healthcare consumers, especially those with a major illness or injury, often need assistance or advice in finding or using healthcare services. Case management is the natural answer to meeting this need. We use tour guides to lead us through unfamiliar places when we travel; why then should the complex healthcare arena be any different? Case management is the natural method of providing guidance through the healthcare system (Fig. 1–1).

Case management offers services that not only encourage early discharge but also help prevent hospitalization or rehospitalization. How is this achieved? It is accomplished by facilitating communication between persons at all levels of the internal hospital and external post-discharge healthcare team, and then implementing or coordinating care needs with the right alternate levels of care and existing community resources. The levels of care used must not only meet the patient's medical needs, they must also maintain quality while containing costs. More important, if done correctly, case management encourages and empowers the patient or consumer to understand and gain control over his or her own medical care; to become an educated consumer; to be more aware of healthcare costs and seek alternatives when services are limited or excluded from the benefit package; and to become knowledgeable about entitlement to and use of community resources. This empowerment is necessary because many patients in the case management arena are those who may eventually require long-term or chronic care. Thus, the patient may require healthcare or community services during their entire lifespan.

Illnesses or injuries requiring case management have historically been classified as "catastrophic." However, case management is not limited to this type of situation. This is especially true now because, as patients live longer, long-term and chronic care has emerged as a

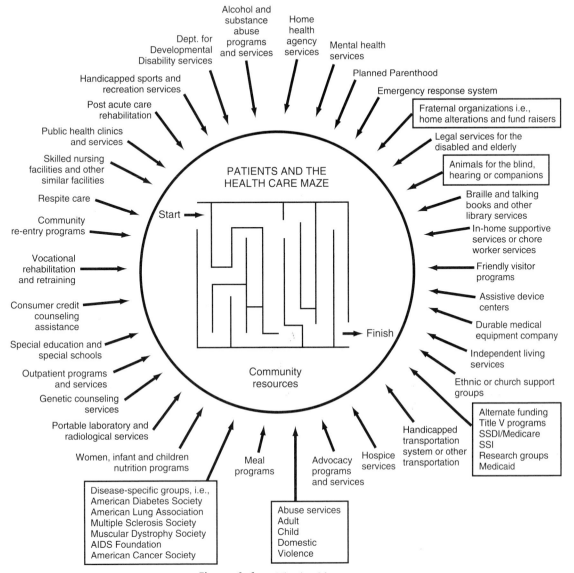

Figure 1–1 • The healthcare maze.

new drain on healthcare resources. Thus, many case management organizations offer their services to patients in this category, whereas others have established referral criteria to capture and screen all patients who have a potential need for long-term or chronic care. Their criteria are set to reflect their realization that if patient education and disease management do not occur in the very early stages of the illness, the end result may be costly long-term care.

Although ideally case management should start while the patient is in the acute or early stages of the illness or injury, this is not always possible. Early involvement may not occur because the patient is making normal progress or

because the family may be aware of community resources and refuses the offer of case management. However, because case management is not required at the onset of the disease or injury does not or should not negate the fact that it may be needed at a later date. Regardless of whether the needs are acute or chronic, referral to case management is highly recommended whenever needs are identified.

Referrals are generally based on high risk diagnostic screening criteria but must not be limited to these criteria.[7] If a problem is suspected, a referral must be made and a preliminary assessment conducted to determine whether case management is necessary.

Ideally, referrals to case management should be made as early in the case as possible or as soon as risks or needs are identified. Experience supports this principle because case management is designed to assist any patient whose care presents issues of quality or financial risk regardless of setting or intensity or severity of the person's medical or psychological condition. It is also designed to ensure a high-quality outcome, educate the patient and family in using their health benefits and resources wisely, assist them in decreasing their out-of-pocket healthcare costs, and assist healthcare payors in controlling or minimizing their costs.

DEFINITION OF CASE MANAGEMENT

What is case management? It was defined in 1992 by the National Case Management Task Force as "a collaborative process which assesses, plans, implements, coordinates, monitors and evaluates the options and services to meet an individual's needs using communication and available resources to promote quality cost-effective outcomes."[8] The American Nurses Association defines case management as "a system with many elements: health assessment, planning, procurement, delivery and coordination of services and monitoring to assure that the multiple service needs of the client are met."[9]

Very basically, case management makes the healthcare system work by ensuring that the patient is at the right level of care at the right time in his or her illness or injury and by encouraging a high quality of care at the correct price.

Case management as we know it today has acquired new meanings because of the multiplicity of organizations offering it and the great number of roles filled by case managers. The role of the "professional" case manager is not found in just one type of organization by virtue of a specific specialty, nor is it limited to one class of healthcare worker.[10, 11] Professional case managers are found in every organization that pays for healthcare services or offers comprehensive case management to its clients. Although their roles are varied, in most cases the title is applied to nurses or social workers. However, the term professional case manager is not limited to hospital professionals, nor is it limited to nurses.

For example, in the nursing profession case management may be done by nurses in the acute care facility. Here their role may be that of the primary care nurse, clinical nurse specialist, nurse educator (i.e., diabetic nurse, respiratory care nurse), or discharge planner. If the nurse is employed in the post-acute care arena, a case manager may be an employee of a home health agency, an infusion agency, a durable medical equipment company, a hospice agency, a disease-specific clinic, a skilled nursing facility, or a healthcare payor, regardless of whether the payor is in the private or public sector. In contrast, a social worker may also be a professional case manager working in either the acute or post-acute care arena.

Thus, today's case managers operate in diverse educational and clinical settings and have broader backgrounds than those found in the typical clinical hospital setting. With this in mind, the National Case Management Task Force developed criteria for the Certified Case Manager as well as a means of testing qualified applicants to become certified in their field. In addition to sitting for an examination, the applicant must have an employment history that validates his or her employment experiences and a job description that must include responsibility for patient advocacy and empowerment; along with the application, the employer must validate the fact that the individual has direct contact with patients in need of case management services. In all, there are six categories for certification. More information on certification can be obtained by writing to the following address:

Certification of Insurance Rehabilitation
   Specialist (CIRSC)
1835 Rohlwing Road
Suite D
Rolling Meadow, Illinois 60008

CASE MANAGEMENT VERSUS UTILIZATION REVIEW

Although many organizations consider case management synonymous with utilization review, they are not the same. On the whole, utilization review and case management are two completely different specialties; each has a different intent, and each requires different areas of expertise. Also, when job duties are combined, results and program goals may be vastly different. Therefore, it is strongly recommended by many case management firms and department directors that case management be separated from the tasks of utilization management. This separation of responsibilities does not mean that the case management nurse and the utilization review nurse are not integral parts of the team in their own right. It means only that both must work closely together if goals are to be reached.

Case management is in many instances a unique variation of utilization review, but it does not involve the duties associated with the normal utilization review processes such as prior authorization, preadmission screening, or concurrent review. Also, the intent of both programs is entirely different. For instance, the purpose of utilization review is to provide a means of monitoring unnecessary services and containing costs, but although the intent of case management may also involve costs, its primary focus is to maintain quality of care as the patient moves through varying levels of care as his condition changes.[12]

Case management is not needed in every case but only in a select few or in those in which quality of care can be or is an issue. It may also be needed for individuals who have the potential to place the healthcare organization at legal or financial risk. In all cases, case management objectives depend on the organization's perspective and on the design of the case management system. They also depend on (1) the population served and the population's health status; (2) the type of case management allowed or offered by an organization (i.e., telephone versus on-site contact, workers' compensation versus large case management); (3) the case manager's level of expertise; and (4) the method by which case management is linked to the organization. The method of linkage involves such factors as who performs case management (e.g., the primary care nurse or the clinical nurse specialist, who may follow the patient only while he or she is hospitalized), whether it is integrated with other healthcare payor departments, whether the duties are contracted out to independent case management organizations, and so forth. Unfortunately, far too often case management is equated and confused with utilization review!

EXPERTISE OF THE CASE MANAGER

The case manager's level of expertise depends on his or her role, the type of case management offered by the organization, and the responsibilities designated to the individual case manager. Clinical expertise is imperative, and this expertise cannot be compromised or minimized.[13] However, because of the changes in our healthcare system and its emphasis on cost containment and alternative care delivery sites, the case manager's strongest assets lie in her or his knowledge of community resources, patient entitlements to these resources, and when and how access to such resources is achieved. Ultimately, this knowledge contributes to the success of each case because patients can be moved expeditiously through the continuum of care once they exhibit readiness to move on.

Movement of the patient through the healthcare continuum of care or system in and of itself makes case management labor intensive. Many labels are used to describe case management services, thus adding to the tremendous confusion that already exists. A search of the literature supports this confusion as it shows the various models of case management. All models vary and this is well documented by such authors as Zander,[14] Weil and Karls,[15] Steinberg and Carter,[16] Ethridge and Lamb,[17] Cohen,[18] and Del Togno-Armanasco et al.[19] As healthcare professionals, we must be careful not to add to the confusion by failing to distinguish between case management services and nursing care delivery models.[10] Such a distinction is necessary because often the nursing care delivery system is short term and episodic; it frequently does not extend beyond discharge from the acute care hospital. In comparison, case management services originating from other sources (e.g., home health agency, insurance company, private case management firm) do follow the patient through the continuum of care. Thus, one of the keys to success is the need for close collaboration among all players.

Case management is labor intensive, plain and simple. The cases followed are "catastrophic" not only in terms of the medical diagnosis but also in terms of costs, both in dollars spent for healthcare and in the diminished quality of life or sacrifices the patient and the family must endure. Many of the cases followed by case managers can consume $100,000 or more in healthcare expenditures in a single episode of care. Additionally, many conditions or illnesses last for the life of the patient, and if the patient is not linked to alternate levels of care or appropriate resources when he demonstrates a readiness or need for them, the benefits offered by the patient's healthcare policy may be exhausted unnecessarily. Because many conditions followed by case managers are chronic or will become chronic, the patient may have limited or nonexistent benefits or financial resources to purchase services for chronic care. Healthcare benefits are precious commodities that must be used prudently.

Experience shows that the success of a case depends on many factors, many of which are related directly to the case manager's clinical expertise and analytic abilities. It also shows that the case manager must be detail oriented as well as knowledgeable about community resources and entitlement programs. Other traits that may be stressed to newly hired or inexperienced case managers include adaptability, flexibility, creativity, resourcefulness, and an ability to find innovative solutions as they go about the tasks of conducting case management, since no two cases are alike.[20]

These skills are vital in managing cases in which specific resources that can augment the care required are not available. For instance, many years ago there was a patient who required pool therapy, but not only was pool therapy excluded from her healthcare coverage, she also lived in a small town where healthcare resources for this service were nonexistent. Through research, several residents of the community were found who did have private swimming pools, and after many phone calls, one family came to the rescue. After negotiations with the owner of the pool, it was decided that in exchange for the use of the pool for the therapy, the patient's husband would assume responsibility for the pool's maintenance and all associated costs. The result? A creative winning solution!

Experience validates the fact that case management is not a job for all persons, especially those who have meek or nonassertive personalities. The ability to assert oneself must rank among the top skills on one's list of assets. The need for this skill will become apparent as one reads this manual and understands the intensity and complexity of the services and care that are necessary for many patients. Other skills required of case managers actually are basic business management techniques. These include the ability to prioritize, organize, and "manage" activities and people (which involves such skills as delegation, conflict resolution, crisis intervention, collaboration, consultation, and negotiation). For instance, the case manager must be able to be diplomatic and must respect and trust his or her peers and others in order to work in a team approach.

Although much of this manual addresses activities associated with case management after the acute care phase, it is nevertheless true that case managers not based in acute care facilities are often not involved in the acute care stages. However, because case management is frequently diagnosis driven, many cases are identified during the inpatient admission process. As a result, much of the initial case management involvement occurs during the patient's hospitalization. It is during this time that many case managers may be involved. When this occurs, the professionals involved must constantly collaborate with each other, keeping one another apprised of case events and variables. Close collaboration and excellent communication during all phases of the case by all case managers is paramount to success. Such collaboration cannot be emphasized enough, and the results are well documented in the literature.[21-24]

A good example of collaboration is seen when, as often occurs, three or more professional case managers are involved (yes, this is common, and it may become common to encounter more in the future), all from different healthcare organizations that are involved in the case. Case managers may be employed by the hospital, the healthcare payor, or the home care agency. All are equally important for various stages of the planning. Their various roles may be characterized as follows:

- For the hospital case manager, becoming an integral part of the healthcare team is important, as is working collaboratively with the facility-based case manager or discharge planner, family, and other pertinent clinicians on details for discharge (i.e., identifying teaching needs, coordinating resources and payment sources, or identifying barriers that can affect the discharge plan).
- For the healthcare payor's case manager, validation of eligibility for all insurances is necessary. This case manager may also identify all limitations, exclusions, copayments, and deductibles, which in turn allows the other members of the healthcare team a chance to develop more realistic plans. It also allows the facility's social worker or case manager to assist the family in exploring alternative funding programs as appropriate.

The healthcare payor's case manager may be useful in assisting with any evaluation of the appropriateness of care (quality, quantity, and level of care) and in making recommendations to the treating team about a move to an alternate level of care, ensuring that the level of care is covered by the healthcare payor and that all prior

authorizations occu...
stance, (1) for a p...
nity hospital who...
actually deterior...
might be to mo...
care center; an...
been hospitali...
now stable a...
recommend...
her back to...
urally, in...
taken in...
must be...
cian.

• For th... lth
  agenc... rom
  the ... that
  all ... tance
  on... ty and
  re... or dis-
  ... valuable
  ... e the one
  ... g that was

... ilities is not
... een from this
... out this man-
... manager can be
... uring the acute
... acility-based case
... lthcare payor's or
... manager during the
... important, but it is.
... pivotal as the patient
... of discharge, and the
... ger's duties will cease
... . In many cases, it is the
... ome health agency's case
... ns actively involved with
... charge or until the patient
... stablished by the team.

...es, case management is a win-
win s... for all: the patient, the healthcare
provider, the healthcare payor, and the organization offering case management services.
There is no textbook answer or "cookbook" to
follow. Each case is individual.

As stated previously, one of the primary driving forces for the certification process for case
managers is the fact that the success of case
management is often directly related to the
skills of the case manager and his or her ability

a team player; his or her knowledge of
...al expertise, treatment modalities, com-
...ity resources, and the patient's entitlement
...heir use; and the ability (and willingness) to
...ke a proactive rather than a reactive ap-
...roach. Equally important is the case manager's
availability to the patients in her or his caseload
in times of crises or as the patient's condition
changes. It also involves the case manager's
employer's interest in cost-effective controls
and also in quality of care.

Additionally, successful case management requires senior management's commitment to the
overall case management program. In most
cases, this means a commitment to ensure that
adequate numbers of highly professional and
adequately trained personnel are available.
Without case management, cases almost always
result in unnecessary and prolonged lengths
of stay or unnecessary use of personnel and
resources. More important, if the case management department is affiliated with a healthcare
organization that pays the claims or one that
has entered into a "risk agreement," payment of
exorbitant or unnecessary sums may be the result.

Senior management of any organization sets
the tone for fostering a sense of commitment
to any program undertaken. As healthcare costs
rise and access to alternate resources becomes
more limited, senior management's commitment to case management activities and cost
containment becomes more critical. This is especially true if the organization is to meet the
stringent quality of care standards imposed by
the various credentialing and accreditation organizations while conserving costs. Senior management must be aware of and understand the
need for and benefits of an effective and well
managed case management program. It must
also understand the potential effect on the overall cost savings potential if adequate resources
are to be allocated for the process.

This awareness and understanding can occur
only through regular communication about case
management activities with those persons actively involved with case management. Commitment of senior management can be attained
through structuring a reporting system that ensures and enhances the integration, collaboration, and communication of any department
associated with case managers or the cases
themselves. The final commitment of senior
management must be shown by the allocation
of sufficient staff to manage case loads.

Certainly, senior management of an organization determines the types of case management

offered. However, it must realize that a lack of success of case management may also be related to such factors as caseloads that are too high or unrealistic to allow case managers to address all details adequately, lack of payor funding, lack of resources or substandard care provided by the facility or agency, and patient-family resistance or noncompliance. Other factors may also be involved, but the foregoing are often the primary culprits for unsuccessful planning.

DEMOGRAPHICS AFFECTING CASE MANAGEMENT

To serve as a management tool for assistance in establishing a new case management program and to determine caseloads and staffing, an informal query was recently conducted by calling several national case management firms and independent case managers and asking their opinion on case management standards and demographics. The following facts were obtained and remain true today:

- Approximately 20% of the insured population uses the benefits of case management, and of this number, approximately 3% to 5% consume 80% of the total healthcare dollars spent because these cases are complex and involve acutely ill or critically injured patients or those with chronic conditions.
- Most cases classified as catastrophic have a potential claim dollar expenditure of more than $100,000 in the initial episode of care.
- Approximately 10% of all births belong in the catastrophic category.
- Although much can be done by telephone, high-quality case management is best accomplished by using a combination of on-site intervention and monitoring and telephone communication and by separating utilization or discharge coordination review responsibilities from case management.
- On-site case intervention and involvement allow greater cost savings and ensure that the patient receives the right care in the right place at the right time, but this type of case management is labor intensive and requires adequate personnel.
- Confidentiality, patient rights, and privacy must be maintained at all times, and only reasonable and lawful means must be used to collect information.
- Caseloads depend on such factors as the type of case management offered, the assigned duties of the case manager, the type of clients or population served by the healthcare organization, the qualifications and expertise of the case manager, the acuity of care and needs of the patient, and any other demands placed on case managers by senior management.
- Case closure occurs when it is thought that the case no longer poses a risk to the healthcare organization. Cases remain open from 2 to 6 months or longer.
- Some mechanism of documentation of case events is of critical importance because of the length of time the cases are open. Also, some form of documentation is required for the protection of the case manager and the organization should the case proceed to litigation.
- Cost savings reports, case time, and case summaries are considered to be three important management tools.
- Finding qualified nurses to serve in the role of case managers is often difficult because most firms require both recent acute care experience and a knowledge of community resources.
- Ongoing inservice training and education of nurses is necessary and must occur on a regular and frequent basis because the staff must be kept abreast of changes in the healthcare system and continuum of care.
- New case managers require monitoring for several months or until they can manage a caseload adequately; the length of time they are actually directly supervised depends on the individual's background and expertise.

CASE VARIABLES AND MOST COMMON DIAGNOSES

Any of the factors in the list just given can affect the success of a case management program. The success of the case and the length of time it is open depend on the intensity and severity of the illness or injury involved. Historically, a review of case management caseloads reveals that the following factors also affect cases:

- Age of patient.
- Family dynamics or problems, marital status, family or support systems.
- Social and ethnic background.
- Recent other life crisis (retirement, divorce, death, empty nest).

- Adequacy of treatment plan, facility, or agency to manage the level of care.
- Medical history and premorbid or personality type of the patient.
- The patient's or family's motivation and compliance with the treatment plan.
- Physical deterioration and level of dependence or independence prior to the illness or injury.
- Psychiatric history, psychological or emotional stability of both the patient and the family.
- Physical or mental ability of patient or family, including ability to understand and be trained.
- Standards of care for the community or region.
- Availability of resources.
- Financial capability to assume out-of-pocket expenses.
- Eligibility for alternate funding programs, as well as the waiting time between application and enrollment into the program.
- Level of acceptance of the condition by both patient and family.
- Number of small children in the home.
- If trauma is involved, the number of persons involved and the severity of their injuries.
- If a small child is involved, the age and maturity of the parents.
- Adequacy, timeliness, and extent of discharge planning and level of expertise of the discharge planner.

Diagnoses encountered in caseloads vary with the type of case management offered by an organization, but again, regular audits of caseloads reveal that the most common diagnoses found in nongeriatric or disease specific caseloads are the following (not necessarily in this order):

- Acquired immune deficiency syndrome (AIDS).
- Terminal cancer or other end-stage disease or diseases that have the potential to result in long-term care.
- Ventilator dependence or dependence on other technologic assistance.
- Neurologic disorders or trauma, spinal cord injuries (SCI), or traumatic brain injuries (TBI).
- Transplants.
- Neonates.
- Technologically dependent children or children with multiple congenital anomalies.

It is absolutely critical that case managers be familiar with medical courses of treatment.

Legally, a case manager must accept only those cases with diagnoses and treatments with which he or she is familiar. However, because of reorganization and downsizing by some healthcare organizations who offer case management, case managers may be required to assume responsibility for patients with diagnoses or conditions with which they may have only a basic familiarity. If there is ever any doubt, the case manager must ask for help or read about the subject to become familiar with its requirements. Familiarity with diagnoses and courses of treatments is necessary because if doubt arises or if a referral to case management does not appear reasonable and customary for the condition, questions must be asked or the issue researched before one proceeds further. This may mean reading on the subject or asking for information from national data sources such as the Center for Healthcare Technology (CHCT), the National Cancer Institute (NCI), or the Food and Drug Administration (FDA).

Experimental or investigational procedures or drugs are common treatment modalities for patients in case management caseloads not only because of the complexity of the illnesses or injuries involved but also because, typical of human nature, hope is a wonderful gift and makes many people willing to try anything that may possibly help.[25] In addition to routine treatments case managers must stay abreast of procedures and drugs that are still experimental but are commonly requested. Such knowledge is necessary to keep patients and families apprised of the fact that if the patient participates in an experimental trial or study without prior approval from the healthcare payor, his or her benefits may be terminated or excluded from coverage. Thus, unexpected out-of-pocket expenses may ensue.

DETERMINATION OF CASELOADS

The best way to determine the number of cases in a reasonable caseload has plagued every case management organization. Although the arbitrary number of 30 to 35 seems to be the best number for some case management organizations, it is not for all. The number fluctuates with the type of case management offered, the type of population served by the organization (i.e., whole populations of Medicaid or Medicare clients), or reductions in the budget. When such events occur, caseload numbers rise. Also, the acuity of particular cases (the intensity and severity of the illness or injury, the intensity and complexity of care, and other variables) also alters the actual number of cases that can be carried by an individual case manager. For instance, if a case manager is assigned only to technologically dependent patients, his or her caseload may be smaller because of the many case variables that affect this category of patients.[26-28]

As caseloads rise, the number of hours spent on each case decreases. If caseloads are not evaluated and efforts are made to keep caseloads reasonable, a decrease in the quality and intensity of the services offered by the case manager is frequently the end result. In essence what may happen is that services are spread so thin that case management occurs on paper only.

Some factors to be considered when establishing caseloads include the following:

- The case manager's level of expertise.
- Senior management's commitment to case management and the resources available for staffing.
- The type of clients or populations served (i.e., Medicaid and Medicare populations may require a different level of case management than a younger and more healthy insured population in a health maintenance organization).
- The type of case management (telephonic or on-site) allowed or offered by the organization.
- The geographic distances covered by the case manager's organization.
- The role of the case manager—either the dual role of utilization reviewer and case manager or the single role of case manager.
- The age of the patients and the intensity and severity of their condition (e.g., ventilator-dependent patients and children with special needs).
- The intensity and complexity of care required as well as the availability of the resources necessary to meet these needs.
- Other factors such as family dynamics, psychosocial factors, and socioeconomic issues.

The more complex the case, the more hours it takes to effectively establish high-quality cost-effective care in an alternative setting. Although the following list of factors contributing to the complexity of cases is not all-inclusive, audits of caseloads reveal that cases with the following characteristics are the most difficult to handle and consume an inordinate number of hours:

- Need for multiple services or care by several agencies.
- Minimal to no family support.
- Infighting and conflicts between the patient and family or within the family unit regarding the patient's care.
- Inadequacy of community resources.
- Inadequacy of healthcare coverage, alternate funding, or personal finances.
- Uncooperative physician.
- Inadequacy of the home or the caregiver if the patient is to be discharged directly home.

Because caseload planning plagues most managers, another study conducted by the author was to assist in determining the components of an "adequate" caseload for staffing. This study concentrated on actual caseloads of case managers. Its intent was to develop an acuity rating for caseloads and a tool to aid in the establishment of appropriate caseloads. The study covered all cases, both open and closed, during a 2-month period. It also covered all ages of patients (the firm insured only a commercial population) and included, in all, 500 cases.

This audit was much easier than one done many years ago of discharge planning. In the audit of a discharge planner's workload, a full 2-week's time study had to be conducted prior to starting the audit. However, the audit of case managers' caseloads was accomplished using preexisting data (including chart data and a monthly tally sheet used by the case managers to summarize the total hours they spent on case activities). The audit was most helpful in planning caseloads and the types of staffing actually required for the unit.

This case management study revealed that approximately 10% to 20% of a case manager's caseload required very intense activity; 30% to 40% required frequent monitoring and changes in the case management plans; and the remaining 40% to 50% required periodic monitoring and adjustments in the plan (patients in this category were more stable and were approaching case closure). It was also found that more than half of the caseload was composed of (1) transplant patients and (2) children, who had the higher acuity rating levels II and III (described later). The study also revealed that the target population that least benefited from case management intervention consisted of those patients (1) whose medical needs were met by their existing healthcare benefit package, and (2) who were progressing at the expected rate of recovery and were expected to be discharged without complications.

The final tally revealed that the actual cases opened to case management fell basically into two categories:

1. Patients who were acutely ill and required multifaceted complex care. Other variables frequently affected these cases. Many patients in this category required care over a prolonged period of time or a whole lifetime. Also, these patients required formal orchestration of services, frequent monitoring, and readjustments to the case management plans to ensure that quality was maintained and costs were contained. In many cases extra contractual processes were necessary if the case manager was to meet the goals established by the team.
2. Patients who had relatively short-term acute care needs. However, these needs were complex and required formal orchestration of services to ensure that quality was maintained and costs contained. This category also included patients in the early stages of their illness, and many required long-term disease management in which linkage to educational resources specific to the disease was very important.

Within each caseload the study further revealed the following levels of case activity:

Level I Activity

These patients had short-term complex needs, but the needs could be met using the normal benefit structure offered by the healthcare payor and community resources. However, because of the complexity of care required, these cases needed formal orchestration of case planning and coordination with multiple agencies to establish their care or ensure that patient education occurred. These cases required 8 to 10 hours to establish the initial case management plan and 1 to 2 hours per month to monitor, reassess the case, and make changes in the plan. Approximately 50% of the cases had this level of activity.

Also found in this level were many chronically ill persons who required the services of a case manager if they were to be linked to services as soon as their specific needs were identified and to maintain quality of care and contain costs.

Level II Activity

In these cases there were many barriers to discharge because of the complexity of care needs or a lack of resources to meet these needs. These cases required 12 to 16 hours to establish the initial case management plan and another 2 to 4 hours per month to monitor, reassess, and make adjustments to the plan. Approximately 30% to 40% of the cases had this level of activity.

Level III Activity

The most complex cases had level III activity. Many of these patients had multifaceted and complex medical care needs, and care was also frequently complicated by psychosocial or socioeconomic issues. These cases were extremely labor intensive; many were neonates or children with special needs, critically ill patients who were dependent on technologic aid, or patients with complex end-stage diseases.

Coordination of care was often further complicated by such factors as family infighting or interference in the decision-making process and complex care needs that made finding resources to manage the care almost impossible. Many of these patients required out-of-area placement or establishment of a "mini-hospital" within the home. These cases required more than 16 hours to establish the initial plan and 8 to 10 hours per month to monitor and reassess the plan. Approximately 10% to 20% of the cases had this level of activity.

The foregoing findings may not provide an appropriate measurement tool for all organizations because clients and populations vary from one organization to another. However, regardless of the type of auditing tool used, auditing of caseloads must be done on a regular basis not only to identify the ongoing educational needs of the case management staff but also to reevaluate and possibly readjust the caseloads. Directors and managers of case management units must keep in mind that the lower the case management activity on a case, the more cases each case manager can assume. Conversely, the higher the case activity, the fewer cases a case manager can assume. The same principle applies to the training and experience of individual case managers: The more training and experience a case manager has, the more cases (either in numbers or acuity) he or she can assume. The important key is to formulate a tool whereby caseloads can be audited or evaluated regularly to ensure that cases are evenly distributed among the staff and that the more stable cases or cases with the least activity are closed. Another important key is to ensure that the staff has access to ongoing education pertinent to the types of cases followed by the organization.

CASE MANAGEMENT PROCESS

There are essentially seven basic components[15] in the case management process (Fig. 1–2). They are:

- Assessment and collection of data.
- Organization of data and planning.
- Service planning and resource identification.
- Counseling, education, and advocacy.
- Coordination and referral.
- Implementation and linkage of patient to needed services.
- Reassessment and monitoring.

Although most of these processes occur in sequential order and appear to be concrete, they are not. Many of these components may continue or may be repeated throughout the duration of the case, or they may be repeated as changes are made to the case management plan. In all situations, the case manager must be flexible and open to changes.

All case management plans must be based on medical necessity and the treating physician's treatment plan or orders. Plans must be comprehensive and must reflect the total needs of the patient (physical, psychological, cultural, financial, social, spiritual, and environmental). Additionally, plans must be changed or modified as the patient's condition progresses or regresses. It is important to determine that the patient's needs are being met satisfactorily at all levels as the patient bridges different resources and moves through the continuum of care and that care is delivered in a timely manner and in the right setting. If this is not happening, corrective action must be implemented immediately. High-quality case management occurs when:

- All members of the team are committed to offering and adhering to ethical case management principles.
- Case management is approached with an open mind.
- Communication is honest and frequent, and there is collaboration between all members of the team.
- Patient and family input, control, and responsibility are promoted.
- Advocacy is undertaken willingly when necessary.
- Specific details are sought.
- The case manager is constantly attuned to problematic issues that can affect the case and takes the necessary steps to ensure that corrective action is implemented when problems are identified.

Case managers are in a perfect position to see that the patient's care continues on a planned basis, that goals are reached, and that the patient is returned to optimal health or to a maximum functional level. There are times when the case manager is in a position to suggest or implement creative, innovative options if these options enhance the benefits of care and do not place the patient at risk. As such, high-quality case management occurs when the case manager is flexible and open to unconventional approaches to accomplish tasks. In many instances, the case manager's creativity and skill at finding or making innovative solutions are the predominant qualities needed when the patient's healthcare benefits exclude or limit services or items.

CASE PLANNERS
Patient and Family

An open-minded approach allows case managers to guide the case, advocate certain mea-

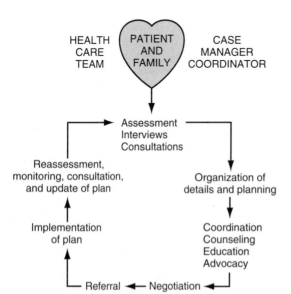

Figure 1–2 • Components of the case management process.

sures, and coordinate different aspects of the plan as the patient's condition changes or remains steady. However, regardless of the organization offering case management, case managers must always remember that the true planners are the patient and the family. To avoid crises, patients and families must be informed and involved in every step of the planning. Also, the final case management plan must focus not only on the patient's needs but on the individual family's needs as well.

Case management plans developed without patient and family input are likely to fail. Also critical to the development of any case management plan is the involvement of the patient's physician and the entire interdisciplinary healthcare team. Case managers must realize that their case management plans are nothing other than extensions of the treatment plans ordered by the physician. When executed, they serve as guides to ensure that goals established by the healthcare team are reached, that resources required by the patient to meet his or her needs are identified, and that linkage with these resources is made.

Physicians

The vital link to planning is the physician. Unfortunately, because of their busy schedules and the many demands made on them, they are often the member of the team that is most difficult to deal with. Not only are physicians difficult to reach, many may have preconceived ideas about case managers because they confuse case management with utilization review. Such physicians view case management as a threat or hindrance whose primary purpose is to deny care. Often the key to working with difficult physicians is getting to know the physician's office nurse in order to work through him or her to gain access to the physician. Once the physician is reached, it is common to find a mutual concern about facilitating the patient's care. Rapport and trust are built as information is shared. Some other keys to working with physicians are as follows:

- *Preparation*: Be prepared to ask questions and have questions prepared in advance.
- *Limits*: Set limits on the number of people who will be calling the physician about the same patient for input into the plan.
- *Knowledge*: Know the resources so that everyone who calls is viewed as an asset and not a hindrance to the patient's care.

Healthcare Providers

The patient and family should have the right to select any healthcare provider used. However, if benefits are linked to such insurers as a health maintenance organization or a preferred provider organization, the conditions for joining the health plan may specifically limit this right. Also, capitation (the insurer and the healthcare provider agree on a prenegotiated reimbursement rate under which the provider provides all services for a specified rate), may limit the patient's right even further. Therefore, specific providers must be used. Unfortunately, because not all networks can manage the level of care required by a catastrophically ill or injured person, a provider that is not contracted must sometimes be used.

In these situations, every effort must be made to advocate on behalf of the patient to ensure that the level of care he or she requires is delivered. Because most negotiations for actual contracts between the payor and the provider occur outside the case manager's arena, case managers can exert an influence on how rates are structured to ensure that providers are willing to accept cases that are more complex and costly. Such influence is gained by ensuring that case managers have input into the contracting process whenever possible. One of the best mechanisms for this is regular meetings between all network development staff and the case management staff. For instance, the case management director or manager should have input into all contracts that are contemplated, or, at a minimum, he or she should review the final contract before it is executed. This is important when the case management services offered will be linking patients to specific resources. A process such as this ensures that not only will the majority of patients benefit from the rates proposed, but so will the small minority found in case management. The final contract achieved in such a process is a win-win situation for all.

COMMUNICATION

Patient or Family

The factor that is possibly most important in the success of a case is communication. The ability to communicate directly, honestly, and positively with all players cannot be emphasized enough. Naturally, the frequency of communication with the various healthcare team players and the patient and family depends on case variables. However, frequent communication with everyone involved in the case is critical, and the patient and family should be kept informed every step of the way.

If receptivity and cooperation between team members are to occur, information and ideas must be communicated and shared. Written communication (i.e., letters and memos) has its place, but the ideal communication mode is speech, either in person or via the telephone.

The timing of any communication to the patient and family, even to provide basic information, must be matched to their emotional readiness to understand. Families vary in their resilience and in their ability to grasp reality. For instance, some families can deal with every situation realistically, whereas others simply fall apart. Some families are intimidated, fearful, and afraid to speak, whereas others remain in denial. In all these situations, the case manager must stay attuned to patient and family differences, communicating in whatever style fits the situation. For families in crisis, it is wise to follow up all verbally communicated instructions in writing because the crisis situation frequently hinders the family's ability to grasp what is said.[29]

In some situations the patient or family simply is not able to communicate their wants, needs, or feelings. In these instances, the case manager must build trust and take on the role of advocate until the patient or family can assume this role for themselves. During this period, the case manager must continually communicate with the patient and family and encourage their questions, input, and presence in the process. When the case manager assumes the role of advocate, he or she must not lose sight of the fact that the patient or family remains the final decision maker and nothing can be implemented until their approval has been granted.

Primary Care Nursing Utilization Review and Case Management

Fostering internal communication and sharing data when primary care nursing or utilization review or case management services are offered by separate entities is of vital importance. One excellent means of accomplishing this is to establish weekly or frequent meetings between the groups. These meetings are an excellent forum for joint sharing of case information. Participants may include the primary care nursing case manager, utilization review and case management nurses, and possibly their department managers. Depending on the type of organization that employs the case manager, other participants may include the medical director, discharge planner, customer service representative, or admission personnel. Similar meetings may be held if case management services are provided by more than one case manager (e.g, an agency-based or alternate funding case manager and the healthcare payor case manager). The goals of such meetings are to:

1. Foster communication, coordination, and support among colleagues.
2. Identify appropriate patients for referral to case management.
3. Exchange patient information to ensure that patients are at the appropriate level of care.
4. Identify discharge planning or ongoing needs.
5. Identify barriers or fragmentation of care that affects discharge or access to resources or services.
6. Allow an opportunity for education.

HEALTHCARE PAYOR TYPES

For ease of writing this manual and because of the multitude of healthcare payor types in our society, the term healthcare payor is used to refer to any type of insurance or organizational entity or alternate funding program that pays the healthcare bill. For instance, there are approximately 20 varieties of healthcare payors, and case managers must be aware of such names and abbreviations as those in the following list:

• Health maintenance organization (HMO): An organization in which the members in a specific geographic area receive health benefits from providers who contract with the HMO to provide services for a set amount. Types of HMOs may include:
  • Closed panel HMO.
  • Staff model HMO.
  • Open panel HMO.
  • Mixed model HMO.
• Administrative services only (ASO): An insurance company that provides administrative services (i.e., claims payments, provider rate

negotiations) but does not assume any risk (often used by self-funded or self-insured groups).

- Preferred provider organization (PPO): An organization that contracts with independent providers for services at a discount.
- Independent practice association (IPA): An organization that contracts with both a managed care company for services and individual physicians and other providers who perform services at either a capitated rate or a fee-for-service rate.
- Exclusive provider organization (EPO): An organization similar to a health maintenance organization that has a limited and very restricted panel of providers.
- Physician hospital organization (PHO): An organization formed by physicians and hospitals that join for the purposes of contracting with managed care plans.
- Third-party administrator (TPA): Companies that handle all the administrative tasks involved with claims processing (often used by self-funded or self-insured groups).
- Management services organization (MSO): Similar to a third-party administrator or administrative services organization in which administrative services such as claims processing, utilization review, and so forth are performed.
- Indemnity insurance: Typical fee-for-service insurance, which, prior to managed care, was the traditional form of insurance available.
- Civilian Health and Medical Program of the Uniformed Services (CHAMPUS): Health entitlement program for all active duty dependents, retirees and their dependents, and dependents of persons killed while on active duty. This program in many areas of the country is called TRICARE. TRICARE is replacing the traditional indemnity benefits historically allowed by the Department of Defense for healthcare coverage; it offers its beneficiaries (the patients) a triple-option choice—an HMO, PPO, and indemnity plan.
- Civilian Health and Medical Program of the Department of Veterans Affairs (CHAMPVA): Program in which the Veterans Administration shares with eligible beneficiaries (the patients) the cost of covered healthcare and services.
- Medicare (Title XVIII of the Social Security Act): Federal insurance for the disabled under the age of 65, persons with end-stage renal disease, and persons over age 65 who qualify.
- Medicaid (Title XIX of the Social Security Act): Federal or state insurance for the poor.

- Children's Medical Services program (Title V of the 1935 Social Security Act): Financial assistance or diagnosis and treatment of any child with a handicapping condition who meets the state's eligibility criteria. All states vary in what they call their specific program, but historically this program has been referred to as Crippled Children's Services.
- Medigap: Medicare supplement plans.
- Supplemental plans: Supplemental insurance policies that pay deductibles and copayments.
- Long-term disability policies (LTD): Income replacement policies for long-term disabilities.
- Cancer policies: Coverage for cancer-related illnesses.
- Long-term insurance: Coverage for skilled nursing facility care (some cover custodial care as well).
- Point of service (POS) plan: Plan in which members can use healthcare providers outside the network without prior authorization, but in exchange they pay higher out-of-pocket costs.

LEGISLATIVE FORCES AFFECTING CASE MANAGEMENT AND THE CONTINUUM OF CARE

In addition to a knowledge of the various types of healthcare payors available, a case manager must have a basic knowledge of the important legislative forces that have shaped the healthcare reimbursement system and the continuum of care. These include the following acts and amendments:

- Social Security Act (1935): Established a system of federal old age benefits.
- Social Security Amendments (1950): Established Aid to Families with Dependent Children (AFDC); Old Age Assistance (OAA); Aid to the Blind (AB); and Aid to the Permanently and Totally Disabled (APTD).
- Social Security Amendments (1963): Improved crippled children's medical services (Title V) and added provisions for mental retardation planning.
- Civil Rights Act (1964): Forbids discrimination and ensures constitutional rights.
- Older Americans Act (1964): Established the Administration of Aging and helped to develop services for gerontology and aging.

- Social Security Amendments (1965): Created Medicare (Title XVIII) and Medicaid (Title XIX).
- Social Security Amendments (1967): Consolidated all maternal and child health and crippled children's services under one authority.
- Social Security Amendments (1972): Established Professional Standards Review Organizations (PSRO) and also, more important, established Supplemental Security Income (SSI) to replace Old Age Assistance (OAA), Aid to the Blind (AB), and Aid to the Permanently and Totally Disabled (APTD).
- Rehabilitation Act (1973): Established vocational rehabilitation services.
- Health Maintenance Organization Act (1973): Established guidelines for HMOs.
- Privacy Act (1974): Established guidelines for protection of personal information that is released between parties.
- Education for All Handicapped Children Act (1975): Mandates that all handicapped children, from birth to age 21, are entitled to a free public education.
- Medicare End-Stage Disease Amendment (1978): Established improvements in renal and kidney disease treatment and services for patients needing these treatments.
- Omnibus Budget Reconciliation Act (1981): Among many other provisions, allows Medicaid waivers for a variety of home care services.
- Developmental Disabilities Act (1984): Requires states to provide services to developmentally disabled persons whose disability occurred before the age of 22; also requires states to meet minimum requirements of care so that the disabled person can live in the least restrictive environment.
- Americans with Disabilities Act (1990): Guarantees the rights of the disabled and ensures equal access and opportunity.
- Ryan White Comprehensive AIDS Resources Emergency Act (1990): Provides emergency assistance to localities that have a disproportionate number of human immune deficiency virus (HIV)-positive persons.
- Patient Self-Determination Act (1990): Mandates that hospitals, home health agencies, and hospices counsel patients of their right to accept or refuse treatment and of their right to use an advance directive (i.e., a living will).
- Individuals with Disabilities Education Act (1991): Replaces the Education for All Handicapped Children Act of 1975.
- Family and Medical Leave Act (1994): Entitles employees up to 12 weeks of unpaid leave to take care of an ill child, parent, or spouse or for birth or adoption and guarantees protection of employment and health benefits during this leave period.

Other acts and amendments have occurred, but those listed are some of the most significant. These are the ones with which the case manager must be most familiar because they have the greatest impact on case management and the continuum of care.

ALTERNATE PAYORS

Although healthcare benefits may be limited or excluded in some cases, in other situations multiple payor sources may be involved in one case (e.g., in the case of a child, the child may have his or her own private healthcare payor as well as alternate payors such as Medicaid, Supplemental Security Income (SSI), services from the state agency responsible for developmental disabilities, and services from the local Title V Children's Medical Services program). In other cases, the patient may be covered by more than one private healthcare payor (e.g., both the mother's and father's insurance, or their own and their spouse's insurance). Whenever there is more than one payment source, it is imperative to identify the healthcare payor that will assume the primary payor role, coordinating all benefits.

Despite the fact that the patient may have healthcare coverage, any patient with long-term needs should be encouraged to explore all alternate funding programs to which he or she is entitled as early as possible. This is necessary to avoid delays in the application and approval processes if the patient's healthcare benefits are limited, excluded, denied, or exhausted.

In cases with multiple payor entitlements it is necessary to establish the proper order of payors. If this is not done, erroneous payments or coordination of benefits and delays in approval or payment for care can result. This issue is sometimes further complicated by the patient's or family's failure to disclose all insurance plans, alternate funding plans, or entitlement programs. Often patients and family members do not understand the concept of coordination of benefits. In some cases, they do not disclose their other insurance plans because they see them as a means to "make money." Therefore, case managers must be prepared to solicit information from the patient and family that identifies all known insurances or alternate funding programs.

Case managers must also be aware that in some instances the patient's injuries are a result of a felonious act or a "third-party injury." When these cases are identified, contact with the appropriate city or county law enforcement agency or insurance company that will be responsible for reimbursement for the care must be made. In some cases, the healthcare payor may assume responsibility for the payment of services, collecting reimbursement of costs through what is known as a "third-party liability" lien. In other cases, they may not. Unfortunately, in some cases, the patient or the family may be required to assume the responsibility for all charges, obtaining reimbursement at a later date or after it has been determined who is responsible for payment. When a law enforcement agency is to assume responsibility for the charges, this entity must be contacted to obtain its consent to payment for any treatment rendered.

COMMON PROBLEMS IN OBTAINING ACCESS TO CARE

One common problem frequently experienced by families who inquire about alternate funding sources or entitlement programs such as Medicaid, Social Security disability income, special education, and the Title V Children's Medical Services program is that they inquire by telephone and get a simple "no" for an answer. In their frustration with the "system," they take this answer for the truth and go no further. As a result, they never complete the formal application, nor do they receive a formal denial from which they can appeal. It is therefore very important for case managers to be knowledgeable about alternate funding resources and the appeal processes because in many cases the patient may have been eligible from the start. However, because a formal application was never made to the agency, a retroactive eligibility determination is made, and consequently, reimbursement for care may not be approved. Thus, the family is required to pay unnecessarily for these expenses or do without.

Not only are alternate funding denials common, so are barriers to access to care. Two of the biggest barriers are lack of resources or fragmentation of resources to meet the ongoing needs of the patient. This is especially true of many patients handled by case managers be-

cause they have ongoing or lifetime needs. Our healthcare delivery system is designed to provide episodic acute care. Rarely does a patient's healthcare benefit coverage (other than in workers' compensation) allow for long-term or custodial care.

Because of the complex nature of some cases, another problem frequently encountered is the use of multiple healthcare providers. When this occurs, it is common to have more case managers than there are services to manage. In such cases, everyone must collectively agree on one "primary" case manager. In many instances, this primary case manager may be the one representing the agency providing the greater number of services (e.g., a home health agency). This appointment of a primary case manager does not mean that the others are not involved, nor does it negate their responsibilities as case managers. The delegation of a primary case manager is merely a mechanism to ensure that one person assumes the responsibility for serving as the primary communication link with all parties, keeping the others informed as changes are made.

Another barrier or problem often encountered is the difficulty of providing care to persons who live in rural areas. These cases are often the most challenging for case managers. Although many rural communities have advantages for most residents, residents needing medical care may experience major difficulties in obtaining access to care or services. Not only are there scarcities in resources, but the patient's distance from what resources there are makes establishment of care most burdensome. For instance, many durable medical equipment companies, which provide respiratory services to technology-dependent clients, require these patients to live within a 1-hour driving distance from their place of business. They find this restriction necessary if they are to successfully manage the care required. For example, in Sacramento there are a number of providers in the immediate area, and many surrounding towns are certainly within the 1-hour driving radius during the summer months; however, fog and sometimes flooding during the winter months precludes these companies (i.e., home health agency, durable medical equipment companies) from accepting responsibility for the management of the case.

The following example illustrates some of the problems encountered by patients in these remote rural areas. In this case, the resources required for the patient's care were found, but there were times when the outcome was in doubt. This patient lived in a small town in the mountains; the closest city was 150 miles away. Snow and ice during the winter months made the roads virtually impassable for weeks or months at a time. The patient required skilled care, and the primary caregiver was to be the wife; unfortunately, she had almost as many medical problems as her husband and was at risk of a stroke or heart attack at any given moment. She would need as much assistance as possible if she was to assume the bulk of his care.

Other factors complicated this case. (1) Financially, the patient and his wife were in the "gray" area; they had too much to qualify for alternate funding but too little to pay privately for all care and services. (2) The husband was very demanding and refused care from others (his primary needs for skilled help included physical, occupational, and speech therapy, skin care for decubitus ulcers, frequent tracheal suctioning [several times per hour], and tube feeding). (3) Despite many hours of counseling from the social worker at the hospital, both husband and wife refused placement. (4) Their children lived out of state. (5) Their home was multi-level. There were positive factors also, and these were the ones drawn on for our plan: (1) both the patient and his wife were well linked with the community and had a multitude of friends; (2) fortunately, this small town did have a skilled nursing facility; and (3) the town had a volunteer fire department.

Once the care needs had been assessed and the initial case management plan had been drawn up, the wife advertised at the skilled nursing facility and in the local paper for assistance. She needed someone to take on the night shift while she slept and another person to assist her in the early morning hours with the patient's initial care, as well as the therapists who would carry out the therapy. Surprisingly, qualified personnel in all professional disciplines were found. A schedule was drawn up for all the friends who volunteered to sit or offer respite while the wife rested during the day. Fire department volunteers assisted in building ramps and parallel bars and installing grab bars in the bathroom; all the labor was free, and the only cost to the patient was for the supplies.

Because the patient's care needs were known to be required for the long term, arrangements were made to purchase the durable medical equipment. This included such items as the bed and side rails, a patient lift, both stationary and portable suction devices, feeding pump, commode, and wheelchair. Because this rural area was plagued by frequent power outages, a portable generator would have been required if the patient did not already own one. Because of his suctioning and feeding needs, a 6-month's supply of all supplies was procured (the wife was taught clean technique before discharge, and this assisted in keeping the costs of sterile supplies to a minimum). Arrangements were also made for the regional medical center's treating team to generate the actual treatment plan, with the local physician implementing all care, consulting as needed with them by phone. All told, the plan took about 4 weeks to orchestrate. However, the final plan was very successful, and the patient remained at home until his death 2 years later.

CAREGIVER BURNOUT

Family caregivers frequently play a pivotal role in providing the care required by disabled or chronically ill patients. This task places a heavy burden on families mentally, physically, and at times financially. This is especially true if care is required over an extended period of time. For these reasons, care of the caregiver is extremely critical, and caregivers must be monitored closely to ensure that they do not succumb to "caregiver burnout."[10]

Caregiver burnout is possibly the number one cause of costly readmissions or nursing home placements. Therefore, all attempts must be made to recruit alternatives to allow respite for the caregiver. Although respite is needed by all caregivers, it is especially necessary for a single person attempting care or for a young mother, who may have not only a child with special needs but also other young children who rely on her as well. All too often what occurs with young mothers is that the mother gives up her career and the father is absent, working extended hours to cover what was once two incomes. As a result, the young mother is faced with giving hours and hours of care without relief. The same thing is true of a spouse who provides care for a loved one without respite. A good example of this situation is the spouse who provides care for a husband or wife with Alzheimer's disease. Depending on the patient's level of care and forgetfulness, the spouse may be a virtual prisoner in his or her own home. Therefore, regardless of the situation, all cases must be assessed for respite needs for the caregiver; if these needs are identified, arrangements should be made to provide solutions.

CASE MANAGEMENT TOOLS

To be successful as guides through the continuum of care, it is crucial for case managers to spend time seeking out and establishing relationships and linkages with key organizations, community agencies, and their staffs. Developing these linkages and relationships is pivotal to success and credibility as a case manager. Networking with other case managers, discharge planners, and other community healthcare providers is also important and is one of the best ways of staying abreast of regulatory changes, standards of care, community healthcare rates, and gaps and problems within the healthcare delivery system or with providers.

Once the case manager has identified and made contact with key resources, a filing system with key names and direct phone numbers helps with future referrals. At a minimum, such a list should include:

- State and county departments of social services, especially the local Medicaid eligibility office and any staff affiliated with the Medicaid waiver programs for the state.
- The state agency responsible for developmental disabilities.
- State department of rehabilitation.
- Title V Children's Medical Services program.
- Local Social Security office.
- Home health agencies.
- Skilled nursing facilities.
- Regional tertiary medical centers.
- Transplant centers.
- Hospice programs.
- Adult or child day health programs.
- Adult and child protective services.
- Shelters for battered women and children.
- Homemaker agencies or private duty nursing agencies.
- Durable medical equipment companies.
- Pain management programs.
- Substance abuse programs.
- Various community and national disease-specific agencies (e.g, American Heart Association, United Cerebral Palsy Association).
- Facilities offering transportation for the handicapped.
- Public conservator's office.
- State and county veterans' services.

Because no two cases are alike nor are the expectations and demands placed on case managers by employers the same, there has been no true "text" for case managers to follow. However, three of the most important books in a case manager's library must be (1) a good nursing practice manual covering nursing procedures for patients from birth to death, (2) a directory of social and health services in the community, and, at a minimum, (3) the telephone directories for all regions covered by the case manager's healthcare organization. In addition, the library should have access to coding books such as the International Classification of Diseases (ICD-9), the Diagnostic and Statistical Manual of Mental Disorders (DSM), and Current Procedural Terminology (CPT), as well as length of stay books (e.g., Diagnostic Related Groups [DRG] and Professional Activity Study [PAS]) as well as other textbooks that describe current diagnoses and treatments. Likewise, there must be access to drug formularies or other pharmacy books, such as the Physicians Desk Reference. Another source of information is handbooks for such alternate funding programs as Title V Children's Medical Services programs, the state agency responsible for developmental disabilities, and all recent publications produced by Social Security.

Because case managers often serve people in various areas of a state or the nation, other books for a case management library might include *The Case Management Resource Guide*. This book is actually a four-volume reference set that divides the United States into four regions: north, south, east, and west. It is updated annually and includes information on home health agencies, mail-order pharmaceutical companies, auto remodelers (for persons needing to retrofit their mode of transportation when they become disabled), and much more. The manuals can be obtained by writing to:

Center for Consumer Healthcare
  Information
400 Birch
Suite 112
Newport Beach, CA 92660

Other books that might be included in a library are directories that list the major national hotlines and clearing houses for the sick and disabled. Also, most states publish manuals that list all licensed facilities within that state. Additionally, if specific healthcare payors or populations are served, case managers must, at a minimum, have access to their manuals or member handbooks. Most important in any case management library are the organization's internal policies and procedures for the case management program.

INTENT OF MANUAL

Although high-quality management, improvement, or performance plays a pivotal role in healthcare, and case management is not exempt, this manual is designed for the day-to-day actions of case managers who actually conduct case management functions. As such, this manual does not cover aspects of case management dealing only with quality improvement because this subject can require an entire manual in itself. Also, despite the fact that quality improvement and performance are the new buzz words, and efforts to standardize qualities are under way, the requirements for an improvement effort vary from employer to employer. Therefore, it is the case manager's responsibility to read and adhere to his or her employer's policies and procedures pertinent to quality improvement. It is also the case manager's responsibility always to keep quality of care foremost in the conduct of his or her daily caseload activities.

This manual is not intended to be a complete medical manual about every illness or medical subject. Its intent is to be a reference guide that provides practical information for any case manager regardless of employer, whether hospital, healthcare payor (e.g., HMO, PPO, independent practice association [IPA], or independent case management company), or any other organization (facility-based, home health agency, or alternate funding or entitlement program) offering case management services. It is also intended for use in any training program for new case managers.

The manual outlines the basic information needed to perform case management activities comprehensively and correctly. It emphasizes the stimulation of ideas that explore all feasible alternatives and resources that can provide or augment care, whether that care is episodic, chronic, or lifelong. It capitalizes on experience, including that of colleagues who edited the book, who, as case managers and discharge planners, were trained in "the school of hard knocks." Learning was accomplished not by reading or taking courses on case management or discharge planning but by trial and error, keeping extensive notes of what worked and what did not. Networking was and still is vital because it is one of the best ways to learn.

⬛ SUMMARY

In conclusion, the case manager is in a position to collaborate with and actively assist the primary healthcare team and family to seek and implement cost-effective alternatives to care. He or she is also in a position to educate not only the patient and family but also other healthcare professionals in methods of using the healthcare system appropriately. Case management is the vital component that empowers the patient and family to assume the role of caregiver, because in many instances care will be needed for the long term or for life. Case management is a vital link between the patient's medical treatment, insurance benefits, and community resources and allows coordination of the needed services without duplication or fragmentation while maintaining quality of care and minimizing costs. Early intervention, on-site capabilities of the case manager, collaboration with other members of the team, and excellent communication with all participants in the care of the patient cannot be overemphasized.

REFERENCES

1. Guiliano KK, Poirier CE (1991). Nursing case management: Critical pathways to desirable outcomes. Nurs Manag 22(3):52-55.
2. Gibbs B, et al (1995). The role of the clinical nurse specialist and the nurse manager in case management. J Nurs Admin 25(5):28-34.
3. Cohen EL, Cesta TG (1993). Nursing Case Management from Concept to Evaluation. St. Louis, Mosby, pp. 3-4.
4. Cohen EL (1996). Nursing Case Management in the 21st Century. St Louis, Mosby-Year Book, pp. 3-9.
5. Hicks L, et al (1991). Nursing challenges in managed care. Nurs Econ 10(4):265-276.
6. Del Togno-Armanasco V, et al (1993). Collaborative Nursing Case Management: A Handbook for Development and Implementation. New York, Springer, pp. 2-5.
7. Cohen EL, Cesta TG (1993). Nursing Case Management from Concept to Evaluation. St. Louis, Mosby, pp. 14-15.
8. Certification of Insurance Rehabilitation Specialists (CIRSC) (1993). Certified Case Manager (CCM) Certification Guide (flyer). Rolling Meadows, IL, Certification of Insurance Rehabilitation Specialists.
9. American Nurses Association (1988). Nursing Case Management. Publication no. Ns-32. Kansas City, MO, American Nurses Association.
10. Lyon JC (1993). Models of nursing care delivery and case management: Clarification of terms. Nurs Econ 11(4):163-169.
11. Cohen EL, Cesta TG (1993). Nursing Case Management from Concept to Evaluation. St. Louis, Mosby, pp. 22-26.
12. Boland P (1993). Making Managed Healthcare Work. Gaithersburg, MD, Aspen, pp. 108-109.

13. Mullahy CM (1995). The Case Manager's Handbook. Gaithersburg, MD, Aspen, pp. 6-13.
14. Zander K (1985). Second generation primary nursing: A new agenda. J Nurs Admin 15(3):18-24.
15. Weil M, Karls JM (eds) (1985). Case Management in Human Service Practice. San Francisco, Jossey-Bass, pp. 1-28.
16. Steinberg RM, Carter GW (1983). Case Management and the Elderly. Lexington, MA, D.C. Heath and Co (Lexington Books).
17. Ethridge P, Lamb GS (1989). Professional nursing case management improves quality, access and costs. Nurs Manag 20(3):30-35.
18. Cohen EL (1991). Nursing case management: Does it pay? J Nurs Admin 21(4):20-25.
19. Del Togno-Armanasco V, et al (1989). Developing an integrated nursing case management model. Nurs Manag 20(5):26-29.
20. Del Togno-Armnasco V, et al (1993). Op. cit., p. 1.
21. Del Togno-Armnasco V, et al (1993). Op. cit., pp. 72-75.
22. Gibson J, et al (1994). CNS-directed case management: Cost and quality in harmony. J Nurs Admin 24(6):45-51.
23. Rheaume A, et al (1994). Case management and nursing practice. J Nurs Admin 24(3):30-36.
24. Phillips CY, et al (1994). Case manager/nurse manager: A blending of the roles. Nurs Manag 24(10):26-34.
25. Thompson RC (1995). Protecting Human Guinea Pigs, 2nd ed. FDA Consumer Report. Washington, D.C., Department of Health and Human Services, pp. 14-18.
26. Case Management Caseloads: How Much Is Too Much (1995). Case Management Advisor 6(5):61-76.
27. CDCP's New Definitions of AIDS Could Increase Case Management Caseloads (1993). Case Management Advisor 4(1):5-7.
28. Determining the Right Caseload Depends on the Type of Case (1993). Case Management Advisor 4(6):73-75.
29. Shapiro J (1983). Family reactions and coping strategies in response to the physically ill or handicapped child: A review. Soc Sci Med 17(4):913-931.

BIBLIOGRAPHY

Bandman EL, Bandman B (1995). Critical Thinking in Nursing. Stamford, CT, Appleton and Lange.
Douglass LM (1996). The Effective Nurse Leader and Manager, 5th ed. St. Louis, Mosby-Year Book.
Erkel EA (1993). The impact of case management in preventive services. J Nurs Admin 23(1):22-31.
Eshwick CJ, Weiss LJ (1987). Managing the Continuum of Care. Gaithersburg, Md., Aspen.
Faherty B (1990). Case management the latest buzzword: What it is and what it isn't. Caring Magazine 90(7):20-22.
Feldman C, et al (1993). Decision making in case management of home health care clients. J Nurs Admin 23(1):33-38.
Hall P (1996). Providing psychological support: A quick rundown of the essential nursing assessments and interventions. Am J Nurs 96(10):16N.
Haynes VL (1996). Caring for the laryngectomy patient. Am J Nurs 96(5):16B-16K.
Hinderson MG, Wallack SS (1987). Evaluating case management for catastrophic illness. Business Health 4(3):7-11.
Joseph IV, Reele BJ (1995). Respite for the caregiver. Am J Nurs 95(5):55.
Katz F (1991). Making a case for case management. Business Health 9(4):75-77.
Lee S (1996). New trends in disease management. Continuing Care 15(7):37-39.
Lilley LL, Guanci R (1996). Educate the patient. Am J Nurs 96(4):14-16.
McKenna H (1990). Which model. Nurs Times 86(25):50-52.
Merrill JC (1985). Defining case management. Business and Health 2(8):5-9.
Milholland DK (1994). Privacy and confidentiality of patient information. J Nurs Admin 24(2):19-24.
Mullahy CM (1992). Ten ways you can improve your working relationship with physicians. Case Management Advisor 3(16):81-82.
Mullahy CM (1995). The case manager IS the catalytic collaborator in managed care. Continuing Care 1(1):7-9.
O'Hare PA, Terry MA (1988). Discharge planning strategies for assuring continuity of care. Gaithersburg, MD, Aspen.
Olis G, et al (1989). Case management: A bottom line delivery model. Part I: The concept. J Nurs Admin 19(11):16-20.
Olis G, et al (1989). Case management: A bottom line care delivery model. Part II: Adaptation of the model. J Nurs Admin 19(12):12-17.
Powell SK (1996). Nursing Case Management: A Practical Guide to Success in Managed Care. Philadelphia, Lippincott, pp. 19-32.
Rogers M, et al (1991). Community based nursing case management pays off. Nurs Manag 22(3):30-34.
Ruppert RA, Sandler RL (1996). Caring for the lay caregiver. Am J Nurs 96(3):40-47.
Siegler EL, Whitney FA (1994). Nurse Physician Collaboration. New York, Springer, pp. 117-121.
Smith MC (1993). Case management and nursing theory based practice. Nurs Sci Q 6(1):8-9.
Tahan HA, Cest TG (1994). Developing case management care plans using a quality improvement model. J Nurs Admin 24(12):49-57.
Winn J, Sierra R (1991). Case management: Cooperation among disciplines—a social work perspective. Case Management 23(4):258-260.
Wolf GA (1986). Communication: Key contributor to effectiveness—a nurse executive responds. J Nurs Admin 16(9):26-28.
Yee DL (1990). Developing a quality assurance program in case management settings. Caring Magazine, July:30-35.
Zander K (1987). Nursing case management: A classic definition. New Definition 2(2):1-3.
Zander K (1988). Nursing case management: Strategic management of cost and quality outcomes. J Nurs Admin 19(5):23-30.
Zarle NC (1987). Continuing Care: The Process and Practice of Discharge Planning. Gaithersburg, MD, Aspen.

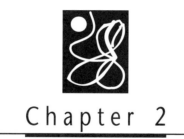

Chapter 2

Case Management Process

Basically, the process used for case management is the same regardless of the employer group (Fig. 2–1). Therefore, the steps or facets of the process listed below apply to any organization that offers case management. The primary differences in case management programs lie in the types of clients served, the intensity of case management services allowed by the case manager's employer, and the type of case management plan that is developed. The case management process also depends on whether the case manager's organization is facility based, community based, or a combination of both or whether these services are provided by the healthcare payor. The basic principles of case management endorsed by the Commission for Case Management Certification are as follows:[1]

Principle 1: Certificants shall endeavor to place the public interest above their own at all times.

Principle 2: Certificants shall respect the integrity and protect the welfare of those persons or groups with whom they are working.

Principle 3: Certificants shall always maintain objectivity in their relationships with clients.

Principle 4: Certificants shall act with integrity in dealing with other professionals so as to facilitate their contribu-

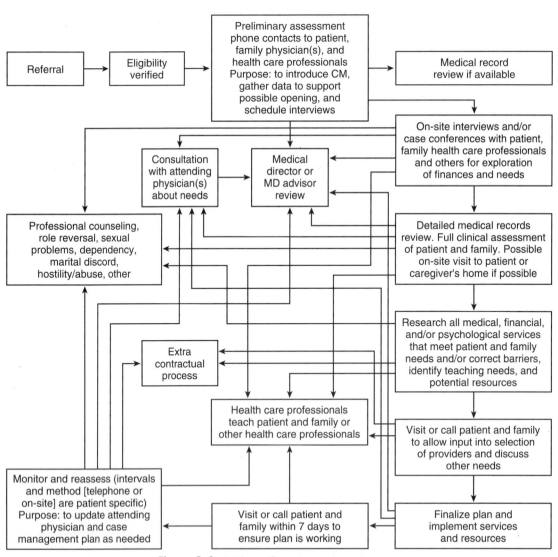

Figure 2–1 • Flow of case management process.

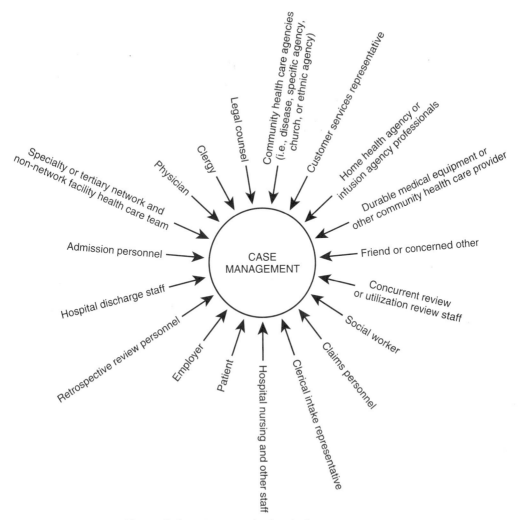

Figure 2–2 • Sources of referrals for case management.

tions with respect to achieving maximum benefits for the client.

Principle 5: Certificants shall keep their technical competency at a level which ensures that their clients will receive the benefit of the highest quality of service the profession can offer that is consistent with the client's conditions and circumstances.

Principle 6: Certificants shall honor the integrity and respect the limitations placed on the use of the CCM designation.

Principle 7: Certificants shall obey all laws and regulations, avoiding any conduct or activity that could harm others.

Principle 8: Certificants shall help maintain the integrity of the Code of Professional Conduct for Case Managers.

REFERRALS

Referrals for case management come from a variety of sources (Fig. 2–2). The most common method of referral is by way of the telephone. Although referral sources are varied, most are healthcare professionals, the healthcare payors, the family, or community agencies. Although computer capabilities can be significantly helpful in finding and targeting cases and can flag potential cases and forward data electronically to the case management division, such automation is not always the best referral mechanism because it may generate a referral after the fact. Also, unless there is a modem link that allows transfer of information between organizations, electronic referrals are limited to internal referrals within a case manager's organization. Consequently, if the referral process is limited to electronic submission, not all referrals can be captured in a timely manner.[2]

Timeliness

Regardless of the referral source, the entire case management process and the success of the case hinge on the timeliness of the referral and the accuracy of the information received, not only at the time of referral but also throughout the duration of the case.[3] There is no cookbook recipe indicating how or what information should be collected or at what point a case must be referred or opened. The key factors are: (1) to have the mechanisms in place to identify patients, (2) to make the referral as early as possible, and (3) to capture as much preliminary and pertinent data as possible. These mechanisms assist the case manager in screening the case to determine whether it should be opened.

Referral Criteria

Each organization using case management has a specific list of cases or types of cases they wish to flag and possibly follow. Naturally, the type of case management offered by the organization is the key to the referral criteria established. For instance, if the organization offers facility-based case management services, the criteria may include a need to see patients much earlier in the course of the disease than if the organization's purpose were to serve persons with chronic long-term needs (as in many geriatric and mental health case management programs). However, as the focus of the healthcare system changes from an illness-driven system to one designed to encourage wellness and prevention, many case management programs may soon redesign their referral criteria to capture this new focus.

When establishing criteria or setting the referral flags, the key is to make the criteria realistic—whether realism is achieved by diagnosis, age, time frames, or dollar amounts. For instance, if the organization is a healthcare facility, the primary criteria for flagging a referral may be patient age, diagnosis, and support system (e.g., any patient over a certain age who has had a stroke and lives alone). In contrast, a healthcare payor or facility that operates on a capitated basis may design their criteria to capture patients by diagnosis as well as by anticipated claims expenditure (e.g., all cardiac patients for whom the stay is anticipated to exceed 10 days or the costs to exceed $75,000—generally the latter limit is set to correspond to the healthcare payor's stop loss or reinsurance policy). However, if the day and dollar referral criteria are too low, the referral numbers may be astronomical. Conversely, if the criteria are not set to capture specific diagnoses for disease management, some patients will not be flagged. Consequently, these cases will not be referred, or valuable time will be spent weeding out inappropriate cases and then delaying services to those patients who are referred appropriately.

The following situations, conditions, and diagnoses comprise some of the most common reasons for referrals to case management:

- Referral (or self-referral) to a nonparticipating provider or to the wrong provider.
- Placement or discharge difficulties.
- Admission to a tertiary care facility or medical center (whether in area or out-of-area) that is not contracted with the healthcare organization paying the claims.
- Absence of a payor source or known insurance.
- Hospital stay anticipated to exceed a specific day or dollar amount (i.e., set days or set dollar amount).
- Claims in excess of specific dollar amounts for outpatient services.
- Repeated hospitalizations or emergency room visits (more than three in 6 months) for the same or similar condition or for drug-seeking behavior.
- Misuse or overuse of services (this includes the overuse of pharmaceuticals).
- Multiple diagnoses.
- Excessive hospitalization or length of stay because the hospital does not have a specialty unit for treatment of the illness or injury.
- Repeated infections or complications of medical conditions.
- Individuals who are dependent on a ventilator or other technology.
- Individuals in a persistent vegetative state.
- Lack of discharge planning.

- Severe burns (i.e., admission to a burn unit).
- Decubitus ulcers (generally, this includes persons whose decubiti are rated at stages three or four; it also includes persons with multiple decubiti, complications, or an underlying catastrophic medical condition).
- Cardiac arrest with hypoxic brain damage.
- Patients with specific diagnoses for whom health education and linkage to community agencies may assist in educating him or her about the disease to prevent future episodes, teach endurance, and handle lifestyle changes better; diagnoses in this category include such disease categories as cardiomyopathy or other cardiac conditions, high-risk pregnancies, respiratory conditions such as asthma and chronic obstructive pulmonary disease, congestive heart failure, and arthritis.
- Patients with new tracheostomies or tracheostomies with complications.
- Persons living alone or those with no family or caregiver or significant other.
- End-stage cancer (or other end-stage illnesses) that require home care or hospice care for a terminal condition, or cases requiring home care that can potentially exceed a specific dollar amount.
- Requests for care that exceeds that classified as intermittent skilled care or usual and customary care for the diagnosis.
- Cases, diagnoses, or conditions referred or designated by contractual agreements between the case management firm and its clients (e.g., Medicaid managed care projects, services to the elderly) or those designated by the legal department, senior management, medical director, or pharmacy director as cases that have the potential to cause added risk to the organization.
- All transplant patients (e.g., bone marrow, liver, heart, kidney, dual, or experimental).
- Multiple trauma patients in whom long-term disabilities are anticipated or for whom ongoing care or hospital costs are anticipated to exceed a specific dollar amount.
- Head trauma patients in whom long-term disabilities are anticipated or for whom ongoing care or hospital costs are anticipated to exceed a specific dollar amount (e.g., $50,000).
- Patients with spinal cord injuries or tumors, with complications or paralysis.
- Patients with amputations.
- Neonates in whom complications, anomalies, or developmental disabilities are identified and care is anticipated to be complex, long-term, or lifelong.

In addition to these reasons, a list of referrals not always appropriate for the case management organization should also be developed. The presence of one of these referrals does not mean automatic exclusion from case management; it only means that cases on this list may be screened last. This list may include such diagnoses, conditions, or situations as the following:

- Learning disabilities.
- Neurologic diseases, meningitis, or communicable diseases involving the nervous system without paralysis or anticipated long-term disabilities or in which the length of stay or treatment course is anticipated to be within the norm for that condition, illness, or injury.
- Fractures with no long-term disabilities or for which the length of stay or treatment course is anticipated to be within the norm for that condition or injury.
- Respiratory conditions (not ventilator or tracheostomy dependent) in which the patient is progressing at the normal rate of recovery or treatment is within the norm for the condition.
- Premature infant who is progressing at the normal rate of recovery, treatment is within the norm for the condition, and long-term care or complications are not anticipated.
- Any case, regardless of diagnosis, that is progressing at the normal rate of recovery or treatment is within the norm for the condition and long-term needs or complications are not anticipated.

Many patients, diagnoses, and case variables can easily fit the characteristics of the "flag." However, by the time the preliminary assessment or the first interviews are completed, it is apparent that case management may not have an impact or effect a change in the outcome.[2] For example, a patient might meet the diagnostic criteria for referral but is progressing well at the expected rate, and the family is already linked to alternate funding sources or community resources. At this point, the case really does not need intervention, so why open the case? The case manager's time may be better spent on another case where everything is falling apart. Certainly, at any time in the first case, if things go wrong, the case can be re-referred for reevaluation to determine whether to open the case. Consequently, referral sources, patients, and families should be made aware of the fact that cases can always be re-referred at any time if there is a change in events.

Good examples of cases that belong in this category are human immune deficiency virus

(HIV), acquired immune deficiency syndrome (AIDS), and terminal cancer. The mere diagnosis of HIV, AIDS, or terminal cancer does not mean that the patient requires case management. In the HIV-positive patient it may be years before he or she actually develops AIDS. In the interim, most of these patients continue working, and their only need may be monthly medications. In such cases, what is the case manager managing? Nothing. So why should such cases encumber a case manager? The same thing is true of the patient with terminal cancer. If the patient receives benefits for hospice care or other skilled nursing services related to terminal care and is linked appropriately to the proper services, and if the family and patient are "coping," what is there to manage? Nothing. The primary question the case manager should ask with each case is, "What is there to manage and will my interventions make a difference?" The cases cited here as examples and similar ones can just as easily be followed by the physician or clinic or the home health agency or hospice nursing staff.

Despite the use of diagnosis and cost flags for referral, not all cases triggering these flags are necessarily appropriate for case management. Also, cases that are flagged and appropriate for one organization or entity may not be appropriate for another. For instance, although the processes of case management are basically the same for most entities, referral flags differ drastically for each. For instance, for case management in workers' compensation, flags are used to trigger injuries by type, patient age, and length of employment. In contrast, a healthcare payor's case management flags may search for acute and chronic "catastrophic" illnesses or cases that are anticipated to use (or actually do use) enormous amounts of high-cost resources, whereas facility-based case management units may set their flags to mark various types of diseases or injuries based on age, financial resources, living arrangements, or a need for early education.

Referral Demographics

As much basic patient demographic information must be captured at the time of referral as possible.[2, 3] A referral form is an excellent means of capturing such data. For ease in screening cases, many case management organizations make every attempt to note, at a minimum, the following elements (workers' compensation may include some additional elements):

- Referral source, name, and phone number.
- Patient's name.
- Patient's address and phone number.
- Patient's date of birth.
- Insured person's name and identification number (often the identification number is the Social Security number).
- Name and identification number of the subscriber of other health insurance.
- Next of kin's name, address, and phone number(s) at home and at work.
- Present location of patient.
- Contact name if hospitalized; if not, contact name from the referral agency or community resource.
- Diagnosis, present medical status, and any identified problem(s).
- Primary care physician's name and phone number.
- Attending physician's name(s) and phone number(s).
- Other pertinent comments.

The information collected during the referral serves as the basis for the preliminary screening assessment and assists in determining the appropriateness of the case for case management services. The more information that can be obtained at this time, the better. This information not only assists the case manager in making his or her decision about opening the case but also, and more important, saves valuable time and eliminates duplicate telephone calls needed to abstract similar information at a later time.

Early referrals allow better case outcomes and closer monitoring of healthcare benefits and also help to prevent wasting of any available benefits. Another reason for early referral is to ensure that the initial period of critical care treatment is provided in the most appropriate setting and by the most appropriate specialty practitioners. Also, as the healthcare system changes to a wellness or prevention model, patient education becomes more important. Early referrals often translate into better outcomes, more lives saved, more appropriate use of healthcare resources, shorter hospital stays, and fewer readmissions. Rehabilitation provides a good example of the benefits of early referral. If the patient is not clinically ready for intense rehabilitation therapy but is admitted to an acute rehabilitation unit anyway, he or she is likely to demonstrate little progress and is not discharged. Rehabilitation benefits from his or her healthcare coverage may then be quickly exhausted. Consequently, when the patient finally does reach a point where he or she can benefit from rehabilitation services, no funds are available, and the patient either is not allowed the benefit of appropriate rehabilitation or must assume the costs privately.

Another good example is a trauma patient. Far too often these patients are stabilized in the hospital's emergency room and then are transferred to the facility's intensive care unit, which may not be equipped or staffed to handle the required level of care. Consequently, valuable time is wasted, the patient's condition may deteriorate, and precious healthcare benefits may be exhausted if the patient is not moved as soon as deficits are identified.[3]

Experience shows that referral intake is best accomplished by a trained clerical staff because professional nursing or social worker time is far too costly. The professional case manager's time is best used for the decision-making processes required in opening and handling cases. However, delegation of this task varies with the organization.

VERIFICATION OF ELIGIBILITY

Although eligibility verification is organization specific and may not seem to apply to a facility-based case management unit, it does. How can services be implemented without knowing who will pay the bill? Therefore, once the case has been referred, the next step is to verify the patient's eligibility for benefits before the case is assigned to a case manager. This step is usually handled by means of a telephone call.

Insurance or payor verification is of critical importance because it allows the case management unit to verify lifetime maximums, limitations, exclusions, deductibles, and copayments and, most important, to determine which insurance is primary. The specific healthcare payors involved and the dollar amounts available are the major factors guiding what can be done. These factors play a key role in the ultimate long-term goals selected and in whether the case management plan can be realized or not.

Despite any dollar amounts that may be available from the healthcare payor, all patients must be screened, not only initially but also continually throughout the case, for their potential need for referral to alternate funding programs and community resources. It is important to add that if anyone on the healthcare team discovers that a patient's benefits might terminate,

immediate communication of this fact to all parties is critical. This is necessary to ensure that the patient and the family are aware of their right to elect their existing insurance benefits under the Consolidated Omnibus Budget Reconciliation Act (COBRA). A good example occurred recently in connection with a kidney transplant patient. Apparently, the renal transplant social worker knew that the patient's wife was to be terminated from her job but never communicated this fact to the other members of the team. The family was encouraged to apply for COBRA coverage; however, this was done on the last day of their eligibility to apply, the reasoning for the noneligibility status. When the patient had a rejection episode, everyone was scrambling because it appeared that the patient was uninsured. Coverage was finally reinstated, but there were many frantic phone calls to the employer, the COBRA service agency, the health plan's member services department, the physician, and the patient, as well as many calls back and forth between the case management staff and the hospital. One simple call, when the initial COBRA need was identified, might have eliminated a wasted morning of desperate phone calls.

PRELIMINARY SCREENING OR ASSESSMENT

Once the referral information has been reviewed and a decision has been made to proceed, the next step is to conduct a preliminary screening assessment. In this phase further details can be obtained that can be used in the decision-making process if it is decided to open the case for case management. The objective of the preliminary assessment process is to elicit enough medical and other pertinent information to make an informed decision about case opening. Most often the information is gathered by telephone and through chart review, medical records review, and patient and family interviews. In addition to any records review, calls may be necessary to such sources as the hospital discharge planner, the physician, other members of the healthcare team, the healthcare payor, and the family.

Documentation of Preliminary Screening Data

Although the preliminary screening process may reveal that there is no need for case management, some form of documenting the data collected must be maintained. At a minimum, such documentation should capture:

- Date
- Person(s) spoken with and phone number(s)
- Brief summary of the case-specific information obtained

Although documentation is an ongoing process throughout the case, it is just as important during the preliminary assessment stage. These notes not only justify any decisions made about opening a case, they also justify the reasons for not opening a case should questions arise at a later date. Documentation is critically important in assisting with one's own protection and recall of events if litigation should occur later. If a decision is made not to open the case, the case must be filed in accordance with the customary procedures for storing records at the healthcare organization.

Reasons for Not Opening a Case

Just because a case is referred does not mean it will be opened. There are many reasons why a referred case is never opened. Some of these factors are as follows:

- Insufficient funds or benefits allowed by the primary or other insurance source, or the patient does not have the ability to pay for services, copayments, deductibles, and other out-of-pocket expenses. This is especially true when benefits are limited or exhausted.

  However, in contrast, this factor may be the decisive one guiding opening of the case for a hospital-based case manager because if the patient requires services on discharge, some payor source must be available to assume this responsibility.
- Attorney on the case hinder effective case management (however, in most cases, if an attorney is involved in a case, the case will be appropriate for case management).
- Extensive and sophisticated family knowledge of community resources and their entitlement to these resources.
- Refusal of patient or family to use any "outside" help or involvement.
- Unwillingness of the healthcare payor to flex benefits or allow an extra contractual process when benefits are limited or excluded.

  However, while such a case may be closed

to a healthcare payor or home health agency case manager, this type of case may require case managers in other organizations (e.g., facility-based case manager or alternate funding case manager) to intensify their case management activity if the patient is to be linked with care.
- Faster rate of recovery than expected, although the diagnosis falls within the referral criteria listing.
- Lack of motivation or compliance of the patient or family, or resistance to change or to the plans recommended.

Based on the initial information received, the referral source must be notified if a decision is made not to open the case. If a case is not opened initially, re-referral at a later date can occur if case variables or circumstances change. If a decision is made to open the case, the next step is to establish interview dates and conduct an in-depth assessment of both the patient and the family.

CLINICAL ASSESSMENTS

Assessment, development, and revision of the case management plan continue throughout the duration of the case. These processes are defined in the flyer issued by the Commission for Case Management Certification[1] and are instrumental if the patient is to be moved through the continuum of care, using resources and healthcare dollars appropriately. The case manager must possess excellent skills of assessment as well as skills related to communication, attention to detail, and the ability to prioritize details.

Accurate and comprehensive assessment of the details of the case is absolutely critical to the development of an effective case management plan. Assessments that are this comprehensive usually require input from a variety of sources and a multidisciplinary team approach. Assessments for case management planning focus not only on the medical needs of the patient but also on the entire picture—family, psychological facets, socioeconomic facets, cultural factors—with all pertinent facts used in the final plan. Although the referral and preliminary screening assessment data can be gathered by phone, the actual clinical assessment is best accomplished during an on-site visit.

On-site visits and assessments allow not only actual review of the medical records but also an opportunity to meet the patient and visualize his or her care needs. The formal evaluation of the case starts with the patient's clinical assessment and an assessment of the family. These are the most crucial steps in developing a case management plan. These assessment phases involve the accumulation of pertinent and accurate data from all parties. It is these data that allow the case manager to begin to identify alternatives and resources.

Data Elements

The data collected must be of sufficient scope and depth to identify the needs of the patient and family and his or her cognitive and physical functional abilities or limitations and barriers. Other data necessary for case management planning include:

- Cultural, ethnic, and religious beliefs or background.
- Daily routines or habits.
- Health perception.
- Dietary habits.
- Values or beliefs.
- Coping ability and the ability to handle stress.
- Role reversal or relationships and the patient's or family's perceptions.
- Sexuality.
- Self-perception.
- Preferences, family dynamics, social and economic background.
- Occupational history and economic abilities.

Although the ideal process is to interview the patient first, this is not always possible, particularly if the patient has sustained trauma or is in a coma. Regardless of who is interviewed, an introductory phone call is necessary to establish a time and date for the actual interview, introduce oneself as the case manager, give a brief overview of the case management role, and allow the person an opportunity to ask questions.[2]

Cultural Sensitivity

Case managers must constantly strive to be culturally sensitive to their clients. Ignorance of cultural beliefs and practices can lead to serious problems that compromise efforts to build a solid relationship between the case manager and the patient or family. Any case manager who works regularly with culturally diverse groups must be extremely familiar with that population's language, customs, folklore, diet, religion, behavior styles, body language, habits, and attitudes as well as the cultural reactions to health and illness. For instance, religious beliefs influence the life styles of most cultures. In many cultures, illness, injury, and death are believed to be "punishments" sent by God for sins. Therefore, whereas persons of one religion may believe that God is punishing the sick person, others may view sickness as a "test of strength."[4-7]

Insensitivity to cultural differences can lead to a potentially dangerous outcome; most commonly, failure of the case management plan. In addition, dishonoring or ignorance of cultural beliefs and practices can result in a perception by the patient or family that they have been harmed or insulted. An attempt by the case manager to impose his or her beliefs onto others accomplishes nothing other than failure.

One of the most difficult aspects of dealing with culturally diverse patients is the need to achieve effective communication. Every effort should be made to assign case managers who speak the dominant language of the patient and family to these cases. If this is not possible, the case manager should arrange for the presence of an interpreter who is familiar with medical terminology. Otherwise, much information can be lost or misunderstood. It is one thing to have access to a general interpreter but another to know that an interpreter can relay comprehensive medical instructions without losing the context or meaning of the message.

If local interpreters are not available, phone companies such as American Telephone and Telegraph (AT&T) can provide a full range of interpreter services. These services can be accessed by calling the local business office of the phone company. Other sources for local interpreters are volunteers from ethnic groups or churches and possibly a community's local information and referral service. Information and referral services are available by telephone. The caller is provided with information about possible local resources along with their phone numbers. Information and referral services are an invaluable resource both for healthcare professionals and the lay public and can be used not only for locating interpreters but also for finding other community resources.

Key to Success

The key to the ultimate success of the case is the assumption by the case manager of a proactive and positive role, which must last throughout the case. Fortunately, most case managers find that they are a welcomed addition to the team because the patient and family are often under tremendous stress and find themselves at a loss about what to do next. Many are intimidated by the complexity of the healthcare system and need an advocate to defend their interests because stressors related to an illness or injury take their toll. Depending on family dynamics, some patients and families go through one crisis after another, whereas others are able to regroup and "go with the flow."[8] The case manager must always stay attuned to the verbal and nonverbal cues that identify the patient's needs and those of the family or caregiver.

Case managers must also keep in mind that if the caregiver goes, the success of the case management plan may go with him. Possibly the most important key to the ultimate success of the plan is good communication with all parties; such communication must be open, honest, and as frequent as case variables dictate. Also, case managers must never promise services without knowing whether they are available or approved. Healthcare professionals must never give the impression that payment for services will be ongoing because this only sets up a "right of expectation" that healthcare benefits will continue indefinitely.

To be effective, assessments must be thorough and systematic. Assessment is defined as "a process by which the nurse collects and analyzes data about the client. Data collection includes gathering information from physical, psychosocial, spiritual, cognitive and functional abilities, and developmental, economic, and environmental dimensions."[9] The Commission for Case Management Certification defines assessment "as the process of collecting in-depth information about a person's situation and function to identify individual needs in order to develop a comprehensive case management plan that will address those needs. In addition to direct client contact, information should be gathered from other relevant sources (patient or client, professional or nonprofessional caregivers, employers, health records, and educational or military records."[1]

According to these definitions, the clinical assessment of the patient and the assessment of the family must be comprehensive enough to reflect their total needs. These assessments must capture details pertinent to the social, financial, cultural, religious, physical, and psychological functioning of both the patient and the family. For instance, the initial and ongoing clinical assessments are used to determine the patient's physical care needs, psychological factors, and functional limits and abilities. Assessments also emphasize the family's and caregiver's physical, mental, and emotional ability to cope with these immediate care needs as well as the stresses and emotional demands of caring for a patient who may have complex or lifelong needs. During the initial assessment, the interview process, and subsequent conversations with the family, the case manager must always strive to get and maintain a clear picture of how the family functioned prior to the illness as well as during the present acute phase.

Assessments are best accomplished by on-site visits using such techniques as chart reviews, visual observation of the patient and family, interviews with the patient and family, case conferences, and consultations with the healthcare team members and the patient's physicians. A case manager who is based in a facility or is a clinical nurse specialist has an advantage because he or she may be able to conduct an actual physical examination of the patient, which can be a real advantage in planning.

On-site visits not only allow the case manager to see and communicate directly with the patient and family, they also allow an opportunity to visualize the personal dynamics operating in the case and a chance to "bond" with the patient and establish a level of trust. More important, on-site assessments allow the case manager to view the actual facts of the case without third-party interpretations. Unfortunately, because of budgetary constraints, senior management directives, or remote geographic territories covered by the case management organization, on-site assessments and reassessments are not always possible. This capability varies with the organization.

Reassessments must be performed at regular intervals throughout the case.[1] These are necessary not only for monitoring purposes but also for making adjustments to the case management plan as the patient's condition progresses, slides backward, or stays the same; the Commission for Case Management Certification describes this process as evaluation.[1] These adjustments in the plan are made as the treating physician alters his or her orders to correspond to the changing needs of the patient. The frequency and type of reassessments made and whether they are accomplished by telephone or on-site depend on many factors. Among these are the intensity and severity of the patient's condition; the quantity, quality, and complexity of the resources necessary to manage the patient's required level of care; and the patient's and family's emotional and coping abilities, to name only a few.

Assessment Components

Assessments involve a continuous process of gathering information to ensure that the patient's needs are being met. They also include a monitoring process to ensure, at a minimum, that the patient's healthcare benefits are not exhausted, that the patient is always at the appropriate level of care, and that the caregiver is following the techniques as required and is not becoming worn out by the demands of the tasks. Monitoring is defined by the Commission for Case Management Certification as the ongoing process of gathering sufficient information from all relevant sources about the case management plan and its activities or services to enable the case manager to determine the plan's effectiveness.[1] Consequently, the assessment phase of case management is never completed.

The initial assessment process should cover at least the following components:

- Demographic information on the patient and family.
- Patient's past and current physical health.
- Patient's current functional status.
- Patient's mental health status, memory, and behavior.
- Patient's psychosocial function and perception of the illness or injury.
- Financial data.
- Caregiver capabilities.
- Home environment.
- Resources and providers.
- Actual physical assessment of the patient and his or her physical care needs, medications, and feedings.[10]

Most case management organizations have established standards that require case managers to complete the clinical assessment phase within a specified period of time after referral. For instance, although a facility-based or community-based case management program may start the assessment process at the time of admission, a healthcare payor's or independent case management program may specify a 7- to 10-day time frame after referral in which to complete the initial assessment. The time frame should be realistic enough to allow the case manager to capture as much relevant data as possible, since the primary purpose of the assessment phase is to determine needs and the corresponding resources to meet these needs.

Even if the patient is hospitalized, the family assessment is best accomplished, if possible, in the home environment. Case managers have a big advantage over discharge planners in that the latter never see at first hand the actual home environment and the family's interactions with each other. Final case management plans can be far more detail oriented than is possible in discharge planning. If on-site visits are allowed, the case manager has a dual advantage—he or she can assess the family and the home simultaneously. Home interviews allow the case manager an opportunity to see such things as:

- Actual environmental risks and barriers.
- The true living situation.
- Environment in which activities of daily living occur (bathroom, bedroom, kitchen).
- Interactions between all parties.

Regardless of where they are conducted, family assessments should determine at minimum the following details:

- Names, addresses, and phone numbers (including work phone numbers).
- Work history of spouse.
- Family health problems and limitations.
- Perception of the patient's illness or injury.
- Emotional status of family.
- Transportation availability and mode.
- Identification of potential barriers within the home, if the home is to be the discharge destination.
- Identification of the person who will be the caregiver.
- Caregiver's physical, emotional, and mental capabilities and availability.
- Cultural, ethnic, and religious beliefs.

Sources of Data

During any part of the referral or assessment phase, solicitation of facts from the family, patient's physicians, and other healthcare team members is vital for the success of the plan. To ensure that all data are collected and recorded properly, a questionnaire that has been specifically developed for the various parties who are to be interviewed is an excellent method for recording data.

As mentioned in Chapter 1, one of the greatest challenges facing a nonfacility-based case manager is to personally meet or speak by telephone with the patient's physician. Most contact with physicians is handled by telephone via his or her nurse. Although some physicians allow their staff to schedule a time and date for a telephone call from a case manager, others will speak directly with the caller if they are available. In some cases, physicians require a letter from a case manager that specifically outlines the intent of the conversation. In any event, the case manager must always have questions prepared before placing a call to the physician.[11]

Physicians treating patients in large tertiary care facilities or teaching institutions present their own challenges. Among these, possibly the most important is their rotation and shift schedules. Also, they may have had little exposure to the business side of healthcare. In such instances, a case manager's best ally is the clinical nurse specialist, head nurse, discharge planner, or specialty department head. For instance, if one works in a large tertiary care center, the best time to catch the physicians may be to join them on "grand rounds." Case managers have to be flexible enough to reschedule their time if access is to be gained to the important link in the case management plan—the physician.

In addition to the physician, contact must be made with the other healthcare professionals involved in the case. The Commission for Case Management Certification and the standard of practice for case management support this contact in the following terms: "Case management is not a profession in itself but rather an area of practice within one's profession. It is collaborative and trans-disciplinary in nature."[1, 12] The entire team's input is invaluable because they have the day-to-day responsibility of providing care to the patient and can provide insight into family or caregiver dynamics. This information can be gathered through personal conversations, interviews, or case conferences. For patients admitted to case management who are not inpatients, contact with the community agency that served him or her prior to referral may be helpful in capturing information that will be pertinent to the final case management plan.

Another source of data that is useful in the assessment phase is the patient's medical records.[12] Hospital-based case managers have an advantage here because they have ready access to the records. Gaining access to the patient's records for a non-facility-based case manager can range from a formal and complex process

(i.e., calling ahead and making all the necessary arrangements) to one that is informal and simple. In any event, if the case manager has a signed consent form, he or she does have a right to review the record.

Attorneys

Because case management often involves patients who have survived severe or catastrophic injuries, it is common to encounter attorneys, and their presence may not be known at the time of referral. If an attorney is involved, the case manager may have to review the case with his or her organization's legal counsel before proceeding. However, this process varies with the healthcare organization. The presence of an attorney poses its own set of issues and challenges.[13] If the case has proceeded to litigation and the patient is represented by an attorney, all contact with the patient may have to be approved by the patient's attorney, who has the right to deny a case manager's involvement with the case. When an attorney is involved, it is also common for direction in the case to come from the organization's legal counsel, and this direction frequently overrides any of the usual case management procedures.

Case managers should not be intimidated by the presence of an attorney. He or she should be contacted in the same manner used to contact others on the case. Many attorneys may be skeptical of the case manager's intent, but the case manager should merely state his or her reasons for involvement in the case. Put simply, a case manager's purpose is to assist the patient and the family to gain access to care while ensuring that the quality of this care is maintained.[13] Like physicians, most attorneys are a delight to work with. As with all interviews, the case manager should have questions prepared for the interview. Although the following scenarios are case specific, it is common for attorneys to:

- Allow involvement and services to proceed without stipulation.
- Set specific stipulations.
- Allow involvement in the case but no access to the patient unless the attorney is present during every contact with the patient.
- Require approval for any phone or personal contact with the patient and family.
- Tape all conversations between the case manager, patient, or family.

Some attorneys, once they understand the

case manager's role and purpose, allow the case manager to work with the patient and family. However, if the attorney poses too many stumbling blocks or denies access to the case, the organization may finally decide to close the case. If case closure does occur, the case manager must always carefully document the reasons for the closure in case questions arise at a later date.

Documentation of Clinical Assessment

Once the clinical assessment process is completed, all information captured must be documented in some written form.[14] The final written data serve as the basis for the case management plan. Although actual formats vary from organization to organization, the final summary must include and identify the following minimum information:

- Date of assessment
- Date of referral
- Patient's name and identification number
- Name of primary physician
- Diagnosis and prognosis
- Summary of medical procedures that have been carried out
- Current level of care and specialty unit, if applicable
- Planned date of discharge, if applicable
- Summary of pertinent past and present medical history
- Summary of special needs (e.g., intravenous therapy, oxygen, suctioning, wound care)
- Medications (frequency and dose)
- Allergies
- Summary of mental status and memory deficits
- Summary of neurological status and functional deficits
- Summary of problems related to skin integrity
- Summary of mobility status and deficits
- Pain and pain control, route, frequency, and type
- Elimination or bowel and bladder status and deficits
- Feeding and nutrition status (type and mode)
- Communication abilities and deficits
- Behavioral characteristics
- Sensory, visual, and auditory status and deficits
- Safety concerns

- Summary of capabilities in activities of daily living
- Amount and type of teaching required and teacher (caregiver, patient, professional)
- Level of care anticipated
- Agencies thought to be needed
- Equipment anticipated
- Type of facility anticipated for placement, if patient is not to be discharged home
- Person who is to assume financial responsibility for costs, or, if assistance is needed from alternate payor sources, the status of the application and eligibility of the patient
- Other (i.e., known barriers)

Not every patient has problems in each category. However, whenever a problem area is identified, a full description is necessary to ensure that an effective plan can be developed and implemented. In some instances, all the information cannot be gathered in one visit. If this occurs, it may be possible to collect most of the remaining data by telephone; if not, subsequent home or hospital assessment visits may be warranted.

INTERVIEWS

Purpose

The purpose of an interview in the case management process is to gather specific information from the patient, family, healthcare team member, or significant others using both verbal and nonverbal interactions. Interview data serve as the basis for the case management plan.

Because of time constraints, dates for actual interviews are often established by telephone, and this contact is then followed by a confirmation letter if time allows. Letters serve two purposes: (1) to confirm the date and time of the planned meeting, and (2) to reiterate the purpose and role of case management. Written confirmation of interviews is helpful because families are frequently in crisis or exhausted and may not hear all that is said.

A proactive approach used in the request for the initial interview serves to promote positive interactions.[15] As stated earlier, in the initial call the case manager should identify herself or himself, explain briefly the role of case management, state the purpose of the request for the interview, and explain basically how the data from the interview will be used.

Keys to Success

Interviews must be planned to be successful. Prior to the actual interview, questions must be prepared that direct the interview toward specific areas, capturing the information required. Careful preparation of questions decreases any chance that key information will be missed. Another effective tool is a questionnaire that is completed by the patient or family before the visit and can be used to elicit key information. However, when use of a questionnaire is not possible, specific questions must be the guide during the interview.

The approach and attitude of the interviewer and the questions asked set the pace for future interactions and rapport. It is a well-known fact that first impressions are lasting, and a second chance is often lost when the first impression is a bad one![16] Patients and families must be made aware of the importance of their contribution to the case management process. During any interview, both parties, the interviewer and the interviewee, make judgments about each other. Consequently, the first few minutes of an interview set the tone for future relationships and rapport between the nurse and the interviewee.

Although it is wise to have questions prepared in advance, the case manager should also listen for key answers and clues that can lead to other questions or areas to be considered. During an interview it is important to know when one should redirect questions or bring the conversation back to the original issue. This ability is especially important when one is exploring some of the more sensitive issues such as marital status or discord, financial issues, abuse, sexuality, or other personal issues. During the interview the case manager must stay attuned to both verbal and nonverbal clues that indicate that the area under discussion is more sensitive than anticipated and that questioning should cease.

Keen interview skills and an ability to listen, a knowledge of the patient's condition and clinical indications, wide contacts with community resources, and a knowledge of the patient's entitlement to these resources enhance the trust and confidence of the patient and family in the case manager and promote a positive relationship and success in the case.

The important key during any interview is to take written notes. Once the case manager has been introduced, the patient or family must be informed that notes will be taken during the course of the interview to ensure that nothing is forgotten that may affect the final plan.

Attire and Location

After the time, date, meeting place, and attendees for the interview have been agreed upon, the case manager must in some cases consider his or her attire for the event. Attire can set the tone for proactive interaction.[16] Certainly it is important to look professional. However, if the interview is to be in the patient's home and that home is in the country or a section of the city that is unfamiliar to the case manager or is in a location where one may not feel secure, showing up in a suit may set the case manager apart. It may also set a tone for the interview that is different from the one anticipated. If the patient's home is in a section of the city that is not safe or is not conducive to an on-site interview, arrangements should be made either for a partner to attend the interview or for a new central location that is convenient to all parties.

Not all homes are comfortable, nor are they clean and tidy. In fact, some are filthy. Case managers should expect to see it all! Differences in lifestyle exist, and case managers cannot impose their lifestyles or beliefs onto others. To do so is asking for disaster. All a case manager can do is to make every effort to educate and advocate. In addition, in some situations there will be findings that must be reported to public officials. If these situations are mandated by law for reporting, the case manager, as a healthcare professional, must report them. Unfortunately, continuation of case management in such cases may require transfer of the case to another case manager. In extreme situations, case closure may be the ultimate outcome.

Length of Time for Interviews

Experience shows that most interviews last a minimum of 1 to 2 hours. The actual length of time varies depending on who is being interviewed, the intensity, severity, and acuity of the illness or injury, the facts that must be elicited to plan care needs, the number of persons present, and other case variables. Also, discharge-planning interviews and case conferences usually last longer than other interviews because so much information and facts must be shared by all.

Case Conferences

Because of time constraints, possibly one of the best ways to interview or communicate with the healthcare team is through case conferences. Many hospitals or other facilities and home health agencies hold patient-specific case conferences on a regularly scheduled basis. If it is not possible to attend every conference, the case manager must make arrangements to ensure that any important data or information shared at these conferences is obtained as soon as possible. Case conferences not only allow an avenue for education and open communication, they are also one of the best forums for mutual sharing of specific patient information.

CASE MANAGEMENT PLAN

As stated earlier, just because a certain diagnosis meets referral criteria does not guarantee that a specific case will be opened; particular case variables dictate which cases are actually opened. Once the decision has been made to open a case and the interviews and assessments have been completed, the next step is the actual writing and development of the case management plan.

A written case management plan (which may be referred to as a care map, map, critical pathway, or similar term by a facility-based case manager) must be developed for every patient followed. These plans must be updated and changed as the patient's condition shows evidence of progression, regression, or failure to change, or as goals are reached. Like assessments, the frequency of these changes depends on the changing needs of the patient.

Focus of Plan

To be effective, the case management plan must be centered on the patient and family and should be developed using an interdisciplinary healthcare team approach. Involvement of the patient and family not only meets any patient rights laws, it also helps to reduce their anxieties and alleviate crises. In addition, it encourages their positive participation in the plan and contributes to a positive outcome. Case management plans cannot be created without input from the physician, the healthcare team, the

patient, and the family. This involvement is the main value underlying case management as outlined by the Commission for Case Management Certification. They list the values of case management as follows:

Recognition that case management is guided by the principles of autonomy, beneficence, nonmaleficence, justice, veracity, and distributive justice.
Belief that case management is a means for achieving client wellness and autonomy through advocacy, communication, education, identification of service resources, and service facilitation.
Recognition of the dignity, worth, and rights of all people.
Understanding and commitment to quality outcomes for clients, appropriate use of resources, and the empowerment of clients in a manner that is supportive and objective.
Belief in the underlying premise that when the individual reaches the optimum level of wellness and functional capability, everyone benefits: the individuals being served, their support systems, the healthcare delivery systems, and the various reimbursement systems.[1]

Data Elements

Although documentation formats vary with the organization, most case management plans are written in narrative form. In all cases, case managers must document their work.[14, 17] Most organizations have developed a format that can be used to summarize the details of case management plans and document the data elements captured. At a minimum, these data elements must include:

- Patient's name or, in some cases, his or her identification number
- Diagnosis and date of illness or injury
- Date opened to case management
- Healthcare payor or other healthcare coverage or alternate funding programs
- Brief overview of the patient's medical history and care
- Identified problems, recommendations, and time frames for resolution
- Types of providers and community resources to be utilized
- Necessary teaching and identification of the person who is to do the teaching and the time frames for completion

- List of all equipment required and sources of procurement
- Long-term and short-term goals

Documentation for the final case management plan is frequently several pages long if all facets relating to the patient, family, and caregiver are assessed and summarized. All case variables and demographic information must be identified and researched because the data collected serve as the foundation for the case management plan.

Some cases are overwhelming, even for experienced case managers, and the problems and amount of data reported are astronomical.[18] However, regardless of the amount of data, it is important to list all problems, possibly numbering them in the order of their importance. Although the ideal goal is to identify recommendations for each problem, this is not always possible. For example, problems may have been present before the case manager came into the picture, and as such, they may never be resolved. The key to success of the case management plan is to list all pertinent problems, list recommendations for solutions for each problem, and then list realistic, achievable, and specific long- and short-term goals. Ideally, the case management plan should be shared with all involved, including the patient. However, distribution of the plan to others outside the treating team varies with the organization.

Second Level Review

At any given time during either the initial development or reassessment of the plan, consultation with the medical director, physician advisor, or the organization's legal counsel may be warranted before proceeding. Some case management organizations have formal mechanisms for this review process. When this type of review occurs, information pertinent to the issue is submitted in writing to the reviewer. In contrast, others allow more informal interactions. Regardless of which review process is used, all sessions and review outcomes must be documented and maintained in the patient's case management record. There may be times when the case manager may believe that a second medical opinion is necessary before proceeding. Although some healthcare organizations allow their case managers the authority to establish such services, others do not, and all such requests must be approved by the medical director.

Developing the Plan

To develop the case management plan the case manager must first formulate the data captured in the assessment and interview phases and then develop it into the data base. All planning must be action oriented and time specific.[19] The Commission for Case Management Certification defines planning as "the process of determining specific objectives, goals, and actions designed to meet the client's needs as identified through the assessment process. The plan should be action-oriented and time specific."[1] The assessment data then serve as a guide for researching and selecting the providers and resources that are required. In today's healthcare arena many healthcare organizations have their own provider network; however, use of these providers is not always possible in the more complex cases. Some healthcare providers cannot meet the needs and level of care required by some patients. If they cannot, the case manager must research the provider community to discover those who can. Once a provider has been found, either the healthcare payor's case manager or someone from the organization's network negotiating team must negotiate an acceptable rate between the proposed rendering provider and the payor. This rate must be agreed upon before the patient is actually moved to the care of the new provider.

Even though the patient may be able to use the services provided within a healthcare organization's network, the case manager must make every attempt to allow the patient and family an opportunity to select the providers that are to be used. One of the best ways of doing this is to give them several provider choices. Case managers must always remember that the patient and the family have the right to chose the healthcare providers they wish because they are the ultimate decision makers.

However, because of the way some healthcare organizations are organized (e.g., healthcare payor plans such as health maintenance organizations (HMOs), exclusive provider organizations (EPOs), and preferred provider organizations (PPOs) or capitated arrangements between a payor and a facility) or because an appropriate provider is not available, it is not always possible for the patient to exercise this right. In all cases, one of the best ways of protecting oneself is to give patients and families the lists of providers. If case managers, discharge planners, and home health agency staff continually recommend, endorse, or steer patients to one particular provider, serious legal implications can result if problems arise with that provider. Another way to establish legal protection is to document why certain providers are constantly utilized or recommended.

If healthcare providers are unknown to the patient or family or if more than one provider is available, the best way of informing the patient and family about their choices is to list at least three providers for their review. There is nothing wrong with listing the three in the order preferred by the case manager, nor is there anything wrong with saying, "this provider is known for his or her excellence." Definitely, if the patient or family selects a provider that is less desirable, the case manager must be careful to protect himself or herself against accusations of defamation of character when taking action to guide the patient and family to a provider with higher standards of care. The important key is that the choice must be theirs. However, if there is a difference of opinion between the case manager and the patient or family, the case manager must document clearly the reasons for the difference.[20]

In some situations the patient and family may not understand the situation well enough or be in a frame of mind that allows them to make an informed decision or contribute to the development of the plan. In such cases decisions are frequently deferred to the case manager or others. In these situations the case manager must document the reasons for the choices made. Additionally, there may be times during the case when the patient and family may not have all the information they need to make an informed decision.[8] When this occurs, the case manager must act as an advocate and obtain the information, which must then be relayed to them in a way they can understand. In other situations, the case manager may be required to pose leading questions to the patient or family that allow them to take part in the decision-making process and acknowledge the issue and the steps they wish to have taken.

Keys to the Final Plan

Keys to the development and implementation of any case management plan are the healthcare benefits available from the patient's individual health insurance coverage and the exclusions and limitations that apply, the patient's or family's financial resources and ability to pay out-of-pocket expenses, and their level of motivation to participate. In the economic climate of today's healthcare system, costs are important, but costs must not be the most important driving factor for the final plan. Quality of care must be. However, the emphasis in many companies today on the bottom line—cost outlays and cost avoidances—affects all other decisions. So case managers must continually juggle not only what is best for the patient but also what is best and expected by his or her employer. In any event, quality of care must be paramount because if it is not, unnecessary costs can accrue.

Although some case managers can augment their case management plans by using free community resources (e.g., the American Cancer Society), for the most part, the healthcare payor will be the "deep pocket" that pays for the majority of the healthcare and services provided. Alternative levels of care vary greatly in price as well as quality and in their ability to render care. Also, some alternative care sources are not available locally, particularly for the cases found in case management caseloads, which require specialized care that is available only at select facilities throughout the state, region, or nation. In these cases, out-of-area placement is necessary. This poses additional strains on the family, and the case manager must then be able to proactively assist the patient and family in making their decision.

When evaluating services and costs for the final plan, case managers must frequently ask themselves many questions, for example:

• Is the patient in the right setting, or can more cost-effective treatment be provided elsewhere?
• What will be the cost for each service? Is the rate charged the usual and customary rate, or is it possible to obtain a better one?
• What frequency of services and level of intensity will be required?
• Are the necessary providers available locally or within the network?
• What training is required, not only for the primary caregiver but also for volunteers and, yes, for some of the healthcare professionals as well? How long will the training take?
• What type and amount of equipment and supplies are required?
• Are there any architectural barriers that have to be corrected?
• Is a second opinion needed before any further action is taken?
• What ultimate outcome can be anticipated, what will be the final cost, and will this move

or service be more cost effective than the current level of care?

This list is not all-inclusive, and additional questions one may ask include:

- If no case management occurred, would the result for the patient be the same?
- Can case management make a difference, especially when the patient has habits and a lifestyle that will not change?
- Are the patient and family at the point where improvement or changes to the situation are unlikely?
- Are the patient and family educated and sophisticated enough to know how to access resources or help?
- Are other case managers involved (e.g., healthcare payor, facility-based, home health agency, alternate funding programs) who have a more active role? Is it possible to delegate a "primary case manager" as the point of contact for the flow of communication?
- If services have been established or linked to a hospice or home health agency for a patient with a terminal illness, and more than one case manager is involved, what more can the others do?
- What happens if the cost of the alternate level of care (e.g., acute rehabilitation, subacute care, or even some plans providing post-acute care at home) will be more expensive than the current level of care? Who will make the decision to allow the patient to remain at this level? Can this decision be made by the case manager, or must it be made by senior management? Who?

Once the case management plan has been implemented, the initial plan may have to be revised numerous times. Revisions will occur as the patient's condition progresses or regresses or reaches a plateau, as goals are reached, or as services are decreased. If goals are not reached, it may be necessary to increase the level of services to meet the patient's needs. Similarly, revisions are necessary as the caregiver becomes more familiar and proficient in the patient's care or as symptoms of caregiver burnout are recognized. Modifications may also be needed if problems occur with the healthcare provider. In essence, the case management plan is modified or revised on an ongoing basis throughout the case.

IMPLEMENTATION

As the case management plan is coordinated and implemented, many different scenarios can occur; they vary as much as the variables in one's cases and caseloads. What worked or is required for one may not work or be required for another. There is no cookbook to follow. Implementation of the plan is accomplished by coordinating and achieving timely transfers of the patient to appropriate cost-effective providers or levels of care in lieu of more costly care. The Commission for Case Management Certification defines coordination as "the process of organizing, securing, integrating, and modifying the resources necessary to accomplish the goals set forth in the case management plan"[1] and implementation as "the process of executing specific case management activities or interventions that will lead to accomplishing the goals set forth in the case management plan."[1]

Transfer and Implementation

There are three key requirements as discharge approaches and implementation of services begins. These requirements are as follows: (1) transfer and implementation can only be accomplished with the consent and support of the family and the physician; (2) implementation of services cannot occur until the patient is medically stable enough for discharge; and (3) the alternative care providers are prepared to accept the patient and render the treatments ordered by the physician.

In most cases, providers can accept the patient only if they are informed well in advance of the actual implementation date that the patient can be expected on that day. Ideally, this advance notice occurs during the developmental stages of the case management plan. More specifically, as the case manager identifies the appropriate resources, he or she must work closely with the providers selected to ensure that time frames and all provider requirements are agreed upon. Therefore, although excellent communication between all parties is critical during all phases of the plan,[21] it is vital during the preimplementation stages because the alternate care provider must be ready and prepared to accept the patient.

Standing Firm

Because of shorter stays in healthcare facilities and the various methodologies associated with the review process, services for some patients may have started before the written case management plan has been finalized. However, in light of recent legal cases against review companies and healthcare organizations for disastrous outcomes associated with denied care and forced discharges, the case manager must be prepared and assertive enough to say no if all conditions for a safe transition are not in place.[22] This factor is supported by the Commission for Case Management Certification in their definition of beneficence as "the obligation or duty to promote good, to further a person's legitimate interests and to actively prevent or remove from harm."[1] Other definitions by the Commission that apply here are those for distributive justice: "deals with the moral basis for dissemination of goods and evils, burdens and benefits";[1] justice: "the maintenance of what is right and fair";[1] nonmaleficence: "refraining from doing harm to others";[1] and veracity: "telling the truth."[1]

To prevent the case management staff from being held accountable when problems arise or disaster occurs it may be necessary at times for case managers to hold their ground and review any actions with their organization's medical director, senior management, or legal counsel. Also, despite the fact that the patient may be ready for discharge, if the proposed agency or provider encounters difficulties and there are indications that they are not prepared or able to accept the patient, implementation of the final plan must be delayed or terminated. This may mean waiting until the provider makes the necessary changes, or, in some instances, it may mean finding another provider. In any event, the reasons for the delay must be clearly documented.

Right of Expectation

As services are implemented, case managers must never imply that the patient has the "right of expectation" that the services will continue. All members of the healthcare team must continually educate the patient and the family that the patient's healthcare coverage for the care or services will not continue indefinitely. The best method of preventing this expectation from arising is to set specific time limits for the actual provision of care, using short-term goals and documenting everything in writing for the patient and family as services are sought or approved. Also, the members of the healthcare team must remember never to promise ques-

tionable services or coverage until it is known that such services have been approved by the healthcare payor.

If services are established via the healthcare payor's extra contractual process, the healthcare payor as a rule finalizes the arrangement in writing and sends copies of the letter to the physician and provider. This letter generally states the exact services allowed, the time span approved, any conditions associated with the approval, and the steps necessary to obtain ongoing approval if the patient requires services beyond the approved period.

MONITORING AND REASSESSMENTS

Once the plan has been implemented, evaluations must occur at regular intervals to ensure that the plan is effective and that goals are being met. Reassessments are necessary to monitor the patient's, family's, and physician's satisfaction, reveal problematic areas, and identify the need for revisions in the plan.[23] Reassessments occur periodically throughout the duration of the case.

Given the complex and frequently unpredictable nature of many illnesses and injuries, case managers must maintain regular contact with the healthcare team.[23] This is necessary to ensure that appropriate modifications to the plan are made. More important, the case manager must monitor both the patient's progress and the caregiver's abilities to ensure that the level of care remains appropriate and of high quality. Because of case variables, case managers must always allow for unforeseen events or extenuating circumstances, and action plans for these must be included in the case management plan. Possibly the events that occur most frequently are caregiver burnout and staffing problems encountered by the healthcare agency or facility. These alone are reasons for maintaining regular contact with the patient, especially if the patient is receiving hourly skilled care or is dependent on technologic assistance.

Frequency of Reassessment

There is no set rule for the frequency of monitoring and reassessments. However, in most cases in which the level of care is high after discharge and the illness is severe, experience shows that an evaluation should be performed at least every 30 days.[24] Other cases may require weekly or bi-monthly evaluations. In long-term cases in which the patient is medically stable, an evaluation every quarter is generally sufficient.

Because what works well in a hospital or facility may not work at home or in an alternative setting, the frequency of case monitoring and reassessment varies from case to case and depends on factors such as:

- The intensity or severity of the illness or injury.
- The agency's or facility's reputation and staffing patterns.
- The frequency and complexity of the care required.
- The patient's and family's emotional stability.
- The abilities of the caregiver.
- Communication patterns.

In some situations, although placement in a long-term care facility is the most realistic option, the family or patient adamantly opposes such placement. What is frequently happening in these situations is that families must ease any guilt associated with long-term care placement and prove to themselves that "they tried." These cases are among the most difficult to manage because a contingency plan for placement must be designed and ready for immediate implementation if the case management plan fails. These cases also require more frequent monitoring to ensure that unnecessary costly acute hospitalization is avoided, deterioration of the patient is prevented, and the contingency plan is implemented immediately should it become necessary. In such situations, documentation to protect oneself is of critical importance, and the attending physician must agree with the discharge.

Techniques of Reassessment

Monitoring techniques for reassessment vary from organization to organization. Facility-based case managers may be allowed to manage cases of patients only while they are hospitalized, and any ongoing post-acute care monitoring required on discharge must be transferred to another case manager involved in the case, possibly a case manager with a home health agency. In other situations, facility-based case managers may remain involved even after the patient's discharge. However, these rules vary with the facility. The same is true of case management offered by healthcare payors: Some allow continued case management after discharge, either on site or by telephone, and others do not.

In the case of case management by the healthcare payor, the decision for or against continued case management may actually rest with the policyholder. Some policyholders are unwilling to allow any monitoring or follow-up intervention once the patient has been established in the alternative level of care. This is especially true when the policyholder contracts and pays separately for case management services. In these situations, every interaction by the case manager costs money because the policyholder pays hourly for case management services, and these expenses may ultimately affect future premium rates. Unfortunately, because patients today tend to be sicker and more dependent on technology, the lack of on-site monitoring may invite potentially disastrous outcomes. Ultimately, these may lead to higher costs for healthcare payors or policyholders for care.

One of the best ways of capturing details and identifying problems between visits is to maintain telephone contact with all parties.[23] This method of monitoring maintains open lines of communication and allows regular contact with the key players in the case, especially the physician, the patient, and the family. If onsite visits are not possible and telephone contact leaves doubt, another method of reassessment conducted for reimbursement purposes is to request copies of the actual nursing or therapy progress notes from the post-acute care providers; such notes should be reviewed at least monthly. Even for case managers who work in a capitated environment, it is a good rule to request 7 consecutive days of notes because this allows them to review the case for the presence of skilled or custodial care, for example, or to identify whether the patient has reached a plateau.

A word to the wise. Most healthcare payors do not pay when the patient reaches a plateau or requires custodial care. As long as there is flux (progression or regression), the treatment course can be justified. Therefore, it is important to establish regular contact with the patient and providers to identify the presence of skilled versus custodial care or plateau details. Also, because of the various laws and regulations affecting healthcare, any identified problems must be acted upon, and healthcare professionals can be held accountable if problems arise as a result of nonaction on an issue.

CASE CLOSURE

General Documentation

To meet professional and legal demands for accountability, charts or some form of documentation must be maintained on all open cases. Documentation on charts must be clear and concise. All actions must be briefly summarized (i.e., events, phone conversations, interviews, and conferences should be summarized, and dates and parties or individuals involved should be noted). The frequency of documentation and contacts with patient, family, and healthcare team varies with each case.

In today's litigious society, case managers, like all healthcare professionals, are required to document, document, and document again. More important, facts must be recorded as promptly as possible to avoid losing details. Because case management charts are discoverable, meaning that they can be requested by a court, documentation must be pertinent and accurate. The key to documenting or compiling reports is to keep information honest, concise, and nonderogatory.

Documentation Elements

To protect oneself and his or her organization, documentation on charts must not include any derogatory personal comments or opinions about the patient, family, case management organization, or other departments. Documentation should be specific and complete enough to capture the specifics of the case and allow ease of interpretation should others need to read the material and take action on the case.[14, 17] Most healthcare organizations have prepared documentation forms available that allow documentation of such case activity as

- Intake referral
- Preliminary assessment
- Family interview
- Clinical assessment
- Interview with physician and other healthcare team member (e.g., therapists, respiratory therapy, dietitian)
- Attorney interview
- Case conference summary
- Verbal communique (used to summarize phone or verbal conversations)
- Monthly cost-avoidance reporting
- Extra contractual recommendations

- Physician advisor or medical director consultations
- Case closure
- Reports used for the various clients served by the case management organization

CASE MANAGEMENT REPORTS

Once a case manager becomes familiar with the type of reports required by his or her employer or the employer's clients, reports must be generated and specific to these needs.[14, 17] If specific requirements are not outlined, individual reports on patients often contain the following information:

- Patient's name, address, phone number, and date of birth
- Insured's name and identification number
- Policyholder (usually employer group)
- Diagnosis, prognosis, and date of illness or injury
- Name of treating physician
- Medical summary to date
- Suggested alternative levels of care or settings and community resources or alternative funding
- Proposed cost of care in the alternative setting in lieu of present costs
- Cost savings to date

In contrast, when reports are required for specific groups or aggregates of a population served by the case management organization (e.g., Medicare, Medicaid), the reports and the details to be reported are specified in any contractual agreements between the two groups (e.g., between the case management organization and Medicaid; between the case management organization and a health plan; between a hospital and a health plan). These reports may be generated monthly, quarterly, or yearly and often include such specific details as:

- Days or visits per 1000 members or lives
- Admissions per 1000 members or lives
- Procedures per 1000 members or lives
- Average length of stay or average number of visits
- Top diagnoses seen
- Top procedures conducted
- Types of admissions

If reports do include actual costs and costs saved, references to any costs and cost savings must not be emphasized in routine case documentation.[17] If costs are emphasized and the case goes to court, the case manager may have to defend references to these. Despite the fact that the case manager focused clearly on quality of care or the expertise of the provider, this intention can be lost as the attorneys hammer away at references to cost. Consequently, case managers are wise to mention costs and negotiations of rates only in cost savings forms, keeping these forms separate from the reports used for day-to-day documentation.

🦋 S U M M A R Y

The case management process is described in detail, covering the many aspects of preparation required if the final plan is to be implemented without delay, duplication, or fragmentation. The same detailed preparation is required if the final plan is to be of high quality and cost effective and if it is to keep the patient at the appropriate level of care at all times as his or her condition shows progression or regression or reaches a plateau. Possibly the most critical "management" skill of all is the ability to communicate. Excellent communication between all members of the healthcare team and the family is paramount throughout a case. Not only is verbal communication critical, so is written communication. Documentation of case events and actions is vital throughout the case, not only to ensure the success of the case but also to provide an important management tool that summarizes case management activity for senior management.

REFERENCES

1. Certification of Insurance Rehabilitation Specialists (1996). Commission for Case Management Certification (flyer). Rolling Meadows, IL, Certification of Insurance Rehabilitation Specialists.
2. Mullahy CM (1995). The Case Manager's Handbook. Gaithersburg, MD, Aspen, pp. 108-120.
3. Mazoway JM (1987). Early intervention in high cost care. Business and Health 4(3):12-16.
4. Grossman D (1996). Cultural dimensions in home health nursing. Am J Nurs 96(7):33-36.
5. Kohn S (1995). Dismantling socio-cultural barriers to care. Healthcare Forum J 38(3):30-35.
6. Leninger M (1995). Transcultural Nursing: Concepts, Theories, Research and Practice. New York, McGraw-Hill.
7. Pachter LM (1994). Culture and clinical care. Folk illness, beliefs and behaviors and their implications for healthcare delivery. JAMA 271(9):690-694.
8. Mullahy CM (1995). Op. cit., p. 126.
9. American Nurses Association (ANA) (1991). Standards for clinical nursing practice. *In*: Phillips CY, et al (1994). Case manager/nurse manager: A blending of roles. J Nurs Admin 24(2):26-34.
10. Weil M, Karls J (eds) (1985). Case Management in Human Service Practice. San Francisco, Jossey-Bass Publications, pp. 1-28.
11. Mullahy CM (1995). Op. cit., pp. 132-138.
12. Mullahy CM (1995). Op. cit., pp. 148-150.
13. Mullahy CM (1995). Op. cit., pp. 102-103, 151-156.
14. Mullahy CM (1995). Op. cit., pp. 99-100.
15. Mullahy CM (1995). Op. cit., pp. 111-161.
16. Mullahy CM (1995). Op. cit., pp. 103-105, 120.
17. Mullahy CM (1995). Op. cit., pp. 161-169.
18. Mullahy CM (1995). Op. cit., p. 160.
19. Mullahy CM (1995). Op. cit., pp. 170-171.
20. Mullahy CM (1995). Op. cit., pp. 156-161.
21. Mullahy CM (1995). Op. cit., pp. 85-107.
22. Southwick AF (1988). The Law of Hospital and Healthcare Administration, 2nd ed. Ann Arbor, MI, Health Administration Press, pp. 52-100.
23. Mullahy CM (1995). Op. cit., p. 173.
24. Mullahy CM (1995). Op. cit., p. 172.

BIBLIOGRAPHY

Ackley BJ, et al (eds) (1995). Nursing: A Guide to Diagnoses Planning Care Handbook, 2nd ed. St. Louis, Mosby-Year Book.

Arras JD (1995). Bringing the Hospital Home: Ethical and Social Implications of High Tech Home Care. Baltimore, Johns Hopkins University Press.

Barry PD (1996). Psychosocial Nursing Care of Physically Ill Patients and Their Families, 3rd ed. Philadelphia, JB Lippincott.

Betts VT (1995). Helping caregivers in long term care situations. Am Nurs 27(4): 24.

Carpenito LJ (1995). Nursing Care Plans and Documentation, 2nd ed. Philadelphia, JB Lippincott.

During CG (1996). Learning to Say No. Am J Nurs 96(4):14-16.

Ethridge P, Lamb G (1989). Professional nursing case management improves quality, access, and costs. Nurs Manag 20(3):35.

Falvo DR (1994). Effective Patient Education: A Guide to Increased Compliance. Gaithersburg, MD, Aspen.

Haggard A (1989). Handbook of Patient Education. Gaithersburg, MD, Aspen.

Ignatavicius DD, Hausman KA (1995). Clinical Pathways for Collaborative Practice. Philadelphia, WB Saunders.

Iyers PW, Camp NH (1995). Nursing Documentation: A Nursing Process Approach, 2nd ed. St. Louis, Mosby-Year Book.

Lilley LL, Guanci R (1996). Educate the patient. Am J Nurs 96(4):14-16.

Loeb S (ed) (1992). Teaching Patients with Chronic Conditions. Springhouse, PA, Springhouse Corporation.

McCubbin HI, et al (1982). Family Stress, Coping and Social Support. Springfield, IL, Charles C Thomas.

Mcquire SL, et al (1996). Meeting the diverse need of clients in the community: Effective use of the referral process. Nurs Outlook 44(5):218-222.

Murray RB, Zentner JP (1993). Nursing Assessment and Health Promotion Strategies Through the Life Span, 5th ed. Norwalk, CT, Appleton-Lange.

Rorden JW, Taft E (1990). Discharge Planning Guide for Nurses. Philadelphia, WB Saunders.

Shiparski L (1996). Successful interview strategies. Nurs Manag 27(7):32F-32H.

Smith MC (1993). Case management and nursing therapy based practice. Nurs Sci Q 6(1):8-9.

Snyder B (1996). An easy way to document patient education. RN 59(3):43-45.

Tahan HA, Cesta TG (1994). Developing case management plans using a quality improvement model. J Nurs Admin 24(12):49-58.

Ulrich SP, et al (1994). Medical-Surgical Nursing Care Planning Guides. Philadelphia, WB Saunders.

Wolf GA (1986). Communication: Key contributor to effectiveness—A nurse education executive responds. Am J Nurs Admin 16(9):26-28.

Chapter 3

Financial Considerations in Case Management

PROVIDERS

Selection of Provider

The case manager or members of the health-care team must make every attempt to use or guide the patient to healthcare providers who can meet the patient's needs safely and adequately. If the patient's healthcare benefits are associated with a health maintenance organization (HMO), preferred provider organization (PPO), or other such healthcare payor, use of other than network providers may be precluded merely by the structure of the healthcare payor's contracts with providers. In some cases the provider simply cannot administer the care required.[1, 2] On other occasions the patient or the family may refuse to allow care by a specific provider, and in some extreme instances the provider may refuse to accept the patient (this may happen at the time of a readmission or when the patient is known to the provider). In these or similar situations, the case manager must search the provider community (network and non-network) for providers who can meet the patient's needs.

If a non-network provider is found, use of its services may be restricted or allowed only with approval obtained through the extra contractual process. In other cases, the organization's network or contract negotiators may be required to negotiate an acceptable rate between the payor and the provider before the patient is transferred; other organizations may allow their case management staff to negotiate a rate on a case-by-case basis. In any case, use of a non-network provider can be time consuming.

Consequently, all case managers must work closely together to ensure that the patient is not moved prematurely until all arrangements are in place and are accepted by all. The key point is that if the required service is a benefit covered by the patient's insurance and the provider network is inadequate to supply it, arrangements must be made to ensure that care is rendered appropriately and safely.

Accuracy of Information

Information supplied to providers must be accurate, honest, and of sufficient scope to allow them to develop their plan of care and assume the case without disruption. Case managers must be very cognizant of the fact that transfer of medical information is protected under the Privacy Act as well as other laws that protect patient rights and confidentiality. Therefore, information must be pertinent and must not contain unnecessary personal information that is not pertinent to the provision of care.

One of the best methods of protection is to have the patient or his or her legal representative sign a form agreeing to the release of information before any information is disclosed. Even with a signed consent form, however, information must be kept to the medical specifics of the case.

Costs

If the provider's quoted price appears to be higher than the usual and customary price range in the community, it is wise to obtain price quotes from other providers in the region for comparison. It is common for prices to vary among different healthcare providers. Also, sometimes the rates quoted by the contracted "network" provider may be higher for certain items or services than those quoted by a non-network provider because contracts are frequently developed to serve the majority of patients covered by an organization, with the final contract a win-win situation for both the provider and the healthcare organization.[3]

In general, contracts are developed to cover equipment or services that are frequently used, and the global or volume-based rates in the contract reflect this usage. This means that infrequently used services or equipment, such as that often required by case-managed patients, can often be obtained outside the network at a lower rate. Although some healthcare payers allow use of non-network providers for various situations, others do not.

As a result, case managers must be familiar with the use of providers and restrictions imposed on them by their organization if they are associated with a healthcare organization that is at "risk" or one that is responsible for reimbursement. Case managers with other healthcare organizations must not select or recommend providers until all details have been cleared with the healthcare payor responsible for paying the claims. If patients are linked to a provider in error, the patient or family may be held financially responsible for all charges.

General Criteria for Selecting Providers

If a noncontracted or non-network healthcare provider must be used, the following questions may be helpful in eliciting information about the provider and assisting in the final choice. Experience as a discharge planner and case manager sharpens one's skills in selecting providers. Appropriate questions might include the following:

- Is the agency or provider staff certified, licensed, or registered as required by state law?
- Does the provider offer prompt access—same day or next workday response—with set-up of equipment or service and provision of all necessary teaching at no extra cost?
- Does the provider offer regular service during working hours or on-call capabilities that can serve clients regardless of the time of day or day of the week (i.e., 24 hours a day, 7 days a week)?
- Does the provider offer specialized trained personnel to meet the patient's needs and is the staff willing to conduct any training the patient or family may require without charge?
- Does the provider agree to return any requested paperwork promptly?
- Is the provider Medicare certified?
- Is the provider accredited?
- Is the provider open to submitting written progress notes or clinical progress notes as requested or to attendance by the case manager at case conferences and on-site review of progress notes?
- Is the provider open to negotiation for discounts or other rate reductions?
- Is the provider open and flexible in response to possible changes?
- Will the provider agree to deliver and set up the equipment in the hospital for teaching purposes 7 to 14 days prior to discharge without additional charges?
- Will the provider agree to on-site visits by their staff to assess the patient prior to discharge if necessary and at no additional charge?
- Does the provider have policies and procedures in place that recognize patient rights and are these enforced?

For services provided by a *home health agency* or *infusion company*, additional questions may include these:

- Will instruction and teaching be provided by a qualified professional at no additional charge?
- Will a licensed professional make the initial home visit within 24 to 48 hours after the patient arrives home if the patient requires services that involve specific skills?

- Will a licensed professional be in attendance during the initial dose of the infusion therapy?
- Will the licensed professional make home visits as often as necessary to ensure that the patient and the family can adequately perform the prescribed therapy or treatment? Is this service provided 24 hours a day, 7 days a week?
- If infusion services are required, is the infusion agency under the direction of a licensed pharmacist who compounds drugs and fluids in accordance with state laws and the standards of the American Society of Pharmacists? Is he or she available to assist the patient and answer pharmacy-related questions?

For equipment provided by a *durable medical equipment company*, additional questions may include these:

- If rental equipment requires repairs, will the provider supply replacement equipment at no additional cost until the repairs are completed?
- If the equipment that requires repairs has been purchased previously, will the provider lend equipment at a prorated rental price until repairs are made?
- Are oxygen cylinders refilled in accordance with Food and Drug Administration (FDA) standards? Is a back-up tank provided for patients who require oxygen?
- Will equipment be inspected regularly, at least every 30 to 45 days?
- When equipment is purchased, will a service agreement be made available? If so, what will be the cost and what services will be included? Can all service cost be included in an all-inclusive monthly service agreement?
- If the patient requires a respiratory therapist, will such a therapist be available 24 hours a day, 7 days a week?
- When applicable, will the appropriate professional staff (e.g., respiratory therapist) be available to perform all treatments until the patient, family, or caregiver can demonstrate proficiency?

Because of the number of mergers of facilities and because not all network facilities can manage all levels or types of care, a case manager may have to apply certain criteria in selecting an appropriate facility. Questions useful in formulating these criteria may include the following:

- Are the services available locally? If not, where is the closest facility that can provide the level of care required?

- Is the facility licensed or accredited appropriately to offer the level of care required?
- Are state surveys or accreditations current? Have any infractions been noted, have they been corrected or are they being corrected, how serious are they, and is the facility habitually cited for the same infractions?
- Does the facility have adequate staff, both in numbers and expertise, to treat the patient and provide the service at the intensity and frequency required by the patient? This question may trigger others about the facility, such as the types of staffing available on all shifts, their numbers, and the types of patients requiring heavy care.
- If staffing is inadequate, is the administrator of the facility or provider willing to hire additional staff? If additional staff is not hired, is the administrator willing to subcontract with an agency that can provide the necessary staff, and if so, who will pay the additional rate charged by the subcontracted agency?
- If training of the staff is required, is the administrator willing to allow the additional training and assume the cost?
- Are alternative programs available in the immediate area that can accomplish the same outcome at a reduced cost?
- If state statutes or administrative codes set the hours of care at a specific minimum number and the patient requires more, is the administrator willing to accept the patient regardless without compromising quality by adding additional staff to increase the hours of care?
- Does the facility offer on-going peer or support groups for patients and families?
- What is the average length of stay?
- To maintain quality, does the staff actively participate in continuing education sessions pertinent to their level of expertise?
- Does the facility compile and maintain outcome studies that attest to successes in patient care, the quality of the program, and the cost effectiveness of the program?
- Will the facility administrator agree to allow review of the patient's medical records, either on-site or by telephone, by the case manager?
- Is the facility administrator open to allowing the case manager to participate in case conferences to facilitate case planning?
- If the facility quotes a fee-for-service rate, is it willing to negotiate a reduced rate, whether discounted, per diem, or capitated?
- What is the ratio of staff to patients per discipline (i.e., therapists, nurses)?

- How often is therapy provided, and how many hours per day is it given? If a skilled nursing facility is under consideration, is therapy provided by staff therapists, or is it subcontracted to a community therapy provider at which most of the therapy is actually administered by the facility's nursing staff or therapy aides?
- Does the facility provide infusion therapy using infusion techniques and standards established by the Intravenous Therapy Association and the American Society of Parenteral and Enteral Nutrition?
- Does the facility have an active performance and quality improvement program that monitors adherence to standards and an established process for continuous improvement and correction if infractions are found?
- Does the facility have adequate equipment and supplies to meet the patient's needs? If not, is it willing to procure such equipment at its expense? If not, will costs be included in a per diem rate or will separate reimbursement at a fee-for-service rate be charged?
- Does the facility maintain a transfer agreement with the nearest local hospital for emergency treatments?
- Does the facility have arrangements in place for portable radiologic and laboratory services? If not, what arrangements exist with local acute care facilities for such services? If the patient requires transportation for these services, who assumes the cost of this transportation—the facility, healthcare payor, family, patient? If the patient requires oxygen en route, will the cost be assumed by the facility? If the patient requires an attendant or nurse en route, will the facility assume costs for this as well?

Certainly, there may be other questions that apply to different types of providers. The key is to formulate patient-specific questions before calling providers. Unfortunately, because of the complexities of care required by many patients, the selection of providers is often limited. Therefore, case managers should maintain a directory of both local and regional providers, along with the types of services they provide. This directory should be kept current and updated as new information is obtained.

SUMMARY

Use of healthcare providers that can provide the level of care required by patients must always be the foremost consideration when arrangements are made for the patient's care. Unfortunately, the use of some providers may be restricted because of the contractual limitations of the healthcare organization paying the bill. Because of these or any other restrictions, providers may not be able to provide the care required. Case managers must be prepared to work together to ensure that an acceptable rate for care is in place before the patient is transferred to the next level of care.

STEPS IN NEGOTIATING REDUCED RATES

Why Negotiate

Many case managers work with or for healthcare organizations that have established provider networks. Unfortunately, as stated earlier, this provider network has usually been established to serve the majority of the insured population, and it may not fit the needs of all patients. In many instances, the contract between the provider and the healthcare payor excludes or "carves out" specific areas. These exclusions create voids in service for the minority of patients classified as having a "catastrophic" illness or injury or for those needing case management. When this occurs and the provider network cannot be used, securing a non-network provider will be necessary. Unfortunately, because a contract for reimbursement is not in place in such cases, a fee-for-service rate will be charged unless a reduced rate can be agreed on.

If one is not careful, costs can rise sharply when care is allowed to proceed at a full fee-for-service reimbursement rate. Thus, it behooves the case manager to know how to negotiate a reduced rate or to have access to a professional who can because many providers are open to discounts or reductions in their rates. If a rate must be negotiated, the best rates are those termed capitated, per diem, or all-inclusive. To be certain that the discounted rate is appropriate, case managers must be keenly aware of the community's or region's usual and customary ("normal") rates for various specific services.[4]

When a non-network provider must be used in cases in which both a facility-based case manager and a healthcare payor case manager are involved and care is not capitated to the hospital, communication and coordination are vital to ensure that the patient is not moved until acceptable rates are agreed on by both the healthcare payor and the receiving provider. In such situations, the healthcare payor's case manager may take the lead in coordinating the case. If arrangements are not made ahead of time, the patient or the family may be held responsible for the charges.

Steps to Follow

Responsibility for rate negotiations varies from organization to organization. Although in some healthcare organizations all rate negotiations fall within the range of responsibilities delegated to their contracting or network development staff, others allow these negotiations to be handled on a case-by-case basis by their case managers. When the case manager is allowed to negotiate a rate, the following steps may be helpful for new case managers unfamiliar with the process:

1. Prior to negotiating any discounts, an attempt must be made to ascertain the "normal" course or standard of care expected for the patient's diagnosis (i.e., normal length of stay, common types of services provided) and to determine the rates of some providers in the local region that can be used for comparison. One of the best ways to discover rates that can be used for comparison is to call providers directly and ask them their rates. In other cases, the case manager may be able to discuss rates for similar services with his or her organization's network development staff. This process provides a baseline from which negotiations can start. If rates are quoted by the case manager's organization, these rates are considered proprietary and confidential information. Consequently, under *no* circumstances should these rates be revealed as discussions ensue for an acceptable rate.
2. Depending on the organization, it may be necessary to contact the claims personnel to ascertain how quickly they think the claim can be processed. This is necessary because many providers may request a 30-day claims turnaround in exchange for the discount or the final rate agreed on.
3. Contact must then be made with the potential provider rendering the service. Here the case manager must speak directly with the person responsible for contracting or discounting the rate. In many cases this may be the administrator, the business of-

fice, or the finance officer. Once the appropriate person has been reached, discussion must concentrate on the level of care required and the provider's normal rates for this type of care. If these rates are higher than the baseline rates quoted, there is nothing wrong with asking if the provider is willing to negotiate a reduction in rate and, if so, what type of reduced rate structure may be available. Providers often are willing to offer a percentage discount or an all-inclusive or per diem rate.

4. If a discounted rate is in order, case managers should not be afraid to start their negotiated discount request at 25% to 30% or higher. If the rate is started high, one can always come down, but the process *never* works in reverse.

5. If a per diem rate or all-inclusive rate is agreed on, all services that are to be included in the rate must be specified in great detail and must be clear to both parties. If specific services are to be excluded, the rate for reimbursement for these must likewise be agreed on.

6. All agreements and conditions must be verbally summarized before the conversation is terminated.

7. All agreements and conditions must then be stated in writing; the letter must state:[5]
   a. The type of rate agreed on (discounted, per diem).
   b. The terms agreed on that could affect the final rate (e.g., claims processing).
   c. How the rate is to be reflected on the claim.
   d. Where to send claims (specify name in claims).

Requirements for Rate Reductions

No matter what type of negotiations occur and how the final rate is agreed on, it is wise to follow any verbal agreement with an agreement in writing. Most healthcare organizations have "standard" letters composed for this purpose. If they do not, a case-specific letter is necessary that outlines the final terms of the agreement. Not all organizations allow their case managers to write case-specific letters about rate negotiations. In these situations, this responsibility is delegated to the network negotiator staff or legal counsel.

It is common for rate reductions to be made

in exchange for timely claims processing. In such cases, the case manager must make every effort to ensure that the claim can be processed within the time frame agreed on. If not, all efforts are worthless and nothing is saved. If a rate is agreed on and is attached to terms for a 30-day claims turnaround, for example, the final letter must contain the following specific details:

- A statement to the effect that the discounted rate will occur in the turnaround time only if the claim submitted is a "clean claim."
- The claims processing time frame agreed on (e.g., 7 days, 14 days) once the clean claim has been received.
- A statement describing the components of a clean claim, which may be:
  - The patient's name, address, identification numbers, and date of birth.
  - The facility's name, address, and tax identification number.
  - All diagnoses.
  - All International Classification of Diseases (ICD) and all Current Procedural Technical (CPT) codes.
  - All billed charges as well as those discounted and the final amount to be paid.

In exchange for any reduced rate the case manager must never *promise* that the claim will not be subject to a retrospective bill review or audit. This is important because there are occasions when it may be in the best interest of the organization not to seek a discounted or reduced rate. In these situations the provider "unbundles" the services and then bills separately for all charges. In the long run, a retrospective bill audit can disclose thousands of dollars of "unbundled" charges, and these must now be paid. These hidden charges may far exceed any discounted savings, and consequently in the end, all efforts at achieving a reduced rate were for nothing.

☙ SUMMARY

Although the person responsible for negotiations for rate reductions varies with the organization, sometimes this process is delegated to a case manager on a case-by-case basis. The basic steps necessary in conducting a rate negotiation are included for new case managers who are unfamiliar with the process.

COST SAVINGS, COST AVOIDANCE, OR COST BENEFIT ANALYSIS REPORTING

The old days when fee-for-service payments dominated as the primary method of reimbursement are long gone. Today the focus is on managed care and on containing costs. Because case management frequently centers on high-cost cases, it is no wonder that some mechanism for reporting and communicating information about cost savings is recognized as an integral part of the case management process. This is true because case management is involved with ensuring not only high-quality outcomes for patients but also is closely intertwined with financial outcomes for healthcare organizations. Therefore, some method of documenting the actual charges incurred and the charges saved must be used. Additionally, reports of cost savings analysis serve as important management and reporting tools.

Cost avoidance reporting is a useful tool because it formally documents the benefits of case management efforts.[6] Just as factors associated with the case management process vary from company to company, so do formats and requirements for cost saving reporting. Unfortunately, because some healthcare organizations are concerned with numbers and number crunching, the real emphasis of case management (i.e., maintaining quality patient care) is frequently lost. If an overemphasis on cost savings occurs, case managers must find some method of documenting case actions for the period reported, even if it is only for internal use.

Format

Although formats and time frames for cost savings reports vary, several key elements must be included. These are:

- Name of patient, file, or case number
- Insured person's identification number
- Diagnosis
- Date on which case was opened or closed
- Actual charges incurred for all levels of care
- Number of days, weeks, or months at each level of care
- Costs avoided (whether reduced through negotiations, reductions of services, or a shift to an alternative funding source) for all levels of care
- Case management fees, if applicable

- Summary of case management interventions, including any community resources used to augment the plan
- Recommendations (e.g., for ongoing case management services, transfer to another level of care, continue care and services at present level)

Frequency of Reports

Not only do formats vary, so does the frequency of reporting. Most reports are done monthly or quarterly and must be completed for every patient followed during the reporting period. Quarterly reports are by far the most preferable because monthly reports are burdensome and frequently unmanageable. The same is true of cost savings reports completed annually. In these cases, too much time has elapsed, and if careful notes have not been made, the actual costs saved will not be reported because they are forgotten. Similarly, if these reports are done annually, they have the potential to become an unmanageable burdensome task.

Not all cases result in saved or avoided costs. This is true especially when the healthcare organization operates a network of providers with discounted or capitated rates and the network is adequate, offering services for all levels of care. If cost savings reporting is not a requirement, it is wise to at least summarize case activity. Such a summary documents case management interventions for the reporting period and serves, if nothing else, as a management tool. Case costs or outcomes could have been worse without case management intervention, and a summary of the case substantiates this fact.

Hard Versus Soft Savings

In preparing cost savings reports, the task of quantifying and then separating hard from soft savings is possibly the most difficult. Hard savings are the most important because they comprise the primary selling point of any case management program to new clients or to senior management. Basically, *hard savings* are best described as savings wherein the case manager's actions directly result in true savings. Examples include:

- Negotiated rates.
- Transfer of care to an alternate funding source.

- Implementation of the alternative plan before the originally planned day of discharge.
- Reduction of care or hours.
- Shift of care from a noncontracted or network provider to a network provider.
- Use of free services from a community agency.

Hard costs are calculated only if a savings occurs or a cost is avoided because of case management intervention. To maintain accuracy in the report it may be necessary to contact providers to ascertain the actual charges or number of visits of practitioners in each discipline (e.g., occupational therapy, physical therapy, speech therapy, registered nurse) that occurred during the month. Additional costs that must be included in the cost savings total include all equipment and supplies, both rented and purchased, physicians' charges, ambulance trips, laboratory and radiologic studies, and so forth. Without these charges, the reports would be skewed because many of the same costs would have been included in a capitated or per diem rate if the patient had remained as an inpatient. If services are denied because they are not covered by the patient's insurance plan, this denial and any costs associated with it cannot be counted as either a hard or soft savings.

Soft savings are "what if" or "could have been" savings and are more difficult to quantify. These savings are certainly important in case management but are not as readily accepted by senior management or clients of the case management organization. Soft savings can best be described as actions that result in the absence of costs that have occurred in the past. In reality, soft savings are what case management is all about because they result from actions that ultimately save hard dollar expenditures. Also, reports of soft savings may be useful for specific patient populations in which certain situations can be captured (i.e., readmissions, emergency room usage) and monitored and the results quantified. In aggregate populations, costs may drop merely as a result of consistent application of case management approaches.

A good example of a case showing soft savings may be a cardiac patient who prior to case management had frequent hospital admissions and emergency room visits. During the assessment phase the case manager found that both the spouse and the patient had little understanding of the disease process. In addition, interview questions revealed that the patient was noncompliant with the medication regimen, and both the patient and the spouse were ignoring the dietary restrictions ordered.

Once the case was opened to case management, the case manager referred the patient and spouse to formal nutrition and diet counseling and had the home health agency nurse or an outpatient clinic nurse set up a medication regimen and a teaching plan. Free literature was obtained from the American Heart Association, and the patient and spouse were linked to a cardiac support group. Within months it was noted that the patient had no more "revolving door" admissions or emergency room visits.

In this case, despite the absence of hospital admissions and emergency room visits, *nothing* supports the fact that admissions or emergency room visits would have occurred. Case activity can be shown in the summary, but how is it possible to calculate savings? There are no actual numbers—only possible ones! However, the foregoing example shows clearly the actions a case manager often undertakes to ensure the success of a case while helping to decrease the financial risk of his or her organization.

The important thing is to link case management actions and savings efforts, whether these efforts resulted in hard or soft savings, and then to transpose them into some type of reporting format. Both types of savings, when presented to group meetings, client sales presentations, or senior management, document the "win-win" benefit of case management. Also, despite the fact that cost savings reports can be a burdensome task, they are a wonderful management tool. They are a means of showing the "bottom line" successes of case management in terms both clients and management understand because they show the money actually saved through case management interventions.

🐌 SUMMARY

Despite the burden of reporting cost savings, these reports are a useful tool for documenting case management interventions. Unfortunately, in today's healthcare arena, where costs are often the bottom line, not all healthcare administrators and organizations desire any cost savings reports except those that show hard savings. However, it is just as important to document soft savings because these also support the win-win benefits of case management.

OTHER CASE MANAGERS

Reasons for More Than One Case Manager

At times, geographic distances preclude cost-effective on-site monitoring, case conferences, interviews, and other case management duties. Although much can be done by telephone, sometimes an on-site visit is needed, and when circumstances prevent this, involvement of another case manager in the patient's geographic locale may be warranted. The decision to use case managers other than those associated with the primary case manager's organization rests with senior management and the policies formulated by them for this situation.

If outside case managers are allowed, the major responsibility and direction for the hired case manager rests with the primary case manager's office. This includes the number of hours authorized for case management intervention or services, directions for intervention or establishment of services, instructions for written summaries or other reports, and the frequency of telephone updates on the case. Likewise, it entails verification of the appropriate credentials and licenses of all personnel involved.

Multiple Case Managers

Although there are many reasons for using other case managers, the most common involve situations in which a patient requires many services and thus many case managers.[7, 8] In these situations, the case managers, patient, and family must confer to decide who among the case managers will serve as the "primary" case manager. The case manager selected for this role is often the one most involved with the patient on a day-to-day basis (e.g., home health agency or infusion therapy agency case manager). The one selected serves as the clearinghouse for communication between all parties.

Regardless of who is selected, it is the primary case manager's responsibility to keep the others apprised of case events. Selection of a primary case manager does not eliminate the others nor negate their responsibilities to their employers or their case management duties. It also does not mean that they are not involved. The primary intent of appointing a primary case manager is to assist in better communication among all parties in the case. Other advantages include:

- Better coordination
- Avoidance of duplication and prevention of possible fragmentation
- Less confusion by the patient and family because they have one person to communicate with instead of many
- Prevention of game playing by the family, when the family may try to play one case manager against another
- Ease of communication by the physician, who has one contact instead of several

Other situations requiring another case manager occur when a case manager and the family, for whatever reason, do not "hit it off." If this occurs, the case must be transferred to another case manager as soon as possible. This helps to avoid an adversarial atmosphere, prevents litigation, and allows the case to continue with direction. This process is critical because although the success of the case manager's intervention depends on many factors, the key factor is the establishment of a good relationship with the patient.

SUMMARY

On some occasions more than one case manager is involved with a case. In most instances this occurs when multiple agencies are involved, all of which offer various degrees of case management services. In cases involving more than one case manager, one means of avoiding duplication and errors is for all case managers to decide who will serve as the primary case manager. Other situations involving multiple case managers include those in which geographic distances preclude on-site case management interventions by the first case manager. In such cases, another case manager in the patient's immediate vicinity must be found to assume some or all of the case management tasks delegated to him or her.

EXTRA CONTRACTUAL PROCESS

What It Is

Basically, the extra contractual process allows the healthcare organization to establish cost-effective services or supplies when they are excluded from the patient's healthcare coverage. This process is commonly used for extending services that are excluded or limited by the patient's healthcare policy. Examples of situations requiring use of this process include post-acute care rehabilitation for traumatic brain-injured patients who continue to need a structured therapeutic environment, private duty nurses for patients who need skilled care when home health benefits are limited or exhausted, specialized equipment for patients who need it but have a limited equipment benefit, and so forth. As a general rule, if the extra contractual request is denied, there is no appeal process, and the decision is final.

Who Allows It

The extra contractual process (also referred to as a waiver of benefits or a benefit modification process) is allowed by healthcare payers who offer comprehensive case management services and realize that the extra contractual process is necessary if costs are to be contained and quality maintained. However, it is not always recognized by all healthcare payors. Although this process varies with the healthcare payor, all case managers must be knowledgeable about the process (i.e., who to contact, what each person's role is) if delays in securing care or services are to be avoided.

Documentation for Extra Contractual Consideration

Prior to a request for extra contractual care, the case manager must document the fact that every effort was made to find alternatives that provided care equal to that provided by the services or item requested or to keep the benefits within the written guidelines or policy limits. Justification for extra contractual arrangements is based on medical necessity for the level of care or services required, the quality of care, the cost effectiveness of the proposed plan of care, and the fact that it is "in lieu" of hospitalization or will prevent rehospitalization or deterioration of the patient's condition.

The extra contractual process varies with each case. It is performed on a case-by-case basis and is a labor-intensive process. This labor intensiveness is true for all case managers involved because it is necessary to capture as much data as possible that supports the request. The request for this process frequently requires both the facility-based case manager and the healthcare payor's case manager to work closely together to collect the data necessary to support the request. To ensure that the extension of benefits is truly necessary, many healthcare payers use the following criteria:

- The alternative option replaces or subsidizes other similar benefits in the policy.
- All options and alternatives have been found to be either unsuitable or unavailable, and chart documentation substantiates this.
- The proposed option is more cost effective than continuing care in an acute care hospital.
- The same treatment or service would be deemed medically necessary in a hospital setting.
- Without the service or item the patient will be placed at risk and the healthcare payor will be at risk for a costly outcome.
- The specific policy has been reviewed carefully and the full liability coverage (both fiscal and legal) has been considered.
- The attending physician, the patient, and/or the insured person (and at times the policyholder) agree to the alternative option, and the attending physician has submitted his or her justification in writing.[9]

Approval Process

Although the approval process varies with the healthcare plan, approval for extra contractual care is above the realm of case managers and results from second-level review, most often the medical director of the healthcare payor. In addition, many healthcare payers require their legal counsel to review the request also, issuing the final approval in a formal letter. Regardless of the approval method, the case manager's responsibility for this process rests with the documentation of need and the accumulation of sufficient data to enable the second-level reviewer to make an informed decision. Most healthcare payors require documentation for the recommended treatment or services to be submitted in letter form with the following information included:

- Patient's name and identification number
- Policy number
- Insured's name
- Insured's Social Security number
- Policyholder's name
- Diagnosis
- Attending physician's name and phone number

- Hospital (if applicable)
- Hospital admission date (if applicable)
- Brief summary of case history to present
- Brief description of the services required but excluded
- Services covered and not covered relating to the existing condition or treatment (brief summary of patient's policy)
- Date services are to begin
- Proposed treatment and service provider for implementation
- Cost comparison justifying recommended alternative
- Physician's statement justifying recommended alternative, signed and dated

Key points to be remembered by case managers:

- Never promise services or supplies that have not been authorized.
- Never give the patient or provider the "right of expectation" that benefit coverage is indefinite. This principle is true regardless of any extra contractual agreement. Therefore, specific time frames for the approved service or item must be included in all written communications.
- Know or inquire whether the extra contractual process is allowed by the patient's healthcare payor or policyholder.
- Review all documentation before submitting it for second-level review to be sure that all information is present and that the attending physician has clearly stated and documented the medical justifications for the services requested.
- Always send an approval letter that clearly states the level of care or services allowed and includes all limitations. The approval letter must also contain such information as:
  - Patient's name
  - Patient's identification number
  - Patient's policyholder name
  - Specific time frame during which the approval will be in effect

If the patient continues to need the services, renewal of the benefit may be warranted. However, as with the initial process, the mode of this extension process varies with the healthcare payor. For instance, in some cases when the services initially approved by this process continue to be required beyond the approval date, all steps in the extra contractual process must be repeated; in others, review by the medical director may be sufficient to extend the benefits. In other cases, no further coverage may be allowed because the initial benefits were agreed to as a one-time benefit allowance.

Private healthcare payors are not the only ones that allow benefit modifications. Medicaid has a similar process, and if the patient meets eligibility criteria, a Medicaid "waiver" may be allowed.[10] Case managers must be very familiar with the Medicaid processes for waivers in their state, the types of patients covered by these waivers, the application process, and the time frame specified for approval. As with any extra contractual process, the Medicaid waiver process is just as labor intensive (or more so) as the process required by a private healthcare payor. Case managers can obtain information about Medicaid waivers by calling their state's Department of Health Services or the United States Department of Health and Human Services or similar agencies.

Currently, the Civilian Health and Medical Program of the Uniformed Services (CHAMPUS) allows applications for waivers to benefits through either the Home Healthcare Demonstration, the Expanded Home Care Case Management Demonstration, or a private CHAMPUS contractor in the immediate region. Information about these waiver projects can be obtained by calling the Project Care Office at the Office of the Civilian Health and Medical Program of the Uniformed Services (OCHAMPUS) in Aurora, Colorado. The main number can be obtained by calling Colorado's telephone directory assistance.

SUMMARY

The extra contractual process allows coverage for benefits that are excluded or limited from the patient's existing healthcare policy. Preparation of the supporting documents and cost calculations for the extra contractual process is an arduous task; approval is granted only after second-level review. Not only is this process available to many insured patients, it is also available to persons on Medicaid and to those covered by CHAMPUS.

CASE CLOSURE

Cases Appropriate for Closure

Case closure, like case opening, is a subjective decision on the part of the case manager.

However, case closure occurs most often because

- The patient is discharged to another level of care, and the case management function is transferred to another case management entity.
- Case goals were reached, and the patient is medically stable.
- Benefits have terminated.
- The patient has died.
- Alternate care plans are inappropriate.
- The patient has reached a level that requires custodial care. This factor is organization specific because there are many organizations in which the primary focus of case management is on custodial care and how to prevent the patient from using acute care services. The same is true of those organizations in which the case management program is designed to offer disease management.
- The patient or family refuses intervention.
- The patient or family has been trained to be the case manager and will call the professional case manager as needed.

Steps in Closing a Case

When a case is closed, documentation must be prepared that briefly summarizes the case events, the present level of care, and the status of the patient. This serves as a guide for reopening the case, if this is required at a later date.

All healthcare providers on the case must be notified of the closure, both verbally and in writing. If the case is closed for reasons other than death, the patient and family must be prepared well in advance to alleviate fears or feelings of abandonment. Also, the patient and the family must know how to reach the primary case manager if problems arise or if they experience any difficulty in accessing services.

Because final case reports are commonly required, these and any cost avoidance forms must be compiled. Because of the catastrophic and long-term care needs associated with many

cases, some form of record retrieval system must be in place to allow easy access to closed cases should the case require reopening at a later date. Closed cases must be stored according to the organization's policy on retention of records, and most records must be maintained for at least 7 years.

SUMMARY

Case closure, like case opening, is in many instances a subjective decision. It may occur for any number of reasons; however, the patient and family must be prepared for it in advance. Additionally, all parties involved in the case must be notified of the fact that it is to be closed. At the time of case closure, all reports must be finalized and all records stored for easy retrieval should the case require reopening at a later date.

REFERENCES

1. DiPrete RS (1987). Impact of capitated finance systems on the continuum of care. *In* Ewashwick CJ, Weiss LJ (1987). Managing the Continuum of Care. Gaithersburg, MD, Aspen, pp. 225–242.
2. Boland P (1995). Making Managed Healthcare Work. Gaithersburg, MD, Aspen, pp. 392–393.
3. Kongstvedt PR (1993). The Managed Healthcare Handbook, 2nd ed. Gaithersburg, MD, Aspen, pp. 70–87.
4. Mullahy CM (1995). The Case Manager's Handbook. Gaithersburg, MD, Aspen, pp. 236–245.
5. Mullahy CM (1995). Op cit., p. 241.
6. Mullahy CM (1995). Op cit., pp. 248–257.
7. Gibbs B, et al (1995). The role of the clinical nurse specialist and the nurse manager in case management. J Nurs Admin 25(5):28–34.
8. Lyon JC (1993). Models of nursing care delivery and case management: Clarification of terms. Nurs Econ 11(3):163–169.
9. Civilian Health and Medical Program of the Uniformed Services (1996). Operations Manual, Vol 2. Home Health Care Demonstration and Expanded Home Health Care—Case Management Demonstrations. Aurora, Colo., Office of Civilian Health and Medical Program of the Uniformed Services.
10. California Department of Health Services (1993). Fact Sheet: In-Home Medical Care (IHMC) Waiver Program. Sacramento, Department of Health Services.

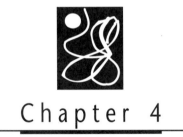

Chapter 4

Funding

FINANCIAL RESOURCES

The financial resources listed in this chapter are presented here only as a quick reference because each funding organization is described in more detail in the following chapters. For every service established for a patient it is important to verify what forms of insurance and insurance benefits the patient has to ensure that the benefits are there and that, if benefits are coordinated, the patient is allowed the maximum benefits. It is just as important to explore all alternate funding programs, unemployment benefits, and other income or healthcare policies to which the patient may be entitled; these are described in detail in subsequent chapters. It is common for patients to require funds from a variety of sources if their needs are to be met and the quality of their care maintained.

When the patient is covered by a private healthcare insurance plan and is also eligible for benefits allowed by an alternate funding program such as Medicaid, the Title V Children's Medical Services program, or the state program for the developmentally disabled, the patient's private insurance always serves as the primary insurance coverage. This rule does not apply to the Civilian Health and Medical Program of the Uniformed Services (CHAMPUS), which, like other alternate funding programs, is always secondary. Also, alternate funding programs will not pay for services if the healthcare payor denies payment because the services are not available in the healthcare payor's network. If the alternate funding program provides reimbursement, it will do so only if benefits are truly limited or excluded from coverage and the patient meets the eligibility criteria of the alternate funding program.

With the exception of Medicare, for which eligibility for coverage is always the same throughout the United States, eligibility for all other alternate funding programs varies drastically from state to state and, in some instances, from county to county within a state. Variations occur not only in eligibility but also in the actual benefits allowed. For instance, although some Title V Children's Medical Services programs cover such services as acute care or care for patients with acquired immune deficiency syndrome (AIDS), others do not.

With the foregoing in mind, it is imperative for case managers to be very familiar with their state's alternate funding programs and any county variations that apply. More important,

they must know how and when to make referrals and be familiar with the basic eligibility requirements. This minimum knowledge is necessary because delays in the actual referral process can make a difference between the patient's qualification for the program and failure to qualify.

Constraints on Coverage

Most healthcare payors place constraints, either dollar or day limits, on benefit coverage for services or supplies. Rarely are funds "limitless." Therefore, case managers from all levels must be creative as they seek and implement services because most services required by the patients found in case management are costly if only because care is frequently required for the long term or lifelong.

Due to the high cost of healthcare and premiums, many employers (policyholders) have decreased the benefits offered by the healthcare policies they provide for their employees. Likewise, to keep premiums affordable, deductibles and copayments have been increased. In fact, two people insured by the same healthcare payor may have two entirely different policies because their employers have selected different policies to fit the financial needs of the company.

Just because a patient has healthcare coverage and benefits at the start of an illness or injury does not mean that he or she will have these benefits throughout the illness. Therefore, case managers must continually verify the existence of benefits and their amounts before any services are implemented. The easiest way to do this is to call the healthcare payor directly. Typically, termination of benefits occurs when a patient:

- Cannot afford to pay his or her premiums (this includes payments due to the Consolidated Omnibus Budget Reconciliation Act [COBRA]).
- Has exhausted the benefit.
- Reaches his or her lifetime maximum for the policy.
- Reaches a plateau.
- Reaches a point when the disease or condition becomes chronic.
- Requires custodial care.
- Requires a treatment or service that is considered investigational or experimental.

Making Use of All Coverage

When benefits or dollars are limited, exhausted, or excluded, the case manager must continually search for alternate funding sources that can augment the plan and help pay for the services the patient requires. It is the wise case manager who consistently searches for means that conserve the patient's healthcare benefits, especially if they are limited. Certainly, if the patient has other health insurance (regardless of type—auto, disability, Medicaid, Medicare), exploration and coordination of any benefits available from these plans are imperative. Other ways to augment benefits are to utilize community resources and to teach the patient and family the care required whenever possible.

Case managers must also encourage patients and families to explore their eligibility for all disability income policies or any unemployment or state disability income or general assistance programs. Although these programs do not pay for medical care, they provide a source of income.

Even when the patient has two or more insurance policies, gaps can exist. It is in filling these gaps that the case manager must be creative. He or she should always ask, "Have all the funding sources for this illness or injury been identified and explored?" For example:

- If the patient is a child or young adult under the age of 21, is he or she eligible for the state's Title V Children's Medical Services program?
- If the child or young adult is under the age of 21, is he or she eligible for any services available in special education programs?
- If the patient is developmentally disabled and the disability occurred before the age of 22, is he or she eligible for services offered by the department or agency responsible for helping people with developmental disabilities?
- If the patient is trainable and motivated to work, is he or she qualified for vocational rehabilitation or any Department of Rehabilitation monies or services?
- If the patient is totally disabled and under the age of 65, has he or she applied for Social Security Disability Income (SSDI)? After 24 months on SSDI, he or she would receive Medicare Part A and become eligible to enroll in Medicare Part B.
- If the patient has a low income or is blind or disabled, he or she can apply for Supplemental Security Income (SSI). Medicaid is given automatically to people receiving SSI, and

they may also be eligible for the services of a chore worker or attendant care.
- If the patient has a low income, has he or she applied for Medicaid or any of its programs? Also, has an application been made for food stamps, general assistance, or, in the case of a single parent with a child, Aid to Families with Dependent Children (AFDC)?
- If the patient has a low income, has multiple needs for skilled services, and has exhausted his or her healthcare coverage benefits, is he or she eligible for Medicaid or a Medicaid waiver program?
- If the patient is a veteran, is he or she eligible for any veterans' services? Is this episode of illness related to any injury incurred during past active duty, which may possibly increase the veteran's disability rating? Thus, he or she may qualify for a different level of care allowed by the Veterans Administration, or will this increase the person's income?
- If the service or treatment needed is investigational or experimental, are any research programs available that offer this service, and if so, is candidacy for the patient feasible?
- Are any fraternal organizations, church groups, or ethnic groups available that could possibly assist with fund raisers or volunteer help or other services such as building ramps and making repairs or corrections to architectural barriers in the patient's home?
- If the patient requires duplicate equipment that is excluded from his or her healthcare coverage (especially diapers and incontinent supplies), can loan closets (i.e., volunteer organizations, disease-specific agencies or churches that offer medical equipment, supplies, and other donated items that can be reused and are provided at no cost) or other organizations in the vicinity assist with procurement of the items?
- If medical supplies are required, can these supplies be "clean" rather than "sterile," or can any of the items be "homemade"?
- If the patient requires care or the caregiver requires respite, are there any organizations available that can provide volunteers or assist with these needs?
- If the patient has been denied services from a public agency, was the denial performed formally, and if so, has the formal appeal process been started?

Certainly, other questions can be asked as well. The key is to be knowledgeable about funding sources, the patient's entitlement to services, and the best way and the best time to gain access to resources. At any given time in any case management plan one or more alternate funding programs or community resources may have to be involved if services are to be supplied to the patient in the frequency and amount required.

POTENTIAL FINANCIAL RESOURCES FOR FAMILIES

Aid to Families with Dependent Children (AFDC). Although this program is currently undergoing major changes, it does exist at the time of this writing. It is included in this section because financial assistance, medical care, and food stamps are available under AFDC as specified in the Social Security Act. Eligibility extends to children and their parents or caregivers who live in their own homes or the homes of relatives. (AFDC as a rule covers children and mothers in homes where the spouse or father of the children is absent from the primary residence.) AFDC is also available to children in foster homes and to those who are wards of the juvenile court or have been referred to the social welfare department for placement. AFDC is a federal and state program that is administered by counties. Application is made at the local Social Service Welfare Department. This program is an income program and does not specifically cover healthcare services except when the family is also eligible for Medicaid.[1]

Children's Medical Services Program (Title V). Title V, or the Children's Medical Services program, was formerly known as Crippled Children's Services; it is part of the Social Security Act. It is jointly funded by federal, state, and county funds but is administered by local state and county offices. This program is available in every state. The money available through this program is used to pay for healthcare services for persons under the age of 21 who meet diagnostic and eligibility criteria and are in need of medical care. Eligibility for care and services is based on diagnosis, income, and state or county of residence. This is not an income program but one that provides payment for medical services to persons who qualify. Retroactive payments are not allowed, and private insurance must be used before any payment is made by this program. Consequently, the Title V Children's Medical Services program is always a payor of last resort. Benefits vary from state to state and from county to county. Each state's name for the program also varies

(for a full list of the names of the programs in each state, please see discussion "Title V of the Social Security Act of 1953: Children's Medical Services" in this chapter.) Application is made in the county or state where the patient lives, not the county or state in which care is supplied.[2]

Fraternal Organizations. Fraternal organizations are many and varied but may include such organizations as the Lions, Shriners, Elks, Masons, Rainbow Girls, DeMolay, Soroptomists, and so forth. Contact can be made with these organizations to obtain specific details about their programs or ability to help. Groups like these often support one-time needs of patients. Examples of services provided include help in deferring medical costs by providing free services or care or offering volunteer help in building ramps or making home alterations. The specific services and money available depend on the organization and the actual fund raising events that are held. One exception to this is the programs offered by the Shriners. These programs are free, can be ongoing, and are designed primarily to assist any child with an orthopedic condition or burn.

Medicaid. Medicaid is part of Title XIX of the Social Security Act. It is a federal-state program that is administered by the local county welfare or social services office. Medicaid pays for medical care for public assistance recipients and other low-income persons. Persons eligible may be deemed low income and medically needy, or they may be receiving SSI or AFDC. Benefits and eligibility vary from state to state, but federal law establishes minimum criteria for eligibility for benefits. Application is made in the person's county of residence to the local welfare or social services department. In California, the program is called Medi-Cal.[3]

Medicare. Medicare, which is part of Title XVIII of the Social Security Act, is a federal health insurance program that has uniform eligibility criteria and benefits throughout the United States. The program covers most individuals entitled to Social Security benefits who are over the age of 65, persons under age 65 who have received federal disability benefits for 24 months, and certain individuals with end-stage renal disease. Under certain circumstances, patients with end-stage renal disease can qualify for benefits from the first month of their renal failure; however, most such patients are on hemodialysis, and coverage for them begins after the third month of dialysis. Coverage is available to persons without regard to income or assets. Medicare is not intended to provide or support long-term care; coverage is focused primarily on acute care and the recovery period. Application should be made at the local Social Security office.[4]

Research Grants. University or teaching hospitals or drug companies may have research grants available to assist certain patients or fund specific types of patient care. If the patient is hospitalized in a university hospital, application and information about the availability of funds can be obtained from the hospital administrator or business office manager. Funding from such programs is extremely limited, and they are available to only a small percentage of the patients who meet the requirements for candidacy.

Sliding Scale. Although a sliding scale is rarely used, many visiting nurse, respite, well baby, immunization, and other public agencies or clinics offer services payable by a sliding scale. The formula is based on the income and size of the family. Information about the feasibility of using a sliding scale can be discussed with the agency administrator.

Social Security Disability Insurance (SSDI). SSDI is a federal income program that is paid from the Social Security trust fund. It is available to totally disabled workers, the blind, or certain dependents under the age of 65. To be eligible, the worker (whether this is the patient, parent, or spouse, or, in some instances, a grandparent or lawfully admitted alien's sponsor) must have contributed the appropriate credits (Federal Insurance Contributions Act [FICA] deductions) to the Social Security trust fund. Application must be made as soon as possible after the disabling diagnosis has been made to the nearest Social Security office because the process takes several months before any benefits are paid. Since this is a federal program, criteria for eligibility are consistent nationally, and recipients of SSDI can move from place to place without losing their benefits. If the applicant is approved and remains on SSDI for 24 months, he or she receives Medicare Part A and is eligible to purchase Medicare Part B.[4]

Special Education—Individuals with Disabilities Education Act (IDEA). Special Education benefits are available to any child under the age of 21 who has not graduated from high school and who meets special education eligibility criteria. The Individuals with Disabilities Education Act (formerly Public Law 94-142) requires school systems to provide those medical services that enable children with disabilities to receive a free and appropriate public education in the least restrictive environment. Services vary drastically from state to state.

Parents or their representative begin the process by filing a written request with the principal of the local school. Once it has been determined that the child needs special education, the school district must complete an individual education plan (IEP) for the child. The IEP must specify what the child requires and how the school district plans to meet the child's needs.[5]

State Agency for the Developmentally Disabled. Each state is required by federal mandate to provide diagnostic services and care for developmentally disabled persons if the developmental disability occurred before the age of 22. Eligibility and services vary from state to state, but the agency's primary focus is on allowing the patient to remain in the least restrictive environment that prevents institutionalization. To accomplish this goal, the agency has the ability to "vendor" necessary services to various healthcare providers.[6]

Supplemental Food Programs for Women, Infants, and Children (WIC). The supplemental food program for women, infants, and children is a federal program that is administered by the county. The program is designed to ensure that the nutritional needs of low-income mothers are being met; the women must meet eligibility criteria. The program serves pregnant women, nursing mothers, infants, and children.[2]

Supplemental Security Income (SSI). SSI is a federal program that is administered by the Social Security Administration. It provides monthly payments to individuals with low incomes who are aged, blind, or disabled. In addition to the monthly payments, recipients of SSI are automatically eligible for Medicaid benefits. A family's income is not counted if the patient is an inpatient in a nonfederally supported facility for 1 full month. Application is made to the local Social Security office.[7]

Veterans' Benefits. Benefits for veterans range from monetary compensation to a full range of inpatient and outpatient medical services. Most of the medical care provided is limited to persons with service-connected disabilities. However, some veterans who are eligible for the Civilian Health and Medical Program of the Uniformed Services (CHAMPUS) are also eligible for services provided at Veterans Administration expense. Information about veterans' benefits is available at any Veterans Administration regional or local service office.[8]

Victims and Witness Program. The Victims and Witness program is a county program that offers some funds to victims of violent crimes. These funds can be used for medical care or to meet temporary unexpected expenses. The local police, sheriff, or district attorney's office is an excellent source of assistance in the application process. Information regarding this program can be obtained by calling local law enforcement agencies.

Workers' Compensation. Benefits (salary and medical care) are available to persons who were injured while working and who have met certain eligibility requirements. There are no payroll deductions because workers' compensation benefits are funded by employer contributions to the State Compensation Insurance Fund. Application should be made to the employer. If a patient is eligible for workers' compensation, he or she is not eligible for regular healthcare benefits for the same condition or for state disability income (SDI [if this is applicable in the state where the patient lives]) or unemployment compensation.

SUMMARY

Case managers must be aware of all financial programs to which patients are entitled. Equally as important is a knowledge of when and where a patient should be referred and the components of the appeal process should services be denied.

Some of the programs listed in this section are intended to provide financial income only, while others cover medical needs and serve as alternate sources of funding for services or care. Benefits must be verified for any patient who has two or more insurance policies, and these various benefits must also be coordinated, thus allowing the patient to gain the maximum entitlement to the services available. This verification process also serves to validate the amounts that have been paid to date and how much remains in the patient's allowable lifetime maximum benefit. Knowledge of this amount allows appropriate referral or re-referral for financial assistance.

There are no hard or set rules about which alternate funding sources are most appropriate for every patient. In certain cases, it may be necessary to combine several funding options to reach the amount required to provide the services identified in the physician's treatment plan or orders and the case management plan. For example, in some cases insurance benefits may be enhanced by the use of benefits available from a special education program, a Title V Children's Medical Services program, the agency responsible for providing developmental disability services, and funds available from a specific disease-related agency. Unfortunately, in other cases patients are not eligible for any additional financial help or alternate medical coverage.

TITLE V OF THE SOCIAL SECURITY ACT OF 1953: CHILDREN'S MEDICAL SERVICES

Medical services for children were established under Title V of the 1953 Social Security Act and are known as Children's Medical Services. Until recently, these programs were referred to as Crippled Children's Services. Title V Children's Medical Services programs are essentially federal-state programs that are governed by the Civil Rights Act of 1964. This act is intended to provide services to low-income children when a need is identified and the child meets certain eligibility criteria. The programs are administered locally by each state.

Under these programs, funding for services is allowed for certain handicapping or disabling conditions if the patient meets eligibility criteria. The programs use a combination of federal, state, county, and family contributions to pay for services. These programs are designed to meet the medical needs of handicapped or disabled persons under the age of 21 whose families are unable to pay, in part or in whole, the cost of recommended treatment.

Purpose and Objectives

Because eligibility criteria vary from state to state, the purpose and objectives of each state's Title V Children's Medical Services program likewise vary. In most states eligibility is based on residency, the family's taxable income, and the child's diagnosis. The key benefit in all programs is that they offer diagnostic capabilities and case management services. Despite the variations in scope, most programs have the following purposes and objectives:

• To locate eligible handicapped persons under the age of 21 who need care.
• To provide diagnostic and preventive services

and early detection of handicapping conditions.

- To enable eligible persons to obtain medical services to maximize their physical, mental, social, and educational development.
- To provide funding for preventive and diagnostic services when funds are not available through private insurance or the family is unable to pay for the services.
- To obtain the highest quality care for persons treated under the program.
- To coordinate these services with those offered by other state and county agencies or departments to ensure that the eligible person receives the benefits to which he or she is entitled (e.g., public health nurses, rehabilitation and vocational retraining, or mental health treatment).
- To serve as the cognizant public official or public official statement (POS) necessary to receive benefits from CHAMPUS and its Program For The Handicapped (PFTH). The public official can be any public official (generally this is someone from the state's Title V Children's Medical Services program, Medicaid, the agency serving the developmentally disabled, or the school district) who can certify that public agencies or services are not available or adequate to meet the needs of the child.
- To work with local Planned Parenthood units to recommend therapeutic abortions when amniocentesis reveals that a fetus has an eligible condition (i.e., known life-threatening anomaly such as micrencephaly) or to prevent AIDS in the newborn.

Typical Eligible Diagnoses

Although the following list of "eligible medical conditions" covered by the Title V Children's Medical Services program is fairly extensive, both eligibility and the level of services provided for the different diagnoses vary from state to state. Thus, a diagnosis that is eligible for services in one state may not be eligible in another (e.g., not all states allow coverage for acute care; some concentrate only on chronic conditions). Occasionally a condition that is not listed below may be eligible. Because of the inconsistencies, it is wise for the case manager to make the referral even if in doubt. Let the experts determine whether the child qualifies or not. Conditions frequently recognized as eligible often include the following:

- Orthopedic conditions due to infection, injury, or congenital malformations.
- Conditions requiring plastic surgery or reconstruction, such as cleft lip, facial anomalies, and burns.
- Conditions requiring orthodontic reconstruction, such as cleft palate, severe malocclusion, or orificial anomalies.
- Eye conditions that lead to loss of vision.
- Ear conditions that lead to loss of hearing.
- Rheumatic fever.
- Nephritis, nephrosis, or nephrotic syndrome.
- Phenylketonuria.
- Hemophilia.
- Hyaline membrane disease (bronchopulmonary dysplasia [BPD]).
- Endocrine or metabolic disorders that pose problems in medical management or problems with the establishment of a diagnosis.
- Convulsive disorders that pose problems in medical management or problems with the establishment of a diagnosis.
- Blood dyscrasias.
- All neoplasms.
- Severe skin disorders such as epidermolysis bullosa.
- Chronic pulmonary conditions such as cystic fibrosis, bronchiectasis, and lung abscess.
- Congenital anomalies causing disabling or disfiguring handicaps.
- Conditions of the nervous system such as inflammatory diseases that produce motor disability, paralysis, or ataxia or other neuromuscular diseases that may include cerebral palsy, muscular dystrophy, or stroke.
- Conditions resulting from an accident or poisoning that are potentially handicapping such as complicated fractures, brain or spinal cord injuries, or stricture of the esophagus.
- Severe adverse reactions to an immunization requiring extensive medical or related care.
- Any disabling or disfiguring condition that may be long term and handicapping.
- AIDS, AIDS-related complex (ARC), human immune deficiency virus (HIV)-positive persons (this category of disease and the services provided for it vary drastically from state to state).

There are times when the case manager may be required to act as the patient's advocate if benefits are to be allowed or if the child has coverage under a health maintenance organization (HMO) but the benefits are limited and there are many exclusions. For instance, many years ago problems occurred in obtaining coverage for a ventilator-dependent infant. No cause could be found for the child's inability to breathe; he had been tested by multiple specialists at a large tertiary center, and he had undergone many tests and procedures that failed to lead to the establishment of a definitive diagnosis. Because of severe limitations and exclusions in his healthcare coverage and because there were no placement or care alternatives, all benefits had to be coordinated with the appropriate agencies before the child could be discharged home with 24-hour care and an inordinate amount of equipment and supplies.

However, without a definitive diagnosis he essentially was not eligible for California's Title V Children's Medical Services program, called California Children's Services (CCS). Similarly, because there was no diagnosis, neither the California Department of Developmental Disabilities nor the Regional Center would assume him as a client! There appeared to be no way to cover the skilled nursing care he would require. The only recourse was to assist the family in seeking assistance from their local congressman. Needless to say, this was done. Eventually, after many meetings with the two agencies, the child was accepted and became eligible for both programs, allowing his medical team to proceed with plans to discharge him to his home.

Referrals

Timeliness of referrals is of critical importance because it is often the key to the time when coverage begins. This is especially true for the technology-dependent child for whom healthcare coverage is limited or benefits are excluded or exhausted. Although the actual medical diagnosis, family income, and place of residence are the three keys to referral, case managers should not hesitate to make a referral if they think the child may qualify for benefits. It is important to remember that referrals:

- Can be accepted from anyone (e.g., healthcare professional or family member).
- Are made to the county or state in which the child lives, not the county or state in which he will receive care (the county or state of residence is determined by the residence of the father or legal guardian).
- Are encouraged regardless of whether the patient has insurance or the family has income.

Eligibility Requirements

Once the child has been referred, his or her financial eligibility must be determined by the county or state agency before authorization for any services is granted. Unfortunately, as a rule, this process may consume several weeks after the referral. If the child merely requires establishment of a diagnosis or referral to a school therapy program, financial screening for eligibility is not necessary. Therefore, if time is important and it appears that the child may be eligible, case managers should not hesitate to make the referral. For all other conditions, as stated earlier, eligibility is based on:

- A medically eligible diagnosis.
- Family income or ability to pay for medical care.
- Place of residence.

When the formal eligibility screening process begins, the case manager may wish to inform the family that they should be prepared to provide the following information:

- Patient's name.
- Patient's (and family's) address and phone numbers.
- Patient's date of birth.
- Proof of Medicaid or eligibility for Medicaid, if applicable.
- State tax records (in some states this is the basis of eligibility and determines the amount of the repayment obligation when appropriate; however, for states without a state tax, this requirement is waived).
- Amount of family income (including, for example, any Social Security payments from a deceased parent, or child support payments from an absent spouse).
- Names of family members earning income.
- Number of persons dependent on family income.
- Employer's name and address.
- Name and address of any company or agency providing healthcare insurance.
- A signed release form allowing release of the patient's medical records, if these medical records have not already been obtained.

Once the eligibility screening process has been completed, the application and any medical information or records supporting the diagnosis or condition are collected and forwarded to the unit responsible for determining the patient's medical eligibility. Medical eligibility is based on the following criteria:

- Evidence of need for care
- Prognosis
- Reasonable expectation for recovery
- Availability of treatment
- Priority of need for treatment

Case managers may want to inform the family about the following facts:

- A referral may be made to Medicaid if the income is such that the family may be eligible for Medicaid benefits. Case managers must keep in mind that all Title V Children's Medical Service funds are secondary to any healthcare payor plan (this includes Medicaid), and if the child is linked to an HMO or other managed care plan, benefits from the Title V program may not be available unless the child's healthcare benefits are limited, excluded, or exhausted.
- If income exceeds the basic standard amount needed by the family to live, the family is responsible for repayment of any portion in excess of this standard.
- If the family moves from one county or state to another during the course of the treatment, benefits cease, and the family must file for a reevaluation and determination of financial eligibility in the new state or county.
- If the family is not eligible for the services, the Title V Children's Medical Services program staff will assist the family in identifying community agencies that can provide assistance.
- All services require authorization before the service is provided; without this authorization the program is not obligated to pay for the service.
- Most programs use only facilities, physicians, agencies, and other providers who have met the Title V agency's standards for care.
- Families with healthcare insurance may be considered eligible for care if it is determined that the insurance coverage or their income is insufficient to cover the needed care.
- For children with a chronic condition, responsibility for payment of medical care services that clearly affect the eligible condition can often be assumed.
- When treatment reaches a plateau or when it becomes evident that treatment is not or will not significantly influence the eventual outcome, healthcare coverage ceases.
- These programs do not pay for custodial care, homemaker services, experimental or research treatments, education, or alterations to the home.

Services Provided

Although the services provided vary from state to state and from county to county, most programs pay for services necessary to establish a diagnosis, provide basic treatment consistent with federal program objectives, or establish a treatment plan. Case management services are a key element in most programs. To ensure that the goals of treatment plans and case management plans are reached, case managers at all levels should work closely with the Children's Medical Services staff. Case *manager collaboration is especially necessary if dual coverage exists (e.g., Children's Medical Services and private healthcare insurance).* Despite the fact that actual services vary from state to state, the following services are commonly authorized for eligible persons:

- Hospitalization
- Outpatient treatment or services
- Physician, dental, optometrist, orthodontist, or other professional physician services
- Blood and blood products
- Medications
- Transportation
- Social worker services
- Nursing services for skilled care
- Braces and other prosthetics
- Laboratory or radiologic services
- Radiation therapy
- Physical, occupational, or speech therapy
- Psychological evaluation
- Durable medical equipment and accessory supplies
- Dressings and supplies

Genetic Programs

Although several states offer limited services in the diagnosis and treatment of genetic conditions, the criteria for eligibility vary in each state. The Title V Children's Medical Services programs in California and Nebraska are the only two offices that offer a formal Genetically Handicapped Persons Program (GHPP). This program in these two states offers a full range of comprehensive medical care, diagnostic evaluations, carrier testing, and ongoing case management for persons who have a genetic disorder and meet the state's referral criteria.

The process for referral and eligibility for genetic services is the same as that previously described for any other Title V Children's Medical Services program. However, one key aspect distinguishes the two programs: There may be times when a child is ineligible for Title V services but is eligible for genetic services. Families, therefore, should be encouraged to apply for these services.

Names for the Various Title V Children's Medical Services Programs by State

The following are the names of each Title V Childrens' Medical Services programs by state:

ALABAMA—Children's Rehabilitation Services (CRS)

ALASKA—Healthcare Program for Children with Special Needs (HCPCSN)

ARIZONA—Children's Rehabilitation Services (CRS)

ARKANSAS—Children's Medical Services (CMS)

CALIFORNIA—California Children's Services (CCS)

COLORADO—Healthcare Programs for Children with Special Needs (HCP)

CONNECTICUT—Children with Special Healthcare Needs (CSHCN)

DELAWARE—Children with Special Health Needs (CSHN)

DISTRICT OF COLUMBIA (WASHINGTON, D.C.)—Health Services for Children with Special Needs (HSCSN)

FLORIDA—Children's Medical Services (CMS)

GEORGIA—Children's Medical Services (CMS)

HAWAII—Children with Special Health Needs Branch (CSHNB)

IDAHO—Children's Special Health Program (CSHP)

ILLINOIS—Division of Specialized Care for Children (DSCC)

INDIANA—Children's Special Healthcare Services (CSHCS)

IOWA—Child Health Specialty Clinics (CHSC)

KANSAS—Services for Children with Special Healthcare Needs (CSHCN)

KENTUCKY—Commission for Children with Special Healthcare Needs (CCSHN)

LOUISIANA—Children's Special Health Services (CSHS)

MAINE—Coordinated Care Services for Children with Special Needs (CCSCSN)

MARYLAND—Children's Medical Services (CMS)

MASSACHUSETTS—Family and Community Support Division for Children with Special Healthcare Needs

MICHIGAN—Children's Special Healthcare Services (CSHCS)

MINNESOTA—Minnesota Children with Special Health Needs (MCSHN)

MISSISSIPPI—Children with Special Healthcare Needs (CSHCN)

MISSOURI—Children with Special Healthcare Needs (CSHCN)

MONTANA—Children's Special Health Services (CSHS)

NEBRASKA—Medically Handicapped Children's Program (MHCP)

NEVADA—Family Health Services Bureau (FHSB)

NEW HAMPSHIRE—Bureau of Special Medical Services

NEW JERSEY—Special Child Health Services (SCHS)

NEW MEXICO—Children's Medical Services (CMS)

NEW YORK—Physically Handicapped Children's Program (PHCP)

NORTH CAROLINA—Children's Special Health Services (CSHS)

NORTH DAKOTA—Children's Special Health Services (CSHS)

OHIO—Bureau for Children with Medical Handicaps (BCMH)

OKLAHOMA—Children with Special Healthcare Needs (CSHCN)

OREGON—The Child Development and Rehabilitation Center or Oregon Services for Children with Special Healthcare Needs (OSCHSHN)

PENNSYLVANIA—Division of Children's Special Healthcare Needs

RHODE ISLAND—Crippled Children's Service (CCS)

SOUTH CAROLINA—Children's Rehabilitation Service (CRS)

SOUTH DAKOTA—Children's Special Health Services (CSHS)

TENNESSEE—Children's Special Services (CSS)

TEXAS—Chronically Ill and Disabled Children's Services (CIDC)

UTAH—Children with Special Healthcare Needs (CSHCN)

VERMONT—Children with Special Health Needs (CSHN)

VIRGINIA—Division of Children's Specialty Services (DCSS)

WASHINGTON—Office of Children with Special Healthcare Needs (CSHCN)

WEST VIRGINIA—Handicapped Children's Services (NCS)

WISCONSIN—Children with Special Healthcare Needs (CSHCN)

WYOMING—Children's Health Services (CHS)

SUMMARY

The Title V Children's Medical Services program is a valuable program that can assist with payment for services for an eligible person under the age of 21 who is catastrophically ill or injured. The keys to obtaining maximum benefits are early referrals and an awareness of variations in coverage from state to state. Not everyone qualifies, but those who meet the referral criteria should be afforded the opportunity for assessment for possible coverage.

MEDICAID

One of the most frequently used alternative funding sources is Medicaid, which in California is called Medi-Cal. Because it is used so frequently, case managers must be familiar with the process of application to Medicaid, its restrictions, the criteria for eligibility for services, and the average length of time from application to entitlement. All of these are key elements in the attempt to establish timely care and services for patients.

Medicaid was established in 1965 under Title XIX of the Social Security Act. Not only does the federal government maintain administrative codes that establish the minimum standards, each state also has its own administrative codes (e.g., in California it is Title XXII) that set guidelines for how the state will monitor and regulate the federal requirements established for the program. If information about Medicaid is required, contact should be made with the nearest state office of the Department of Health and Human Services. Information about the actual law is available at any state or county law library.

Although Medicaid is a federal program, it is essentially each state's health insurance program for the poor. Despite the fact that each state receives federal funds for the program, state tax dollars make up the bulk of the money available; this is the reason for the variations in the program from state to state.

Federally Mandated Benefits

Although subject to federal guidelines, each state administers its own program. Federal guidelines require all states to cover, at a minimum, the categorically needy (i.e., recipients of AFDC and SSI, pregnant women and children up to age 6 if the family income is below 133% of poverty level; children under the age of 18 if the family income is below poverty level; and Medicare beneficiaries with incomes below poverty level). Federally mandated Medicaid benefits include the following:

- Inpatient hospital services
- Outpatient hospital services and ambulatory care
- Laboratory, radiologic, and other diagnostic tests
- Physician services
- Home healthcare services
- Early and periodic screening and diagnostic services and treatments for children under the age of 21
- Care in a skilled nursing facility
- Family planning services
- Nurse, midwife services
- Family nurse practitioner services

Optional state services may include:

- Mental health care
- Podiatry service and foot care
- Durable medical equipment and medical supplies
- Vision examination and eye care
- Hearing aids and audiology services
- Dental services
- Hospice care
- Both skilled nursing facility care and custodial care
- Dialysis
- Artificial limbs, braces, and eyes
- Chiropractic care
- Acupuncture
- Family planning services
- Blood and blood derivatives and their administration
- Therapies such as occupational therapy, physical therapy, and speech therapy
- Medications
- Ambulance service (both emergency ambulance and nonemergency transportation such as gurney car or wheelchair car)

Although the list of benefits appears extensive, each state imposes varying levels of restrictions on almost every category. For instance, therapy may be limited to two times per month, home healthcare to one to two times per month, and so forth. Also, most services require prior authorization, and benefits are monitored closely through review processes such as prospective and concurrent review.

Managed Care and Medicaid

As healthcare professionals know, although managed care has been in existence for years in the private sector, it has not been used so far for Medicaid owing to federal restrictions. Until just recently, Medicaid has allowed reimbursement only by a fee-for-service system. Now, as some federal compliance restrictions are released and as states attempt to balance their budgets, Medicaid is moving toward managed care. As such, it is contracting with private sector healthcare payors who provide their services in administering or monitoring Medicaid benefits in one state's program in exchange for money. Usually this money is derived from cost savings gained by managing the healthcare of Medicaid recipients appropriately. Most Medicaid managed care contracts are established as "at risk" contracts, meaning that if the healthcare payor does not manage the healthcare of the individuals enrolled efficiently, it loses money. Therefore, the healthcare payor has a financial incentive to manage the Medicaid enrollees in the same way as it would its own members or the groups traditionally enrolled.

Key Pointers

Case managers must be aware of certain key points regarding Medicaid:

- Medicaid is always the payor of last resort (i.e, if the patient has private insurance and Medicaid, the private healthcare payor is the first payor and Medicaid reimburses only if the primary payor's rates are lower than those of Medicaid).
- The only exception to the secondary rule is the state's Title V Children's Medical Services program, which is always the payor of last resort; Medicaid is primary to this program.
- The person must have applied for and been determined eligible for Medicaid services.
- Copayment and deductibles for Medicaid are generally nonexistent or extremely low.
- Many' healthcare providers will not treat or accept or are not certified to accept Medicaid patients (this is especially true of specialty physicians and skilled nursing facilities. It is imperative to ask providers if they are certified and if they accept Medicaid before a patient is moved into the facility because if the patient is eligible for Medicaid and the provider is not certified, transfer to another provider must ensue).

Once a person has been declared eligible for Medicaid, emergency out-of-state care is covered if an emergent health situation should arise while the patient is traveling. However, routine care or other medical care received out-of-state requires prior authorization.

Medicaid, like any other healthcare payor, has an appeal process, and any person who disagrees with an adverse decision has the right to appeal and request a hearing. All requests must be made within a specific date of the county action or inaction (e.g., 30, 60, 90 days). Requests can be made verbally or in writing at the local county welfare department.

It is also important to note that when a service is denied by Medicaid for reasons of medical necessity or "reasonable and customary," the patient is not responsible for the charges and cannot be pursued by the provider for payment.

Reasons for Variations from State to State

Generally speaking, there are several reasons for the variations in Medicaid coverage that occur from state to state. Most often these involve the following basic factors:

- The state's tax base and subsequent availability of federal matching funds (remember that not all states have a state tax).
- The state's regulations and codes that determine how they administer the program while adhering to the basic requirements imposed by the Health Care Financing Administration (HCFA) regulations for Title XIX.
- The state's eligibility requirements (e.g., income, residence in a state versus intent to reside and so forth).
- The benefits allowed versus the limitations imposed (as a rule, Medicaid benefits are comprehensive, covering such services as dental care, eye examinations and glasses, and chiropractic care; however, in contrast, Medicaid may also impose major restrictions on such services as therapy, home health nursing care, and so forth).
- Provider contracting requirements.
- Reimbursement methods.
- Barriers to access to care (including lack of transportation, communication or language barriers, geographic distances, lack of a primary care physician to manage the patient's medical needs, providers that are willing to accept Medicaid reimbursement rates, and so forth).

All these factors can potentially affect the outcome of a catastrophically ill or injured person in need of long-term care. However, access to care, benefit limitations, and low reimbursement methods have the most serious consequences. These are the primary reasons for delayed or nonexistent care.

Eligibility for Medicaid

Other than the absence of any healthcare coverage, the most common reasons for eligibility for Medicaid are exhaustion of healthcare benefits or termination of insurance coverage when the patient still needs care and services. When this occurs, the patient may or may not have enough money to pay privately for the needed services. Hence, the ultimate payor is Medicaid, which has extreme limitations on benefits; also, if application has not been made at the appropriate time, delays in care can result. Patients who are eligible for Medicaid services are those who are:

- Categorically needy persons.
- Blind or disabled persons of any age.
- AFDC recipients.
- SSI recipients.
- Medically needy or indigent patients (includes both persons requiring medical care and those requiring mental health care who cannot afford to pay for their care; however, not all states have this criterion).
- Catastrophically ill or injured persons under the age of 21 who qualify for Title V Children's Medical Services.
- Refugees (legal or illegal).

Application Process

As with all other patients in case management, the case manager must ask the patient and family about their financial resources and must continue to ask as the case proceeds. This is not a pleasant process, but it must be done! The most successful discharges and case management plans are those developed after the case manager has realistically performed a "nitty gritty" financial assessment. Patients and families must be queried about their finances, and the case manager must honestly explain to them what may be expected of them financially throughout the course of the illness.

It is only with this type of approach that the case manager can correctly refer the patient and family to the welfare department for eligibility screening. Unfortunately, Medicaid has a negative connotation, and it is frequently necessary to take a proactive approach to the family to support the fact that Medicaid is not a "welfare" program but a form of insurance.

As soon as the patient is identified as a potential candidate for Medicaid, the patient or family should apply to the nearest medical assistance unit at the county welfare or social services department. Despite a timely referral, the eligibility process can take weeks or months before a final determination is made.

Once contact has been made, the patient is given an appointment with a Medicaid eligibility worker. In some instances, a preliminary screening for eligibility can be conducted by telephone, but as a rule the person must go directly to the social services department or welfare department for this process. To expedite the process, whether it is conducted by phone or in person, patients or families should be prepared to provide such items as:

- Proof of identity, which may include:
  - Valid driver's license
  - Alien card
  - Photo ID (available at the Department of Motor Vehicles)
- Social Security (SS) card or proof of receipt of Social Security funds; this may include:
  - Original Social Security card
  - Official statement from the Social Security Administration that the Social Security card is not available
  - Social Security number of spouse even if patient is widowed or divorced
- Verification of place of residence, which may include:
  - Property tax statement
  - Rent receipt
  - Utility bill
  - Memo from landlord, parent, or roommate indicating location of the patient's residence
- Proof of income, which may include:
  - Wage stub
  - Tax return
- Proof of current bank accounts, which may include:
  - Bank account numbers
  - Checking statements
  - Savings statements
  - Stocks or bonds

- Proof of value of real property, which may include:
  - County tax identification number or receipt of property owned (including rentals)
- Proof of value of motor vehicles (boats, cars, or recreation vehicles) owned, which may include:
  - Owner registration or loan receipt
- Insurance policies, which may include:
  - Health and medical insurance policies
  - Hospital insurance policies
  - Dental insurance policies
  - Life insurance policies (especially whole life)
- Other details
  - Place of birth (of both patient and spouse or parent)
  - Marital status
  - Names and dates of birth of all family members within the household
  - File containing any medical receipts (in some states Medicaid can be issued retroactive to 3 months prior to application)

Persons eligible for Medicaid are allowed a maximum amount of liquid assests. Liquid assets are defined as cash, savings, checking accounts, stocks, cash value of life insurance, and sometimes an automobile or paid cemetery plot (if costs are above the allowed limit). Allowable amounts of liquid assets are adjusted yearly; they vary and depend on the number of persons in the household.

If the patient is deemed eligible for benefits, he or she is issued a card or some form of identification as proof of eligibility. The card or eligibility letter contains many identification numbers, which are codes indicating the type of services to which the person is entitled. It is wise for case managers to be familiar with these codes or at least to know where to obtain the information relating to them should the need arise. For instance, the numbers on the card can indicate:

- Valid date of eligibility.
- Whether the person also has Medicare, SSI, or AFDC.
- Whether the person is blind, disabled and under age 65, disabled and not receiving SSI, a foster child, an adopted child, or is eligible for a pilot Medicaid project or waiver.
- Whether the coverage is limited, restricted, or linked to other programs.

Program Administration

Medicaid administration rests with the state's Department of Health and Human Services or a similar state agency. Day-to-day operations and responsibilities for prior authorizations, reviews, and inspections generally rest with the various field offices, and day-to-day determinations of eligibility are performed by the county social service or welfare offices located throughout each state and county.

Waivers

Medicaid has now established in-home programs for persons eligible for Medicaid. These programs, referred to as Medicaid waivers, are intended for patients who have suffered a catastrophic illness or injury. These waivers are similar in intent to the extra contractual or waiver-of-benefit process allowed by private healthcare payors.

Medicaid waivers were established by the Omnibus Budget Reconciliation Act of 1981. This act specifically allows Medicaid to authorize waivers for a variety of home- and community-based services for individuals who, without the services, would require institutionalization at a minimum in a skilled nursing facility. Case managers at minimum should be familiar with:

- The in-home waivers that allow hourly skilled nursing care for persons who are technologically dependent.
- The AIDS in-home waiver that allows in-home care for terminally ill AIDS patients.

A Medicaid waiver is established only if:

- The patient's health insurance has limitations or exclusion for the services, or the third party payor has denied the services.
- Without the waiver, the patient would continue to require hospitalization for a minimum of 90 days.
- The cost of the in-home care has been documented to be less than the cost of continued inpatient care.
- The care can be provided in a barrier-free and safe environment, and the family is willing and supportive of the home care plan.
- The care is to be provided by a licensed and certified home health agency.

Prior to the establishment of in-home care, intensive evaluation is conducted on all factors that affect the case. The following factors or situations are evaluated:

- The patient's medical condition, including careful calculation of the number of hours, costs, and the frequency and types of services

and equipment needed to ensure continuity of care.
- The home and environmental situation.
- Ability of the family or caregiver to care for the patient.

Documentation must support the facts that the home plan is cost effective, that its quality remains high, and that it is accepted by both the patient and the family. Prior to the implementation of the plan of care the Medicaid physician or consultant must review the case and issue a statement of approval.

Once the care is established, a nurse reviewer is responsible for conducting on-site evaluations every 90 days at minimum. This evaluation or assessment report must cover the following areas:

- Changes in the patient's condition.
- Changes in equipment, supplies, and ancillary services or nursing care.
- Documentation of continued need for licensed nursing staff, adequacy and quality of the nursing staff and its supervision, quality of the care provided, adequacy and timeliness of nursing documentation, and treatment plan changes.
- Family's relationship with the patient and nursing staff.
- Family and home health agency responsibilities for out-of-home activities.
- Cleanliness, organization, and relative safety of the home environment.
- Name of attending physician and level of participation.

Skilled Nursing Facilities and Medicaid

By far the largest portion of public expenditures for skilled nursing facilities, nursing homes, and long-term care is financed by the Medicaid programs. Any patient who exhausts his or her healthcare benefits but must remain hospitalized in a skilled nursing facility or nursing home because of a classification of "total care" or "custodial care" must either pay privately or apply for Medicaid for this level of care. If the patient cannot pay, Medicaid will finance the care if the patient meets certain financial criteria for eligibility. If the patient does not qualify, arrangements must be made for an alternate level of care at the patient's or family's expense.

SUMMARY

Medicaid is the most frequently encountered alternate funding source. However, only those with very limited assets and property qualify for this program. Basically, Medicaid is insurance for the very low income person or the person who has limited assets and cannot afford medical care. Unfortunately, because not all patients qualify, they may "fall through the cracks" or be in the "gray area"—they have too much income to qualify but too little to pay the high cost of medical care themselves. Coverage for most services is greatly limited or excluded in Medicaid. Also, some patients may be responsible for paying part of the cost before Medicaid pays its allowed amount. States and counties vary in their ability to provide services to eligible recipients. For this reason, case managers must be familiar with state and county benefits and restrictions and with special programs.

Medicaid is one of the few alternate insurance sources that allows retroactive coverage without penalty. However, to avoid delays in initiating services, application must be made as soon as possible.

SPECIAL EDUCATION

Public Law 94-142, the Education of All Handicapped Children Act of 1975, now the Individuals with Disabilities Education Act (IDEA) of 1991, declares that all individuals in whom exceptional needs have been identified have a right to a free and appropriate public education. This includes any special instruction, services, or adaptive environment necessary to provide the education. The programs covered by this act are frequently referred to as Special Education.

Purpose

Special Education is specially designed instruction or schooling that is provided at no cost to the parent to allow children with exceptional needs to obtain an education if their needs cannot be met by modifying the regular school program. Information about the program is available from the state or county Department of Education. Because many case management caseloads are composed of a significant number of children with special needs, case managers must be familiar with Special Education processes and understand what the program can and cannot provide for the child. Depending on the needs of the child and the problems the parents are experiencing in establishing services for the child, case managers may be invited by the parents to assist in the process. The process includes an independent evaluation of the child for services, often called individual educational plan, or IEP.

Benefits for Special Education vary from state to state. However, because this is a federal act that protects all children from birth to age 21, it is important for case managers be aware of the benefits allowed. Also, because some families may be intimidated by the complex processes involved, it may be necessary for the case manager, if requested by the family, to act as an advocate for the patient, assisting the family when problems arise in relation to gaining access to services or when the patient is denied benefits inappropriately.

The Individuals with Disabilities Education Act (IDEA) protects all persons from birth to age 21 who need Special Education and stipulates basically that:

- Education shall be offered at no cost in the most appropriate and least restrictive environment possible.
- Once a person has been referred, an assessment and IEP must be developed within a specified period of time (ranging from 50 to 90 days, depending on the requirements in the individual state).
- Noneducational public agencies cannot reduce eligibility for medical or other assistance due the person under the Title V Children's Medical Services program or Title XIX (Medicaid) of the Social Security Act.
- All state and federal resources must be used when necessary to provide the education, and all benefits must be coordinated to ensure that there is no duplication.

Criteria for Eligibility

Persons with exceptional needs are those who have a low-incidence disability or a chronic or severe handicapping condition (autism, blindness, deafness, severe orthopedic impairment, or severe emotional disturbance). A low-incidence disability is defined as a severe handicapping condition that has an expected incidence rate of less than 1% of the total state-wide school population from kindergarten through grade 12.

Special Education is not intended for persons whose educational needs are due primarily to unfamiliarity with the English language, a temporary physical handicap, or maturational, environmental, cultural, or economic factors. Special Education is intended for individuals afflicted with problems associated with:

- Function below the normal level for the child's chronologic age
- Impaired fine or gross motor control or a severe orthopedic impairment
- Abnormal receptive or expressive language development
- Abnormal social, emotional, or psychological development
- Impaired cognitive development
- Deafness or impaired hearing development
- Blindness or impaired visual development
- Disabling medical or congenital syndrome

All services needed by children with these disorders are performed by qualified professionals and may be of many types:

- Referrals and assessments
- Any special instruction the pupil requires
- Consultation
- Coordination with other agencies or individuals

Services Provided

To enable the person to participate in a Special Education program, the school district must provide any related services at no cost if these related services are not covered by insurance. However, if coverage by a healthcare payor is available, school districts have the right to seek reimbursement from such a payor to cover the cost of the related services to the extent permitted by federal law or regulation.

The direct and related services that may be available under Special Education programs vary from state to state.[9] Case managers must keep in mind that healthcare payors generally do not pay for speech therapy or occupational therapy if such therapy is required for a learning disorder rather than a medical disability. Consequently, once a diagnosis has been made and a need is identified, parents must be informed of this fact and encouraged to apply for Special Education for the child. If the child is accepted as a client, he or she may be entitled to "direct" or "related" services. Direct services are those specifically designed to address the educational component, but related services may be therapeutic, medical, or physically necessary "healthcare"-type services. Related services are generally provided by such healthcare professionals as:

- Occupational, physical, or speech therapists
- Nursing aides (who provide personal care or assistance)
- Special nurses (who provide such services as gavage feedings, suctioning, catheterization, or other medically related services)

Other related services that may be provided if the child is deemed eligible for Special Education may include:

- Assistive technology or specialized equipment (e.g., computers)
- Transcribers, readers, or interpreters
- Transportation between home and school

As with so many state programs, the person who is designated to perform the actual care also varies from state to state. One state may allow a higher level of care and related services for the child than another. For instance, in one state the care and related services may be performed by training teachers how to administer the care; in another the state may contract with qualified individuals or a home health agency to provide the services; and in still another the state may rule that care is limited to personal care only (i.e., helping the child use the toilet). Thus, in these states the family or healthcare payor must provide the bulk of any skilled care needed.

In addition to providing Special Education within the confines of a specially designated classroom or public school, the local school district or county Department of Education is responsible for providing schooling in a full range of other locations. This continuum of responsibility covers all persons placed in a licensed children's institution, foster family home, special center or state hospital, psychiatric hospital, or other health facility located within or functioning under the district's jurisdiction.

A school district is also responsible for providing instruction to a pupil confined to a hospital or home with a medical condition related to surgery, an accident, a short-term illness, or medical treatment for a chronic illness. When home teaching is required, it is not classified as Special Education. It is home tutoring. Tutoring is available by calling the school district and making the necessary arrangements.

Special Programs

Children receive Special Education instruction and services according to their specific needs. Children are placed in Special Education programs only after the resources of the regular education program have been considered, used, and deemed inappropriate. The following is a brief description of some of the Special Education programs that may be available:

Severely Handicapped. These programs are for children who have severe disabilities in learning or behavior that may be related to the following diagnoses:

- Mental retardation
- Developmental disability
- Multiple handicaps
- Developmental disorder with autistic-like behavior
- Serious emotional disturbance

Physically Handicapped. Children placed in this program have a physical condition that interferes with learning. These conditions include:

- Orthopedic impairments
- Other health conditions
- Visual handicaps

Communicatively Handicapped. Children in these programs have a language disability that interferes with their academic achievement. Such disabilities include:

- Severe language disorders
- Deafness and hearing impairments
- Speech disorders

Learning Handicapped. This program is for children who have a significant disability in learning, such as:

- Learning disabilities
- Mild mental retardation

Special Education students may be served in a variety of settings depending on their needs as determined by the IEP team. Settings and services may include the following:

Special Day Classes. Special day classes are provided for students with more intensive educational needs. Students in these classes spend most of the school day in this setting. The pupils are grouped according to similar instructional needs. They are mainstreamed or integrated into the regular educational program as much as possible; decisions about this capability are based on the individual student's ability and on input from staff members involved in the student's education.

Resource Specialist Program. Students in this program remain in the regular classroom for most of the day. They attend the resource class for intensive work in specific areas in which they show need. These areas are determined by observation and test results. The teacher provides instruction to each student either individually or in small groups. Instruction can be delivered within the regular classroom or on a "pull-out" basis.

Nonpublic Schools. These services may be provided to a student who has exceptional needs that cannot be met by public education. School districts are required to try all appropriate Special Education settings within the public school environment before recommending nonpublic school placement. On placement in a nonpublic school, the parents are notified that they are responsible for notifying their local school district of any change of residence.

State Special Schools. Residential schools for the blind and deaf are located throughout the United States. If a case manager routinely works with blind or deaf children, it behooves him or her to maintain lists of these schools. Decisions about placing students in these programs are based on the IEP team's recommendations if no appropriate placement is available in the local area.

Extended School Year. This program is available to students who require a special day class setting to achieve the best educational benefits. This service is offered to help students maintain their educational progress by attending school during the summer recess. The extended school year program lasts for a minimum of 20 days.

Infant Development Program. Children with exceptional needs from birth to 3 years of age are eligible to receive these services, which are offered in a variety of ways to accommodate each family's unique needs. Parent involvement is a strong component of the "infant program." A team of trained specialists provides an individualized program designed to meet the needs of the infant and the family.

Vocational or Transitional Program. This program provides job readiness experiences in diversified occupations. Classroom experience and on-the-job training opportunities are carefully planned according to each student's abilities. There are times when children as young as age 14 may be considered for this program.

Least Restrictive Environment (LRE). Special Education is an integral part of the total public education system. It provides education in a manner that promotes maximum interaction between children with disabilities and those who are not disabled in a way that is appropriate to the needs of both.

Referrals

Referrals for Special Education should be made in writing to the local school district or county office of education in which the pupil is enrolled. The school district must complete the needed assessments and tests and develop the individual education plan within a relatively short period of time (on average, 50 to 90 days) from the date of referral. The referral should include:

- The type of illness or disability.
- The possible medical side effects, complications, or treatments that could affect school function.
- The educational and social implications of the disease and its treatment, including the likelihood of fatigue, absences, changes in physical appearance, amputation, or problems with fine and gross motor control.
- Any special considerations for a child with an infectious disease.

Assessments

After the referral has been made, assessments and testing must be completed within a specified period of time from receipt of the request for Special Education. These assessments and tests are performed at no charge to the parent. Parents should be aware that they must grant written consent for the tests or assessments and that they may have to obtain medical records and a written report from the child's physician.

At no time is a single test procedure used as the sole criterion for determining the appropriate educational program. Testing, assessment materials, and procedures used must:

- Cover all areas of function related to the suspected disability.
- Be performed by competent credentialed persons.
- Be selected and administered to avoid racial, cultural, or sexual discrimination.
- Be provided in the person's primary language or mode of communication.
- Be selected and administered to ensure that

the test results accurately reflect the person's aptitude, achievement level, or other factor purported to be measured by the test.
- Not measure the person's impairment unless this is indicated.

To ensure that the IEP is tailored to the pupil's needs, the assessments must cover the following areas:

- Relevant health and development or medical condition
- Visual ability (including low vision)
- Hearing ability
- Motor, self-help, and mobility abilities
- Interests (including social interests)
- Emotional and psychological status
- Language functions
- General ability
- Academic performance
- Orientation
- Vocational abilities and interests

Any person who fails to meet predetermined criteria for the area assessed is further tested by another specialist who has credentials in the same area. Parents have the right to request retesting at the Department of Education's expense. Parents also have the right to obtain, at their expense, independent educational assessments as long as these assessments are performed by qualified specialists.

Regardless of who conducts the assessments, the written assessment report serves as the data base for the final IEP and the specific instruction and services that are eventually designed for the child. The assessment report must include:

- A summary of the medical, physical, developmental, or psychological findings
- A statement regarding whether the pupil needs Special Education or related services
- The basis for making the determination
- The relevant behavior noted during the observation of the pupil
- The relationship of that behavior to the pupil's academic and social function
- A determination about the effects of environmental, cultural, or economic disadvantage on the pupil
- Recommendations for specialized services, materials, and equipment necessary to provide the education

Assessment reports for pupils with learning disabilities should state whether there is a discrepancy between the child's achievement and his or her ability and information supporting the fact that the disability cannot be corrected without Special Education or related services.

Individualized Education Plan (IEP)

Once the tests and assessments have been completed, the findings are presented at an IEP meeting. This meeting must include qualified persons who can develop the pupil's IEP. The team members selected often include:

- A school representative who is knowledgeable about program options appropriate for the pupil and is qualified to provide or supervise the Special Education program.
- The pupil's teacher or a Special Education teacher who is qualified to teach pupils of this child's age and level of impairment.
- One or both parents or their representative.
- When appropriate, the pupil.
- If approved by the parents or school district, any other individual who possesses expertise or knowledge about the development of the pupil's individual education plan.
- The person or persons who conducted the assessment.
- A representative from the county mental health department if the child has a severe emotional disturbance and the recommendation is residential placement.
- A representative from the county welfare department if the child is placed in an out-of-home setting; this person must help in identifying a facility suited to the child's needs.

The team is responsible for reviewing the assessment results, determining eligibility, and reviewing the contents of the IEP plan. In making their recommendations, the team also must consider any transportation needs and needs for related services and, when appropriate, make placement recommendations.

The individual education plan, once developed, is a written statement that serves as the data base for the designed instruction and any services the pupil requires. The plan must be maintained at each school site where the pupil is enrolled. Parents must be aware that they have a right to obtain a copy for their records and should be encouraged to keep such a copy. Case managers likewise should request a copy for the child's file; it is helpful in establishing the case management plan because it can help to ensure that gaps, fragmentation, and duplication of services do not occur. At a minimum, the IEP must note or describe:

- The present level of the pupil's educational performance.
- A list of annual goals, including short-term objectives.
- The Special Education program and any related services required.
- The extent to which the pupil is able to participate in regular educational programs.
- The date for initiation and anticipated duration of the Special Education program or services.
- Appropriate objective criteria, evaluation procedures to be used, and a schedule or time frame with which to determine whether the goals are being achieved.

When appropriate, the plan should also include:

- Recommendations for prevocational career education for pupils in kindergarten through grade 6.
- Recommendations for vocational education or work experience or a combination of both for pupils in kindergarten through grade 12.
- Linguistically appropriate goals, if the pupil's primary language or mode of communication is other than English, and an outline of the programs and services necessary to reach these goals.
- A description of the specialized services, material, or equipment necessary to reach the outlined goals if the pupil has a low-incidence disability.

Once the initial plan has been developed, future planning meetings are held annually or

- When the pupil receives or requires any subsequent formal assessment or testing.
- When the pupil demonstrates lack of anticipated progress.
- When the teacher or parent requests a review or revision of the plan.

Designed Instruction and Services

From the IEP, specifically designed instruction and services (DIS) are developed that are intended to meet the unique needs of the pupil. Prior to actual implementation of the pupil's Special Education program, the designed instruction plan must meet standards established by the local school board. The designed instruction and services may include the following:

- Language and speech development and remediation
- Audiologic services
- Orientation and mobility instruction
- Instruction in the home or hospital
- Adapted physical education
- Physical or occupational therapy
- Vision services
- Specialized driver training
- Counseling and guidance
- Psychological services other than those necessary for the assessment and development of the IEP
- Parent counseling and training
- Health and nursing services
- Social worker services
- Specially designed vocational education and career development
- Recreational services
- Specialized services for low-incidence disabilities such as readers and transcribers
- Transportation

Special Education classes or centers or state schools are used only when the nature and severity of the handicap are such that education in a regular classroom cannot be achieved satisfactorily by modifying the classroom or using supplementary aids and services. If the pupil is placed in other than a regular classroom, nonacademic extracurricular services and activities must be provided that allow the handicapped pupil to participate with nonhandicapped pupils to the maximum extent possible considering the pupil's condition.

In the United States there are approximately 60 special schools for the blind and more than 60 public residential schools for the deaf. In the schools for the blind, courses include Braille and instruction in skills of daily living, orientation, and mobility in addition to the full range of regular academic curricula offered by other schools. Schools for the deaf accept children from infancy through grade 12; the children receive educational training as well as speech therapy, lip reading, use of hearing aids, and sign language. Parents who need information about these schools should contact their local state Department of Education.

Parents should know that if their child cannot be placed in a regular classroom and there are no other provisions for Special Education in the local public school district, the child can be placed in a private school designed to handle persons with exceptional needs. Pupils placed in a nonpublic, nonsectarian school are deemed to be enrolled in a public school. The school district in such situations is responsible for paying full tuition. However, before state funds are used for this purpose, it must be documented that attempts were made to place the pupil in an appropriate alternative public setting, either within or outside the state, and fund usage must be approved by the state superintendent of schools.

Early Education Programs

As a condition of receiving state aid under the federal law, each school district must operate early education programs. These programs are intended for (1) individuals with exceptional needs who are younger than 3 years of age, and (2) preschool children between the ages of 3 and 5 years. In the programs for children under 3 years old, the infant's parent is the primary teacher. Here the early education program may be provided as a home-based service. For preschool children, the program must be provided in the most age-appropriate environment conducive to learning. Again, because case management caseloads often include children who are dependent on technology or children who need special education, it is important for case managers to be familiar with the early education programs in his or her area because these programs are vital to the development of children.

Standardized tests are considered invalid for children under age 5. Alternative means, such as scales, instruments, observations, and interviews, must be used for the assessment report or data base, the development of the early education or preschool IEP, and the development of the program itself.

An early education or preschool program includes specially designed education that will meet the unique needs of infants or children and their families. The programs consist of either a home-based program or a variety of group services. The primary purpose of these programs is to enhance the development of the infant or preschooler and ready him or her for kindergarten or first grade. Professional services and consultations for both these programs are provided by a multidisciplinary team.

This multidisciplinary team is composed of professionals from various disciplines or specialties and parents who share their expertise in child development and education. In addi-

tion to the family, the team consists of specialists in:

- Early childhood education
- Speech and language
- Professional nursing
- Social work, psychology, or mental health
- Occupational or physical therapy

The consultation services provided by the team include advice on nurturing, stimulation, positioning, feeding, the neurologic system and its impact on learning, adaptive equipment, possible limitations in movement, strength, and endurance, and appropriate handling techniques.

Services at home are often provided at least one or two times a week and include such services as:

- Observation of the infant's behavior and development in his or her natural environment.
- Presentation of activities that are developmentally appropriate and based on the infant's needs.
- Modeling and demonstration of developmentally appropriate activities for the infant to the parents, siblings, and other caregivers.
- Interaction with the family and other caregivers to enhance and reinforce the skills necessary to promote the infant's development.
- Discussion of parental concerns related to the infant and family and support for the parents in coping with their infant's needs.
- Assistance for parents in solving problems, seeking other services in their community, and coordinating the services provided by various agencies.

Activities recommended in early education programs, whether home-based or in a group, must be designed to conform with the infant's needs or the child's IEP, ensuring that the activities do not conflict with his or her medical needs. These activities may include:

- Opportunities to socialize and participate in play and exploration.
- Opportunities to receive services from the individual transdisciplinary team members.
- Opportunities for family involvement, parent education, and support groups.

Family involvement activities may include:

- Educational programs that present information or demonstrate techniques that can assist the family in promoting the infant's development.
- Parent education and training to help families

understand, plan for, and meet the unique needs of their infant.
- Instruction in making toys and other appropriate educational material.

Early education and related services are based on the needs of the infant or preschooler and the family. These services are specified in the IEP along with recommendations about the frequency, type, and duration of each service. Arrangements for this type of education are made using one of the following methods:

- Direct provision of the services by a local educational agency.
- Interagency agreement between the local educational agency and another public agency.
- Contract with another public agency such as the state Department of Mental Health, the state agency responsible for developmental disability services, state Department of Social Services, state Department of Rehabilitation, state Department of Youth Authority, state Department of Unemployment, or the Title V Children's Medical Services program.
- Contract with a nonsectarian school or a nonpublic or nonprofit agency.

Before the preschooler makes the transition to kindergarten or first grade, an appropriate reassessment must be conducted to determine whether he or she continues to need Special Education services or is now able to participate in a regular classroom setting.

Career and Vocational Education Programs

Under the Rehabilitation Act of 1973 federal funds are made available to the states for use in career and vocational programs that serve individuals with exceptional needs. The goal of this program is to allow the person to obtain gainful employment and to maximize his or her economic and social independence in the least restrictive environment. Planning for this transition from school to the adult life environment should begin well before the pupil leaves the public school system. Programs such as this are intended to support independence rather than dependence.

Transitional career or vocational educational programs must include in-service training programs and resource materials that provide the following:

- A definition of transition and the major components of an effective school-based program.

- A definition of the roles of other agencies in the process.
- A description of the role of the family in actively participating in the planning and implementation of transition-related goals and activities.
- A list of resources and model programs in existence.

Additionally, these programs must provide:

- Training in work skills in a variety of vocational settings in the school or community.
- Assistance in developing multiple employment options to facilitate job or career choices.
- Training for job trainers and employers to familiarize them with the unique needs of the individuals.
- Collection and analysis of data on the student once he or she leaves the school system and enters the adult world.
- Vocational and career education in the elementary grades for students who can benefit from it.
- Instruction and experiences that reinforce core curriculum concepts and skills and prepare the student with learning difficulties or severe physical or mental disabilities to make a successful transition to self-supporting employment in the community.
- Development of a network of model demonstration sites.
- Coordination with other specialized programs or the state Department of Rehabilitation, state agency responsible for developmental disability services, state Department of Unemployment, or other agencies designed to serve students who face barriers to the transition process.
- Assessment of work-related skills, interests, aptitudes, and attitudes.

Complaints and Appeals

As with all state, federal, and other healthcare services, any individual or agency who disagrees with any decision made by the individual education plan has the right to file a complaint or appeal.

✒ S U M M A R Y

This section has briefly summarized the Special Education programs available and the provisions of the Individuals with Disabilities Education Act of 1991 (formerly Public Law 94-142) as they relate to persons with a low-incidence disability or a severely handicapping condition.

Families often describe the process necessary to establish Special Education as confusing, lengthy, and frustrating. However, a free public education is a right for all persons from birth to age 21. This includes early education, preschool education, elementary and secondary school education, and career and vocational programs.

Before a child is enrolled in a Special Education program, an assessment is completed, called an individualized education plan (IEP). From this plan, specifically designed instruction and services are developed, tailored to meet the unique needs of the individual. The plan is based on the findings of the initial assessment and any reassessments performed and is developed or modified as often as the child shows progress or lack of progress.

Persons who disagree with any issue in Special Education have the right to appeal and attend a mediation conference. If they disagree with the first-level appeal decision, they have the right to request a due process hearing. Case managers must encourage families to exercise their right of appeal, especially if their child has a handicapping condition that can qualify the child for services allowed by Special Education.

Case managers must be very familiar with the Individuals with Disabilities Education Act and any state regulations pertinent to this law because a large percentage of patients in a case manager's caseload are composed of infants or children under the age of 21 who qualify for services provided by Special Education.

VETERANS BENEFITS

Overview

The Department of Veterans Affairs (Veterans Administration, or VA) is responsible for overseeing and administering its programs, which are available to eligible veterans. Approximately one of every three persons living in the United States is a potential Veterans Administration beneficiary.

The Veterans Administration operates healthcare facilities in 50 states, the District of Columbia, Puerto Rico, and the Philippines, making it the nation's largest healthcare system network and the fifth largest insurance program. Almost all of the Veterans Administration's 150+ medical centers are affiliated with medical schools. In addition to the medical centers, the Veterans Administration's healthcare system includes nursing homes, domiciliary care facilities, readjustment counseling centers, outpatient clinics, and contracts with specific agencies for home healthcare and other services.[10]

All Veterans Administration benefits payable to veterans or their dependents, with the exception of some insurance programs and certain medical benefits, require the veteran to have served in one of the armed forces. Entitlement to the scope of services is based on an honorable or general discharge and the person's disability rating. Further information about benefits is available by writing or calling any Veterans Administration regional or service office. All 50 states have toll-free numbers to their state's regional VA office.

Although the Veterans Administration benefit programs are national, medical benefits vary from region to region. The actual scope of services provided depends on the Veterans Administration resources available for that region. For this reason, case managers must be familiar at least with the Veterans Administration medical center responsible for their "catchment" area or region. They should maintain that medical center's phone number as well as the current phone number of the Veterans Administration regional office in their phone listing when information or a referral is needed.

Referrals

To file a claim or make a referral for veterans' services, it may be necessary to contact the nearest Veterans Administration office and identify the veteran by submitting his or her full name, date of birth, and Social Security number. If the person has ever filed a claim before, he or she will have a "C" identification number on file. To expedite the process of referral, the C number should always be referred to when known. To further expedite the initiation of services, the veteran or his or her family is advised to keep the following information in a safe and convenient location:

• Death certificate (if applicable)
• Marriage license or certificate (if applicable)
• Birth certificates
• A statement regarding burial preferences
• Discharge papers

Veterans who are disabled by injury, disease, or a condition aggravated during active duty, whether wartime or peacetime, and who have been honorably discharged may be eligible for service-connected disability benefits. Disabilities are classified in terms of percentages and range from 0% to 100%. Monetary compensation is based on this disability rating. Veterans who are classified as 30% or more disabled are entitled to additional dependent allowances. Veterans with the same classification are entitled to further allowances if they have a spouse in need of aid and attendant care. Veterans aged 65 or older, whether working or not, must meet income criteria and be classified as totally disabled to be granted a pension.

Medical Center Care

Entrance of a veteran into a VA hospital is based on the veteran's service disability rating, regardless of whether he or she may also have Civilian Health and Medical Program of the Uniformed Services (CHAMPUS) coverage. Many patients with a disability rating of less than 100% are medically retired from military service; these patients are entitled to both CHAMPUS and VA benefits.

Veterans classified as disabled are eligible for hospital benefits and are issued a medical card that identifies them and categorizes their eligibility for these services. Eligibility for hospital services and nursing home care is divided into three categories—A, B, and C. Within these three categories, assessment procedures based on income levels are used to determine whether veterans with nonservice-connected disabilities are eligible for free medical care in one of the VA facilities or clinics.

Category A veterans receive full hospital care and outpatient services. Nursing home care may be provided as well as other related healthcare services on a case-by-case basis. Veterans in category B may receive services such as hospital care, outpatient care, and nursing home care depending on the capabilities (e.g., does the facility offer the level of care required by the patient). Category C veterans are allowed care only if space and resources are available. Whether they receive inpatient or outpatient care, veterans in category C must agree to a copayment to the Veterans Administration before they are considered eligible for care. If a patient is hospitalized in a Veterans Administration medical center, they have first priority for

further care in a skilled nursing facility, domiciliary care facility, or home healthcare agency at Veterans Administration expense.

Category A patients are predominantly veterans with service-connected disabilities. However, they can also include former prisoners of war, veterans who were exposed to herbicides while serving in Vietnam or to radiation during atmospheric testing or the occupation of Hiroshima or Nagasaki, veterans who are receiving a VA pension, veterans of the Spanish-American War, veterans serving during the Mexican Border period or World War I, and veterans eligible for Medicaid.

Veterans with nonservice-connected disabilities can only be classified in category A if their yearly income is less than the level set by the Veterans Administration to determine eligibility for benefits. Nursing home care is provided to these patients only when space or resources are available.

Care Outside a Veterans Administration Medical Center

If a veteran with a service-connected disability is hospitalized in other than a Veterans Administration hospital, contact must be made with the nearest VA hospital within 72 hours of admission to obtain authorization of medically necessary care or transfer. Normally, the patient's attending physician must speak with the Veterans Administration's Admitting Officer of the Day or with the VA physician responsible for the medical service most pertinent to the patient's condition and reason for current hospitalization.

If the VA physician or admitting officer agrees that care is their responsibility and the Veterans Administration hospital is unable to admit the patient, authorization must be obtained if the patient is to remain at the civilian hospital at Veterans Administration expense. If continued attempts to transfer the patient fail and the patient is to remain entitled to care at Veterans Administration expense, approval for care in the civilian hospital must be obtained as often as directed by the Veterans Administration personnel or until the patient is either transferred to a VA facility or discharged.

If a transfer is agreed to, the necessary arrangements often can be made only through physician-to-physician discussion. If the patient requires travel arrangements, these too must be discussed by the physicians; at this time, the mode and time of pick-up will be given to the patient's attending civilian physician. This discussion is necessary because travel payments or reimbursements for care are made only for certain veterans and in connection with their medical care, which is related to their service-connected disability.

If the Veterans Administration cannot provide transportation itself, it will make the necessary arrangements for an ambulance or other form of transportation at its expense. At times, the mini-van at the nearest Veterans Administration clinic may be used to transport the patient to the medical center. This mode of travel is used primarily when the person encounters difficulty in getting to the Veterans Administration medical center by private car. If the mini-van is used, the patient may be required to report to the local clinic at a specific time and place. Failure to comply means that the patient or family must assume the cost of the transportation.

Skilled Nursing or Intermediate Care Facilities

Admission to a skilled or intermediate care facility requires the same procedure as that used for hospitalization in a VA medical center. Direct admission to these facilities at Veterans Administration expense is provided only to:

- Veterans who require nursing home care for a service-connected disability.
- Persons in an Armed Forces hospital who require continued skilled care and become veterans on discharge from active duty.
- Veterans discharged from a VA medical center who receive home care services paid for by the Veterans Administration.
- Veterans discharged directly from a VA medical center to a skilled nursing or intermediate care facility or a domiciliary care facility.

The Veterans Administration may also transfer a veteran in need of "nursing home" care to a skilled nursing facility at their expense if the patient was confined to one of their medical centers or domiciliary care facilities and was discharged directly to the skilled nursing facility. Authorizations for care in a skilled nursing facility rarely exceed 6 months at a given time. The only exceptions are for veterans whose need for nursing home care is directly related to a service-connected disability. Admission to a skilled nursing facility for a veteran with a nonservice-connected disability, whose income does not exceed the income threshold amount, may be authorized if the veteran agrees to pay the applicable copayment.

Domiciliary Care

Admission to a Veterans Administration domiciliary care facility requires prior approval, and the application process is started at the nearest Veterans Administration regional office. Due to limited space, waiting lists are often lengthy. The average processing time for admission often exceeds 6 months. Entrance into a domiciliary care facility is limited to veterans who:

- Were discharged for a disability or receive disability compensation and suffer from a permanent disability.
- Have no adequate means of support, are unable to work to earn a living, and meet certain other requirements.
- Have a nonservice-connected disability that prevents them from earning a living but is not severe enough to require hospitalization.

Outpatient Medical Treatment

Outpatient medical treatments are the most common services provided. These treatments include examinations and related medical services, drugs and medications, rehabilitation therapy and training, consultations, professional counseling, mental health services, and any other services that are necessary.

Outpatient services include home health services when they are medically necessary or appropriate to maintain effective and economical treatment of a disability. Home health services may also include home improvements and structural alterations that are necessary to ensure continuation of treatment or provide access to the home or to essential lavatory or sanitation facilities. Cost limitations apply to these improvements and structural alterations. Information about these improvements can be obtained by calling the nearest Veterans Administration regional office.

As a rule, outpatient medical services are furnished without limitation to:

- Any veteran with a service-connected disability.
- Any veteran with a combined service-connected disability rating of 50% or more.

- Any veteran in a vocational rehabilitation program approved by the Veterans Administration.
- Any veteran with a service-connected disability rating of 30% to 40% or whose annual income does not exceed the applicable rate for attendant care and who otherwise needs pre- or posthospital care necessary to prevent deterioration of his condition or hospitalization.

In most other cases, outpatient medical services are furnished without limitation (depending on the availability of resources and facilities) to:

- Any veteran who is a former prisoner of war.
- Any veteran of World War I or the Mexican Border period.
- Any veteran receiving aid and attendant care or homebound pension benefits.
- Any veteran in the following groups who needs pre- or posthospital care that is necessary to prevent hospitalization or to maintain the patient until the condition stabilizes or the patient is admitted. This category includes veterans who have been:
  - Exposed to toxic substances, herbicides, or defoliants in Vietnam or to radiation exposure as a consequence of participation in the test of a nuclear device or during the occupation of Hiroshima or Nagasaki, Japan prior to July 1, 1946.
  - Identified as category A for hospitalization purposes whose income is more than the pension rate of another veteran in need of regular aid and attendant care.
  - Identified as category B for inpatient purposes.
  - Identified as category C for inpatient purposes.

Dental Care

Outpatient dental services are also available to eligible veterans with service-connected disabilities. Dental services include the full spectrum of modern diagnostic, surgical, restorative, and preventive techniques. In some situations, dental care is comprehensive whereas in others the type and extent of treatment are limited. The amount and type of treatment are determined by the veteran's specific service-connected eligibility or the correlation between the dental condition and the veteran's medical problems.

Alcohol and Drug Treatment

Veterans who have completed a course of treatment as an inpatient at a Veterans Administration drug and alcohol treatment facility may be eligible to receive continued outpatient care. These veterans are also eligible for treatment or rehabilitation services in facilities such as halfway houses or therapeutic communities at Veterans Administration expense.

Durable Medical Equipment and Prosthetics

Durable medical equipment and prosthetic appliances necessary for any condition are available to veterans receiving care in a hospital, domiciliary care facility, or nursing home under the direct jurisdiction of the Veterans Administration. Veterans who meet the basic requirements for outpatient medical treatment (as listed above under outpatient services) may be offered such equipment when it is required.

Services for the Blind

Veterans in any of the eligible categories of veterans listed under outpatient services can receive authorized aids for the blind. Veterans with a best-corrected vision of 20/200 or less in the better eye or with a field defect of 20 degrees or less are considered legally blind. Blind veterans need not be receiving compensation or a pension to be eligible for admission to a Veterans Administration Blind Rehabilitation Center or clinic. Benefits available to a blind veteran include:

- Annual review by a visual impairment team.
- Training in adjusting to blindness.
- Home improvements or structural alterations to the home.
- Aids for low vision and training in their use.
- Approved electronic and mechanical aids for the blind, including repair or replacement of such aids.
- Guide dogs, including the expense of training the veteran to use the dog and the cost of the dog's medical treatment when indicated.
- Talking books, tapes, and Braille literature.

To apply for blind benefits the veteran should contact the coordinator for the blind at any Veterans Administration medical center.

Medical Care for Dependents or Survivors

The Civilian Health and Medical Program of the Department of Veterans Affairs (CHAMPVA) is a medical benefits program through which the Veterans Administration helps to pay for medical services and supplies obtained from civilian sources to eligible dependents and survivors of certain veterans.

Once a person's eligibility has been determined by the Veterans Administration, benefits are cost-shared in the same way as they are for recipients of Civilian Health and Medical Program of the Uniformed Services (CHAMPUS) benefits. However, the policies of CHAMPVA are determined by the Veterans Administration, not CHAMPUS.

The following persons are eligible for benefits from CHAMPVA provided they are not eligible for care under CHAMPUS or Medicare:

• The spouse or child of a veteran who is totally disabled from a service-connected disability.
• The surviving spouse or child of a veteran whose death resulted from a service-connected disability or who at the time of death was totally disabled from a service-connected disability.
• The surviving spouse or child of a person who died while in the line of active duty.

Care under the CHAMPVA program is normally provided in civilian facilities. In general, the program covers most healthcare services or supplies that are medically or psychologically necessary. Veterans Administration facilities are used only when they are equipped to provide such care or when the use of these facilities does not interfere with the care and treatment of veterans. Under the program, special rules or limitations apply to certain services.

Clarification of what is and what is not covered can be obtained by calling the toll-free number for the CHAMPVA office located in Denver, Colorado or from a social worker at any Veterans Administration medical center.

Persons eligible for CHAMPVA benefits are not eligible for the Program for The Handicapped (PFTH) offered under CHAMPUS, nor can they receive care in a military treatment facility (MTF). Likewise, they cannot be included in any special programs such as Project Care (a case management demonstration project), the Home Care Demonstration (HCD—a demonstration for home care "in lieu" of hospitalization for active duty dependents), or any of the managed care programs offered by CHAMPUS and its civilian healthcare payors.

Overseas Benefits

Reimbursement is available for fee-for-service care rendered outside the United States to veterans with adjudicated service-connected disabilities and conditions related to the rated disabilities. Prior to treatment, authorization must be obtained from the nearest American Embassy or consulate. In emergency situations, treatment must be reported to these agencies within 72 hours. Nursing home care is not a benefit.

Appeals

Claimants have 1 year from the date of notification of a denial of care to file an appeal if they disagree with any determination. An appeal is initiated by filing a notice with the Veterans Administration facility responsible for issuing the determination. Further information about the appeals process and the relevant time frames can be obtained by contacting any Veterans Administration regional office.

Other Veteran Organizations

Services from community veterans' groups or organizations vary from community to community. The willingness of the organization or its members to assist the veteran usually depends on the veteran's membership status or commitment to the group. Services available are often limited to a one-time use or request. Services available from individual veterans' organizations may include requests for fund raising, equipment, respite care, or assistance with home modifications or repairs. Veterans' organizations with regional offices include the following:

• American Legion
• American Red Cross
• American Veterans (AMVETs)
• Blind Veterans Association
• Catholic War Veterans
• American Ex-POWs
• Fleet Reserve Association
• Jewish War Veterans
• Military Order of the Purple Heart
• Paralyzed Veterans Association

- Veterans of Foreign Wars
- Veterans of World War I

Other veterans' organizations include:

- Air Force Sergeants Association
- Allied Council of Veterans Home
- Armed Forces Retirees Association
- Council of the Vietnam Veterans of America
- Congressional Medal of Honor Society
- Marine Corps League
- United States Submarine Veterans of World War II
- Vietnam Veterans (state or specific area)
- Women's Army Corps Veterans Association
- National Maritime Union or Administration

✿ S U M M A R Y

Most veterans and their families know whether they are eligible for Veterans Administration benefits. However, in some situations family members may not know whether their loved one is eligible for services at Veterans Administration expense. Also, occasionally a patient receiving CHAMPUS benefits is admitted to a local hospital for an emergency procedure, and it is then discovered that this patient may be eligible for Veterans Administration services because he or she has a service-connected disability that has been rated by the Veterans Administration. In these situations, the nearest Veterans Administration medical center must be notified within 72 hours of the emergency admission if the civilian hospital is to be reimbursed at Veterans Administration expense.

In addition to services provided at Veterans Administration expense, specific services may also be available on a one-time only basis from local or regional veterans organizations or groups. These groups also offer emotional support to the veteran in need.

As with other community and regional resources, the case manager must be familiar with the Veterans Administration regional office in the region in which he or she practices. This is necessary if the patient's benefits are to be enhanced.

CIVILIAN HEALTH AND MEDICAL PROGRAMS OF THE UNIFORMED SERVICES

The Civilian Health and Medical Program of the Uniformed Services (CHAMPUS) is a health benefits program that offers benefits to the seven branches of the uniformed services.

- Army
- Navy
- Marine Corps
- Air Force
- Coast Guard
- Public Health Service
- National Oceanic and Atmospheric Administration

TRICARE

In certain areas of the country the Department of Defense (DOD) has conducted experimental demonstrations or health projects in which private insurance companies or health maintenance organizations (HMOs) offer a triple option plan to persons eligible for CHAMPUS benefits. Therefore, the CHAMPUS program as most people know it has undergone multiple changes. Within the next few years the program is expected to become similar to any managed care program offered by traditional healthcare payors. In addition, the program will have a new name—TRICARE.

Not only has the name changed, so have many other features. Eligible persons now have a "triple option" choice in selecting their healthcare coverage. This triple option includes an HMO model called TRICARE PRIME, a preferred provider organization (PPO) model called TRICARE EXTRA, and an indemnity option called TRICARE Standard.

TRICARE PRIME

Under the PRIME program a person enrolls in the program, pays a yearly enrollment fee, and selects a primary care manager (PCM)—either a civilian or a military physician. The primary care manager agrees to treat the patient for specific routine medical conditions. The patient must then follow rules similar to those used by an HMO managed care organization. Under the PRIME program, the person must seek prior authorization to receive certain services (most services, especially specialty care, require prior authorization). In addition, he or she is also required to use either the nearest military treatment facility or the healthcare payor's network of providers when medical care is required.

All care is provided in exchange for a small

out-of-pocket copayment for each service (i.e., if the patient is a dependent of an active duty employee, the amount he or she is required to pay is based on the rank of the military employee; if the covered person is retired, the copayment is a specific dollar amount for each medical service required). In 1998 there was no enrollment fee for all active duty personnel, whereas for the retiree and his or her family the fee was $460 per year for a family and $230 for a single person. Copayments for most services were $12.

Also featured under the TRICARE PRIME program is the option to use point of service (POS) payments, which may be chosen by patients who desire to use providers outside the PRIME network. Point of service requires no prior authorization from the managed care organization. However, the beneficiary (patient) is responsible for paying a large percentage of the charges and a separate deductible (i.e., a $300 deductible and a copayment of 50% of the remaining charges after payment by the fiscal intermediary [same as a claims processor]).

The keys to the PRIME program are appropriate use of military treatment facility (MTF) services and the need for prior authorization for services. Therefore, for any person enrolled in the PRIME program, all requirements for the use of military treatment facilities and nonavailability statements (NAS) remain in effect (for more details on NAS, see below).

TRICARE EXTRA

The second option available in the Department of Defense demonstration regions is the EXTRA program. Essentially, this program makes use of a preferred provider organization (PPO). The patient who chooses this option does not enroll in the PRIME program but elects to use the PRIME network. In exchange for using this network, the patient's out-of-pocket expenses are reduced by a small percentage (i.e., 20% versus the standard CHAMPUS deductible of 25%). In the EXTRA program the patient is not issued a TRICARE card but merely uses his or her military identification card to gain access to services. However, because PRIME providers are used, all requirements for prior authorization and military treatment facility use remain in effect.

TRICARE STANDARD

The third option is to remain as a CHAMPUS Standard patient. This program is essentially an indemnity insurance plan and is the plan, known merely as CHAMPUS, previously available in most regions of the United States. Persons using the Standard program are not required to enroll, nor are they required to use predetermined providers. They gain access to care by using their military identification card (only TRICARE PRIME has the extra healthcare coverage card). If the patient has a current and valid military identification card (this military card is issued to all military personnel, whether active duty or retired, and their dependents) and is enrolled in the Defense Enrollment and Eligibility Reporting System (DEERS), he or she is entitled to seek care from any provider he or she desires.

There is one stipulation to the foregoing: the person is free to use any provider of his or her liking as long as the provider is certified by the regional fiscal intermediary selected to pay claims for CHAMPUS. This certification process is similar to that used by Medicare. Persons electing the Standard program remain responsible for all deductibles and copayments (at present this copayment is 25% of the allowable amount), and if he or she uses a provider that does not accept assignment, any balance remaining between the amount paid by the fiscal intermediary and that billed by the provider is the responsibility of the patient.

ACCESS TO INFORMATION AND PRIOR AUTHORIZATION

In TRICARE regions, most referrals, whether issued by the military treatment facility or by the patient's primary care manager, must have prior approval by the local TRICARE office. These offices are staffed by registered nurses who are experienced in utilization review and managed care. These nurses are called healthcare finders (HCF). Not only do they conduct normal utilization review functions, they also play a pivotal role in directing patients to the appropriate provider for care and answering any questions asked by the beneficiary (patient) about the three TRICARE programs.

In regions where the military maintains an active duty base, these nurses and other TRICARE personnel are located in or near the military treatment facility. In other regions where a base is closed, access to the healthcare finder is gained by calling a toll-free number that is operational 24 hours a day, 7 days a week.

Who Is Eligible

The Civilian and Medical Program of the Uniformed Services does not cover the healthcare needs of the active duty person (this will change October 1998); currently needs are met by the nearest military treatment facility. If care is not available there, the beneficiary (patient) is directed by the military treatment facility to appropriate civilian care, which is then paid for by the military.

However, CHAMPUS does cover the healthcare needs of spouses and unmarried children of active duty personnel; retirees and their unmarried dependents; unmarried spouses and children of active duty personnel or retirees who have died under hostile fire; spouses and unmarried children of reservists ordered to active duty for more than 30 consecutive days (dependents of reservists are covered only during the time the reservist is on active duty); and former spouses of active duty or retired military personnel who were married to the service member for at least 20 years, have remained unmarried, are not covered by their own employer-sponsored healthcare plan, are eligible for Medicare Part A (a few exceptions), and are not former spouses of a North American Treaty Organization (NATO) member. The program does not cover parents or parents-in-law of active duty personnel.

Services Provided

Generally speaking, CHAMPUS covers most types of healthcare that is deemed to be medically or psychologically necessary. Much of the policy pertaining to healthcare benefits follows the guidelines developed by Medicare, traditional healthcare insurance companies, or managed care organizations.

The program differs from most other health insurance programs because it is exempt from all state and federal laws that traditionally govern healthcare payors. As such, it is always secondary to any other insurance (this includes Victims of Violent Crime programs; also, it does not follow the birthday rule when determining which parent's insurance plan is primary). (The birthday rule is a rule used by healthcare payor when coordinating benefits, especially when children are covered by both parents' health plans. The parent whose birthday falls first in the year is then considered the "first payor.") The only exception to the secondary rule is

Medicaid; it is very important for case managers to be aware of this fact because if it is thought that CHAMPUS is primary when another insurance is actually primary, serious financial consequences and appeals can ensue. The rules of the patient's actual primary insurance must be followed exactly.

Military Treatment Facilities and Their Responsibility

If the patient resides near a military treatment facility, certain types of care must be obtained there. This is especially true for TRICARE PRIME members. Contrary to popular belief, military treatment facility care is not substandard. Many of these facilities, depending on their capabilities, compare favorably with any center of excellence in the civilian medical community. The other important aspect of care provided by the military is that it is provided free to all eligible CHAMPUS beneficiaries (patients). These facilities are also the primary source of care for active duty personnel. If the proper care is not available, the facility issues a disengagement form that allows the patient to gain access to civilian care.

Nonavailability Statement

The disengagement form (often referred to as a 2161, referral for disengagement for civilian care, or nonavailability statement) allows the patient to obtain both access to civilian care and reimbursement for such care. Elective admissions and many outpatient procedures in civilian care centers require proof of a nonavailability statement before the claim is paid. This statement merely validates that the particular level of care or services was not available at the time the service was needed. A nonavailability statement is not required in life-threatening emergencies or for admissions that are the result of a life-threatening event.

Reimbursement and Copayments

Payment or reimbursement occurs only if the services were provided by healthcare providers certified by CHAMPUS. Claims are reimbursed at a certain rate called the CHAMPUS maximum allowable charge or CMAC. Under this program, if the patient is a dependent of an active duty sponsor, the yearly cap for catastrophic care is limited to $1000, but retirees and their dependents and all other persons eligible for the program have a much higher catastrophic cap.

Persons not enrolled in a TRICARE PRIME program are responsible for a yearly deductible, any copayments, and any balances remaining between what is paid and what is billed if the provider does not accept assignment of benefits. Case managers must therefore be familiar with this program if they practice in an area where there are large numbers of persons eligible for CHAMPUS.

Demonstration Changes

Not only is the entire CHAMPUS Program undergoing change as it makes the transition to a managed care health benefits program, many of the current demonstration projects under its wing (see later discussion) are expected to become obsolete. Thus, benefits that are currently available only under the demonstrations are expected to become policy. Two important demonstrations undergoing this change are the Home Health Care demonstration (HHC) and the Home Health Care–Case Management (HHC-CM) demonstration project. When this change occurs, benefits now allowed only under these demonstration projects, such as traditional case management services and waivers to policy, will be allowed under the basic benefits.

Other Important Programs

CHAMPUS offers several other programs and demonstration projects with which case managers should be familiar, especially if they practice near an active duty military base. Information about the following programs can be obtained by calling the nearest military treatment facility, the health benefits advisor (HBA), a healthcare finder (HCF), or OCHAMPUS (Office of CHAMPUS, located in Aurora, Colorado). These special programs are described in the following paragraphs.

PROGRAM FOR THE HANDICAPPED (PFTH)

This program is essentially a financial assistance program for dependents (including spouses) of the active duty person. Retirees and their dependents are not eligible. To qualify for this program a person with a serious handicapping condition must enroll in the program. The intent of the program is to offer assistance with the long-term care needs of the person with the handicap or challenging condition.

Benefits are limited to $1000 per month. All services require prior authorization. Prior approval guarantees that if public funds and programs are available or adequate, they will be used first. However, if public funds or programs are limited, insufficient, or nonexistent, PFTH funds can be used to make up any difference (for example, if the school district can provide 1 hour of speech therapy per week for a child but the child requires 2 hours of therapy per week by physician's orders, the school district in this case would provide 1 hour of therapy and PFTH the other).

To ensure that funds from public entitlement programs are used before PFTH funds, the application must be accompanied by a public official's statement (POS), which certifies that the services are unavailable or insufficient. This statement can be signed by any responsible representative in the public programs. This person basically attests to the fact that public funds or programs are inadequate or unavailable. Typical officials include school superintendents or representatives from the welfare or Medicaid office, the local Title V Children's Medical Services program, or the state agency responsible for developmental disabilities.

The Program for the Handicapped also helps to pay for hearing aids (which are not included under the basic medical benefits offered by CHAMPUS), transportation, eyeglasses, communication devices, and private duty nursing care either in the home or in a facility. Unfortunately, as stated earlier, total expenditures per month are limited to $1000. Any amount over this becomes the sponsor's responsibility.

WILFORD HALL MEDICAL CENTER (WHMC)

This project offers help to all recipients of allogeneic bone marrow transplants. Any CHAMPUS beneficiary (patient) who needs an allogeneic bone marrow transplant must be evaluated by the Wilford Hall Medical Center before care or reimbursement at a civilian transplant center is allowed. If services are provided by a civilian transplant center, a nonavailability statement from Wilford Hall stipulating that care was not available there is necessary before claims from the civilian center can be honored.

Wilford Hall Medical Center and Brooke Army Medical Center (BAMC) are located in San Antonio, Texas. Both are comparable to any civilian transplant center of excellence in their level of expertise and success in transplantation. Like other major military treatment facilities (e.g., Walter Reed Medical Center), Wilford Hall and Brooke Army Medical Center are also capable of performing other types of transplants such as liver transplants, heart-lung transplants, autologous bone marrow transplants, and so forth. If the patient elects to have the transplantation procedure performed at Wilford Hall or another military treatment facility, most costs associated with the transplant and its subsequent care are assumed by the facility.

Any arrangements needed for evaluation or coordination of patient care can be made by calling the social worker, admission coordinator, or the appropriate transplant service physician. Case managers can also seek assistance from any of these individuals if the patient requires an air ambulance for transportation once he or she has been deemed eligible for the transplant. In most cases, if the military's air medical evacuation unit is available, this mode of transportation is used if the patient requires immediate care. Otherwise, the social worker at the military transplant center will assist in making arrangements for a civilian air ambulance or commercial air travel.

The Office of the Civilian Health and Medical Program of the Uniformed Services (OCHAMPUS) currently allows autologous stem cell recovery, high-dose chemotherapy, and bone marrow transplantation for some breast cancer patients who meet certain criteria for candidacy. At this writing this procedure is allowed at either Brooke Army Medical Center or Walter Reed Medical Center. Further information about this program is available by calling OCHAMPUS in Aurora, Colorado.

HOME HEALTH CARE DEMONSTRATION (HHC)

This program is a case management demonstration project intended for dependents of active duty personnel who are catastrophically ill or injured and have ongoing acute care needs. Primary emphasis is placed on establishing the acute care patient at home "in lieu" of hospitalization as soon as the patient is medically stable. All services require prior authorization. Further

information about the Home Health Care demonstration project can be obtained by calling the Project Care office at OCHAMPUS, the HBA at the local military treatment facility, or a local HCF.

HOME HEALTH CARE-CASE MANAGEMENT DEMONSTRATION (HHC-CM)

A similar case management demonstration is the expanded home healthcare demonstration project, referred to as the Home Health Care-Case Management (HHC-CM) project. This project is similar to the Home Health Care demonstration; however, it differs in that it is available to all eligible CHAMPUS beneficiaries (patients), which includes retirees and their dependents.

The emphasis in this demonstration is placed not only on the catastrophically ill or injured patient, and allows services to be established in lieu of hospitalization. In contrast, the expanded home healthcare demonstration allows care for patients with chronic illnesses regardless of their location. The primary focus of the services allowed is to keep the patient out of the hospital.

All care for both demonstration projects requires prior authorization. Again, information about this demonstration can be obtained by calling the Project Care office at OCHAMPUS, the local health benefits advisor, or a healthcare finder.

ADJUNCTIVE DENTAL CARE

Routine dental care is not included as a benefit under CHAMPUS. However, if the patient has a dental condition that is related to a medical condition, coverage can be obtained under the adjunctive dental benefit if the care and services needed have received prior authorization. Conditions often covered under this program include cleft palate repair, temporomandibular joint problems, and dental problems related to chemotherapy or radiation therapy. Any local health benefits advisor or healthcare finder can explain the program in detail or direct the caller to the appropriate fiscal intermediary claims processor for answers or information about the requirements for the program.

MENTAL HEALTH

CHAMPUS offers a full range of mental healthcare. This care includes inpatient care, outpatient services, partial hospitalization, use of residential treatment facilities, drug and alcohol rehabilitation, individual and group psychotherapy, family therapy and marriage counseling, diagnostic evaluation services, pharmacotherapy, psychoanalysis, and psychological testing.

Information about the mental health benefits available can be obtained by calling OCHAMPUS, the local health benefits advisor, or any mental healthcare finder if a TRICARE managed care project is in the immediate area.

AEROMEDICAL SYSTEM

Another important program is the military aeromedical system. This military air ambulance is a state-of-the-art service and comprises the most sophisticated air ambulance system in the world. Although active duty personnel and their dependents have first priority for use of the system, it may be available to any person who is eligible for benefits under CHAMPUS. The aeromedical evacuation program is based at Scott Air Force Base in Illinois. However, information about it can be obtained from the local health benefits advisor, the patient administration office at the nearest military base, or a healthcare finder.

Terminology Used in the Civilian Health and Medical Program of the Uniformed Services

In addition to terms associated with other healthcare payors, the following terms relevant to CHAMPUS can be helpful to a case manager. Full lists of definitions and other terms are found in the CHAMPUS Regulations and Operations manuals or can be obtained by calling the local military treatment facility.

Adjunctive Dental: Dental care that is necessary for or enables treatment of a medical condition, not a dental condition. This type of procedure requires special or prior authorization.

Aeromedical System: A highly specialized military air ambulance. This ambulance is based at Scott Air Force Base, Illinois, and its use is free of charge to military personnel and their dependents. It can be used for civilians, but approval for this use must be obtained from Washington, D.C.

Beneficiary: The patient.

Catchment Areas: Geographic areas determined by the assistant Secretary of Defense. These areas designate which five-digit zip codes fall within an approximately 40-mile radius of a military treatment facility (MTF) that has inpatient capability. If the MTF is capable of providing the service, the patient is required to receive his or her care at this facility. If care is not available, a nonavailability statement (NAS) is issued; this form allows the patient to seek care offered by a civilian provider.

CHAMPUS (Civilian Health and Medical Program of the Uniformed Services): The medical benefit entitlement program available to all dependents of active duty personnel, dependents of deceased active duty personnel, and retired military personnel and their dependents. It is intended to supplement the benefits available from the military hospital or clinic. Since this program is not an insurance program, it is exempt from laws governing the insurance industry. The program has undergone many changes and is now called TRICARE and offered nationwide to all persons who are eligible.

Contractor: Private healthcare organization, fiscal intermediary, or healthcare payor under contract to deliver healthcare, offer managed care, or pay claims for the Department of Defense at minimum.

CHAMPUS Maximum Allowable Charge (CMAC): The amount recognized as the lowest national prevailing charge or national appropriate charge level and the maximum amount that is allowed to be reimbursed regardless of what the provider charges.

CHAMPUS Reform Initiative (CRI): A 5-year demonstration in California and Hawaii that provided a managed care and triple option concept; it was operational from 1988 to 1993.

CHAMPVA or Civilian Health and Medical Program of the Department of Veterans Affairs: The Veterans Administration shares the medical bills of the families and survivors of certain veterans. Once a person's eligibility has been determined by the Veterans Administration, benefits are cost shared in a manner similar to that used by CHAMPUS. However, CHAMPVA policies are not determined by CHAMPUS; the latter program's only involvement is to process the claims. Information about this program can be obtained by calling the CHAMPVA office in Colorado, a local

Veterans Administration medical center, or the local Veterans Administration office.

Cooperative or Supplemental Care: Coordination of civilian care or supplies that are medically necessary but are unavailable at the military treatment facility. The patient is disengaged to receive this care, but the military pays the bill, not the CHAMPUS fiscal intermediary.

Defense Enrollment Eligibility Reporting System (DEERS): The data base used by the armed forces that validates whether a person is eligible for military benefits and privileges.

Disengagement: The process used to allow nonactive duty persons access to civilian providers when services are not available at a military treatment facility. Payment is made either privately or by a CHAMPUS fiscal intermediary.

Health Benefits Advisor (HBA): A person employed by the uniformed services who is located at the military medical facilities to offer information and answer any questions.

Healthcare Finder (HCF): A professional nurse employed by a Department of Defense contractor and assigned to a military treatment facility. This person is responsible for granting prior authorization for services and directing the caller to the appropriate provider for medical care, whether it be the military treatment facility or local community resources.

Home Health Care—Case Management Demonstration (HHC-CM): A case management demonstration project available to any eligible beneficiary (patient) in which the emphasis is on preventing rehospitalization. Information about this demonstration can be obtained by calling the Project Care office at OCHAMPUS in Aurora, Colorado.

Home Health Care (HHC) Demonstration: A demonstration project offered by OCHAMPUS for dependents of active duty personnel whose care would otherwise result in a continued or prolonged hospital stay. For information, calls can be directed to the Project Care office at OCHAMPUS in Aurora, Colorado.

Military Treatment Facility (MTF): The military hospital or clinic. Patients should always try to obtain their care from a military treatment facility before using a CHAMPUS provider. Patients who reside in specific zip codes within a 40-mile radius of the MTF must use this facility when it provides the care and services needed.

Nonavailability Statement (NAS): A statement number issued by the base commander or designee indicating that the needed inpatient or outpatient care is not available at the military treatment facility. This statement is necessary for certain groups of patients who reside in the zip codes specific to the military hospital and must be attached to the claim if payment is expected. Without this form or number the claim is denied. Certain outpatient procedures also require a nonavailability statement. Outpatient services require an outpatient nonavailability statement (ONAS), and inpatient care requires an inpatient nonavailability statement (INAS).

OCHAMPUS: The Office of Civilian Health And Medical Program of the Uniformed Services located in Aurora, Colorado. Basically, this is the administrative arm in which all policies and procedures are developed.

Primary Care Manager: Same as primary care physician and may be a civilian or military treatment facility physician.

Program for the Handicapped (PFTH): A program designed for active duty military families who are restricted from using public resources when residency laws apply. The intent of the program is to provide "habilitation" and services to the handicapped person. It is only open to active duty dependents, and the total benefits payable are limited to $1000 per month. To qualify for the program, the patient must apply for benefits, submitting medical records along with the application, which justifies the requested care or service. The patient must have a public official's statement (POS) on file stating that the services requested are either inadequate or not available from alternate funding or entitlement programs such as Title V Children's Medical Services program, Special Education, or Medicaid. All services require prior authorization.

Public Official's Statement (POS): Statement made in writing by a cognizant public official (generally the superintendent of schools or a designated person from the Medicaid program or the local Title V Children's Medical Services program) that public funding or community healthcare programs are not available or are inadequate to manage the patient. This statement must be secured prior to obtaining authorization for coverage under the Program for the Handicapped.

Residency: The beneficiary's (patient's) physical residence in the state that determines which fiscal intermediary is responsible for payment of the claims.

Resource Sharing Providers: Civilian providers who agree by contract to provide healthcare services at the military treatment facility to military dependents and retirees.

Special Authorization: Authorization required for services or supplies necessary to treat a person who is receiving care under the Program For The Handicapped or the adjunctive dental care program. Special authorization is also needed when a mental health inpatient stay is anticipated to exceed 60 days or when a child needs care at a mental health residential treatment center (RTC).

Sponsor: Active duty, deceased active duty, or retired military personnel whose status determines their eligibility for benefits, copayments, deductibles, and catastrophic capitated limits.

TRICARE EXTRA: A program similar to that offered by a PPO, in which the patient does not enroll in the HMO version of TRICARE. The person then has the right to select or make use of the providers that contract with the HMO, thus minimizing out-of-pocket expenses.

TRICARE PRIME: An HMO type of medical benefit in which the patient is not responsible for filing claims or making copayments other than predetermined amounts (e.g., $5.00 to $12.00). To take advantage of TRICARE PRIME the sponsor must enroll in it and use only those healthcare providers that are under contract with or are utilized by the Department of Defense's contracted managed care organization.

TRICARE Standard: A program similar to an indemnity plan in which benefits are payable without regard to the provider used, the expense of care, or the length of stay. However, the beneficiary (patient) pays 25% of the maximum allowable amount plus other charges as determined by the program.

Wilford Hall Demonstration: A demonstration project offered to those who need an allogeneic bone marrow transplant. All potential candidates for this type of transplant must be evaluated by Wilford Hall Medical Center (WHMC) in San Antonio, Texas, prior to the transplant. Wilford Hall allows the patient to choose a civilian transplantation center for the transplant, but such a choice also requires the patient to obtain a nonavailability statement issued by Wilford Hall. Care in a civilian center is not always the most cost advantageous method. If the transplant is done at Wilford Hall, all costs associated with the transplant and many costs associated with its subsequent care are assumed by the military.

SUMMARY

The Civilian Health And Medical Program of the Uniformed Services is the health benefit coverage offered to military personnel and retirees and their dependents. The program recently underwent many changes and is now called TRICARE, assuming a managed care focus nationwide.

Case managers who work near an active military base must be very familiar with the program because it does not always follow the traditional rules established for other types of insurance. Also, a knowledge of where coverage is allowed is vital; otherwise, the patient could be responsible for the charges associated with any care. Information about the many programs offered under CHAMPUS can be obtained by calling the Office of the Civilian Health and Medical Program of the Uniformed Services (OCHAMPUS), located in Aurora, Colorado, or by speaking with a local health benefits advisor or a healthcare finder.

SOCIAL SECURITY PROGRAMS

Possibly the most complex alternate funding programs for catastrophically ill, injured, or disabled people under age 65 are those offered by the Social Security (SS) system. This section highlights the basic information that must be relayed to the patient or family when he or she has been identified as potentially eligible for a Social Security program.

Full details about the programs and eligibility can be obtained at the nearest Social Security office or by calling the toll-free teleservice number, 800-234-5772. Calls or messages are routed to the appropriate Social Security office nearest the caller. Social Security also publishes many pamphlets about the various programs available. In most cases, these pamphlets are updated yearly and are available free of charge. It is wise to keep copies of all such publications in one's case management library for reference because they are an excellent source of information.

Because Social Security is a federal program,

criteria for enrollment are consistent nationwide. The primary eligibility requirements for cash benefits as well as for Medicare, Social Security's health insurance program, are as follows:

- Age over 65.
- Disabled or blind and under the age of 65.
- Citizen of the United States, resident of the Mariana Islands, or lawfully admitted alien who has resided in the United States for a minimum of 5 years.
- Contribution of the appropriate number of credits to the Social Security fund or to the Railroad Retirement System.

Four major programs are paid from the Social Security trust fund and administered by Social Security:

- Retirement benefits to persons over the age of 62
- Disability insurance or income for disabled workers under age 65
- Survivor's insurance or benefits
- Health insurance (Medicare)

Social Security offices also administer a fifth program, Supplemental Security Income (SSI). This program offers additional cash benefits or supplemental income to low-income blind, disabled, or aged persons. Payments are not based on any individual employee contribution to the Social Security trust funds. The funds used for benefit payments are paid from the general tax fund, not the Social Security trust fund. Despite the fact that SSI is also a federal program, benefits vary from state to state.

To quality for Social Security benefits or the four Social Security programs, the appropriate credits must have been contributed to the trust fund by the worker. A person earns one credit for each quarter worked during the year if the earnings meet the quarterly amount established by Social Security or the Railroad Retirement System. No more than four credits can be accumulated per year regardless of income or the number of jobs held during the year.

Persons are not enrolled automatically into any program for which they may be entitled; they must apply and be accepted. One example is the Medicare program for those over age 65. A person must apply 3 months prior to his or her 65th birthday. Failure to do so causes a delay, and the person will not be eligible to enroll until January first of the next year or the next general enrollment period. More important, Medicare coverage will not be effective until July of that year.

Case managers must be familiar with the major federal Social Security programs to which disabled patients in their caseloads are entitled. These programs are:

- Social Security Disability Insurance (SSDI)
- Medicare
- Supplemental Security Income (SSI)

Social Security Disability Insurance (SSDI)

Social Security Disability Insurance (SSDI) is an income and insurance program available to disabled workers, the blind, and certain dependents under age 65 who meet the Social Security's or the Railroad Retirement System's criteria for total disability. In some cases government employees and certain members of their families can obtain benefits if they have been disabled for more than 29 months. However, the best way to obtain information about this category of disabled persons is to call the Social Security office directly. Despite the fact that a person may qualify for SSDI and receive income, he or she will not be eligible for Social Security's insurance, Medicare, until he or she has received SSDI for 2 years.

Social Security's definition of disability is related to work, and persons are considered disabled only if they are physically or mentally impaired or both and have been prevented from obtaining "gainful" employment for at least a year, or if the condition is expected to result in death. To receive SSDI a person must be totally disabled as defined in the Social Security Act as opposed to the definitions accepted by state disability programs, which are established to provide benefits to persons temporarily disabled from an illness, injury, or pregnancy.

Persons eligible to enroll in SSDI are:

- Disabled workers under the age of 65
- Unmarried children under the age of 18 (disability is immaterial and Medicare is not available to this group)
- Unmarried persons over the age of 22 if the disability occurred before the age of 22
- Disabled widows or widowers
- Disabled divorced spouses if the marriage lasted more than 10 years

Disabling conditions must be supported by documented medical evidence and must result in significant loss of function, cognitive abilities, or judgment. The most frequently recognized disabilities are:

- Diseases of the heart, lungs, or blood vessels
- Severe arthritis
- Brain abnormalities
- Cancer that is progressive and not under control or cured
- Diseases of the digestive system that result in serious weight loss or malnutrition
- Loss of motor function
- Serious loss of kidney function
- Total inability to speak
- Legal blindness

Application should be made as soon as possible after the disabling condition has been diagnosed because the application and determination process takes approximately 5 months, the longest processing required for any Social Security program. Benefits start after the sixth full month of disability if the person is approved and meets the eligibility criteria. To assist with expediting the application, case managers should inform the patient or family at their intake application appointment with the staff at SSDI that they will be required to provide:

- Social Security number
- Proof of age of the disabled person (original birth certificate or a certified copy of the original)
- Names, addresses, phone numbers, and dates of treatment of all physicians, hospitals, clinics, or institutions
- Work history, summary of duties, and all jobs held over the past 15 years
- Copy of W2 form (or federal tax return if self-employed)
- Dates of military service
- Dates of prior marriage (if divorced)
- If widowed, copy of death certificate and proof of marriage
- For a divorced spouse, proof that the marriage lasted 10 years or more
- For persons disabled before age 22, proof that disability started prior to age 22
- For stepchildren, proof of the parent's marriage
- For adopted children, Social Security will explain what is required
- Any supporting medical records

Once the application has been completed and it has been determined that the person meets the requirements of the law, the packet is forwarded to the Disability Determination Service (DDS) Unit. This team, composed of a physician and a disability evaluation specialist, reviews the records, considers the medical facts of the case, and issues a determination. If the information is incomplete or is thought to be inadequate, the team will request the applicant to undergo further testing, which is paid for by Social Security along with any transportation costs.

A written notice of the decision is issued by the disability determination team. The actual amount of the monthly cash benefit is based on the worker's earnings covered by Social Security prior to the disability and varies significantly from person to person. Benefits continue indefinitely or until the patient can perform substantial gainful employment. To ensure continued payment, periodic evaluations are required to verify that the disability continues.

During the initial time period of coverage by SSDI, coverage for healthcare expenses rests with the patient's private insurance, Medicaid, or the patient's own funds. If the person remains on SSDI for 24 months, he or she is entitled to Medicare.

Supplemental Security Income (SSI)

Supplemental Security Income (SSI) is an income program that pays a monthly income to low-income persons who are aged, blind, or disabled. Since eligibility is based on income and the cash benefits are paid from the general state and federal tax fund, not the Social Security trust fund, benefits vary from state to state. When a person is eligible for SSI, he or she is also eligible for Medicaid. Eligibility is based on:

- Income, assets, and resources
- Blindness or disability
- Citizenship (see earlier requirements under Social Security) or lawfully admitted alien
- Willingness of a disabled person to accept vocational rehabilitation if it is offered

Application should be made as early as possible to the local Social Security office. To expedite the process, the family or patient should expect to supply:

- Social Security number
- Birth certificate (original or certified copy of the original or evidence of lawful admission for permanent residence)
- Property tax records, mortgage, or rent receipts
- Records that show amounts spent for food and utilities, if sharing a household
- Payroll slips, bank books, tax returns, car reg-

istration, and any other information about income or resources
• Medical records and names and addresses of physicians, hospitals, or clinics that treated the disabling condition

Applications for SSI should not be delayed if the required information is not readily available because the Social Security representative may be able to obtain it. However, eligibility cannot be determined until all information is available, and patients and families must be apprised of this fact. Case managers should also be aware that persons eligible for both Aid to Families with Dependent Children and SSI cannot have both and must decide which program offers better benefits or greater income for their situation.

Since the recipient of SSI is also eligible for Medicaid, he or she is often eligible for other social services offered by the local Social Service or welfare department as well. Such services may include chore worker services, meal preparation, shopping, and transportation. Referrals are also made to other appropriate agencies within the community for counseling, work skill training, job placement, or training for independent living. However, in all cases, benefits vary from state to state.

Disabled drug addicts or alcoholics are referred to appropriate agencies for treatment; if they fail to undergo the recommended treatment or comply with the terms and conditions of the program, they are not eligible for SSI. SSI payments made to eligible drug addicts or alcoholics are made only to a representative payee, not to the addict or alcoholic.

Certain other conditions dictate which patients must have a representative payee. The local Social Security Administration office assists in this determination. If the person does not have a family member or friend who can assume this responsibility, the Social Security office will make the necessary arrangements with an appropriate community agency or designee.

Supplemental Security Income is designed to encourage blind or disabled recipients to work, and therefore it allows for certain expenses that permit the person to work. Examples of such expenses may include:

• Attendant care to provide assistance in getting to and from work
• Readers for the blind or interpreters for the deaf
• Special devices such as telecommunication equipment or Braille reading materials and writing devices
• Residential modifications that improve mobility
• Cost of keeping guide dogs
• Special transportation arrangements or modified vans

Medicare

Medicare is federal health insurance for:

• Persons over the age of 65.
• Patients with permanent end-stage renal disease requiring dialysis or transplantation.
• Certain totally disabled persons under the age of 65 who have received SSDI or Railroad Retirement Disability payments for 24 months.

Medicare, unlike other Social Security programs, is administered by the Healthcare Financing Administration (HCFA) under the U.S. Department of Health and Human Services. Local Social Security offices accept applications, provide information about the programs, and assist beneficiaries in filing and completing Medicare claim forms.

Medicare is divided into two parts—Part A and Part B. Part A is financed through payroll deductions or FICA withholdings from workers' paychecks. If a person meets the requirements for entitlement and applies for Medicare, Part A comes automatically if he or she is eligible for Social Security. Enrollment in Part B is voluntary and requires a monthly premium paid by the patient. Like Part B, Part A can be purchased if the person is not eligible and does not have the appropriate credits but does desire the coverage. The monthly premiums for Part A for such a person are adjusted yearly; the cost averages several hundred dollars per month. In both Parts A and B some out-of-pocket expenditures for deductibles or copayments are required, and these amounts are adjusted yearly.

Both Part A and Part B are discussed in more detail in the following pages. In general, Part A, the hospital portion, covers:

• Inpatient care in an acute-care hospital
• Inpatient care in a skilled nursing facility (SNF)
• Care at home by a home health agency (HHA)
• Hospice care

Part B, the medical portion, covers:

• Physician services

- Diagnostic tests
- Outpatient services
- Home health agency services
- Durable medical equipment (DME) and supplies
- Ambulance fees
- Other medical or health services

Claims are paid by contracts established with insurance organizations called intermediaries or carriers. Intermediaries make coverage and payment decisions about services provided under Part A, whereas carriers handle claims for Part B. Regardless of who pays the claim, patients have the right to appeal any coverage decision they disagree with. During the past decade Medicare has established contracts with many managed care organizations, and if the patient is linked to one of these, claims for both Part A and Part B will be paid by this group.

For claims to be paid, providers of services must be certified by Medicare, meet all licensing requirements of state or local health authorities as well as Medicare's conditions of participation, and comply with Title VI of the Civil Rights Act, the Privacy Act, and any other federal acts that protect patients' rights. Additionally, all care provided must be medically necessary, not custodial.

It is important to note that Medicare has specific rules that apply to patients who have Medicare but are disabled under the age of 65 and are also covered by another healthcare plan. This healthcare payor may be available through either their former employer (many people retain their employer healthcare benefits through COBRA or a medical pension type plan) or through their spouse's employer or insurance coverage. In these cases, Medicare is the secondary payor if the employer employs more than 100 people. However, case managers must always check with the insurer to verify this.

Like employer group coverage, Medicare has specific criteria that determine when it will be the secondary payor. For instance, Medicare is secondary when no-fault insurance or liability insurance is available. It is also secondary for 30 months when patients who are eligible for Medicare due to permanent kidney failure have group health insurance through either their own employer or the employer of a family member. Likewise, Medicare has specific requirements governing the eligibility of patients who are disabled veterans. Information about what can or cannot be covered is available by calling the Social Security toll-free phone number.

Persons on Medicare often refer to their card as the "red, white, and blue one," so if the patient is not sure he has Medicare, the case manager should merely ask if he has a card with these colors. Surprisingly enough, many people are unaware that Medicare Part A covers primarily inpatient care and does not cover physician or outpatient services.

If the patient elected not to sign up for Part B at the time he or she was eligible for Part A, he is charged a premium surcharge for a late enrollment. Patients who elected not to take Part B must wait to enroll until the next general enrollment period, which is held January 1 through March 31. Also, their monthly premium will be increased by 10% for each 12-month period they could have had Part B but were not enrolled. Although this surcharge is steep, Medicare does have provisions whereby this penalty can be waived if patients can prove they were not informed about the need for Part B.

Case managers must be aware that Medicare has special provisions for low-income persons on Medicaid. In certain cases a state's Medicaid program may pay the Part B premiums, and in some cases it may also purchase Part A for the patient. These programs are known as Qualified Disabled Working Individual (QDWI), Qualified Medicare Beneficiaries (QMB), or Specified Low-Income Medicare Beneficiaries (SLMB) programs. Information about these programs is available by calling Social Security's toll-free number.

Other points to remember about Medicare are discussed in the following sections.

PART A BENEFIT PERIODS

Benefit periods are associated only with Medicare Part A. If the patient has only Part A and not Part B, there is no coverage for physician services or outpatient care. Also, as stated earlier, Medicare Part A covers four kinds of medically necessary care:

- Inpatient hospital care
- Inpatient care in a skilled nursing facility following inpatient care in an acute-care hospital for the same diagnosis
- Home health agency care
- Hospice care

Medicare sets limits on the number of days it will pay for care in a benefit period. Benefit periods under Medicare are very confusing. It behooves a case manager to be keenly aware of these periods and the deductibles, copayments, and coinsurance charges for each. These expenses can greatly affect healthcare payor expenditures or the out-of-pocket expenses of the patient or family if they are ignored. Medicare typically allows the following benefit periods for Part A inpatient care:

Day 1 through day 60
Day 61 through day 90
Lifetime reserve day 91 through day 150

For each benefit period the patient or healthcare payor is responsible for specific yearly deductibles and coinsurance charges. Because Medicare readjusts these deductibles and coinsurance payments yearly, it behooves case managers to become familiar with these charges. This is done by keeping a current Medicare handbook (published yearly) in the case management library.

Basically, the rules governing a benefit period are as follows: the first day of hospitalization starts the benefit period, and the patient is responsible for a deductible, which covers the first 60 days of hospitalization. Patients who remain hospitalized for the entire 60 days or any portion of the 60-day period pay nothing else for the facility portion of the bill. Patients who remain confined beyond the sixtieth day are responsible for a substantial daily coinsurance payment, which continues for each day of hospitalization up to the ninetieth day. Patients who need medical inpatient care beyond the ninetieth day can then use what is termed their 60 days of lifetime reserve. Patients using these 60 days again pay a huge premium for each day they are hospitalized. If they remain hospitalized beyond day 150, Medicare coverage ceases. At this point, either the patient must pay privately, or the healthcare payor (if the patient's healthcare coverage is other than a Medicare supplement plan) or Medicaid must pay the bill.

Day 1 through day 90 are renewable if the patient remains out of an acute or skilled nursing facility or rehabilitation facility for 60 days in a row. There are no limits on the number of benefit periods a patient can have. However, with the start of each new benefit period the patient is responsible for repeated deductibles and copayments. Once any or all of the lifetime reserve days have been used, they are gone and cannot be renewed.

The following examples may help in explaining benefit periods:

1. Patient A enters an acute-care hospital for a total hip replacement and pays his or her

benefit period deductible. After 7 days the patient is discharged. Unfortunately, 10 days later the patient develops a wound infection that requires readmission. The patient is rehospitalized and the first day of readmission is really day 8 of the first 60-day benefit period. As such, the patient has no further expenses because the deductible for this benefit period has already been paid. If this patient is discharged and remains out of an acute-care hospital, rehabilitation hospital, or skilled nursing facility for 60 consecutive days, the benefit period can be renewed.

2. Patient B also has a total hip replacement but develops serious complications during surgery and subsequent postoperative care. These complications are so severe that the patient remains hospitalized for 180 days before the patient dies. In this case, the patient pays the yearly deductible for the first 60 days and then a daily coinsurance rate (for example, in 1997 the daily coinsurance rate for days 61 to 90 was $190). Then, from days 90 to 150 the patient pays an even higher daily rate (for example, in 1997 this daily coinsurance rate was $380). After day 150, the patient pays privately for his care until he dies.

OTHER PART A POINTERS

Inpatient Care

To receive Medicare coverage in an acute-care hospital, the patient must meet four conditions:

- A physician must prescribe inpatient care for treatment.
- The type of care needed can only be provided on an inpatient basis.
- The hospital participates in Medicare.
- The hospital utilization review department or Professional Review Organization (PRO) does not deny the stay.

When these basic conditions are met, Medicare Part A coverage includes the following specific services:

- Semi-private accommodations
- All meals
- Regular nursing services
- Cost of special care units, operating and recovery rooms, and anesthesia services
- Medications dispensed while an inpatient
- Blood transfusions (after the first three pints)
- Laboratory tests

- Radiologic tests and other radiology services, including radiation therapy, billed by the hospital
- Medical supplies
- Use of equipment, such as wheelchairs
- Rehabilitation services
- Psychiatric inpatient care (lifetime maximum of 190 days)
- Care in Mexico or Canada (only in certain situations)
- Care in a participating Christian Science sanatorium (only if it is operated or listed and certified by the First Church of Christ in Boston)

Medicare Part A does not cover:

- Custodial care
- Personal convenience items
- Private duty nurses
- Private room, unless it is determined to be medically necessary and the fact is documented
- Care outside the United States (Puerto Rico, the U.S. Virgin Islands, American Samoa, and the Northern Mariana Islands are considered part of the United States)
- Care that is not medically necessary

Skilled Nursing Facility

In addition to inpatient care in an acute-care facility, Medicare Part A pays for skilled nursing facility (SNF) or skilled nursing unit (SNU) care if the patient continues to require daily skilled nursing or rehabilitation services. Medicare pays for skilled nursing facility care if the patient meets five conditions:

- Daily skilled nursing care or rehabilitation services that can only be provided in a skilled nursing facility are required.
- The patient has been in an acute-care hospital for at least 3 days (not counting the day of discharge).
- The patient is admitted within 30 days of discharge from the acute-care hospital.
- The admitting condition or diagnosis is the same as the one treated in the acute-care hospital.
- The physician certifies that the patient requires skilled care and services.

During hospitalization in the skilled nursing facility Medicare pays for:

- Semi-private accommodations
- All meals (including special diets)
- Regular nursing services
- Physical, occupational, and speech therapy

- Medical supplies
- Durable medical equipment

As with acute facility care Medicare does not pay for:

- Personal convenience items
- Custodial care
- Private duty nurses
- Private room unless it is deemed medically necessary

Medicare Part A pays for 100 days of skilled nursing facility care per benefit period if the patient's stay remains medically necessary. Under this part of Medicare, 20 days are covered in full, and days 21 to 100 are covered with payment of a daily coinsurance rate (for example, in 1997 the daily coinsurance rate for care in a skilled nursing facility was $95 per day). As with acute care, if the patient remains out of the hospital for 60 consecutive days, this 100-day skilled nursing facility benefit can be renewed.

If the patient remains in the skilled nursing facility for the entire 100 days and still meets the criteria for skilled care, Medicare continues to pay. Once the 100-day limit has been reached, Medicare coverage terminates, and the patient must pay privately or Medicaid must be used as the source of payment for the continued stay. This is necessary despite the fact that the patient may still be classified as requiring skilled care.

Home Health Agency

Home health agency services covered by Medicare Part A include nursing, physical therapy, occupational therapy, speech therapy, part-time home health aides, social worker services, and durable medical equipment. With the exception of durable medical equipment, Medicare covers all charges for medically necessary intermittent care by a home health agency. Coverage of services by a home health agency is allowed when the following four conditions are met:

- The skilled care is required intermittently (generally this care can be provided daily, every other day, or several times a week for as long as the patient requires skilled nursing services).
- The person is confined to the home.
- The physician certifies that the person needs intermittent home healthcare.
- The agency participates in Medicare.

Home health coverage by Medicare does not

cover general housekeeping or homemaker or other services or items such as:

- Medications
- Meal preparation or home-delivered meals
- Shopping
- Services to support activities of daily living
- Hourly or 24-hour skilled nursing care for the technology-dependent patient or highly skilled nursing care

Hospice

Hospice care is allowed under Medicare Part A and is intended for the terminally ill. To be covered by Medicare three conditions must be met:

- The physician certifies that the patient has a terminal illness.
- The patient chooses to receive care from a hospice rather than use standard Medicare benefits for the illness.
- The hospice participates in Medicare.

Under Medicare's hospice program the patient does not pay for any care other than a small coinsurance payment for outpatient drugs; if hospitalized for respite care, the patient is responsible for 5% of the rate allowed by Medicare.

Medicare stipulates that care provided by the hospice agency must be palliative and not curative. Patients entering a hospice program must sign a waiver to indicate that they understand this fact. Under the hospice benefit Medicare pays for:

- Nursing services
- Physicians' services
- Drugs for pain relief or symptom management
- Physical, occupational, and speech therapy
- Home health aide and homemaker service
- Medical supplies and equipment
- Short-term inpatient care, including respite care
- Bereavement counseling

The hospice benefit does not cover treatments that are not related to pain relief or management of symptoms of the terminal illness.

PART B

As stated earlier, when first eligible for Medicare, many people elect not to enroll in Part B. This is unfortunate because this portion covers physician services and outpatient services. These services now comprise the bulk of the care provided because inpatient stays are so limited and hospitalization is nonexistent for some diagnoses. Medicare Part B, unlike Part A, which is free, is obtained only if the person pays a monthly fee.

Case managers must be aware that not every patient who has Medicare coverage has Part B. In addition to the monthly premium for Part B, the person is responsible for a yearly deductible and for 20% of Medicare's approved charges. Also, if the healthcare provider does not accept Medicare assignment, the provider can bill the patient for the difference between the amount actually billed and the amount Medicare paid as its allowable amount.

Unlike Part A, for which certain conditions must be met, Part B covers the following services if they are medically necessary:

- Physicians' services
- Outpatient hospital services
- Outpatient mental health services
- Ambulatory surgical services
- Outpatient therapy (physical therapy, occupational therapy, speech therapy)
- Comprehensive outpatient rehabilitation
- Independent clinical laboratory services, including portable services
- Radiologic services, including portable services
- Ambulance transportation
- Durable medical equipment
- Blood and blood components
- Prosthetic devices
- Medical supplies
- Radiology and pathology services
- Home health agency services
- Drugs that cannot be self-administered
- Second opinions

Medicare Part B does not cover:

- Routine physicals or related testing
- Routine foot care
- Routine dental care
- Eye examinations or eyeglasses
- Hearing examinations or hearing aids
- Most immunizations
- Most prescription drugs
- Cosmetic surgery unless it is related to an accidental injury or to improve a malformed part of the body

Although routine services and examinations are not covered, Part B does cover such services as:

- Chiropractic services for manipulation of the spine to correct subluxation demonstrated by radiologic examination
- Podiatric care for treatment of diseases of the foot, hammer toe, bunion deformities, and heel spurs
- Dental services, if the dental problem is medically related and not routine
- Optometry services for cataract spectacles
- Contact lenses or intraocular lenses required after cataract surgery
- Therapeutic shoes for persons with severe diabetic foot disease
- Pap smear every 3 years
- Mammography screening every 2 years

Although historically Medicare has not covered the cost of drug prescriptions, it does cover the following prescribed drugs:

- Antigens
- Hemophilia clotting factors
- Hepatitis B vaccine
- Immunosuppressive drugs
- Oral cancer drugs
- Vaccines for flu and pneumonia (and for these neither the yearly deductible nor the 20% coinsurance rate apply)

If home health agency services are required, the patient must meet the same conditions as required for Part A coverage (listed previously in this chapter) for such services. If the patient requires outpatient therapy, three conditions must be met:

- The physician prescribed the service.
- The physician or therapist established the plan of treatment.
- The plan is periodically reviewed for appropriateness.

Mental health benefits under both Part A and Part B are extremely limited. For instance, patients are covered for only 190 inpatient psychiatric hospital days per lifetime. Other care is limited to day treatment programs and individual psychotherapy.

MEDICARE AND THE END-STAGE RENAL DISEASE PATIENT

Persons with end-stage renal disease are entitled to Medicare beginning the third month after the month they start hemodialysis. Home dialysis can be accomplished using one of the following methods: hemodialysis, home intermittent peritoneal dialysis (IPD), home continuous cycling peritoneal dialysis (CCPD), or continuous ambulatory peritoneal dialysis (CAPD). If the patient starts a self-dialysis or CAPD program or is admitted for a kidney transplant, he or she is eligible immediately. If the patient is already covered by Medicare for another condition, he must still apply for the end-stage renal Medicare program.

To receive Medicare reimbursement, all facilities used by the patient must be specifically approved for dialysis or transplantation even if they are already approved for the provision of other health services. In addition, they must meet any health, safety, professional, staffing, and minimum utilization standards developed by other federal, state, or local community licensing bodies that directly relate to dialysis and kidney transplantation. Facilities that participate in the Medicare end-stage renal program must accept assignment (Medicare's allowable amount).

Once the patient's condition has stabilized and he or she no longer requires inpatient care for the shunt or dialysis, most of the coverage is paid by Part B or the medical insurance portion of Medicare. Medicare Part B for end-stage renal dialysis patients pays for:

- Outpatient dialysis treatments
- Laboratory tests
- Equipment (rented or purchased, and maintenance costs)
- All supplies associated with dialysis
- Physicians' services
- Training for self-dialysis (by the patient or person who will perform the dialysis if the patient is incapable of doing it)
- Heparin, the antidote for heparin when this is medically indicated, and any topical anesthetics
- Facility-based home health agency care or other facility support services or personnel needed for intermittent monitoring of the equipment, assistance if an emergency arises, installation or maintenance of the equipment, and testing and appropriate treatment of the water system
- Blood and packed red blood cells (after the first three pints)

Medicare (Parts A and B) for end-stage renal disease dialysis patients does not pay for:

- Ambulance or other transportation
- Dialysis aides to assist with home dialysis
- Drugs and medications other than heparin and typical anesthetics
- Inpatient acute care or care in a skilled nurs-

ing facility when chronic long-term dialysis is the only reason for this care
• Lodging costs incurred because an outpatient dialysis facility is not near the patient's home
• Wages lost owing to training
• Kidney purchase (NOTE: organs cannot be sold—this is illegal)

Once a kidney transplant has been planned and the patient has been admitted to the hospital, Medicare Part A will be used. In addition to the normal inpatient care covered by Part A, Medicare pays for the following charges relating to transplantation:

• All inpatient care if it is provided in a Medicare renal-approved facility.
• Kidney registration fees.
• Any laboratory tests or other tests required to evaluate the patient or potential donor for the transplant.
• Costs associated with procurement of a suitable kidney if a suitable donor is not available.
• Full cost (with no deductibles or copayments) of care for the donor, including any costs incurred should complications arise with the donor.

End-stage renal disease Medicare Part B for kidney transplantation pays for:

• Physicians' services for preoperative care, the surgical procedure, and follow-up care for both the patient and the donor.
• Immunosuppressive drugs for 1 year after the transplant.
• Laboratory tests.

Coverage for end-stage renal disease patients ends 12 months after the month they no longer require dialysis or 36 months after the month of a successful kidney transplant. Should Medicare benefits terminate and problems occur requiring dialysis or another transplant, coverage is resumed immediately.

Patients who disagree with a Medicare determination about their eligibility or coverage have the right to appeal. The local Social Security office will explain the appeal process, its time frame, and all necessary requirements.

☙ S U M M A R Y

The purpose of this section is to highlight the basic programs available under the Social Security system. Many people confuse Social Security with welfare, and thus this program and its benefits are overlooked. They are overlooked because it is assumed that these programs are only for those over age 65 or for the "needy." For these reasons, many people never apply.

Case managers must be familiar with the programs to which patients are entitled and keep abreast of changes. Likewise, because of the large copayments and deductibles required for persons on Medicare, case managers must assess patients for potential referral to alternate funding programs such as Medicaid whenever possible. Because of the complexity of the programs and to avoid misinterpretations, families should be directed to the local Social Security Administration office for answers to any questions.

STATE DEPARTMENT OF REHABILITATION

The state Department of Rehabilitation or, in some states, the Office of Vocational Rehabilitation or the Rehabilitation Commission is the department responsible for providing vocational rehabilitation services. This department offers the services of trained vocational rehabilitation counselors to physically or mentally challenged people who wish to prepare for gainful employment.

By the time many patients reach the level of vocational rehabilitation their cases are closed to the healthcare payor, facility-based, or community-based case management program. However, this does not mean that case managers should not be familiar with vocational rehabilitation programs. Similarly, case managers should be familiar with the application and testing procedures that determine whether the patient is an appropriate candidate for vocational rehabilitation.

Because of the importance of vocational rehabilitation, it is common for vocational counselors to be included in head trauma and physical medicine and rehabilitation teams. Their purpose is to identify patients who are appropriate candidates for vocational rehabilitation and to guide the patient into a program as soon as feasible. Vocational rehabilitation programs accept patients with any handicapping physical or mental condition; the key to acceptance is the patient's motivation and determination.

Eligibility Requirements

To be eligible for vocational rehabilitation certain basic requirements must be met. For example, the patient must:

- Have a physical or mental disability that constitutes or results in a substantial handicap and prevents employment.
- Be motivated to participate.
- Show reasonable evidence that he or she can obtain and hold a job once vocational training is completed.

Goals

The goal of vocational rehabilitation is to return the patient to gainful employment. Fortunately, many patients can return to their previous employment. For those who cannot, vocational rehabilitation makes use of various modalities in retraining the person. In addition, the program uses "training sites" found throughout any given community (generally these are larger cities or towns). Here the person can be given any type of vocational retraining he or she requires. Many of these training sites are provided through such organizations as the Salvation Army, Desert Industries, Purple Heart, and so forth.

The types of retraining offered vary from site to site and from program to program. In all cases, clients are placed in the most appropriate site or program that matches their impairment level and capability for learning.

Referrals

Ideally, patients refer themselves for services. However, referrals can be accepted from any source. Referrals must be made when active participation is acceptable, when the patient's participation has been approved by his or her attending physician, and when the patient is medically stable. A medical release for partial or complete participation is usually required.

After referral, a delay of several weeks usually ensues until actual on-site assessment and testing are performed. When the initial assessment and tests are scheduled, patients should be apprised that they must provide the following mandatory information:

- Name
- Social Security number (copy of Social Security card)
- Address and county of residence
- Birth date and age
- Copy of alien card, if appropriate
- Copy of driver's license with picture

- Proof of any public assistance received
- Monthly amount of public assistance
- Number of months on public assistance
- Proof of Supplemental Security Income (SSI), unemployment verification, Social Security Disability Income (SSDI) status, or other special federal programs providing income resources
- Work status at time of referral
- Weekly earnings at time of referral
- Primary source of support
- Any previous contact with the Department of Rehabilitation (when, where, and how long)
- Highest grade of schooling completed (school records)
- Number of dependents
- Total number of people in family unit
- Total family monthly income
- Names of previous employers
- Copy of medical records
- Current psychological information
- Veteran status
- Type of available transportation

Assessment and Testing

Once all the data from the above sources have been compiled, the patient undergoes the actual vocational testing, which consists of a variety of components from which his or her transferable skills can be identified and used in training. Some typical test components include:

- Situational evaluation (five days of observation while the patient completes tasks)
- Psychological testing
- Oral interview and questioning
- Written test questions

The following factors are taken into consideration before a disabled patient returns to work or is placed in a training site:

- Physical capabilities, especially endurance and the ability to sit for extended periods of time or to walk
- Frustration level and tolerance to noise
- Perceptual abilities
- Speech and communication skills
- Accessibility and maneuverability to areas such as work space, bathrooms, break rooms, cafeteria, parking lot, elevators, ramps
- Temperature and circulation of air in the work environment (e.g., quadriplegics and burn patients have difficulty with body heat regulation)
- Appropriateness of equipment to be used or

evaluation of adaptive devices that will be required to operate any equipment. In addition, the existing equipment the person will be using is evaluated to determine whether it will require modification

After the vocational rehabilitation counselor completes the assessment and the various tests, the packet of information is submitted to the vocational rehabilitation medical consultant for a recommendation. Medical review of the case varies from state to state and can take several days to several weeks. If the patient is accepted as a client of vocational rehabilitation, an individual written rehabilitation plan (IWRP) is developed with the client present. The IWRP outlines goals and objectives and the expected completion date for the training.

If the client is denied rehabilitation or disagrees with the IWRP, he or she has the right to appeal. The person has 1 year from the date of notification of any denial to appeal. In addition to the right to appeal, the rights of the disabled are protected by the Federal Rehabilitation Act, Titles VI and VII of the Civil Rights Act, the Americans with Disabilities Act, and in some cases, the Individuals with Disabilities Education Act. Complaints of discrimination should be filed within 100 days of the alleged unlawful act with the civil rights officer from the Department of Rehabilitation, the Department of Education, or the Department of Fair Housing.

Services Provided

If the patient becomes a client of vocational rehabilitation, the following services or supplies are commonly provided:

- Diagnostic services and services related to diagnosis
- Counseling
- Physical restoration
- Placement at a rehabilitation training site
- Books and training supplies
- Supplemental allowance
- Actual purchase of tools, equipment, initial stocks, or supplies that enable the person to work
- Transportation allowance (which sometimes includes modification of vans or the fees associated with testing and certification for driving)
- Management and supervisory services for those placed in small business enterprises

- Payment of fees for occupational licenses
- Reader services for the blind
- Interpreter services for the deaf
- Job placement assistance
- Postemployment services
- Services to family members
- Other services deemed necessary to encourage gainful employment

Should the patient move to another part of the state for any reason during rehabilitation, coordination of the program with other state offices is possible. However, if the patient moves out of state, the entire application process must be started from the beginning in the new state of residence.

SUMMARY

The final step in the rehabilitation process is returning the disabled person to work. The disabled have made considerable strides during the past several years in their attempts to show that they can be contributing members of the everyday work environment. The state department responsible for vocational rehabilitation services is often the driving force behind a person's return to work.

Despite the fact that many cases are closed to case management by the time vocational rehabilitation occurs, case managers must be familiar with the application process and the services provided by his or her state of practice. This knowledge assists in guiding the patient to the appropriate sources that encourage a return to work and the development of self-esteem and worth.

STATE AGENCY FOR DEVELOPMENTAL DISABILITIES

The rights of the developmentally disabled are protected under federal legislation and the Developmental Disabilities Act of 1984. In addition, they are protected by other federal acts such as the Americans with Disabilities Act, the Rehabilitation Act, the Privacy Act, and others. Under the Developmental Disabilities Act, states are required to provide specific services that will meet the needs of the developmentally disabled. Case managers must be very familiar with these laws and the agency responsible for administering developmental disability services to patients in their caseloads.

Because the developmentally disabled constitute a large percentage of many caseloads, case managers must be familiar with the requirements for aid to these patients in the state in which they practice. If the state agency's name is unknown, one of the best resources for locating it is the state capitol's telephone directory service.

Definition

The federal law defines a developmental disability as "a substantially handicapping disability which originated prior to an individual attaining the age of twenty-two and continues or is expected to continue indefinitely. These handicaps include such conditions as mental retardation, cerebral palsy, epilepsy, autism, stroke, traumatic brain injury or any condition which is attributable to a mental or physical impairment and results in substantial functional limitations." It further states, "to be considered developmentally disabled, the functional limitations must be in three or more of the areas which affect major life activity. These are areas such as self-care, receptive and expressive language disorders, learning, mobility, self-direction, capacity for independent living and economic self-sufficiency."[7]

To meet the patient's needs and allow him or her to function as independently as possible in the least restrictive environment, services can be provided in any combination. These services may include diagnosis, evaluation, treatment, personal care, day care, domiciliary care, special living arrangements, training of the parents, education, sheltered employment, recreation and socialization, counseling for both the patient and the family, protective services and other services, information and referral, transportation for delivery of services, and any other services that promote and coordinate the activities and services required by the person with a developmental disability.

Responsible State Agency

The actual names of the state agency responsible for administering services to the developmentally disabled vary from state to state. However, in most states the point of entry is often the state Department of Mental Health, the Department of Mental Retardation, or whatever state department or agency is responsible for delivery of developmental disability services. Like the variations in name, the processes required for application to the program, services, or access to care from this state agency vary greatly from state to state.

Unlike other states, California's point of entry into the state's continuum of care system for people with developmental disabilities (DD) is a network of 21 private nonprofit units called regional centers. These centers are contracted by the state Department of Developmental Services and are legislatively funded.

Regardless of which agency is responsible for providing services, the intent of such agencies is to provide services to any person regardless of current age (as long as the developmental disabling condition occurred before age 22). Services are also intended to reach persons who are believed to have a developmental disorder or are at high risk of parenting a developmentally disabled infant.

Referrals

Referrals must be made as soon as a developmentally disabling condition has been identified. Not all persons will be eligible for services. Developmental disability counselors are in a position to offer assistance with information and referral. The important thing is to refer the patient and allow the developmental disability staff to determine whether the person meets the state's eligibility requirements. Once a referral has been made, an initial data intake session is scheduled, at which the person or parents should provide the following information:

- Name
- Address
- Social Security numbers of both patient and parents
- Birth dates of patient and those of the parents
- Disability status of the parents, if applicable
- Whether the parents are living or deceased
- Any insurance coverage
- Proof of receipt of SSI or other state or federal aid or other income
- Proof of residency
- Copies of any medical records, psychological or intelligence evaluations, or individual education plan (IEP)

During this initial session the counselor may provide the patient or family with information or advice on the following:

- The nature and availability of the services

provided by the developmental disabled programs and other community agencies (e.g., Title V Children's Medical Services program, any services from mental health)
- The conservatorship process
- Exploration of income maintenance, money management, and financial programs or funding sources
- Training to which they, volunteers, or professionals are entitled
- Supportive services to which the person is entitled
- Housing or placement services to which the person is entitled (e.g., board and care, residential care, intermediate care facility, domiciliary care facility, home care)
- Education entitlement
- Work opportunities and training
- Medical and dental services
- Recreational activities within the community
- Preventive services for high-risk parents and patients
- Other services as determined by need

Many children referred to this program are also eligible for benefits from the Title V Children's Medical Services program. Therefore, many children receive services not only from this program but also from the healthcare payor as well as the agency responsible for developmental disability services. However, in all cases, the healthcare payor is the primary payor if the requested service or item is a benefit of the child's healthcare coverage.

Because many persons with developmental disabilities are receiving services or input from a number of different agencies, coordination of case management activities is imperative, especially since many organizations now offer case management services for the clients they serve. As stated in several sections of this manual, when multiple agencies are involved in the care of one patient, it is imperative for all case managers to confer and develop a joint case management plan.

It is equally important for case managers, especially those associated with a healthcare payor, to advocate proactively that providers used by either the agency responsible for developmental disability services or the Title V Children's Medical Services program be allowed to provide care by the healthcare payor. Such providers are "vendors" for these programs but are not part of the healthcare payor's network. If the same provider is allowed to provide care, there is a greater opportunity for open communication, and simultaneously, the chances of confusion, fragmentation, and duplication of services are decreased or avoided.

Assessment

Once referred, a complete medical and psychological assessment is required. This assessment includes:

- Collection and review of historical, medical, and diagnostic data.
- Provision or procurement of necessary tests and evaluations from which a determination for coverage can be made. These tests often include intelligence or psychological tests, and occupational, physical, and speech therapy evaluations.
- Summary of the developmental disability levels and recommendations for services.

"Habilitation" Plan

If after the initial data intake and assessment procedures the person is found to be eligible for developmental disability services, a "habilitation" plan is developed. This plan must be completed within the state's specified time frame after the initial eligibility assessment has been completed. (For example, in California this habilitation plan, referred to as an individual program plan [IPP], must be completed within 60 days of the assessment.) This plan is prepared jointly with one or more representatives from the developmental disability staff, the patient, and, when appropriate, the parents or conservator. The final habilitation plan must contain the following information:

- Summary of the person's specific capabilities and problems.
- Time-limited goals and objectives.
- The type and amount of services and, if known, identification of the providers of services necessary to achieve program objectives.
- Scheduled dates for review and reassessment to determine whether the planned services have been provided within the time frames established for the goals and objectives.
- Identification of the person responsible for program coordination. This may be a developmental disability staff member, a qualified individual or employee of an agency contracted by the department to provide program coordination, and, at times, the parent or legally appointed conservator.

Services Provided

To achieve the stated objectives of the habilitation plan, the agency or department handling people with developmental disabilities can contract for services from local providers or "vendors." As with all state agencies, this ability to vendor services varies from state to state, but the following services are commonly provided:

- Training of parents, volunteers, or healthcare professionals as required.
- Purchase of and referral for services.
- Collection and dissemination of whatever information is necessary to coordinate and establish the programs.
- Placement in a licensed community care home or other healthcare facility.
- Monitoring of services for any person placed out-of-the home.
- Advocacy and protection of the patient's civil and legal rights.
- Termination of services, if the provider is ineffective or noncompliant.
- Identification, maintenance of listings, and use of every appropriate and economically feasible alternative for care available within the region. If services are not available in the immediate area, services outside the region are provided and coordinated.
- Authorization of medical, dental, and surgical treatment if the patient's parent or conservator does not respond to the request or if he or she has no parent or conservator, or if the patient himself or herself is mentally incapable of authorizing such treatment.
- Initiation of conservatorship proceedings when appropriate.
- Referral for SSI and Medicaid or SSDI and Medicare.
- Identification and use of all governmental or other income or insurance sources available and necessary for payment of the person's care. This includes school district funds allotted for special education for handicapped pupils.

All habilitation plans are reviewed and modified if necessary at least annually by the developmental disability counselor, the program coordinator, the patient, the parents, or the conservator.

To establish or maintain the person at the appropriate level of care, the developmental disability counselor has the ability to purchase services that allow the person to live outside of an institution. Priority is given at all times to supporting the patient at home if this is feasible and acceptable to the parents. Supportive services for the patient living at home may include:

- Advocacy
- Specialized medical or dental care
- Specialized training for parents or caregivers
- Infant stimulation programs
- Respite care for parents or caregivers
- Homemaker services
- Babysitters
- Camping or outings
- Day care
- Short-term out-of-home placement or care
- Psychological counseling
- Behavior modification programs
- Special equipment and accessories or other self-help devices
- Adult vocational training programs
- Placement in a community day care program

If the person cannot be maintained at home services may include placement in a facility such as a:

- Community care home (board and care)
- Residential care facility
- Intermediate care facility (ICF); in California these facilities are referred to as intermediate care facilities—developmental disability (ICF-DD), and in other states they might be referred to as intermediate care facilities—mental retardation (ICF-MR)
- State institution

In all cases, the patient is placed in the least restrictive facility that can manage the level of care and provide the services required. Persons are placed in an intermediate care facility when they cannot be managed at home or in a community care facility (i.e., a home providing board and care). Patients placed in an intermediate care facility frequently have problems with self-care skills and require a structured environment that permits behavior modification or training.

Patients placed in residential or intermediate care facilities often cannot participate in any day program activities because of the severity of their disabilities. Actual licensed nursing care in these facilities ranges from less than 1 hour per day to 8 hours per week. Although short-term placement is the goal, developmental disability facilities are primarily designed to provide long-term care.

If the patient is self-destructive or unmanageable in a board and care or intermediate care facility, placement options are limited. Generally, this type of patient is placed in a state developmental center, a state-operated facility, or a state hospital. Entrance into a state facility requires a court order if the person is over age 18; if he or she is under 18, the parents or legal conservator must grant permission for entrance, or a referral must be generated from the developmental disability counselor responsible for the case.

Payment and Alternate Funding

Most of the care and services provided by the developmental disability agency is free of charge. However, in some circumstances parents can be required to pay a fee for a child under age 22 who is placed out of the home. This fee is based on a sliding scale or the ability to pay and cannot exceed the cost of provisions of care for a normal child living at home. Many developmentally disabled patients, especially those placed in a facility, qualify for SSI and Medicaid.

As with most alternate funding or entitlement programs, all developmental disability services require that insurance benefits or other funds be utilized before departmental funds can be released. However, this stipulation must never negate a referral because there is always a possibility insurance benefits may be limited, exhausted, or excluded.

Appeals

Anyone who does not agree with an adverse decision by the developmental disability agency has the right to request a hearing or appeal within 30 days of the decision. Developmentally disabled persons and parents classified as high risk for parenting a developmentally disabled infant are protected by the Federal Rehabilitation Act of 1973, Titles VI and VII of the Civil Rights Act of 1964, and the Americans with Disabilities Act (ADA) of 1990. Complaints of discrimination must be filed within 180 days of any infraction of these rights with the civil rights officer from the Department of Developmental Services, the Department of Education, or the Department of Fair Housing.

SUMMARY

Developmentally disabled clients should be referred as early as possible to identify and obtain the appropriate resources necessary to manage them. This is important because most persons in this category frequently have long-term or lifelong needs. The prime intent of these agencies is to allow the person to function in the least restrictive environment and keep him or her out of an institution whenever possible. To do so, those services that are necessary to keep the person at home or in the least restrictive environment are "vendored" to various providers that can accomplish this goal.

Case managers must make every effort to coordinate benefits when working with this agency to ensure that all services established allow the patient to function in the least restrictive environment. Therefore, they must be very familiar with the services provided by these agencies because developmentally disabled patients make up a large percentage of many case management caseloads.

California is the only state that offers regional center services to developmentally disabled clients. In all other states the point of contact is the Department of Mental Health, the Department of Mental Retardation, the Department of Developmental Disabilities, or the agency or state department delegated to provide services to the developmentally disabled.

REFERENCES

1. United States Code Service (1985). Title IV. Grants to states for aid and services to needy families with children and for child welfare services. 42 USCS §601-676.
2. United States Code Service (1985). Title V. Maternal and child health services block grant. 42 USCS §701-731.
3. United States Code Service (1993). Social Security Act. Title XIX. Grants to states for medical assistance programs, appropriations. 42 USCS §1396.
4. United States Code Service (1993). Social Security Act. Title XVIII. Health insurance for the aged and disabled: Prohibition against any federal interference. 42 USCS §1395.
5. United States Code Service (1989). Chapter 33. Education of the handicapped. 20 USCS §1400-1485.
6. United States Code Service (1994). Chapter 75. Programs for persons with developmental disabilities. 42 USCS §6000-6083.
7. United States Code Service (1993). Social Security Act. Title XVI. Supplemental security income for the aged, blind, and disabled. 42 USCS §1381-1385.
8. United States Code Service (1992). Veterans benefits. 38 USCS §101-8528.
9. Sacramento County Department of Education (1993). Sacramento County SELPA Presents. A Parent's Guide to Special Education. Sacramento, Department of Education.
10. United States Department of Veterans Affairs (1996). Federal Benefits for Veterans and Dependents. Washington, D.C., Department of Veterans Affairs.

BIBLIOGRAPHY

California Department of Health Services (1988). AFDC Recipient Handbook. (Department of Health Services Publication 62). Sacramento, Department of Health Services.

California Department of Health Services (1993). Fact Sheet: In-Home Medical Care (IHMC) Waiver Program. Sacramento, Department of Health Services.

California Department of Health Services (1993). Fact Sheet: Model Waiver Program. Sacramento, Department of Health Services.

California Department of Health Services (1993). Fact Sheet: Skilled Nursing Facility (SNF) Waiver Program. Sacramento, Department of Health Services.

California Department of Health Services (1994). Medi Cal: What It Means to You. Department of Health Services Publication No. 6/n94. Sacramento, Department of Health Services, p. 68.

Civilian Health and Medical Program of the Department of Veterans Affairs (1996). CHAMPVA Handbook. Washington, D.C., Department of Veterans Affairs, U.S. Government Printing Office.

Civilian Health and Medical Program of the Uniformed Services (1994). CHAMPUS Handbook (1994). Washington, D.C., U.S. Government Printing Office.

Civilian Health and Medical Program of the Uniformed Services (1991). CHAMPUS Regulations Manual DOD. 6010.8R. Washington, D.C., Department of Defense.

Clark MM (1996). The many forms of function. Case Review 2(1):72–78.

Clemen-Stone S, et al (1995). Comprehensive Community Health Nursing: Family Aggregate and Community Practice, 4th ed. St. Louis, Mosby-Year Book, pp. 116–124.

Foundation Health Federal Services (1996). TRICARE PRIME. Member Handbook.

Health Care Financing Administration (1996). Medicare Hospice Benefits. (Publication No. HCFA 02154). Washington, D.C., U.S. Department of Health and Human Services.

Health Care Financing Administration (1992). Medicare and Other Health Benefits: Who Pays First? (Publication No. 110 HCFA 02179). Washington, D.C., U.S. Department of Health and Human Services.

Health Care Financing Administration (1996). Your Medicare Handbook. (Publication No. HCFA-10050). Washington, D.C., U.S. Department of Health and Human Services.

National Association of Insurance Commissioners and the Health Care Financing Administration (1996). 1996 Guide to Health Insurance for People with Medicare. (Publication No. HCFA-02110). Washington, D.C., U.S. Department of Health and Human Services.

Reis J (1990). Medicaid maternal and child health care: Prepaid plans vs. private fee-for-services. Res Nurs Health 13(3):163–171.

Smith SM, Maurer FA (1995). Community Health Nursing Theory and Practice. Philadelphia, W.B. Saunders, pp. 124–131.

Social Security Administration (1984). When You Get SSI: What You Need to Know. (SSA Publication No. 05-11011). Washington, D.C., U.S. Department of Health and Human Services.

Social Security Administration (1990). Understanding SSI. (SSA Publication No. 17-008). Washington, D.C., U.S. Department of Health and Human Services.

Social Security Administration (1993). A Guide to Social Security and SSI Disability Benefits for People with HIV Infection (SSA Publication No. 05-10020). Washington, D.C., U.S. Department of Health and Human Services, Social Security Administration.

Social Security Administration (1993). If You Are Blind: How Social Security and SSI Can Help. (SSA Publication No. 05-10052). Washington, D.C., U.S. Department of Health and Human Services, Social Security Administration.

Social Security Administration (1993). Medicare for People Who Have Permanent Kidney Failure. (SSA Publication No. 05-10013). Washington, D.C., U.S. Department of Health and Human Services.

Social Security Administration (1993). Retirement. (SSA Publication. No. 05-10035). Washington, D.C., U.S. Department of Health and Human Services.

Social Security Administration (1993). SSI. (SSA Publication No. 05-11000). Washington, D.C., U.S. Department of Health and Human Services.

Social Security Administration (1993). Survivors. (SSA Publication No. 05-10084). Washington, D.C., U.S. Department of Health and Human Services.

Social Security Administration (1994). Disability. (SSA Publication No. 05-10029). Washington, D.C., U.S. Department of Health and Human Services, Social Security Administration.

Social Security Administration (1994). How Social Security Can Help With Vocational Rehabilitation. (SSA Publication No. 05-10050). Washington, D.C., U.S. Department of Health and Human Services, Social Security Administration.

Social Security Administration (1994). Social Security...What Every Woman Should Know. (SSA Publication No. 05-10127). Washington, D.C., U.S. Department of Health and Human Services.

Social Security Administration (1994). SSI Fact Sheet. Washington, D.C., U.S. Department of Health and Human Services.

Social Security Administration (1994). Understanding Social Security. (SSA Publication No. 05-10024). Washington, D.C., U.S. Department of Health and Human Services.

Social Security Administration (1995). A Guide to Social Security and SSI Disability Benefits for People with HIV Infection (SSA Publication No. 05-10026). Washington, D.C., U.S. Department of Health and Human Services, Social Security Administration.

United States Code Service (1989). Chapter 33, Education of the handicapped. 20 USCS §1400–1485.

United States Code Service (1997). Chapter 44, Vocational Education. 20 USCS §2301–2471.

United States Code Service (1992). Veterans benefits. 38 USCS §1101–2305.

United States Code Service (1985). Title V. Maternal and child health services block grant. 42 USCS §701–731.

United States Code Service (1993). Social Security Act. Title XVIII. Health insurance for the aged and disabled: Prohibition against any federal interference. 42 USCS §1395.

United States Code Service (1993). Social Security Act. Title XIX. Grants to states for medical assistance programs, appropriations. 42 USCS §1396.

United States General Accounting Office (1993). Medicaid—States Turn to Managed Care to Improve Access and Control Costs.

Veterans Affairs, Department of (1996). Federal benefits for veterans and dependents. (Publication No. 80-96-1). Washington, D.C., Department of Veterans Affairs.

Chapter 5

Barriers to Effective Case Management

QUESTIONS TO BE ADDRESSED PRIOR TO DISCHARGE OF CASE-MANAGED PATIENTS

All too often cases requiring case management are so complex that discharge coordination and implementation of the case management plan are complicated by a variety of problems. Until these can be addressed and resolved, the patient usually requires prolonged hospitalization. If the patient is discharged before the problems are resolved, costly and unnecessary readmission or even deterioration in the patient's medical condition can ensue.

To ensure that all problems are identified, the case manager must interview all parties thoroughly. Certainly the questions need not be limited to the following examples. Case managers must develop their own lists of questions pertinent to the patients they serve and the resources they use. Also, as situations and events change, or as case variables become apparent, different questions may be needed. In general, the following questions are good examples of the sort of information that should be sought at any time for most patients.

1. Does the patient exhibit readiness for a move?
2. Will the quality of care be compromised if the patient is moved?
3. What level of care does the patient require?
4. Can care be provided by the family? If so, who will be the primary caregiver, and is training of this caregiver required?
5. Is a home health agency required? If so, does specialized staff need to be hired or trained, and how long will this process take? If this period will be lengthy, will the patient require interim placement?
6. If teaching is required, can it be completed by the home health agency or other health-care provider once it has been started without interrupting patient care, placing the patient at risk of rehospitalization or decreasing the quality of care?
7. Is out-of-home placement required? If so:
   a. Is it available locally?
   b. What level of placement is required:
      (1) Acute rehabilitation?
      (2) Postrehabilitation?
      (3) Extended care facility (ECF) or subacute facility care?
      (4) Skilled nursing facility (SNF) or skilled nursing unit (SNU)?
      (5) Intermediate care facility (ICF)?
      (6) Residential care?
      (7) Board and care?
      (8) Other (i.e., foster home)?
   c. If placement is not available locally, will the family accept out-of-area placement? If they will:
      (1) Where are the needed facilities located?
      (2) Can the facility accept a patient with the level of care required by this patient?
      (3) Is there a waiting list?
      (4) If there is a waiting list, what is the interim plan?
      (5) If an out-of-area provider is required, will the staff require training? If so, who will do the training and how long will it take? Can the patient remain at the current level of care until all plans are in place? If not, where will care be provided?
      (6) If the provider is a non-network provider for the patient's healthcare payor plan, is it willing to work with the healthcare payor's case manager and accept a negotiated rate?
8. Despite the ultimate placement (home or facility), what other supportive services or agencies are required? If other services are required are they available locally?
9. Does the patient require technologically complex equipment? If so:
   a. Is it available or must it be specially ordered?
   b. If the equipment can only be special ordered, what is necessary, and how much time will elapse from order to delivery?
   c. Can the equipment be secured from the usual durable medical equipment sources? If not, is it available from a loan closet (donated equipment or supplies that are available from a church or service organization or some disease-specific agencies at no cost to the patient) or other source?
   d. Does the patient require customized equipment, and if so, how long will it be before it is available?
   e. If the equipment must be customized and is not yet available, is suitable alternate equipment available for rental or loan in the interim?
   f. Will the family or professionals require training in the use of the equipment prior to discharge?
   g. If training is necessary, how long will it take?

h. If training in the use of the equipment is required prior to discharge, will the durable medical equipment company deliver the equipment to the hospital? (If early delivery is required, the patient and family should be told that reimbursement from most healthcare payors does not start until the day of discharge.)

i. Will the professional staff or the caregiver require training? If so, how much, and what type is required? How long will it take? Has training been started?

10. Is the patient or family accepting of the idea of high-technology home care? If home care is not an alternative, are the patient and family agreeable to out-of-home placement?

11. If the patient is discharged to home:

a. Is it adequate to meet the patient's needs?

b. Are there structural barriers? If so:

(1) What are the actual barriers?

(2) Can they be modified or corrected?

(3) How long will it take to make the necessary corrections?

(4) If barrier correction is extensive, what is the interim plan for the patient's care?

(5) Does the family have the money to make the changes? If not, are fund raisers or donations necessary? If so, how long will this process take before money is available and the barriers are corrected?

(6) If money is available for correcting barriers, who will do the work required, and how long will the process take?

(7) Does the patient or family need special instructions to overcome the barriers if they are minor and require no correction? If so, who will assume responsibility for this teaching to ensure that the barriers are negotiated correctly?

12. To ensure a safe discharge to home, are other arrangements necessary? If so:

a. What are they?

b. Is it necessary to make contact with the utility company in the event of a power outage? Is back-up battery equipment or a power generator necessary? Who must be contacted if a power outage extends over a prolonged period of time? Does the patient qualify for reduced utility rates? If reduced rates are available, who must be contacted to arrange these rates, and what other procedures are necessary to ensure that this reduction occurs?

c. Is it necessary to make contact with the local paramedics if the patient is likely to experience frequent life-threatening situations, and will these events require paramedical attention and transportation?

d. Is it necessary to make contact with the local health officer or public health department to report infectious conditions or to obtain information?

13. Who has been identified as the primary caregiver? If the caregiver has been selected:

a. Has training of this person been started?

b. If training has not been started, who will actually assume the responsibility for the training, and how long will the training last?

c. Once the training has been "completed," what plans have been made for monitoring the teaching-learning cycle and for keeping abreast of any ongoing training needs?

14. Is there a need for a back-up caregiver? If so:

a. Has the alternate caregiver been selected?

b. Has training of this person been started?

c. If not, when will this training begin and how long will it take?

15. If the family is unable to provide care, has a professional agency or nursing staff been selected to provide the care? If the patient or family must assume any out-of-pocket costs, have these been addressed? (This step is necessary because if the patient requires custodial care, most healthcare payors will not reimburse the costs of this type of care. Many healthcare policies require copayments or cost shares that are the responsibility of the patient or family, and many impose limits on the number of home health agency visits or amounts they will reimburse.) When benefits are limited, excluded, or exhausted, the family must be prepared to assume these costs; if this is the case, has the situation been discussed thoroughly with the patient and family to ensure their willingness and ability to assume such expenditures?

16. Are the caregivers mentally and physically capable of assuming the caregiver role?

17. Is respite care required? If so:

a. Who will provide it?

b. How frequently will it be required?

c. Does the respite caregiver require training?

d. What is the cost of such respite care, and who will assume it?

18. Does the patient require medications? If so:

a. Is teaching of administration techniques, side effects, and contraindications required?

b. Are any special steps necessary to procure the drugs (e.g., if the patient is limited to a certain pharmacy network, can the medications be obtained locally)?

c. Are medications required on a short-term or long-term basis? If long-term, can the patient use a mail order pharmacy to obtain the drugs at a discount, with door-to-door delivery and reduced out-of-pocket expenses? If a mail order pharmacy is needed, is one available within the healthcare payor's network? If not, are the cost savings significant enough that it would be worthwhile to undertake the extra contractual process to use a national mail order pharmaceutical company?

19. Does the patient have specific dietary or nutritional needs that require:

a. Teaching of administration techniques (e.g., spoon feeding, self-feeding with assistive devices, tube feeding, special positioning)?

b. Instructions about special diet or formula preparation?

c. Assistance in procuring formulas or solutions?

d. Procurement of the formula if it is excluded from healthcare payor coverage? If so, what arrangements or family education is necessary to ensure procurement (e.g., identification of procurement sources; and can the family make the formula following instructions from a nutritional specialist or dietitian)?

20. Does the patient have special care needs that require teaching for:

a. Treatments or application of medications or ointments.

b. Dressing changes or wound care.

c. Transfers or repositioning.

d. Self-help skills.

e. Restorative therapy.

f. Respiratory or ventilator care.

g. Suctioning.

h. Caregiver body mechanics.

i. Infusion medications, solutions, and site care.

j. Tube feedings.

k. Special diets.

l. Clean versus sterile technique.

m. Care of tubing (e.g., Foley catheter, feeding tubes, intravenous tubing, suction catheters).

(1) If so, what steps are necessary to ensure that the patient, family, and caregiver are trained?

(2) Are arrangements in place to ensure that the patient, family, and caregiver are given adequate time to master the care techniques required?

n. Cardiopulmonary resuscitation.

21. If the patient is to be discharged to another facility (e.g., SNF or SNU):

a. Is it adequate to meet the patient's needs?

b. Is there a designated area for patients in need of skilled care?

c. Are there adequate numbers of professional registered nurses or licensed vocational or practical nurses (RNs, LVNs, or LPNs) and other staff on all shifts to administer the level of care required?

d. Is specialized or patient-specific training necessary prior to the move? If so, how long will it take to adequately train the facility staff? (The cost of this type of training is not always reimbursable by the healthcare payor.)

e. If therapy is required, how often is it available and who provides it—professional therapists or trained therapy aides?

f. Will extra equipment or supplies be necessary? If so, are they readily available when reordering is necessary?

g. Will the facility assume responsibility for billing the healthcare payor directly? If not:

(1) Is the family responsible for paying and submitting claims to the healthcare payor?

(2) If payment is required by the family, are funds available, or is a delay in securing these funds expected? Has application been made for Medicaid?

h. Is it known whether the facility will cooperate with the healthcare payor or case management organization? Is there a case manager available at the receiving facility to coordinate ongoing care?

i. Is the facility open to negotiation of a rate reduction if it is a non-network facility for the healthcare payor?

22. What other financial options or resources must be explored?
    a. Have the patient and family been apprised of all alternate funding programs to which they are entitled, and have they applied for these? Have the patient and family been apprised of unemployment benefits, and have they applied for these? Has the availability of all other healthcare payors been explored?

23. Are there other community resources that must be involved or that the family should be aware of?

24. Have all agencies been given clear instructions or sufficient medical information on which they can base their plan of care?

COMMON BARRIERS TO DISCHARGE

The discharge of many patients with certain diagnoses involves specific barriers that are common to each, and these are described in the various sections of Chapter 10 in this manual. However, in many cases, discharge is specifically linked to deficits in the healthcare delivery system. A wide variety of problems may be encountered in this category, among them:

1. The quality of care may be compromised if the patient is moved, placing the healthcare organization at risk of litigation.
2. Alternate care costs are prohibitive.
3. Out-of-pocket expenses are prohibitive, and delays in screening for eligibility for alternate funding have been encountered.
4. A home is available, but structural or electrical barriers that could be modified are not completed or were not identified in a timely fashion; alternatively, there may be environmental or other conditions or case variables that make discharge to home unacceptable.
5. Problems are encountered pertinent to nursing care and discharge to home, for example:
    a. A caregiver is not available, or is repulsed at the sight of the patient's condition, or is intolerant of the patient's illness.
    b. A caregiver is available, but there is no back-up, and because care is needed over a long term, the primary caregiver will require respite.
    c. The caregiver requires teaching before the patient is discharged.
    d. Barriers have been identified but have not been corrected.
    e. A physician is not available or willing to assume responsibility for the patient's care.
    f. The equipment required is not available for use outside the acute care facility, or the distance between the provider and the patient's home is too great during inclement weather.
    g. Local agencies or resources are not available or are unwilling to assume responsibility for managing the level of care required.
    h. An agency is available, but:
        (1) Staffing is limited.
        (2) Nurses are available but require specialized or patient-individualized training.
    i. The patient's or family's emotions, perception, stress or role reversal, inability to read and comprehend, visual impairment, altered coping abilities, or physical limitations inhibit or preclude discharge.
    j. The level of care recommended for the patient is beyond that considered by the medical community as the standard of care for the condition or that considered the standard of care outside the acute care facility.
6. Problems are encountered pertinent to placement, for example:
    a. No alternative facility is available (due to lack of beds, lengthy waiting list, inadequate staffing, severity or acuteness of patient's condition, or presence of contagious disease or condition).
    b. The move will impose social isolation on the patient.
7. Other barriers frequently encountered include the following:
    a. Because a conservator is required prior to any move and the conservatorship proceedings have not been started or completed, the patient cannot be moved until a final or temporary conservator has been appointed.
    b. The patient or family refuses placement alternatives.
    c. The physician refuses placement alternatives.
    d. The patient is in an abusive situation that requires intervention or investigation.
    e. Cultural, ethnic, perceptual, or language barriers are present that preclude or delay

the move or an understanding of the situation.

f. The patient or family has other responsibilities or priorities.

g. The patient lacks motivation for compliance or follow through.

h. The patient or family has had an unpleasant experience with a specific provider or agency, and another must be located.

SUMMARY

Other problems or barriers than those previously mentioned may be present because each case has its own variables. However, as these various issues are identified, their impact on case planning must be taken into account and included in the case management plan as it is developed and implemented. Because the greatest challenge to implementation of timely services and resources is the presence of discharge barriers, it behooves the case manager to stay constantly attuned to ways to minimize

or eliminate them whenever possible. If such barriers or difficult situations are not dealt with or corrected, costly delays and, more important, a compromise in the quality of care may result.

OVERCOMING BARRIERS TO CASE MANAGEMENT

Some of the most common barriers encountered are included in this section, which can be used as a guide in working through the kind of problems facing case managers (Fig. 5-1). The examples given by no means constitute an all-inclusive list, nor will the suggestions given here work in all situations. In fact, in some cases no solution may be possible (e.g., long waiting lists, nonexistent providers, family conflicts, nonexistent financial alternatives or ineligibility of patient or family for alternate funding, resulting in inability to pay privately for services). Unfortunately, in such cases the pa-

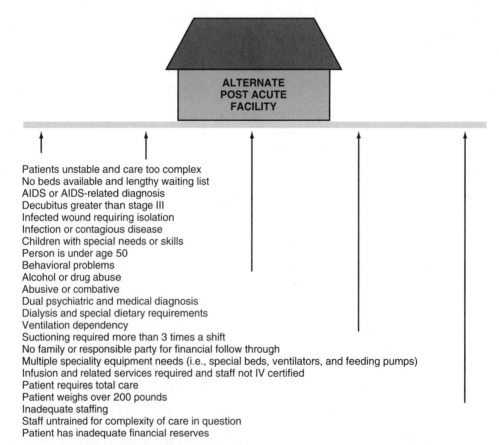

ALTERNATE
POST ACUTE
FACILITY

Patients unstable and care too complex
No beds available and lengthy waiting list
AIDS or AIDS-related diagnosis
Decubitus greater than stage III
Infected wound requiring isolation
Infection or contagious disease
Children with special needs or skills
Person is under age 50
Behavioral problems
Alcohol or drug abuse
Abusive or combative
Dual psychiatric and medical diagnosis
Dialysis and special dietary requirements
Ventilation dependency
Suctioning required more than 3 times a shift
No family or responsible party for financial follow through
Multiple speciality equipment needs (i.e., special beds, ventilators, and feeding pumps)
Infusion and related services required and staff not IV certified
Patient requires total care
Patient weighs over 200 pounds
Inadequate staffing
Staff untrained for complexity of care in question
Patient has inadequate financial reserves

Figure 5–1 • Barriers to placement for high-tech, high-cost patients.

tient's case must be closed to case management because nothing further can be offered.

In all cases, families and patients must be kept informed about all issues and problems and the resolution (or lack of resolution) of these problems. If the ultimate choice is to close the case, the patient and family must be made aware of this decision. In this situation, they must be given the phone numbers of key persons or agencies that can be called when the case is closed and they encounter difficulty in obtaining access to agencies or resources or when the patient's condition deteriorates.

One of the keys to overcoming case management barriers is to keep as current as possible on such matters as the capabilities of the various resources and national standards of care. Case managers must also keep informed about their own organization's position on various important issues (e.g., capitation agreements and which providers can or cannot be used, the extra contractual process, and the use of non-network providers). How does one do this? It may be necessary to:

1. Join a local, state, or national organization involved with continuity of care or case management for networking purposes.
2. Keep an up-to-date list of the names and numbers of key contacts in a personal reference file.
3. Maintain a list of key networking and provider contacts in the community who can provide pertinent and expert information.
4. Maintain a list of key provider agencies or alternate funding program supervisors. This may include their direct phone numbers or those for specific persons in an organization when immediate access is required.
5. Keep abreast of current continuity of care practices, the standards of care for the most common procedures or diagnoses in a caseload, legislation relevant to continuity of care, changes in resources or resource capabilities, and the usual and customary costs of services in the community. The best resources for this information are publications, directories, nursing journals, newsletters, seminars, conferences, interviews with key healthcare specialists, and networking contacts.
6. Participate in local provider or agency boards, utilization review committees, or other key planning committees in the community. These contacts provide opportunities for networking and for identifying (and

eliminating) gaps in the continuity of care process.
7. Learn to be a good listener, taking notes and acting promptly when necessary.
8. Learn how to expect and anticipate the patient's or family's needs and act promptly on identified issues.
9. Learn to be innovative and creative in finding solutions to problems. As long as the end product satisfies the original request, accomplishes the goal, and produces the quality and services required, do not be afraid to try other, more unconventional processes! Likewise, allow the patient to be creative as well.
10. Maintain a resource library (e.g., nursing articles, provider brochures) for reference on pertinent patient care techniques, continuity of care requirements, and resource capabilities.
11. If necessary, encourage or set up brown bag lunches or meetings with various key provider or community healthcare professionals, continuity of care professionals, or other groups to allow information sharing. This process also aids in keeping one's personal reference files current.
12. Remain informed about the facts pertinent to the caseload, primarily by reading and maintaining good communication links with other healthcare team professionals or colleagues.
13. Improve and maintain confidence in the basic case manager's skills, which include, at a minimum, (1) clinical competence, (2) competent knowledge of community resources and entitlements, (3) strong advocacy skills, (4) strong abstract and analytical thinking skills, and (5) an ability to be flexible, creative, and innovative.
14. Maintain a positive attitude about yourself, managed care, your organization, and cost containment.
15. Most important, take care of yourself! How do you do this? Learn a hobby, take up a special project, develop interests outside work, and try to forget about work and the patients in a caseload for a period of time.

There are certainly other ways to overcome barriers. Above all, do not be intimidated by the difficulties or afraid to try new solutions, since no two cases are alike. Therefore, what was successful for one patient may not be possible for another!

The following examples of problems and possible solutions offer guidance in overcoming some of the barriers that are frequently encountered in case management. Although many of the following problems and strategies are pertinent to a healthcare payor's case manager, many others are not and can be used by any case manager involved with the case.

PROBLEM: The provider or family knows nothing about case management and does not understand the role.

Strategy A: Physician or Provider

1. Make contact with all physicians or providers involved with the patient's care as early as possible.
2. Introduce yourself and offer a brief, concise explanation of the organization's case management role.
3. Use a brochure, introductory or explanatory letter, or a business card when appropriate.
4. Make face-to-face contact with all parties as frequently as possible.

Strategy B: Patient or Family

1. Introduce yourself as early as possible in an onsite visit or on the phone if a personal visit is not possible.
2. Explain in a concise manner, using lay terminology, what case management is, what its goals are, and how it works.
3. Write an introductory or explanatory letter and send a business card.
4. Provide a phone number and list the hours of availability of case management services.
5. Use good public relations skills to develop rapport and trust with the patient and the family.
6. Speak in the language of a patient advocate and avoid use of medical terminology and the terms used in utilization review.
7. Establish a schedule for providing updates and making routine phone calls. This is extremely important if the family lives out of the area or is working and is unable to take time off for face-to-face conferences.
8. Encourage the patient or family to become an active part of the team. Again, even for families who live out of the area, teleconferences are a means of including them in the planning.
9. Keep the lines of communication open, honest, and frequent. Most important, continue to use terminology that is at the patient's or family's level (this may include using appropriate interpreters occasionally). No less important as communication is the need to keep the patient or family informed and involved in the decision-making process.
10. Be accessible, returning phone messages as promptly as possible.
11. Teach the patient and family how to use and obtain access to community resources and inform them of their entitlement to specific programs.
12. Be honest, and do not promise or portray services as indefinitely available or foster a "right of expectancy."

PROBLEM: The physician perceives the case manager as the adversary because he or she confuses the case management process with that of utilization review.

Strategy:

1. If at all possible, do not combine the duties of utilization review and case management into one role. If both functions are performed by the same person, carefully identify questions that are being asked for case management planning purposes rather than for utilization review needs.
2. Maintain a positive proactive role.
3. Rely on the case management organization's medical director for direction or assistance if the patient's attending physician refuses to cooperate.
4. Use the primary care physician or family to "sell" case management to the physician when this is appropriate and they are aware of the advantages of case management.
5. Speak in the language of patient advocacy, avoiding the terminology and actions of utilization review whenever possible.
6. Be savvy about patient care needs and community resources.

PROBLEM: The attending physician is inaccessible to case management or is unwilling to cooperate.

Strategy:

1. Be brief, concise, and well prepared in all contacts with the physician; limit calls or contacts to those that are imperative to allow action. Avoid hostile confrontations, making use of public relations skills and keeping calm.
2. Develop rapport with the office staff, if possible, to gain access to the physician.

3. If necessary, case managers can use their organization's medical director for assistance.

PROBLEM: The physician, provider, or family believes that case management can authorize any services to meet the patient's needs because the services they want were offered to another patient.

Strategy:

1. Be savvy about the actual needs of the patient.
2. Clarify the case management organization's philosophy regarding its services, role, and policy guidelines. If necessary, explain how other healthcare professionals can assist in the extra contractual process if this process is required for approval of the desired benefits.
3. Use assessment, abstract, or analytical thinking skills to avoid being unduly influenced by the description of the patient's needs.
4. Request the physician to submit in writing all facts that support the medical necessity and justify the need for the items or services in question.
5. Use good communication skills to present the case details to the healthcare payor's medical director for approval or denial.

PROBLEM: The local physician is unable or unwilling to accept responsibility for care.

Strategy:

1. Ascertain whether there are other physicians in the general vicinity who can possibly assume care. If so, call or discuss the possibility of this with the office nurse or with the physician directly.
2. Ask the specialty physician to call and speak directly with the local physician to clarify the special care required.
3. Call the nearest emergency room and ascertain what their capabilities are if the local physician is unwilling to assume the care.
4. Ensure that the patient, family, or caregiver is trained and proficient in giving all care necessary for any condition that has the potential to trigger the need for a physician or emergency room visit between discharge and the time the patient is seen again by the specialty physician or treatment team.
5. Place the patient in a skilled nursing facility or other facility that can administer the appropriate level of care. Such placement may be either a long-term or short-term situation

(e.g., until the patient is medically stable or until the patient and family have mastered all necessary care techniques).

PROBLEM: Hospital chart is consistently inaccessible, but the information is required to establish the ongoing case management plan and treatment program for the patient.

Strategy:

1. Ask the patient or legal guardian to sign a form authorizing the release of information. Become familiar with the organization's rights to gain access to the chart, especially if the case manager represents a healthcare payor, who has the potential power to deny claims when concurrent review or case management cannot be performed.
2. Call and speak directly with the hospital's head nurse, utilization review nurse, discharge planner, or clinical nurse specialist to arrange a specific time for a review or an onsite visit to collect the necessary details.
3. Call and speak directly with the clinical nurse specialist or other pertinent staff person to discuss the need for the chart or schedule a case conference.
4. If access remains a problem, arrange to have pertinent sections of the patient's medical record copied and either sent or picked up in person.
5. Carry introductory letter, business card, or identification badge at all times.
6. Establish regular communication with and use public relations skills to develop rapport with the utilization review department, discharge planners, and other key departments.
7. Use every opportunity to educate key departments and other staff members about the case management services offered and how these services can expedite the patient's care and increase satisfaction. If necessary, share with them successful case histories of patients in case management.
8. Arrange for an inservice training session with the business office or other staff to educate them about the importance of other case managers on the case, the processes involved in case management, and why data are needed and important in case management.
9. Attend patient care conferences as often as time allows or as needed. If attendance is not possible, ask that notes from these conferences be prepared and submitted for review.

PROBLEM: Too many people are performing the same tasks (e.g., discharge planner, social worker, facility-based case manager, community-based case manager, healthcare payor case manager).

Strategy:

1. Clarify the roles of all personnel involved in the case.
2. Introduce yourself early in the case not only to the discharge planner, social worker, or facility-based case manager but also to other key professionals involved in the case.
3. Demonstrate clinical competence and knowledge of the community, regional or national resources, and the patient's entitlement to services or agencies.
4. Establish regular and frequent communication with the facility-based healthcare team.
5. Determine early and communicate to all involved who will be responsible for discharge planning and the role to be played by each of the others.
6. If case management is conducted by the healthcare payor and the discharge process is conducted by the hospital discharge planner, it may be necessary to render assistance to ensure that all steps occur in a timely manner, that both the healthcare provider and the rates are acceptable, and that all benefits and limitations or exclusions have been communicated to the patient and family.
7. If case management is conducted by a community-based organization, the access capabilities of this organization and the level of involvement of this case manager with the discharge process must be determined as early as possible.
8. Avoid duplication of effort whenever possible by clearly describing each person's duties, especially if a case manager, discharge planner, or social worker is involved.
9. Be flexible and accessible. Demonstrate your value by becoming very familiar with community, state, and national resources and relaying this information as quickly as possible. If employed by a healthcare payor, know the patient's benefits, limits, and exclusions as well as any provider restrictions, and again, relay this information in an expeditious manner.
10. Return phone calls promptly.
11. Be concise and specific if requests are made for additional information.
12. Become familiar with the capabilities of other discharge planners or case managers in the area; share information with them and use them as resource persons as often as necessary.
13. Make face-to-face contact as frequently as possible with the facility staff in the area. If employed by a facility, make contact with the case managers of the healthcare payors or community agencies you deal with regularly.
14. If the case management is conducted by a healthcare payor, have approvals ready for post-discharge needs. If a potential denial is anticipated, communicate this fact early enough to allow the other case managers to explore and prepare alternatives.

PROBLEM: Limited or nonexistent resources pose barriers to discharge or access to care.

Strategy: Facility-Based Case Manager

1. Allow the nonfacility-based case manager to be an active participant in the case management planning process, coordinating case management plans as required to avoid duplication and fragmentation.
2. Keep the lines of communication open to clarify patient care needs to the healthcare payor's or community-based case manager as soon as they are identified to ensure that benefit coverage is possible or that the healthcare agency can assume the responsibility for care.
3. Assist the healthcare payor's or community-based case manager in gathering information to ensure tht all ongoing care needs are met or that the extra contractual process can be used if benefits for the care required are limited or excluded.
4. Schedule case conferences and interviews as necessary to resolve any questionable issues or educate the patient, family, or healthcare team about any problems involving healthcare benefits or patient care needs.
5. Keep the lines of communication open and be honest with the patient and family about any barriers encountered. Include the patient and family in any case conferences whenever possible.
6. Maintain a proactive approach with the patient or family if placement out of the area is required, pointing out the positive benefits of such placement, such as maintaining

the quality of care and meeting the patient's needs.

7. Be honest with all providers and transmit accurate and pertinent information about the patient's care and needs. This allows the provider to make sound judgments about the patient and the case, which ultimately ensure a smooth transition, continuity of care, and maintenance of the quality of care.
8. Early in the case, discuss the possibility of encountering problems in gaining access to resources. Ascertain whether the family is willing and able to assume care at home as an alternate plan if placement difficulties are anticipated. If home is to be the placement objective, start any necessary teaching as soon as this is known. If the original plan for discharge was to have been the home but problems are encountered in achieving this goal, seek the family's approval for placement and their cooperation in achieving it.

Strategy: Healthcare Payor's Case Manager

1. Monitor placement and referral processes closely to discover problems and, when these are identified, to offer alternatives, if this is appropriate and agreeable with the discharge planner.
2. Assist the discharge planner as necessary when barriers to discharge or problems with access to care are encountered.
3. Identify possible barriers as early in the case as possible and work with the family and the healthcare team to identify alternative solutions.
4. Maintain lists of community, regional, and national resources, noting current phone numbers, names of key personnel, and information about their capabilities.
5. Assist the discharge planner as requested by calling providers to discuss the care needs of the patient and the providers' capacity and willingness to assume responsibility for care for the amount that will be reimbursed.
6. Keep communication lines with the healthcare team open so that all parties remain apprised of the actions taken or any barriers to healthcare coverage that are encountered.

Strategy: Community-Based Case Manager

1. Communicate to all parties as early in the case as possible the agency's responsibilities for case management.

2. Be open and honest about the agency's capabilities and requirements.
3. Keep communication lines with all parties open so that everyone is aware of any problems or issues that may affect the discharge planning process.

PROBLEM: The healthcare provider selected does not meet quality standards or issues affecting quality of care arise or are identified after referral.

Strategy:

1. Be savvy about patient needs, and make use of strong analytical skills.
2. Discuss the issues identified with the provider administrator and seek to have a corrective plan of action implemented immediately.
3. In any conversations with the family ask simple questions about their opinion of the care provided, encouraging a frank discussion of the issues identified.
4. Report all details to the quality management or improvement department of your organization so that the problem can be monitored and a plan of action can be drawn up.
5. Discuss major infractions (e.g., abuse, sexual advances, intoxication) with your immediate supervisor, if necessary, taking actions required by law for reporting of certain situations.
6. Research other similar providers to ascertain their capabilities for care. If the family and patient agree, transfer the care to another provider if necessary.
7. Depending on the infraction of the standard of care, make any necessary reports to the appropriate agencies.
8. The quality management or improvement department may desire to conduct random checks or patient satisfaction surveys on all providers used.

PROBLEM: The provider selected is unable to meet the patient's needs.

Strategy:

1. Become familiar with the capabilities of most providers in the community (both network and non-network). This knowledge is often gained through networking with peers.
2. Evaluate the capabilities or availability of re-

sources in the community early in the planning phase.

3. Keep the family or patient apprised of any problems encountered. Educate them and gain their approval for either an out-of-area move, should it become necessary, or its opposite, a plan for discharge to home, if satisfactory placement cannot be found.

4. Be honest with all providers, transmitting accurate and pertinent information about the case. This allows the providers to make sound judgments that will ensure a smooth transition and continuity of care.

5. If applicable, discuss the feasibility of special training of the staff with the provider's administrator. If agreeable, ascertain the length of time the training is expected to take and any other details required to accomplish the task.

6. Search for other providers to ascertain whether they are able to meet and manage the level of care the patient needs.

7. If the provider is unable to provide this level of care, explore the possible use of a non-network provider. Initiate whatever steps are required to allow non-network use (i.e., use of the extra contractual process, review with the healthcare payor's medical director or senior management).

PROBLEM: A caregiver is not available or trainable, or is unwilling to be trained.

Strategy:

1. Assess the patient's needs as early as possible to determine the complexity of care needed and the extent of teaching that will be required. Similarly, assess the family's or caregiver's capabilities (e.g., availability and mental and physical abilities).

2. If there is no one in the family who can assume the role, explore the patient's or family's financial ability to pay privately for these services. Such assessment is necessary when the required level of caregiver services is limited or excluded from the patient's healthcare benefit package.

3. Explore the feasibility of establishing caregiver reimbursement through the extra contractual process. If case management is originating from the healthcare payor, the initiative and direction of the information required may rest with this case manager (all other case managers involved with the case may play a role in the information gathering process, but they will be directed by the

healthcare payor's case manager if their assistance is required). If the extra contractual process is required and the healthcare payor's case manager is not involved with the case, the facility-based case manager must initiate the request to the healthcare payor, following any instructions given by the healthcare payor's personnel.

4. If the patient or family is unable to pay privately for the care required, they should be encouraged to explore all alternate sources of funding for which they may qualify. In cases requiring attendant care, one primary resource the family may wish to explore is Supplemental Security Income. In cases involving children, the family should be encouraged to explore the Title V Children's Medical Services program or the agency responsible for handling services for the developmentally disabled. Also, any other health insurance policies the patient might have should be explored.

5. If the patient is not eligible for alternate funding, the patient or family must be encouraged to seek volunteer caregivers among friends or community resources such as churches or ethnic or social service agencies.

6. If a caregiver still cannot be found, placement in the least restrictive environment that can manage the level of care required may be the only other alternative.

PROBLEM: Family conflicts arise about discharge planning, patient care decisions, or money or the cost of care.

Strategy:

1. Schedule a meeting at which all family members are present.

2. Present the issues and seek to find a solution in an open discussion involving all participants present.

3. Have the family identify one person who will act as spokesperson to convey the family's decisions on any issues that are causing the infighting.

4. At the conclusion of the conference, send a written confirmation of all details to all parties.

PROBLEM: Funds are limited or nonexistent, and the patient or family does not qualify for any alternate funding or public entitlement programs.

Strategy:

1. Explore the family's finances and financial ability to pay for care as early in the case as possible.
2. Be open and honest with the family and the patient about the needed resources, their cost, and the family's or patient's responsibility for payments (e.g., copayments, deductibles, or amounts due when benefit coverage terminates or is denied).
3. Make referrals as early as possible to all alternate funding programs to which the patient is entitled and explore all other known insurance policies.
4. If the patient is deemed ineligible to receive assistance, conduct research of all community resources that could possibly provide the level of care needed—either at no charge or through use of a sliding scale based on the patient's or family's ability to pay.
5. Identify any financial restrictions early in the case, so that the entire healthcare team can explore alternative solutions with the patient and the family.
6. Explore creative options with the patient and family that hopefully may equal any proposed resources and can still meet the patient's care needs.

NOTE: This barrier is frequently the one most commonly encountered. Unfortunately, there are times when, despite all referrals and exploration of resources, no alternative package of financial help is available. In these situations, there is nothing more the case manager can do. In extreme cases, the ultimate choice may be to close the case to case management.

PROBLEM: Respite care is not available or is not reimbursable from the healthcare payor.

Strategy:

1. Explore with the caregiver all options for respite care (i.e., friends, other family members, financial ability to pay privately for such care).
2. Inquire at ethnic, church, and social service agencies for possible volunteers. If any are found, make arrangements to ensure that they are trained.
3. Seek or request approval of respite through use of the extra contractual process.
4. Explore all alternative funding programs to which the patient may be entitled in regard to their ability to provide respite care.

5. Explore with the family the possibility of short-term admission to a skilled nursing facility. If this option is possible, the healthcare payor, the family, or an alternate funding program must agree to the reimbursement of costs for this level of care.

PROBLEM: Delays in eligibility for alternate funding programs occur.

Strategy:

1. Early in the case ascertain the financial ability of the patient or family to pay for the services required.
2. Encourage referrals to all alternate funding programs to which the patient is eligible. If the patient and family are reluctant to make the referral, determine whether they need assistance.
3. Maintain a list of key names and phone numbers of personnel in alternate funding agencies that can be used when delays are encountered. It may be necessary to call to expedite assistance if the situation is urgent.
4. Reaffirm with the family or patient that the referral has been made, or request an update from them on the status of eligibility from time to time.
5. Become familiar with the appeal process and encourage the patient or family to exercise their appeal rights if necessary. Assist them as required in this process.

PROBLEM: The family members are not coping well or do not understand the situation, or they are too intimidated to function and desire the case manager to be their advocate. Advocacy may be warranted in a number of situations, for example, obtaining access to physicians and encouraging them to communicate with the patient and family or in a manner the patient and family can understand; making the initial referral phone call to the alternate funding program; communicating problems and issues to the healthcare team and relaying back to the patient or family any information they may need for decision-making; assisting the patient and family in appeal processes; and so forth.

Strategy:

1. Discuss all problems and issues with the patient and family, documenting their specific desires in the patient's record.
2. Communicate openly, honestly, and fre-

quently with the patient and family about any issues advocated on their behalf.

3. Make every attempt to include the patient or family in any sessions during which advocacy is carried out on their behalf. This allows them an opportunity to see the process at work and participate in the interactions that occur because they have someone who is serving as their mentor or guide until they can assume the responsibility themselves. Despite the fact that they have delegated the advocacy role to the case manager, they are the ultimate decision makers, and this fact must always be remembered by case managers.

4. Any situation in which advocacy is undertaken by the case manager (e.g., issues, results, and discussions with the patient or family and their reactions and instructions) must be documented in the patient's case management chart.

5. Recommend and encourage patients and families to join support groups where they can share experiences and learn first-hand how others have handled various similar issues.

Despite the fact that the responsibility of advocacy may have been delegated to the case manager, one should *always, always* ensure that the patient and family are the final decision makers. Their decisions and instructions must always be documented.

PROBLEM: Because there are too many case managers, care planning is fragmented, or the physicians are irritated by the constant need to repeat orders or instructions, or the patient, family, and physician are confused about who to call and when and for what purpose.

Strategy:

1. Whenever more than one case manager is involved in a case, all case managers must meet to talk about their responsibilities. A plan must be developed stating who will assume responsibility for what and within what time frame (collaboration is critical in effective case management). Also, the plan must include the recommended frequency of communication to apprise one another of any actions taken.

2. Develop the case management plan jointly to prevent fragmentation and duplication of care and actions.

3. Establish a point of contact (decide who will be the primary case manager). This person will pass on communication of new orders and instructions from physicians and will communicate information to and from the patient and family or providers.

4. Ensure that physicians, providers, patient, and family are aware of key case management contacts and phone numbers.

5. Document all actions taken in the patient's case management record.

NOTE: This delegation process by no means negates or minimizes any case manager's involvement; all case managers must continue to perform their duties as outlined by the organization they represent and their job description. This delegation process is strictly a means to ensure that the lines of communication remain open and that care planning actions are not duplicated or fragmented.

PROBLEM: The goals of the case manager's organization pose a conflict with meeting the goals of the patient and caring for his or her needs. Thus, as the patient's advocate, the case manager is in a quandary—on the one hand, he or she must try to do what is best for the patient, and on the other, what is best and expected by the employer.

Strategy:

1. Do not promise any services to the patient or family until clarification of the conflict is obtained from key individuals in the case management organization.

2. If necessary, evaluate community resources or alternate funding programs to ascertain whether there are alternative measures that can be implemented in this case.

3. Prepare documentation that supports the position taken on the issue. Documentation, at a minimum, should cover such areas as:
   a. Issue in dispute.
   b. Discussion of similar services allowed.
   c. Cost advantages to the organization should the disputed issue be approved or allowed.
   d. Cost disadvantages to the organization should the disputed issue be denied or should the organization maintain a firm position on the issue.

4. Schedule a meeting with key officials of the case management organization to present the case and reasoning behind the decision. If the issue remains unresolved, identify

what steps may be necessary to pursue the issue further.

5. In all cases, document the issue in conflict and outline recommendations and expected outcomes.

6. Depending on the nature of the conflict, careful consideration must be given to the level, scope, and frequency of communication with the patient or family during this time of dispute. This is frequently a judgment call; the key is not to place the case management organization in a litigious situation. Many times conflicts in this category (e.g., where organizational goals are different than those of the patient or family) are highly charged and emotional. As such, every precaution must be taken to protect oneself and one's organization and to avoid being placed in an adversarial role. In most situations involving conflicts of this type, the frequency of conversations with the patient and family is reduced, and the conversations themselves are kept very basic.

Unfortunately, in some situations the final decision of the case manager's organization on the issue will prevail. In these cases, the directive is to close the patient's case to case management. In other cases, the organization may require the case manager to continue monitoring the case but avoid any intervention techniques.

PROBLEM: The patient is noncompliant and abuses the healthcare payor's benefits through frequent use of the emergency room for nonemergent medical conditions, or displays drug-seeking behavior or patterns of physical abuse in the hope that the physical abuse will not be disclosed.

Strategy:

In most cases this type of problem is identified by the healthcare payor's case manager, but sometimes the hospital's case manager may discover such episodes as well (especially if the hospital is capitated for services and is responsible for payment of claims because it is "at risk"). In cases such as this the following sequence of events often occurs:

1. Regardless of who discovers the pattern of abusive use of the healthcare payor's benefits or suspected physical abuse, the two case managers must communicate to review the patient's medical record or claims history and prepare an action plan to try to correct the situation.

2. If review of the medical record or claims history supports abuse of benefits, or if the pattern of emergency room usage supports suspected physical abuse, discuss the situation and the action plans devised with a supervisor, medical director, or the organization's legal counsel to obtain their recommendations before taking any direct action with the patient.

   In the case of suspected physical abuse, discussion with the patient's primary care physician may be required. However, in most cases, direct reports to the agency responsible for handling abuse cases and to the case manager's organization's quality improvement department may be the only actions taken.

3. In cases involving overuse of medical services or emergency room care, discuss your concerns and findings with the patient and attempt to determine the reasons for the episodes. Offer assistance in locating other resources or alternative options to care.

4. Contact the primary care physician to obtain his or her cooperation and to discuss options for alternative care solutions and recommendations.

5. Review the findings with your supervisor, medical director, or the organization's legal counsel to obtain their recommendations and clarify the wording of the follow-up letter to the patient informing him or her of action plans. In some cases, the recommendation may be to "lock in" the patient to one primary care physician. In such cases prior approval of ALL medical care needs and pharmaceuticals must be secured by this physician.

6. Contact the claims supervisor or pharmacy director and ask to have all claims suspended to one claims analyst rather than undergoing automatic adjudication. In cases involving patients showing drug-seeking behavior, the automatic approval of drugs allowed at the pharmacy level may be removed, placing responsibility on the pharmacy to call the healthcare payor directly to obtain approval to fill the prescription. In some cases, the patient may be required to pay for the pharmaceuticals himself and then seek retroreimbursement from the healthcare payor for the cost of the drugs. In cases in which the patient is locked in to a specific ordering physician, claims will be paid only if the request is written with this physician's referral or prescription.

7. Call the patient back and discuss the health-care payor's position and the plans requiring prior approval and payment of future medical care needs.
8. Document all plans and expectations of the patient in the form of a written letter, sending the letter by registered mail to all parties.
9. If the patient continues to be noncompliant, the healthcare payor may have to terminate the patient's coverage. In these cases, all actions needed for this process usually rest with the healthcare payor's legal counsel.

PROBLEM: Because the patient's medical care is very complex, treatment planning would benefit from close coordination of care by a designated specialist instead of the family's primary care physician, who in many instances is a generalist. At other times the primary care physician is unwilling to assume responsibility for the patient's care (for example, when the patient has been discharged from a large tertiary care center after a complex procedure). These situations tend to occur in persons with AIDS, ventilator dependency or other complex respiratory care needs, spinal cord injury or other complex neurologic disorder, or in children with special needs.

Strategy:

1. Discuss the need for such an action plan with the current primary care physician and the family. If their consent is obtained, recommend a specialty care physician to the healthcare payor's case manager instead of the current primary care physician.
2. The healthcare payor's case manager may call the specialist most involved with the treatment planning to ascertain whether he or she is willing to assume the role of the patient's primary care physician. If the patient is currently in a tertiary care center and is returning to the immediate local community, it may be necessary to call local specialists to determine whether any of them are willing to serve as the primary care physician and assume the responsibility for the patient's care.
3. If the specialist concurs with the proposed plan of action, discuss the need and reasons for the recommendations with the medical director to gain approval of the action plan to switch primary care physicians on the case.
4. Notify the designee of the member services department of the change. This is necessary to ensure that the correct documentation is made in the patient's eligibility record if claims are to be adjudicated correctly.
5. The patient and all physicians on the case are notified of the change by phone and possibly also by letter.

✖ S U M M A R Y

Although barriers to discharge are addressed in many sections of this manual pertinent to specific diseases or injuries, this chapter was included to outline in more detail some of the more common barriers encountered, together with possible solutions. The barriers described here and the strategies suggested for coping with them are by no means all inclusive. Each case is different, and solutions that worked for one patient may not work for another. The key is to be flexible and maintain a positive attitude despite the number of hurdles one may have to jump as the patient is moved through the continuum of care.

BIBLIOGRAPHY

Anderson A (1996). Nurse physician interaction and job satisfaction. Nurs Manag 27(6):33-36.
Don't ask doctors to do what you can do yourself, physician recommends (1992). Case Manag Advisor 3(3):40-41.
Goka RS, Arakaki AH (1991). Centers of excellence: Choosing the appropriate rehabilitation center. J Ins Med 23(1):66-69.
Guide to Choosing A Nursing Home (1994). Publication No. HCFA-02174. Washington, DC, U.S. Department of Health and Human Services.
Matthews J (1990). Eldercare: Choosing and Financing Long Term Care. Berkeley, Nolo Press.
Matthews J (1993). Beat the Nursing Home Trap: A Consumer's Guide to Choosing and Financing Long Term Care. Berkeley, Nolo Press.
Morgan F, Jorgensen B (1996). Protect yourself with a rehabilitation services checkup. J Subacute Care Nov pp. 124-126.
Mullahy CM (1992). Ten ways you can improve your working relationship with physicians. Case Manag Advisor 3(16):81-82.
National Head Injury Foundation (1992). National Directory of Head Injury Rehabilitation Services (flyer) Washington, DC.
National Head Injury Foundation (1992). What to Look for When Selecting A Rehabilitation Facility: A Working Guide (flyer) Washington, DC.
Siegler EL, Whitney FW (1994). Nurse Physician Collaboration. New York, Springer Publishing Co.
Winn J, Sierra R (1991). Case Management: Cooperation Among Disciplines—A Social Work Perspective. Case Manag 23(4):258-260.
Q and A—Selecting and Monitoring Head Injury Rehabilitation Services (Learning Services flyer).

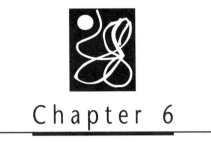

Chapter 6

Utilization Review

PURPOSE

The purpose of any utilization review process is to evaluate the medical necessity, appropriateness, and effectiveness of care while ensuring that all services are provided at the appropriate level of care. As stated earlier (see Chapter 1), case management in some organizations and for some healthcare payors is really nothing more than intensified utilization review. In other organizations, the duties of utilization review and case management are combined, and the staff is expected to perform both functions. This combination is unfortunate because the functions of both processes are separate and specialized fields. The best outcomes are achieved when utilization review and case management are kept separate and are performed by different departments in the organization.

The major difference between utilization review and case management is that utilization review monitors the length of stays, appropriateness of care, and medical necessity of the care rendered. In contrast, case management's primary purpose is to coordinate care across multiple points of service over a period of time. The ultimate goal is to maintain the quality of care by keeping the patient at the appropriate level of care, coordinating all existing healthcare policy benefits and community resources, and keeping costs to a minimum. "The overall goal of case management is to produce a service delivery approach to (a) ensure cost-effective care, (b) provide alternatives to institutionalization, (c) provide access to care, (d) coordinate service, and (e) improve the patient's functional capacity."[1] In addition, the American Nurses Association identifies the goals of case management to include the "provision of quality along a continuum, decrease fragmentation of care across many settings, enhance the quality of life and contain cost."[1] If the healthcare organization employs both a utilization review nurse and a case manager, it is very important for both parties to spend time orienting each other to their various job functions. This process not only helps to clarify roles, it also assists both persons in gaining an appreciation and understanding of one another and the duties required of each.

CASE MANAGEMENT AS INTENSIVE CARE UNIT

As more healthcare organizations "downsize," utilization review may be shifted to the case management department or vice versa. When this happens, little thought may be given to the qualifications and knowledge base needed by case managers to function effectively. Unfortunately, when a shift in duties occurs, one or another process may suffer.

True case management, if it is to achieve the outcomes desired, is a labor-intensive process. It requires a vast knowledge base not only of clinical medicine and treatment modalities but also of community resources, alternate funding programs, standards of care, and alternate treatment settings outside the acute care hospital. In all cases, action must be taken immediately if problems arise; they cannot wait until the nurse case manager or utilization reviewer has completed his or her duties. In today's litigious society, too much is at stake for the case manager and the organization if problems are not dealt with immediately.

To understand the relationship between case management and utilization review, it may be helpful to compare these two functions with the different kinds of hospital nursing. In this comparison, case management is equated with the intensive care unit and utilization review with the general medical-surgical unit. As we know, both units require different levels of expertise, with medical-surgical nursing being more generalized and critical care nursing more specialized. Nurses in both areas function similarly, but they have different emphases. The same statement is true of utilization review and case management.

Senior managers of healthcare organizations, like those in hospitals, must realize that case managers require more expertise if the goals of case management are to be reached and costs contained. To reach these goals, case managers must have the ability and flexibility to see patients and become involved with them as events evolve. Hospital general duty nurses do not just read charts and talk on the phone without seeing the patient—they are actively involved with all aspects of care. The same thing occurs with case managers. Unlike hospital nurses, however, case managers are not giving hands-on nursing care, but they must be able to visualize the actual care if the patient is to be linked appropriately with available resources. Therefore, on-site assessments are strongly advised.

CASE MANAGEMENT INVOLVING TWO COMPANIES

When two companies are involved, one for utilization review and the other for case management, or when one case manager is facility based and the other is employed by a nonfacility-based organization (e.g., healthcare payor or home health agency), two major problems can occur. These are (1) lack of timely sharing of information, resulting in delays in implementation of care, and (2) inappropriate delays in referral.[2]

The earlier the intervention occurs and the case is referred and opened to case management, the greater the opportunities for success. If more than one case manager and one utilization reviewer are involved, it is important for case managers to establish good working relationships with the entire team and to educate the referral sources about the importance of early referral and timely sharing of information.

TYPES AND CATEGORIES OF UTILIZATION REVIEW

Although this manual is not intended for utilization reviewers, the various types of utilization review and some of the criteria used for such review are worth mentioning. In most organizations, utilization review is closely related to quality improvement or performance. Both utilization review and quality improvement rely on review of individual medical records to evaluate and analyze the relationship between the patient's need for medical services and the services actually received. Whereas utilization review focuses on the efficiency of care and its costs, quality improvement focuses on the effectiveness of the services provided as well as on the qualifications of the providers who actually rendered the services. There are three types of utilization review:

- Prospective review (also known as per certification or prior authorization review) is the review that occurs before services are rendered.
- Concurrent review is the type of review that occurs while the services are being rendered.
- Retrospective review is the review that occurs after the services or treatments are rendered.[3, 4]

Utilization review can be broken down even further into four categories—what, when, where, and how much. For instance, when review is conducted (concurrently or retrospectively), the reviewer is looking for answers to the following questions:

- What type of care is or was required?

- Where was or will the care be provided—does or did the patient require inpatient care or outpatient care, ambulatory care or an alternate care setting? Also, for inpatient care, was the care provided (or will it be provided) in a general care facility or a center of excellence or tertiary care facility?
- When was the care provided? What are (or were) the dates of service?
- How much care is or was provided, and is it appropriate for the diagnosis in terms of duration, types of care provided, and frequency? Also included in this category is an estimation of whether services were overutilized or underutilized.

OVERUTILIZATION VERSUS UNDERUTILIZATION

Overutilization and underutilization are two types of costly and inappropriate use of services that must always be watched. Overutilization is best described as care that is of no benefit to the patient (e.g., excessive testing) or that could have been provided in a less costly alternative setting. In contrast, underutilization of services results in inadequate care or services to meet the medical needs of the patient. Underutilization is often found when one reviews the types of care provided and the location, duration, frequency, and intensity of care.

Whereas overutilization results in unnecessary cost expenditures, underutilization results in costly and inappropriate readmissions, deterioration of the patient's condition, or even death. Despite the fact that underutilization may be intended as a means of saving money, it can actually be a double-edged sword and has tremendous long-term cost implications that affect not only financial outcomes but personal and social ones as well. Briefly, underutilization is directly related to the quality of care.

TECHNIQUES AND CRITERIA USED IN UTILIZATION REVIEW

Each organization that conducts utilization review has its own set of criteria and its own methods of conducting the review.[5] Many organizations conduct review using on-site techniques and actual review of the patient's medical records. Others conduct the review by telephone, requesting only selected portions of the patient's medical record when questions arise. Although many organizations use review techniques such as those used by Medicare, others use explicit criteria developed either internally by specific policies and procedures or by recognized leaders in review techniques. Possibly the best known and most widely used criteria are those developed by Medicare. Another source of appropriate criteria is InterQual, which developed the original criteria in 1978 and has revised them frequently since that time. Until recently, InterQual's criteria were strictly designed for inpatient services, leaving a void when it came to outpatient services and care. Fortunately, this void has now been filled, and InterQual offers criteria for multiple services and levels of care. Still another source of criteria may be Milliman and Robertson's Healthcare Management Guidelines, or a combination of many guidelines may be used.

InterQual criteria are designed to measure services by evaluating the intensity of the services provided and the severity of the illness. If the patient fails to meet these criteria, the reviewer moves to the criteria used for discharge. These criteria are referred to as Intensity-Severity-Discharge-Appropriateness (ISD-A) criteria. Basically, they refer to the intensity of the service, the severity of the illness, the stability of the patient for discharge, and the appropriateness of the level of care. If the patient meets the criteria for intensity of services and severity of illness, the admission or continued stay can be approved. If not, the patient's stay is denied, and discharge is expected. In all cases, the appropriateness of the level of care (i.e., specialty units) is continually assessed. In contrast, Milliman and Robertson's guidelines basically focus on length of stay or nonproductive hospital days, alternative care settings, and quality of care issues.

In other organizations, a combination of review techniques may be used. For example, the organization may use its own review techniques or criteria in combination with review criteria from various and specifically selected length-of-stay manuals. In many organizations clinical pathways are taking on new importance as a review tool. Clinical pathways are a multidisciplinary management tool that proactively depicts important events and the total multidisciplinary aspects of patient care that should take place on a daily basis. Throughout the patient's entire stay, key events change daily, moving the patient toward discharge. The overall goal is to achieve high-quality care by paying continuous concurrent attention to variances, minimizing delays, and maximizing the use of resources.

Regardless of the criteria used for review, the results of utilization review are contingent on such factors as the medical care process, patient variables, inaccuracies in the medical record, and differences in practice patterns of physicians in various regions. Results vary depending on the scope and depth of review performed and the level of expertise of the actual reviewer.

LEVELS OF REVIEW

Utilization review, whether accomplished externally or internally, is generally conducted by professional nurses. This is called first-level review. These nurses review for medical necessity, appropriateness of care, place of service, quality of care, and overutilization or underutilization. Their job is to approve services or length of stay. Any review findings that appear doubtful require further review and are forwarded to physicians for second-level review.

It must be kept in mind that nurses cannot deny services; denials are always generated from second-level review. Second-level review is normally conducted by the medical director or by a selected panel of physician advisors. If the case is reviewed by the medical director and no determination on coverage can be reached, he or she may request another opinion from a physician advisor before the final coverage determination is made. If a determination still cannot be made, the case may require review by a committee of physician advisors; this review is called third-level review. Physician advisors play a key role in utilization review and case management processes. As a rule, physician advisors review cases of their "like specialty" when questions arise. They also serve as an internal second opinion for the medical director.

In general, physician advisors are used to resolve such issues as validation of the standards of care, recommendations for treatment alternatives, validation of denials made by the review organization's medical director, and review of cases in which the patient's attending physician requests another review. Most review organizations require their physician advisors to be active practitioners of their specialty (local, statewide, or nationally), and these physicians agree (by contract or by a specific letter of agreement) to review questionable cases when they arise.

SECOND OPINIONS

One tool used frequently in both the utilization review and case management processes when the current treatment program raises doubt is the second opinion. Case managers often use a second opinion to validate treatments before proceeding with the treatment course or allowing the present treatment course to continue.

A second opinion is a medical, surgical, or psychiatric consultation provided by another physician (generally one with a similar [or like] specialty). His or her opinion is sought to validate the proposed treatment plan or recommend alternative methods. Although many healthcare organizations offering case management services delegate the ability to seek second opinions to their case managers, others allow them only at the direction of the medical director.

REFERRAL FLAGS

Most healthcare payors and case management organizations use some form of flagging system that triggers cases at any point in the review process for referral to case management. Depending on the type of case management organization, most referrals originate from several sources, the most common of which are utilization review, claims processing, admission personnel, discharge planning personnel, and home health agency staff. As such, these referral sources as well as certain other key departments in the healthcare organization must be educated about:

- What the flags are.
- How the referral information is communicated (formally or informally, by phone or in writing) and to whom.
- What type of information is required and how much time should elapse from the time of identification to referral and making the decision for case management.

If utilization review and case management are offered by the same organization, the various departments in that organization must be educated about the different goals and emphases of these two functions. This education should consist not only of basic knowledge of one another's job duties but also typical cases, diagnoses, and costs and the value of an integrated system and case management approach. Some of the best cases to present during such educational sessions are those that arrived too late; examples of these case outcomes can be contrasted with similar cases that were successful.

Just as important as early referrals and a flagging system is open, honest, and frequent communication between the utilization review staff, the case management staff, and the healthcare team. The simple task of communication is the critical link if all departments are to function as a team. To foster this process, weekly staff meetings, in which all participants can compare notes and share pertinent information, are an excellent modality. If communication is not open and frequent, disastrous outcomes and a crisis atmosphere can ensue. For example, the utilization review staff may not approve an extension of a patient's inpatient stay, yet unforeseen barriers surface, precluding a safe discharge. What happens? The patient or family may receive an unnecessary letter of denial and file an appeal, whereupon the denial is overturned. Thus, they (and often the entire healthcare team as well) are subjected to a crisis situation for nothing.

✏ SUMMARY

Although case management is a variant of utilization review, the processes are totally different, and each discipline requires different types of expertise. Utilization review is designed to monitor services for medical necessity and appropriateness of care. In contrast, case management is designed to coordinate the patient's care with the appropriate providers and resources, monitoring the patient's treatment plan to ensure that high-quality care is rendered. Both processes are integral to one another, and the ultimate goal for both is quality and cost-effective care. Education, early referrals, and excellent communication cannot be overemphasized.

Unlike utilization review, in which most, if not all, duties can be fulfilled through telephone contact or chart review, case management often requires on-site observation of the patient and family if appropriate and timely actions are to be taken and goals reached.

REFERENCES

1. Lyon JC (1993). Models of nursing care delivery and case management: Clarification of terms. Nurs Econ 11(3):163-169.
2. Mazoway JM (1987). Early intervention in high cost care. Business and Health 4(3):12-16.
3. Boland P (1995). Making Managed Healthcare Work. Gaithersburg, MD, Aspen, pp. 172-175.
4. Kongstvedt PR (1993). The Managed Health Care Handbook, 2nd ed. Gaithersburg, MD, Aspen, pp. 182-188.
5. Boland P (1995). Op. cit., pp. 401-414.

BIBLIOGRAPHY

InterQual, Inc. (1997). InterQual clinical support criteria. Marlborough, MA, InterQual, Inc.
Milliman & Robertson, Inc. (1997). Healthcare Management Guidelines.® San Diego, CA, Milliman & Robertson, Inc.
Powell SK (1996). Nursing Case Management: A Practical Guide to Success in Managed Care. Philadelphia, J.B. Lippincott, pp. 77-142.

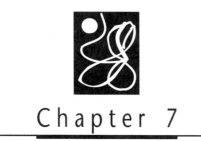

Chapter 7

Legal Aspects of Case Management

Because case management activities center around expensive, high-risk cases, case managers must be aware of legal issues that can affect caseloads and their handling. This chapter highlights some of the basic issues affecting the continuity of care process with which case managers should be familiar.

More specific information pertinent to legal issues should be obtained from the legal counsel that represents the case management organization. At a minimum, it is wise for case managers to be familiar with (1) the laws governing patient rights and entitlements, (2) any standards of practice by which case management or discharge services are judged, (3) the timing relevant to setting appeal processes in motion, (4) the laws governing patient confidentiality, (5) the laws governing patient abuse, and (6) the various types of conservatorship and power of attorney processes.

This advice does not mean that case managers should be walking texts on each of the foregoing topics, nor must the legal aspects that affect case management discourage case managers from taking action. Case managers should use common sense, make use of their legal counsel, and possibly consult a law library whenever necessary. Should this latter resource not be available, the library maintained in any state capitol is an excellent source of information when questions about law arise. However, the legal counsel employed by the case manager's organization is in the best position to offer advice about sensitive legal issues or legal defense guidelines. Guidelines to effective legal defenses often include the following pointers:

- Information supplied to other agencies is confidential.
- Documentation should be sufficient and legible.
- Knowledge of community agencies and their capabilities is essential.
- The patient should be involved in decision making and in the selection process for treatments and place or agencies that will render the care.
- Development of rapport and a strong successful relationship with the patient and family is important.
- Education of the patient and family should be maintained continuously.
- Signed release of information forms and consent forms should be used.
- Letters should be used to document coverage determinations and limitations.
- Quality issues should be reported to the qual-

ity improvement or contracting or network development department as well as to the case manager's immediate supervisor.
- Legal counsel should be consulted when questions arise.[1]

CONFIDENTIALITY

The rights and confidentiality of the patient are protected not only by state and federal statutes but also by the Joint Commission on Accreditation for Healthcare Organizations (JCAHO) and the American Nurses Association (ANA), among many other organizations. Case managers, like all healthcare professionals, are ethically charged to maintain confidentiality concerning health, financial, sexual, and any other personal matters for all parties involved. The federal Privacy Act and the administrative codes of all states pertinent to the federal act specify in detail the terms required for disclosure of medical information, medical records, addresses, phone numbers, race, Social Security numbers, and photographs.

The intent of these statutes is to preclude unauthorized disclosure or misuse of all personal information relating to a patient.[2, 3] Regardless of the healthcare provider used or the reason for sharing information, the giving and receiving of personal information must not be taken lightly, nor should it be an arbitrary or capricious procedure. Before releasing any information, case managers should always ask themselves: (1) what is the basic information I need to disclose to get the results needed, and (2) what should not be disclosed? The Privacy Act closely protects four subjects in particular:

- Drug or alcohol abuse and its treatment
- Mental health
- Acquired immunodeficiency syndrome (AIDS)
- Sexually transmitted diseases and abortions

Although these topics are protected by law, states vary in their requirements for mandatory reporting of certain events, such as births, deaths, communicable diseases, or abuse. Certainly, if state laws require reporting of specific conditions or situations, they must be obeyed. Case managers must therefore be familiar with the mandatory reporting requirements for all situations in their state. To assist in this process, it is wise to maintain a list of current names and phone numbers of persons and organizations that can accept such reports as well as notations about when reporting is necessary. Despite the need for mandatory reports to outside agencies, many case management organizations also require notification of their legal counsel or quality improvement department as well when a case is reported to an outside agency.

Providers at all levels of care are also protected by these privacy laws. Common sense plays a key role in maintaining confidentiality. However, it is best to disclose only the information needed by the provider or agency to develop its plan of care. Sensitivity and respect for the patient's wishes are necessary, yet it is also necessary to supply complete and truthful information that will allow the receiving provider to make its healthcare decisions.

One of the best ways to safeguard oneself when disclosing information is to use a form signed by the patient that permits the release of information. Without a signed release form, penalties can be severe if information of a personal or sensitive nature is disclosed or misused and the patient seeks recourse. This release of information must be signed by either the patient or his or her legal guardian. If the patient is a child, the parents or the legal guardian must sign the form. A signed release by the patient or his or her legal guardian is also useful when the medical record must be reviewed.

PATIENT RIGHTS

The existence of a policy guaranteeing certain patient rights is a condition of application for Medicare certification and JCAHO[3] accreditation for acute care hospitals, skilled nursing facilities, hospice programs, and other healthcare organizations. All hospital and healthcare organizations maintain, as a matter of public record, their "Patient's Bill of Rights," and case managers have the right to view this document. If patients continue to be discharged "sicker and quicker," and more continuity of care agencies and providers seek accreditation, patient rights will soon be protected at all levels of care.

As stated in the provider section (Chapter 3) of this manual, patients or their legal representatives have the right to be involved in decisions that affect their care, and this includes the selection of the facility or agency that will be providing the care. Case managers serving in an advocacy and advising role thus are responsible for ensuring that the patient and family

are allowed to participate in all such decisions. However, in this era of managed care, many patients sign away the right of choice of providers when they enroll in a health maintenance organization (HMO) or similar healthcare payor. Despite this requirement, case managers must still make every attempt to keep the patient and family in the decision-making loop, and whenever possible, more than one provider name should be presented to them during the selection process.

Patient rights are also enforced and advocated by such agencies as the agency responsible for administering developmental disability services, the department of rehabilitation, the department of mental health, adult and child protective service agencies, and the local ombudsman programs, to name a few. Failure to comply with the rules governing patient rights can have serious consequences for any healthcare professional who disregards these requirements.

CONSERVATORSHIP VERSUS POWER OF ATTORNEY AND DURABLE POWER OF ATTORNEY

Questions about the ability of a patient to give informed consent regarding his or her treatment are frequently encountered. Although in many states laws pertinent to informed consent clearly indicate that only the patient or his or her legally appointed representative has the right or authority to refuse treatment, in other states the issue remains unclear. Therefore, case managers must be familiar with the laws of consent for treatment in the state in which they practice.

Likewise, case managers must be familiar with the differences in (1) a conservatorship (person or estate), (2) a general power of attorney process, (3) a durable power of attorney process, and (4) advanced directives and living wills, as well as the impact of each of these processes on decisions affecting healthcare.

Conservatorship

A conservator may be indicated if the patient appears to be substantially incapable of making appropriate decisions, providing for personal and basic needs, managing his or her financial affairs, and appropriately protecting himself or herself against fraud and undue influence or loss of property.[4]

A conservatorship can be a condition of a person or an estate and is issued as either temporary or final. The process requires a psychiatric evaluation to determine the patient's level of competence and understanding. Once this is completed, the process is then usually referred to a public or private agency or a private attorney who specializes in the conservatorship process. In case management it is common to find, once the proceedings have started, that the patient cannot be relocated until a "temporary conservator" has been appointed because any relocation voids the process. One of the most frequent barriers to discharge involves problems associated with the conservatorship process; among these delays are the following:

- Resistance of the physician or family or refusal to cooperate.
- Backlog of requests at the public agency designated to handle the public conservatorship process.
- Heavy workload of public conservator case workers.
- Backlog in the court system for the actual conservatorship hearings.

The process of evaluation and the final decision making for conservatorship is time consuming and difficult. It involves accumulating sufficient data from which a decision can be made and a person competent to handle the patient's person, estate, or both can be appointed by the court. Due to the length of time this process takes, many states have laws that provide protection of the proposed conservatee's rights and property during the process. The steps necessary to establish a conservatorship are:

- Evidence about the proposed conservatee's mental ability is gathered.
- A petition with the evidence is submitted to the court.
- A hearing date is established, and notices of the hearing are sent to the patient (the conservatee has the right to be present) and any known blood relatives.
- The court examines the evidence and determines the result.

A public conservator is a person in a county agency who has been designated by the court to serve as the conservator for elderly or disabled persons within the agency's jurisdiction. Public conservators are also used for persons who have no families or whose families refuse to cooperate. Due to the backlogs of caseloads and court hearing dates, public conservatorship is by far the most time-consuming method, although it costs the patient nothing. Its biggest drawback is the waiting time, which is often 3 to 6 months on average. If a public conservatorship is required, the case manager must be familiar with the basic processes required, the time frames that apply, and the alternatives for care in his or her region.

A private conservator can be a family member, friend, attorney, or private agency who assumes this responsibility. The filing process needed to appoint a private conservator is generally handled by a private attorney. Although it is not common, banks often assume conservatorship of an estate but rarely of an individual "person." The cost of a private conservatorship varies depending on the agency or attorney used but usually averages several thousand dollars. Depending on the court schedule and the attorney's time, the waiting time for a private conservatorship is shorter than that required for a public conservator.

Durable Power of Attorney, Living Will, and General Power of Attorney

A durable power of attorney is a process whereby a person who is still competent and capable of planning ahead signs a document designating a certain person to act as his or her "attorney in fact." This person acts as the decision maker if the patient becomes incapable of making informed decisions.[4] To be recognized, the document must be signed by two witnesses.

Durable power of attorney should not be confused with a living will, advanced directive, or general power of attorney. A living will is executed while a person is still healthy (or shortly after a terminal illness has been diagnosed) and capable of planning ahead. This form merely states the person's desires and the conditions under which he or she wants treatment to be terminated. An advanced directive merely states the patient's wishes for care. This form is often provided at the time of admission to a hospital and is signed by the patient and a witness. The durable power of attorney, on the other hand, is a document that appoints a proxy agent, usually a relative or friend, to make medical decisions on the patient's behalf if he or she can no longer make such decisions for himself. This type of document is preferred to a living will because it has a broader application and can include treatment preferences.

A general power of attorney is issued only when a person is competent but for some reason is unable or unwilling to assume responsibility for conducting his or her financial affairs. This is a formal written document in which the person appoints someone to manage his or her finances.[5] General power of attorney forms are available at local banks or stationery stores. However, to be recognized by law the written appointment must be notarized.

ANTITRUST LAW

The Sherman antitrust law until recently was not enforced in the healthcare field because it was believed that healthcare professionals were exempt from the law. This position has radically changed because of court cases decided since 1984. Therefore, case managers should become familiar with the provisions of the law.[6]

The antitrust law has two important features that pertain to healthcare. Section I prohibits the restraint of trade in the form of tying arrangements for healthcare to specific providers or dealing exclusively with specific healthcare providers, and Section II prohibits the formation of a monopoly. Violation of Section I occurs when a hospital or healthcare provider owns or controls agencies to which it refers its patients. Violations of Section II occur when a hospital or healthcare provider is a competitor in the healthcare market yet possesses sufficient market power to exert control over referrals. Consequently, a case manager's best defense against violations of this law is to guard against making inappropriate referrals or discharges to a single facility, agency, or other provider owned by a hospital or healthcare provider.

PATIENT ABUSE

All healthcare professionals are mandated by state law to report abusive situations that come to their attention; failure to report such abuse is punishable by law. Therefore, case managers must be familiar with the law relevant to reporting abusive situations in their own state or the state where the patient is receiving care.

Any patient, regardless of age, who is found during case management intervention to be in an abusive situation must be referred to the appropriate agency mandated by the state to investigate such cases. In most states a verbal report must be made within 24 hours of knowledge of the abuse; this must be followed within 24 hours by a written report. Abuse or neglect can occur in a variety of forms; however, it typically appears in one of the following four categories:

- Emotional or verbal abuse accompanied by threats of violence or harassment.
- Sexual abuse involving inappropriate touching, fondling, or sexual acts that occur when the patient is forced, unable to understand, or threatened.
- Physical abuse that is witnessed or is apparent by unexplained bruises, welts, fractures, abrasions or cuts, or burns from cigarettes, ropes, or other hot surfaces.
- Physical and mental abuse that is assumed if the patient is found confined or locked in a room or tied to a bed or chair.

Financial exploitation is another form of reportable abuse. This occurs when family members or others misuse or withhold funds, neglect to purchase food, clothing, personal items, or medical care and supplies, or grossly overcharge the patient for services. Theft of property or funds is certainly included in this category.

Neglect is also reportable and includes such situations as:

- Filthy, unsafe, or hazardous housing environment or patient hygiene.
- Lack of medical care or failure to administer prescribed medications or treatments.
- Unexplained weight loss, malnourishment, or failure to thrive.
- Absent parents or caretaker and inappropriate supervision.
- Irregular school attendance.

Agencies mandated to investigate reports of abuse include the following:

Child Protective Services (CPS) for all children under age 18. This service is available through the local social services department or similar state or county agency.

Adult Protective Services (APS) for all adults (over age 18). This service is also available through the local social services department or similar state or county agency.

Local ombudsman offices for all adults over age 18 who are confined to a facility (e.g., skilled nursing facility, board and care, intermediate care facility, residential treatment center, and so forth). These services are frequently provided by the local department of aging or agency on aging, social services department, or a similar state department or agency. These offices provide staff members, either paid or volunteer, who follow up issues or complaints filed either by the residents of the facilities or family members.

WICKLINE CASE

The Wickline case is the first case decided under California law in which a healthcare payor was tied to a malpractice suit.[7] This case has elements pertinent to both case management and discharge planning practices and is possibly the most well known case nationally that deals with these issues. As such, it is frequently referred to by attorneys and other experts who speak on malpractice at national or local case management meetings.

This case involved a Medicaid patient who was, on the medical evidence, eligible for continued hospitalization. However, the patient was discharged prematurely when the attending physician failed to seek an additional extension because he believed that the Medicaid (Medi-Cal) consultant put the state's interest above the patient's welfare. The court ultimately found Medi-Cal not liable because of the fact that the final decision for discharge rests with the attending physician.

As patients become more knowledgeable about their rights and more willing to challenge and appeal adverse decisions, it is anticipated that such suits will become more common. Third-party payors will be held as legally accountable as physicians who comply without protest when inappropriate medical decisions result from cost containment efforts and pressures.

Because of the present emphasis on cost cutting and cost containment and because case managers can be held accountable for the patient's care and ultimate welfare, case managers should not comply with any unreasonable demands by employer groups, policyholders, managed care organizations, or third-party payors without formally protesting or stating their position in writing. Copies of such statements should be placed not only in the patient's chart but also in the case manager's personal file. If such a situation occurs, either the legal counsel employed by the case manager's organization or private legal counsel should be consulted for direction.

ABANDONMENT

Abandonment of a patient requiring care most often arises in the home environment and usually involves such issues as noncompliance by the patient with the regimen, lack of safety of the environment, or ineligibility by the patient for reimbursement of services. In such cases it is often the family, caregiver, or provider agency that abandons the patient, often without prior notification of others on the healthcare team. One of the best ways to ensure that charges of abandonment are not filed against a healthcare professional is to send a written notification of impending termination to all parties involved. This letter must include a list of alternate resources or other pertinent information that can assist the patient or family if alternate arrangements are required. The key to a successful termination is to allow adequate time for education of the patient or family about alternate resources or provision of alternate arrangements before the termination takes effect.

STANDARDS OF CARE AND NEGLIGENT REFERRAL

Standards of care are written guidelines that advocate quality care and set the ground rules for practice for newly hired staff.[7, 8] Case managers should familiarize themselves with the standards of care required for specific diseases, illnesses, and injuries, as well as any standards associated with the medical condition, discharge into the community, and the continuity of care process. In reviewing standards of care, the case manager must be sure to look not merely at the standards in his or her own medical community but also at the national standards of care, since these are used to judge the case should it end in the hands of the legal system. Equally important is a knowledge of what duties are allowed to be performed by post-acute care nurses. A state's nurse practice act clearly outlines the duties that can be performed by both registered nurses and licensed vocational or practical nurses. Likewise, it is important to be familiar with treatment modalities and settings and what can and cannot be provided or allowed in the post-acute care arena.

When referring a patient to an alternate level of care, case managers, as healthcare professionals, are responsible for acting in good faith and using reasonable care in making referrals. The case manager's best defense is to be open and honest with continuing care providers and to offer multiple choices to patients and families, allowing them to make their own selection of the provider or providers to be used. It behooves case managers to continually investigate the certification, licensure, and qualifications of providers and to keep current with technologic advances and how they relate to the standard of care.

One of the best ways of keeping current is to make personal visits to facilities and providers both during business hours and after hours (skilled nursing facilities and rehabilitation facilities, for example, are open 24 hours a day, and in most cases a case manager can go in unannounced during visiting hours or at meal times; in this way, the ambiance and mood of the patients can be observed without having to take a formal guided tour that is limited to the areas the administrator wants one to see). These unannounced visits allow an opportunity to truly see what patients are experiencing.

A formal tool that can be used to judge a provider's compliance and capability of offering high-quality care is the inspection reports issued during the state health department's licensing survey. These reports and surveys are a matter of public record. As such, facilities or provider groups usually post their most recent survey results in the lobby of their main building; if not visible, case managers should not hesitate to ask or call for the results. These reports should be reviewed for evidence of nursing care deficiencies and whether or not corrective actions have been taken or completed.

Another tool is networking with peers. The importance of this simple process cannot be underestimated. Among other things, networking allows case managers to collaborate and keep current about providers, changes in standards of care, reimbursement rates, the availability of new services, and so forth.

PROVIDER AND PATIENT FRAUD AND ABUSE OF THE SYSTEM

Healthcare fraud is a healthcare expense that costs several billion dollars annually and is best described as billing for services that were not rendered or altering or falsifying records.[9] Provider abuse comprises overutilization and underutilization of services and issues pertaining to quality of care and performance of medically necessary services for specific conditions. Patient abuse and fraud generally center around the submission of fraudulent claims and failure to report other insurance coverage. Regardless of the perpetrator, most healthcare payors, including public programs such as Medicare and Medicaid, have units whose primary function is to monitor and report suspicious provider activity. An excellent resource for combating fraud and abuse is the National Healthcare Anti-Fraud Association, in which most major healthcare payors are active participants.

Catastrophically ill or injured patients are vulnerable to the temptation for patient abuse, and the chronicity of their illness allows opportunities for providers to defraud or abuse the system. Therefore, it behooves case managers to stay attuned to the details of their cases, especially when suspicions of fraud or abuse arise.

Large expenditures and multiple providers encourage opportunities for fraud and abuse. Whenever money is involved, there are always people who attempt or succeed in defrauding or abusing the system. As stated in the chapters of this manual dealing with home health care and durable medical equipment, cases found in case management are high dollar and tend to last for the long term or the lifetime of the patient. Expenses that are reimbursed for services provided can be the bread and butter (or even gravy) for the provider, so all catastrophic cases must be monitored closely to ensure that claims payments are accurate and that the healthcare payor or organization is not being exploited.

As case managers or, more important, as healthcare professionals, it is part of the job to be alert to potential or actual fraud and abuse, to report it, and ultimately to stop it. Anyone can commit fraud. Although this section primarily addresses provider fraud and abuse of the system, patients and their families are not exempt, nor are the employees of healthcare organizations.

What are some of the processes used to detect fraud and abuse of the system? Certainly, first-hand observations and conversations can be a tip-off, and these should be reported. In most cases, however, fraud and abuse are identified through claims processing. Most claims processors use prepayment and postpayment utilization review processes to detect provider fraud and abuse.

Prepayment and postpayment review programs are similar to the prior authorizations and retrospective review processes that are used for "front end" utilization review. In a prepayment utilization review program, claims are reviewed for medical necessity before they are paid, utilizing what are termed claims edits. If a claim fails to pass this edit, it is suspended and is forwarded to a person who reviews the information and decides whether the failure was due to clerical error or to the probable cause. If there is any doubt, the claim remains suspended, and the actual medical records are requested from the provider and reviewed. If the medical records do not support the medical necessity for the claim, it is denied and, depending on the findings, may be sent to the appropriate department that investigates fraud and abuse.

Postpayment utilization review units focus their attention on claims already paid. Additionally, they concentrate on review of specific studies of services or providers. Whenever providers or patients are suspected of fraud or abuse, a special flag is used as a marker, and all claims from this patient or provider are suspended for what is termed manual review. This process assists in identifying trends, billing practices, and fraudulent use of services.

Healthcare payors may be defrauded in several ways. For example:

- Other health insurance (including private health insurance and automobile insurance) is not reported, and the patient or provider bills separately and collects from both insurance companies.
- Large bills are submitted several months after the services are rendered, which triggers suspicion because most providers want their receivables current and do not deliberately withhold claims for payment.
- Claims contain "white-out" or blank areas that would normally be completed. Additionally, review of the actual hard copy claim may show different type styles or colored ink, all of which are indicators of other health insurance coverage.
- Unusual dollar amounts beyond those considered usual and customary or reasonable for the region or provider specialty are claimed for specific items or services.
- Unusual billing practices are used, such as daily charges that include holidays and weekends when the provider is known to operate normally from Monday through Friday.

- Claims are filed for services not rendered; this can be detected in one of two ways:
  - Actual review of the claim against the medical record.
  - Questions from the patient, who has received an explanation of benefits (EOB) statement for services not rendered, prompting him or her to report this to the healthcare payor.
- Equipment or medical supplies are billed but never received.
- Some families or patients "physician or provider hop" to get prescriptions for items and then stockpile them, thus, excessive ordering of durable medical equipment supplies or drugs can be noted.
- Patients may file all claims all under one patient's name to avoid annual deductibles or cost shares. Again, these can be detected through actual review of the hard copy, looking for whited-out areas or different ink colors and type styles. This type of fraud can often be detected through claims edits, which are set to review claims for medical necessity for diagnosis, age, or sex groups.
- Providers may bill repeatedly for the same services for all their patients; examples include patients confined to specialty care centers such as post-acute care rehabilitation centers, skilled nursing facilities, and special schools for children with mental health conditions (i.e., state schools, residential treatment centers).
- The claim is unbundled when the test or service should be paid as one unit—for example, chemistry or other laboratory panels that should be billed as a unit but instead are billed individually.
- Primary care managers who have excessive numbers of patients should be watched closely; often their services are nothing more than a "referral mill" that does the least while collecting a specific rate for doing more.
- Overutilization of specific services or referral patterns should be watched closely. Investigation may reveal that the provider has a financial interest that could benefit him or her personally.

For all healthcare professionals, the key to preventing provider and patient fraud and abuse is to keep one's eyes and ears open at all times and report all suspicions.

SUMMARY

The purpose of this chapter is to highlight some of the common legal issues that affect case management and the continuity of care process. This is especially important because we work in a litigious environment. Because so many cases in case management are "catastrophic" in nature, there is a strong possibility that many will result in some form of litigation. For this reason, case managers must take care that all their actions follow legal defense guidelines.

One of the best legal defenses is documentation and the use of signed release of information forms. If in doubt, the case manager must always consult his or her organization's legal counsel.

Two major areas that must always be watched by case managers are patient neglect and abuse and provider or patient fraud and abuse of the healthcare payor or healthcare system. Although patient neglect and abuse are reportable by law, provider or patient fraud and abuse are not. Fraud and abuse by both patients and providers contribute unnecessarily to increased healthcare costs. Therefore, it behooves case managers as healthcare professionals to report any suspicions of abuse or fraud situations.

REFERENCES

1. O'Hare PA, Terry MA (1988). Discharge Planning Strategies for Assuring Continuity of Care. Gaithersburg, MD, Aspen, pp. 142–143.
2. Southwick AE (1988). The Law of Hospital and Healthcare Administration. Chicago, Health Administration Press.
3. Mullahy CM (1995). The Case Manager's Handbook. Gaithersburg, MD, Aspen, pp. 52–63.
4. Fraley AM (1992). Nursing the Disabled Across the Life Span. Sudbury, MA, Jones and Bartlett, p. 210.
5. O'Hare PA, Terry MA (1988). Op. cit., pp. 146–147.
6. O'Hare PA, Terry MA (1988). Op. cit., pp. 136–137.
7. O'Hare PA, Terry MA (1988). Op. cit., pp. 138–139.
8. Southwick AE (1988). Op. cit., pp. 52–53.
9. Kongstvedt PE (1993). The Managed Health Care Handbook, 2nd ed. Gaithersburg, MD, Aspen, pp. 228–230.

BIBLIOGRAPHY

Andrews M, et al (eds) (1996). Nurse's legal handbook, 3rd ed. Springhouse, PA, Springhouse Corp.
Annas GJ (1992). The Rights of Patients, 2nd ed. Totowa, NJ, Humana Press.
Berrio MW, Levesque ME (1996). Advanced directives: Most patients don't have one. Do yours? Am J Nurs 96(8):24–28.
Chez N (1994). Helping the victim of domestic violence. Am J Nurs 94(7):33–37.
Clemen-Stone C, et al (1995). Comprehensive Community Health Nursing: Family Aggregate and Community Practice, 4th ed. St. Louis, Mosby-Year Book, pp. 105–137.
Confidentiality: The case manager's role in respecting the client's rights (1993). Case Manag Advisor 4(9):117–120.
Guido GW (1997). Legal Issues in Nursing, 2nd ed. Stamford, CT, Appleton and Lange.
Hall JK (1996). Nursing Ethics and Law. Philadelphia, W.B. Saunders.
Helvestine WA (1991). Legal issues in case management and utilization review. Presented to Case Management Society of America, April 17, 1991.
Iyer PW, Camp NH (1995). Nursing Documentation: A Nursing Process Approach. St. Louis, Mosby-Year Book.
Lampe SS (1985). Focus charting: Streamlining documentation. Nurs Manag 16(7):43–46.
LaRooco SA (1985). Patient abuse should be your concern. J Nurs Admin 15(4):27–31.
Milholland DK (1994). Privacy and confidentiality of patient information. J Nurs Admin 24(2):19–24.
Mullahy CM (1995). The Case Managers Handbook. Gaithersburg, MD, Aspen, pp. 52–79.
Powell SK (1996). Nursing Case Management: A Practical Guide to Success in Managed Care. Philadelphia, J.B. Lippincott, pp. 143–168.
Powers AM (1990). Current legal issues in psychiatry. Presented to Foundation Health Utilization Review/Case Management staff, September 13, 1990.
Smith CM, Maurer FA (1995). Community Health Nursing: Theory and Practice. Philadelphia, W.B. Saunders, pp. 88–109.

Chapter 8

General Services

CARE OF THE CAREGIVER

Anyone who actively practices case management is aware of the fact that case managers deal with the more complex cases. So do the families. Healthcare professionals can say at the end of their 8- to 12-hour shifts that they are tired, often exhausted, and can go home and rest. Why is the situation not the same for caregivers? The answer is that the healthcare payor system places limits on what is considered a reimbursable benefit. The result is the need for care that must be provided by someone. Unfortunately, the healthcare profession expects caregivers (1) to perform the same tasks as professionals, (2) to perform these tasks unassisted by others, and (3) to perform these tasks with little or no training. More important, there are times when the caregiver is expected to perform all these tasks without rest or any break from the day-to-day care.

As a result, case managers must be as alert to the needs of the caregiver as to the needs of the patient. All too often care of the caregiver is overlooked. The result is not only that all these factors take a toll on the caregiver but also that they cause an inappropriate use of resources, because caregiver burnout may be the primary reason for costly deterioration in the patient's condition and a subsequent poor outcome.

To be effective as a caregiver, a person must be thoroughly trained in all aspects of care. To ensure this result, training must be started at the time of admission and must continue as the patient's needs change and additional training needs are identified; usually it continues throughout the duration of the illness and recovery period.

In addition to any initial training, the caregiver also requires supervision by the healthcare team until he or she is proficient in all aspects of care. In addition, whereas much attention is placed on the equipment needs of the patient, the caregiver also must be assessed for any equipment needs that will make caregiving tasks easier (e.g., patient lifts, slideboards), since in many instances the caregiver will be alone. One critical aspect of planning for caregiver training is the need to ensure that the therapy team teaches the caregiver the use of proper body mechanics; remember, the caregiver will be useless if he or she is injured while trying to complete the required tasks.

Respite

In any long-term care case regular breaks or respite for the caregiver must be scheduled. What is respite? Respite is the process that allows the family or primary caregiver a chance to take a break or a rest or just to get away for a while. Respite is a necessity, not a luxury. Caregivers are of little help to anyone if they are physically or emotionally drained or if they injure themselves.

In many cases, care by the caregiver is a job that continues 24 hours a day, 7 days a week, all year long. Due to the demands of the care they are giving, many caregivers forget, ignore, or neglect their own physical and emotional needs. This is especially true if no one is present to relieve them of their duties.

With this in mind, case managers should remember that whenever care is assumed by a nonprofessional caregiver, he or she must be trained not only in all aspects of the patient's care but also—and just as important—in the importance of caring for themselves. Thus, periodic assessments of the caregiver are just as important as the monitoring and reassessment of the patient. This process must be included in the schedule established for monitoring the patient's progress.

Respite is especially important for single caregivers and mothers with a chronically ill child or a child with special needs. Not only does the mother need respite, but, if there are other children in the home, she needs to spend time with these children as well.

Respite Services

Formal respite care units and their capabilities vary from community to community. Unfortunately, in many communities formal respite care is often not available. In such situations, back-up caregivers or volunteers must be recruited and fully trained for the respite care required. If volunteer caregivers are not available, factors to be considered include the healthcare payor's policy for respite reimbursement and the family's financial ability to pay privately for respite care. Depending on this assessment, arrangements for respite care may be made through the use of such providers as home health agencies or skilled nursing facilities.

Respite services can range from care that is given by the hour or day or overnight, to care that lasts for several days or weeks. If a respite unit is available in the immediate vicinity, families should be encouraged to arrange well in advance for any planned respite because long waiting lists are common.

Respite care for an ill child, with few exceptions, is limited to the care offered by skilled sitters because respite services and other facilities are nonexistent in many communities. Skilled sitters are available from licensed home health agencies or agencies that specialize in providing hourly or shift care to children with special needs. If such sitters are not available, case managers must help the family in identifying volunteers, friends, or relatives who can be trained to assume this function.

In light of the foregoing information, case managers should maintain current lists of all known respite services within the region of practice. It is vital to share such information with any person who assumes a caregiver role.

Reimbursement

Unfortunately, reimbursement for respite care or skilled sitters frequently occurs only through private funds because respite is often excluded from healthcare benefit coverage. If so, the case manager must know how and when to seek possible coverage from the healthcare payor through the extra contractual process.

Peer Support Versus Professional Counseling

The need to assume too many roles (especially those of nurse, therapist, wage earner, and head of household) and the occasional presence of complete role reversal frequently threaten the caregiver's emotional well-being and ability to cope. Likewise, changes in plans, lack of personal free time, restrictions on freedom, and even the need to provide care when it is totally disagreeable take a toll. These feelings must be dealt with rather than ignored because they may then escalate and begin to fester.

Not only can feelings fester, in many cases the caregiver also may feel guilty if he or she needs help or cannot cope, so emotional or psychological support must be given as required. Caregivers who deal with technologically dependent or long-term care patients commonly experience such feelings as

- Guilt
- Depression
- Resentment
- Stress
- Anger
- Bitterness
- Frustration
- Despair
- Loneliness and isolation

Caregivers must always be allowed an opportunity to express such feelings. If necessary, they can be referred for possible counseling or linked to support groups when stressors are identified.

Counseling, whether professional or offered by peer support groups, is a necessary component of case planning. One of the best and most economical means of support is the use of disease-specific, community, church, or ethnic support groups. Such groups should not be underestimated for the peer support they provide. However, at times it may be necessary to encourage caregivers to seek professional counseling from a psychologist, psychiatrist, or licensed clinical or medical social worker. If the caregiver does require professional counseling, the case manager may need to assist him or her in pursuing any mental health authorizations required.

SUMMARY

Far too often, the caregiver's needs are overlooked in the management of the catastrophically ill or injured. When this happens, the result is caregiver burnout, which can in turn lead to a multitude of other problems. The consequences are not only costly to the healthcare payor, they are just as costly to the patient and the patient's quality of life. In many cases, the patient's condition deteriorates, and he or she must be rehospitalized until alternate plans can be made.

The caregiver's needs for respite care are commonly not included in the patient's healthcare coverage. For this reason, families must be aware of their resources and must understand the importance of the need to establish backup resources to prevent burnout.

HIRING HELP FOR HOME CARE

Often, one of the first arrangements patients and families must make when they decide to plan for home care is to find qualified help. This is especially necessary when care will not be reimbursed by the healthcare payor. Because of the high charges associated with hiring help from a home health agency or nursing registry, many patients and families prefer to recruit their own help. However, this has pitfalls and in many instances can result in higher costs than if the family had elected to use an agency. As a discharge planner and case manager, the author often heard families react negatively to the high rates charged by professional agencies. However, with education, they were better able to make an informed decision about whether they should make this choice. If they do their own recruiting, there are several factors that must be considered. This chapter is written to explain these factors so that families can understand the many pitfalls of hiring help for the home as well as the advantages.

Employer Responsibilities

As a potential employer, the patient and the family must become familiar with their new responsibilities. For instance, if they are unfamiliar with paying wages they must contact the Internal Revenue Service to discuss the requirements for this process. They are also responsible for:

- Contacting the Social Security office to obtain Social Security reporting forms and the amount of wages they must report each quarter.
- Reporting any wages greater than the quarterly amount specified for Social Security to the state agency responsible for unemployment benefits.
- Keeping detailed records on each employee, including:
  - Name
  - Address
  - Social Security number
  - Hours worked
  - Amount of wages paid
- Distributing W-2 forms.
- Maintaining workers' compensation insurance coverage in case the employee is injured.

The major disadvantage of hiring help directly rather than using an agency is the lack of appropriate supervision of the employee. Also, despite the fact that the patient may require only custodial care, the employee may not have a clear understanding of the physician's orders, leading to confusion and inappropriate care. More important, when help is hired directly by the patient or family, there are no provisions for back-up help if the person quits, becomes ill, or takes time off.

Recruitment Methods

Although the following lists of suggestions for recruiting attendants appear lengthy, the actual time needed to elicit a response to an advertisement and hire the attendant varies from a few days to months. Consequently, it is advisable for families to advertise in several sources at once. Such sources include:

- Newspapers
- Social service agencies
- Vocational schools or other work training programs
- Church-sponsored or ethnic agencies
- Bulletin boards (e.g., at churches, hospitals [both skilled nursing facilities and acute care facilities], and senior centers)
- Employment agencies
- Friends and other word-of-mouth discussions
- Centers that serve the disabled and offer independent living skills and referral services
- College placement centers

In writing the advertisement, it is best to use a post office box instead of a phone number. This allows the patient and family to screen the resumes and references before they make any actual contact with the applicant. The advertisement should include the following information:

- Type of services or specific duties required.
- Number of hours required per day, week, or month.
- Rate of pay.
- Statement requiring resumes and references.
- Post office box number to which applicant should reply.

Interviews

The patient or family should be advised to prepare a list of questions or issues they desire to cover during the interview. This list should be prepared in advance. The questions serve as a guide during the interview and prevent the interviewer from forgetting to raise important questions or issues. Interview questions must be broad enough not only to cover the specific requirements of the job but also to give some insight into the applicant's personal characteristics. Due to the Privacy Act, certain questions of prospective employees are illegal, and patients and families must be advised of this fact. Questions must be phrased in such a way that the maximum information about the person can be gained without violating this act. However, questions should be directed to the following areas:

- Job qualifications, training, and certification
- Recent work history, length of employment, reason for leaving, and specific tasks performed
- Any medical problems that limit the employee's ability to perform any tasks that require strength or physical labor
- Criminal record, including arrests or convictions
- Personal habits such as smoking that might be annoying
- Transportation mode and dependability
- Personal likes and dislikes that the employee would like to share or have known

It is advisable for a second person to be present during the interview to validate the family's impressions and to ask additional questions. The patient and family should keep in mind that the person they hire will be coming into their home and they must feel comfortable with him or her. Key personal characteristics to look for during the interview include:

- Compatibility
- Reliability
- Promptness
- Honesty
- Willingness to learn
- Good listening skills
- Ability to grasp details
- Neat, clean appearance

Other key points the patient or family might wish to consider during the interview are (1) proposal of a 2-week trial for training purposes, and (2) agreement of the applicant to accept payment by check because this verifies that the person was paid if questions arise at a later date. To avoid any misunderstanding, families should be encouraged to draw up a contract for the new employee that outlines the duties, rate of pay, pay dates, and time off. In addition, families should maintain a list of nursing registries and agencies that can render the required

care if problems arise and help is needed immediately.

Verification of References

References must always be checked! Remind families that when checking references they should look for the following details:

- Length of previous employment
- Reliability
- Dependability
- Specific tasks performed and competence with which they were performed
- Employee's reaction to suggestions and criticism
- Other problems or situations the previous employer would like to share

Common Problems

Although problems among employees can be many and varied, families must be aware that when hiring help they must be alert to signs of the following common problems:

- Thievery
- Abuse
- Sudden termination without notice
- Substitute help during periods of illness or absence of the employee
- Alcohol or drug use
- Criminal record

Hiring Help Using a Nursing Agency

If continuous private duty nursing is necessary and an agency is used, the following factors should be considered before the final selection is made:

- What are the capabilities and availability of the agency staff to manage the care required? Will any needed training of staff be done at no extra charge?
- How do the rates of the chosen agency compare to the rates of other agencies in the area?
- Is the agency willing to discount services and work with the family for possible reimbursement by the healthcare payor?
- Is the agency certified or accredited and licensed appropriately?

• What is the contingency plan for back-up staffing if problems occur?

Even when the healthcare payor is reimbursing the family for the cost of private duty nursing, the patient and family must understand that they must assume final responsibility for the hiring of the individual. Also, they must be informed of the fact that the actual contract is between them and the agency, not the healthcare payor.

SUMMARY

This section highlights the basic information that must be shared with patients or families who are considering the possibility of hiring attendants or home healthcare workers. Although the rates charged by a nursing or home healthcare agency may appear high, the disadvantages of being the employer often outweigh the advantages. The patient and family must be aware of these issues prior to their decision for help in the home.

RECREATIONAL ACTIVITIES

Because of our society's emphasis on rehabilitation and wellness, many communities now have a full array of recreational opportunities available for use by disabled individuals. Information about the types of activities available can often be found by calling the local department of parks and recreation or a national, state, or local agency focused on a specific disease or injury. In all cases, catastrophically ill or injured persons should be encouraged to continue to live as active a life as possible, since such activity is essential to their physical and mental well-being. Unfortunately, for a variety of reasons, many patients do not wish to or will not participate in such activities. Nevertheless, case managers must be familiar with the recreational activities available in their communities should patients inquire about them.

In some cases, before the patient will participate in any social or recreational activities, peer or group support or counseling will be necessary to build self-esteem or acceptance of the person's limitations or body image changes. Persons with a disability or disfigurement commonly feel embarrassed or shamed and, therefore, seek isolation or activities where public contact can be avoided.

Types of Recreational Activities

For patients wishing to participate in some form of physical activity, most large communities offer a variety of sport or recreational activities for the disabled including:

• Hiking
• Mountain climbing
• Camping
• Dancing
• Football
• Basketball
• Bowling
• Skiing
• Softball
• Swimming
• Tennis
• Track and field
• Weight lifting

In addition, for those who prefer less active or organized recreational events, many support groups offer outings and other social events that can at least provide some "fun" time or a social outing if the patient or family desires.

Informational Sources

Patients and families should be encouraged to contact the following agencies for information about recreational opportunities in any given community:

• City parks and recreational departments
• National Park Service
• Chamber of Commerce
• Centers that serve the disabled and offer independent skills
• Disease-specific and other community service agencies
• Easter Seal Society
• Disabled groups at local colleges
• Special Olympics

SUMMARY

To enhance their mental well-being, patients and families should be informed of recreational activities in their community that offer programs for disabled or seriously ill individuals. Lists of agencies and the opportunities they provide should be maintained by case managers. In certain cases, counseling, whether by a professional or a peer support group, may be necessary before a disabled person will participate in activities. This occurs when the person feels shame or embarrassment because of changes in his or her body image or functioning.

TRANSPORTATION AND TRAVEL

Because so many patients found in case management caseloads are disabled or physically challenged, case managers must be familiar with transportation services for this category of persons. If transportation resources are unknown, three of the best resources are the rehabilitation unit's adaptive driving program, the local department or agency on aging, or the Department of Rehabilitation.

General Information

If the patient is disabled, he or she can apply to the state Department of Motor Vehicles for a handicapped placard or a disabled persons (DP) license plate. Generally, there is a nominal charge for the plastic disabled placard, which is transferable to other vehicles. However, there is no additional charge for a license plate designating the person as disabled.

Disabled persons are covered by the following transportation laws:

• Car insurance rates cannot be increased, the policy canceled, or insurance denied when a person is determined to have a disability.
• At gas stations, health and safety codes allow the disabled the right to receive minimum service at self-serve islands for the self-serve price. The patient should carry a copy of the law in the glove compartment of the car should problems occur. If the station refuses to honor the law, the patient or family can contact the local office of consumer affairs of the District Attorney's office to initiate court action.

Adaptive Driving Programs

Disabled persons can drive legally if their previous driving record is good and they are capable of passing a road test conducted by an occupational therapist from a certified adaptive driving program. For information about current training programs and locations, the patient or family can call their state's Department of Rehabilitation, the nearest independent living center, or any acute care hospital that offers physical medicine and rehabilitation services.

As a rule, most adaptive driving programs are located at regional spinal cord rehabilitation centers. The average time needed for an evaluation and test is approximately 5 hours at a cost of $75 to $100 per hour. The fee for the certification is not paid by traditional healthcare payors. However, it is paid by workers' compensation or, if the patient has vocational goals, the state Department of Rehabilitation may consider paying the fee. Otherwise, the cost must be assumed by the patient or family.

The driving program consists of two sessions. The first session consists of a clinical assessment, and the second one is spent behind the wheel. To be evaluated, the patient must have:

• A physician's prescription for the occupational therapist driver evaluation.
• A valid driver's license or permit.
• A prearranged appointment with the program.

At the end of the evaluation the patient is supplied with written specific details regarding:

• Specific information on how to transfer into and out of the vehicle.
• Correct positioning while behind the wheel.
• Vehicle modifications or driving equipment required.

Modified Vehicles

The cost required to equip a van or car varies from person to person depending on the individual's needs. The cost of equipping a vehicle is excluded from healthcare payor coverage and must be paid privately. In some cases, these costs are paid by workers' compensation or occasionally by the state Department of Rehabilitation if the patient has a vocational goal. Costs for such equipment vary, for example:

• $500 or less for hand controls.
• $7000 to $15,000 or more for modifications to vehicles or vans (excluding the cost of the vehicle).

Bus Services

LOCAL HANDICAPPED BUS SERVICES

Many cities offer local bus services for the disabled or mentally or physically challenged at a nominal cost. The local public transportation office should be contacted for specific details. The application process takes 3 to 4 weeks. In the interim, other systems of transportation must be explored and utilized.

Once accepted as a participant in the public handicapped transportation system, a person desiring a ride must register several days in advance of pick-up. He or she should reconfirm the pick-up by calling 24 hours in advance of the pick-up time. Because delays are common, participants should be reminded to alert the physician or therapist to the fact that they will be arriving via public handicapped transport. Most providers are willing to adjust their schedules to accommodate the patient if they are informed about the problem.

To assist in determining eligibility, functional and therapeutic classifications as well as medical statements from the attending physician are used. Conditions that indicate eligibility for use of handicapped transportation systems are divided into three categories—physical, developmental, and mental. For instance, the following are examples of some physical conditions that can qualify a person for the service:

- Ambulatory disabilities or disabilities in coordination
- Use of mobility aids
- Arthritis
- Amputation
- Stroke or other neurologic disorder
- Pulmonary problems
- Cardiac problems
- Dialysis
- Sight difficulties
- Hearing disabilities

Examples of developmental disabilities include:

- Mental retardation
- Cerebral palsy
- Epilepsy
- Autism
- Neurologic handicap

Examples of mental disorders include:

- Emotional disturbance
- Participation in an activity workshop or training center
- Residence in a boarding house or group home
- Mental disorders as recognized by the American Psychiatric Association

LOCAL SCHOOL BUS SERVICES

As stated earlier, the Individuals with Disabilities Education Act ensures access to a free education for all children. If the child requires transportation to reach the site of the school or classroom, the school district is required to provide such transportation free of charge. To use this benefit, transportation needs must be identified and included in the individual education plan (IEP) developed for the child. Every school district is required to develop such an individual educational plan, but if delays are encountered, other arrangements must be made in the interim to transport the child to and from school.

COMMERCIAL BUSES

Commercial bus travel is the most economic mode of transportation for persons who need to travel long distances, but it is also the most restrictive and least favored mode of travel. Bus travel is very restrictive when it comes to providing accommodation and accessibility for the disabled. Most of these problems are encountered when boarding and unboarding the vehicle, using the bathrooms, and obtaining access to meals.

Airlines

COMMERCIAL AIRLINE SERVICES

Most commercial airlines can accommodate travelers with minimal to moderate disabilities, but regulations vary from airline to airline. If the patient travels by air, it is advisable to contact the airline at least 48 hours in advance of the departure time to arrange for a wheelchair or escort service.

Few commercial airlines can accommodate severely disabled travelers or those who require oxygen en route. In these cases, the family or patient's physician must contact the airline's medical department (located at the airline's central headquarters) well in advance of any scheduled travel to discuss the patient's medical needs, requirements, and restrictions. The Federal Aviation Administration (FAA) has specific requirements relating to the transportation of disabled persons in pressurized cabins.

AIR AMBULANCE OR MILITARY AIR MEDICAL EVACUATION SYSTEM

If the commercial airlines are unable or unwilling to transport a patient who is severely disabled, it may be necessary to arrange for a commercial air ambulance. If the patient is a military retiree or dependent of either an active duty sponsor or retiree, arrangements can made with the military Aeromedical Evacuation Unit, which is dispatched from Scott Air Force Base, Illinois.

Although the military air medical evacuation system is intended for use by active duty personnel, it can also be used by their dependents and by military retirees and their dependents at no charge. Civilians can use this system also, but there is a charge and approval for use must be granted from the Department of Defense in Washington, D.C.

Details of the military air medical evacuation system can be obtained by calling Scott Air Force Base or any military treatment facility. For those who are unaware of it, the military air medical evacuation system is the most sophisticated air ambulance in existence. The Aerovac plane itself is very large, and not all landing strips can accommodate it.

When use of an air ambulance or the military air medical unit is medically indicated, it is usually necessary to coordinate use of a land ambulance at the sites of both departure and arrival. Provisions for this are often included in the service provided by the air ambulance company. However, to avoid confusion and possible fragmentation of care, the case manager must ascertain, when the initial arrangements with the air ambulance representative are made, who is to assume responsibility for this coordination—the air ambulance service or the case manager.

In some situations, it may be necessary to coordinate a "life flight" helicopter service from the departure point or at the point of arrival when the air strip necessary for landing is some distance from the patient and the patient cannot tolerate long-distance land travel. Most "life flight" helicopters are located at large tertiary medical centers or trauma centers.

The cost of commercial air ambulance service averages several thousand dollars. Medical necessity is the determining factor for healthcare payor reimbursement. When the cost of an air ambulance is excluded from coverage (e.g., most often this service is used when the patient is moved for the sake of convenience rather than medical necessity), it may be necessary for the family to pay the cost of the air ambulance themselves.

When a move closer to the family or for convenience is desired and the patient's finances are limited, the family should be encouraged to contact private plane owners about the feasibility of using their plane and pilot. Before making this suggestion, the case manager should obtain the attending physician's consent to this type of transportation. In these instances, the family is responsible for reimbursement of any costs agreed on. Depending on the extent of the illness or injury, equipping the plane to handle the patient may take several days to weeks, but private planes, like most post-acute care settings, can be equipped and staffed to handle most conditions or to simulate an air ambulance. Again, the cost of any equipment required for this mode of transportation must be borne by the family.

Ambulances and Other Modes of Medical Transportation

AMBULANCE VERSUS NONEMERGENT TRANSPORTATION

The use of an ambulance (an emergency-equipped vehicle) is, in most instances, not an appropriate method of transporting the majority of patients who are ready for discharge. Far too often an ambulance is used merely for convenience or because it is a "covered benefit."

All decisions related to use of an ambulance must be made on a case-by-case basis and must be based on medical necessity. The most common reason for reimbursement by the healthcare payor for ambulance transportation is that few communities offer nonemergent gurney or stretcher services and the patient is unable to be transported in a private vehicle because of a medical reason, such as a need for oxygen, suctioning, or restraints during transport. Other reasons for use of an ambulance may be that walking flights of stairs at home poses a risk or physical activity itself places the patient at risk.

Case managers must keep in mind that a trip of only one block in an emergency-equipped ambulance can cost several hundred dollars. In contrast, the same trip in a nonemergent vehicle or a wheelchair-accessible car costs half to one-third that amount if this type of transportation is available and medically acceptable. However, nonemergent transportation is not a covered benefit by most healthcare payors. For patients covered by the Civilian Health and Medical Program of the Uniformed Services (CHAMPUS) or veterans whose healthcare needs are being met by the Veterans Administration, every effort must be made to use the military or veterans ambulance systems or transportation services.

Trains

Contact the national headquarters of Amtrak by calling their toll-free number for information about the accessibility to departure and destination sites as well as the accessibility to and accommodations on the trains, including the bathrooms. Because of the limited and cramped aisles and bathroom capabilities, train travel, like bus transportation, is less than ideal for a disabled traveler. Families should be aware that Amtrak does offer discounts for the disabled and senior citizens if the ticket price exceeds a certain limit.

Ship or Cruiselines

Services for the disabled vary on ships and cruiselines, so it is best to inquire far in advance of the desired travel date. Motorized wheelchairs are not allowed on most ship or cruiselines, and many ships require that the disabled person use their equipment. Few ships or cruiselines can accommodate disabled travelers owing to lack of accessibility because of the lack of ramps, narrow doorways, and small bathrooms.

Rental Cars

All major car rental companies in most major cities offer rental cars with hand controls. In most cases, the companies require a 2-week notice to install the hand controls, which is done at no extra cost.

Fast Food Restaurants

For the visually impaired, the major fast food chains have printed or braille menus that are available on request.

SUMMARY

Application for use of public handicapped transportation must be made as soon as the patient is identified as a potential candidate for its use. This will avoid delays or fragmented arrangements if alternative arrangements are necessary while eligibility is established.

Costs associated with transportation or modification of vehicles are often not a covered benefit, and families must be prepared to assume these costs or make alternative arrangements. Case managers must be familiar with policy guidelines and should be prepared to educate the patient and family about the proper use of the emergency transportation benefits that are covered by their policy. If other modes of transportation are possible, these alternatives must be shared with the patient and family.

Ambulance transportation is often abused. It is common for patients to assume that since ambulance transportation is covered by their healthplan, they are entitled to use it even when other more cost-advantageous methods can be used and are available.

BIBLIOGRAPHY

Aldape VT (1994). Home caregivers make the difference (tips for screening and hiring). Paraplegic News 48(12):40.

Begany T (1996). Care for the caregiver. Patient Care 30(18):108–114.

Betts VT (1995). Helping caregivers in long term care situations. Am J Nurs 27(4):24.

Directory of Information and Referral Services in the United States and Canada (1995–1996 Edition). Alliance of Information and Referral Systems and United Way of America.

Falvo DR (1991). Medical and Psychological Aspects of Chronic Illness and Disability. Gaithersburg, MD, Aspen Publishers.

Gaynor SE (1989). When the caregiver becomes the patient. Geriat Nurs 10(3):120–123.

Glass C, Boling PA (1996). Collaborative support for caregivers of individuals beginning mechanical ventilation at home. Crit Care Nurse 16(4):67–72.

Hall SE, Marshall K (1996). Enhancing volunteer effectiveness. Am J Hospice Palliative Care 13(3):22–25.

Joseph IV, Reele BJ (1995). Respite for the caregiver. Am J Nurs 95(5):55.

McDonald TP, et al (1996). The impact of major events on the lives of family caregivers of children with disabilities. J Contemp Human Services 77(8):502–513.

McGlaufflin H (1996). Training volunteers and professionals to work with grieving children and their families. Am J Hospice Palliative Care 13(2):22–26.

Miller MS (ed) (1995). Health Care Choices for Today's Consumers. Resources for People with Disabilities and Chronic Conditions, Washington, DC, Living Planet Press.

Mintz SG (1996). Caregiver disorder: Recognizing an unacknowledged illness. Exceptional Parent 26(8):72.

Pillemer JJ (1996). It takes one to help one: Effects of similar others on the well being of caregivers. J Gerontol Series B 51(5):250-258.

Ruppert RA, Sandler RL (1996). Caring for the lay caregiver. Am J Nurs 96(3):40-47.

Shapiro J (1983). Family reactions and coping strategies in response to the physically ill or handicapped child: A review. Soc Sci Med 17(14):913-931.

Susik DH (1995). Hiring Home Caregivers: The Family Guide to In-Home Eldercare. San Luis Obispo, CA, Impact Publishers (American Source Books).

Wallhagen MI (1992). Caregiving demands: Their difficulty and effects on the well being of elderly caregivers. Sch Inq Nurs Pract 6:111-133.

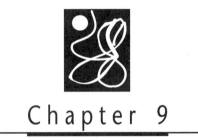

Chapter 9

Ancillary Services

DURABLE MEDICAL EQUIPMENT AND SUPPLIES

The federal Food Drug and Cosmetic Act of 1938 defines the term device as an instrument, apparatus, implement, machine, contrivance, implant, in vitro reagent, or related article including any component, part, or accessory thereof. It further stipulates that these devices must be recognized in the National Formulary or the United States Pharmacopeia or any supplement to these sources. In the definition, devices are intended to be used in the diagnosis, cure, mitigation, treatment, or prevention of disease or malformation and not for any other purpose or person.[1]

Almost every patient followed by case management at some time in the course of the illness or injury requires some kind of durable medical equipment (DME) or medical supplies. Medicare and most other healthcare payors use the categories and definitions used by the Food and Drug Administration (FDA) as a guideline in issuing decisions on coverage of DME.[2]

Definitions

As with devices, the FDA defines DME as "items which can withstand repeated use and are medically necessary for the treatment of the covered illness or injury." In contrast, medical supplies are "disposable or expendable items that cannot withstand repeated or prolonged use." A prosthetic device is defined as "an artificial substitute for a missing body part," whereas an orthotic device is "an external device to restrict or enhance motion or support a body part."[1]

Examples of medical supplies include such items as incontinent pads, catheters, Ace bandages, elastic stockings, adhesive tape, solutions, diabetic syringes, colostomy supplies, and irrigation sets. Many DME items, such as ventilators and oxygen delivery systems, regardless of whether they are rented or purchased, require the purchase of medical supplies. Such supplies are required on an ongoing basis and comprise an additional expenditure each month.

Although spectacles, eyeglasses, contact lenses, other optical devices, and hearing aids meet the definition of DME, most of these items are excluded from coverage by traditional health care payors. Additional exclusions may include prosthetic and orthotic devices, dupli-

cate DME items, educational items, home and transportation modifications, and environmental controls. In addition, any type of durable medical equipment that is considered merely "convenient" and not medically necessary is excluded from coverage.

Community Resources and Alternate Funding Sources

Most healthcare payors use lists of the types of DME they allow as well as those they exclude. Case managers must be familiar with both lists. If equipment is necessary to carry out the case management plan but is denied or excluded from coverage, the case manager must explore loan closets and any other possible sources of supply for the equipment. Community agencies that are known sources of assistance for DME supplies include:

- American Cancer Society
- Easter Seals Society
- Church, ethnic, or social service agencies
- American Lung Association
- United Cerebral Palsy Association
- National Multiple Sclerosis Society
- Other disease-specific organizations
- Make-A-Wish Foundation or similar organization

Examples of alternate funding sources that may help with equipment or supplies are:

- Other health insurance policies bought by the patient.
- Medicaid.
- Title V Children's Medical Services program.
- State Agency responsible for developmental disability services.
- Donations from fraternal organizations or private sources.
- Special Education program (this program is available only to those children who are eligible for services; equipment will be supplied only if it contributes to the general learning ability of the child).

If the required equipment is not available from any alternate source but is medically indicated and critical to the overall plan, the case manager must make every attempt to gain approval for it using the extra contractual approval process.

As indicated earlier, some equipment associated with learning is available through the school district if the patient is under the age of

21, is enrolled in school, and meets the eligibility criteria for the school's Special Education program. Unfortunately, even when the child meets these criteria and the equipment is approved, many school districts restrict its use to school hours. Because each state varies in the services it allows for children who qualify under the Individuals with Disabilities Education Act, case managers must be familiar with the various school districts and the policies applicable in his or her region when equipment is required.

Healthcare Payor Requirements

In addition to requiring patients to use their network of providers to obtain medical equipment, most healthcare payors allow reimbursement only for DME that has been approved by the FDA. In addition, they require that the equipment be used within the realm for which the FDA granted its approval. Just because a physician orders the equipment does not make it a benefit or a medical necessity. Also, a letter does not necessarily justify the equipment unless the letter and the medical information supporting it testify to the medical necessity of the item.

Excluded or Frequently Denied Items

Due to the types of patients enrolled in case management, the extra contractual approval process for DME may be used almost daily by case managers (this is not necessarily true with workers' compensation as benefits are more flexible). Such approval is needed because many of the patients require duplicate items, "deluxe" items, or items classified as "convenience" or "comfort" items if they are to function as independently as possible.

Although these so-called deluxe, convenience, or comfort items may be classified in such a way and denials for their use may be justified for the majority of the insured population, they are commonly considered a medical necessity for a person with quadriplegia or paraplegia or a child with cerebral palsy. Without such items, the patient may be at risk of costly complications. Consequently, the extra contractual process is used as a mechanism for validating the reasons for using these items and justifying their cost.

A variety of DME items are often excluded or denied, but most can be categorized, with examples, as follows:

- *Convenience items:* duplicate pieces of equipment, bed pans, overbed tables, shower chairs, and chair lifts.
- *Environmental equipment:* heating devices, air conditioners, electronic sensory devices for turning lights and appliances on or off, and air filters and air cleaners.
- *Exercise equipment:* exercise bikes, weights, and treadmills.
- *Nontherapeutic items:* fully electric beds (which are convenient rather than medically necessary), hand controls in automobiles, and van lifts.
- *Comfort items:* spas, water mattresses and pads, and hydromassage bath devices.
- *Hygienic equipment:* shampoo trays and wigs.
- *Education devices:* braille teaching texts and certain computers or electronic equipment used for speech or communication.

Commonly Ordered Equipment

The following is a list of the DME and orthotic devices used for a person with quadriplegia. These items are recognized as medically necessary for this condition and comprise the standard of care for such patients. As can be seen, many of the items are considered deluxe or convenience or would be so considered for other patients. The items required by a person with quadriplegia may include:

- Fully electric wheelchair with tongue, chin, or breath or mouth stick control (customized)
- Custom wheelchair pads (this item is required for patients with all levels of spinal injuries with paralysis)
- Wheelchair trunk supports or seating systems (customized)
- Slide boards
- Lumbar sacral orthotics
- Lapboards
- Arm supports
- Wrist and hand supports
- Adapted grooming and feeding equipment
- Semi-electric hospital bed
- Bed rails
- Patient lift and sling
- Standing frame

Of the foregoing, the only items that are truly not medically necessary are the lapboards and adapted grooming and feeding equipment. All the others are medically necessary if the patient is to have proper support and mobility. Certainly, the list is not limited to these items. In all cases, the final list of equipment ordered depends on the level of spinal cord injury in the particular patient.

In other patients, again depending on the diagnosis, DME items ordered may include:

- Semi-electric hospital beds, bed rails, and trapezes
- Bedside commodes, toilet rails, shower or tub benches
- Standard wheelchairs with removable arm and leg rests
- Transfer benches or slide boards
- Specialty beds (i.e., air beds, fluidized beds; these are generally used for persons with multiple and severe decubitus ulcers and persons confined to bed)
- Continuous passive motion (CPM) devices
- Glucometers (for insulin-dependent diabetics)
- Canes, walkers, and crutches
- Apnea and cardiac monitors
- Oxygen systems (varying from combinations of oxygen concentrators, liquid oxygen, and oxygen cylinders, to air compressors) and their related supplies
- Ventilators and all related supplies
- Feeding pumps, stationary poles, and all feeding supplies
- Infusion equipment and all related supplies
- Continuous positive air pressure (CPAP) devices and supplies
- Suction devices and related supplies
- Urinals and bedpans

Of the foregoing, often the toilet rails, shower or tub benches, and many bathroom devices are commonly excluded by healthcare payors. Believe it or not, most bathroom items, adaptive feeding and dressing devices, and some special items are excluded by healthcare payors or individual health benefit packages because they are considered not medically necessary! Additional bathroom and sleeping devices that are often not covered include:

- Raised toilet seats
- Grab bars for shower or tub
- Bath lifts
- Whirlpool equipment
- Special pillows (cervical or wedge)
- Air or gel mattresses
- Handheld shower heads

Ongoing Medical Supply Costs

Even when a DME item is purchased, it may also require the purchase of monthly supplies to operate the basic equipment. In such cases, case management plans must include provisions for this occurrence. Fortunately, some of these related supplies, which are required monthly and sold as "sterile" supplies, can be homemade. Therefore, whenever possible, the case manager must evaluate which supplies can safely be made at home or eliminated merely by using "clean" techniques instead of sterile techniques. However, the final decision for conversion to clean technique rests with the ordering physician. If the patient's supplies can be homemade or used with clean techniques, significant cost savings will result.

Home Monitors

Although premature infants compose the largest category of patients requiring home monitoring, there certainly are others, for instance, infants who are dependent on technology for a variety of reasons, those who are siblings of sudden infant death syndrome (SIDS) patients, infants with apparent life-threatening events (ALTE), and infants of substance abuse mothers (ISAM). In addition, monitors are frequently ordered for patients who are ventilator dependent or have other severe respiratory disorders. However, because patient stays are now so much shorter and patients are being discharged sicker, the list of persons requiring home apnea monitoring is not limited to the foregoing.

Despite the fact that home apnea monitoring is widespread and is used as a medical management tool, it can also become a "crutch" for the family or caregiver. In these instances, the monitor may be used when body language and other physical clues to ensuing problems could be just as helpful. For this reason, recommendations or authorizations for an apnea monitor must be based on clinical medical necessity. Continued authorization must be based on the actual events recorded for the previous month.

Before any home monitor can be recommended initially and before the authorization can be renewed subsequently, many questions must be answered. Such questions may include the following:

- What are the advantages and disadvantages of home monitoring and has it proved effective for this diagnosis?
- For approximately how long will the monitor be required?
- What are the emotional needs of the parents or family?
- Are there support groups available for families where they can learn from their peers how to cope with the demands of home monitoring and care?
- What additional teaching of the family is required?

Before the patient is discharged the family and any alternative caregivers must be instructed on how to operate the device and how to troubleshoot problems when they arise. In addition, all caregivers must be taught cardiopulmonary resuscitation (CPR). Not only must they be taught these skills, they must be able to demonstrate proficiency in the performance of the skills.

On discharge, there must be, at minimum, regular follow-up contact with the respiratory therapist from the DME company. In addition, care by a home health agency may also be warranted, depending on other needs for skilled care specific to the case. Certainly, if the monitor has been shipped by mail, home nursing visits by the local home health agency are warranted, and the staff must stay involved until the family adjusts to the monitor.

Families who must care for a patient requiring any high-technology equipment, such as a monitor, must have access to medical and technical support that is available 24 hours a day. In addition, whenever high-technology equipment is placed in a home setting it is wise to alert the local paramedics and the local power companies of the patient's condition and the devices used to manage it. If the patient resides in a region that experiences frequent power outages, battery back-ups and a power generator are required equipment.

In most cases, monitors should be rented because most patients require them for a relatively short period of time. Although the actual time frame varies, it commonly runs from 3 to 6 months. If it is evident that the patient will require the monitor for a long term, it may be more cost effective to purchase the unit. However, case variables, the patient's actual diagnosis, the frequency of the apnea episodes, and the healthcare payor's policy on equipment purchase all play an active role in the final determination of coverage. As with any other respiratory equipment, if the unit is purchased, consideration must be given to a service contract that should cover, at minimum, routine maintenance of the unit.

The decision to discontinue the monitor is usually made when the patient has not experienced any episodes of apnea during a specified time frame, generally 4 to 6 weeks. As with all equipment and services, this decision varies from patient to patient and is based on the patient's medical needs and condition as well as on the ordering physician's practice style.

Purchase Versus Rental of Durable Medical Equipment

Patients who require even the most sophisticated equipment can be discharged. The homes of case-managed patients are often converted to resemble mini-hospital units. However, to obtain reimbursement, several factors must be considered before any equipment is rented or purchased. Among these factors are the following:

- Is the equipment available from a network provider?
- Have the specific needs and medical justification for the equipment request been documented?
- What are the rental versus purchase costs of the equipment (including its maintenance)? If the equipment is rented, can the rental price be applied to the purchase price?
- What is the policy for buy-back, trade-ins, or loan of other equipment during periods of routine maintenance or repair?
- How long will the equipment be necessary (this answer will assist in deciding whether it is more cost effective to rent or purchase the item)?
- Is there a need for back-up equipment (i.e., if the equipment malfunctions, to allow the patient some independence, or during periods of routine maintenance)?
- Are alternative suppliers available in the area for purposes of cost comparison or in case the equipment or supplies are not available from the first supplier?
- Can the supplier schedule prompt same-day service or delivery with no extra charges for delivery or set-up?
- Is the provider willing to provide the equipment or training to the patient, family, caregiver, or professional before the patient is discharged at no additional cost?

Decisions about purchase of equipment vary from community to community and must be made on a case-by-case basis. In some cases, it is appropriate to rent the equipment for a brief period before an actual purchase is made. This allows enough time to ensure that the patient can be managed safely at home or indeed that the equipment requested is appropriate.

When considering rental versus purchase (and yes, it is often cheaper to purchase this type of equipment), several factors must be considered before the final decision is made. These factors demand answers to the following questions:

• How long will the patient require the equipment?
• Is the patient stable on the present model or are adjustments still being made that could indicate the need for another model?
• Is a service contract necessary? If so, who will cover the monthly service cost?
• If a service contract cannot be purchased by the patient or family, will the patient be at risk of a costly outcome if the equipment fails and a back-up unit is not readily available?

Although the long-range treatment plan may indicate that the equipment will be used for the long term, it is best to rent the equipment for the first 30 to 90 days or longer. This time frame allows changes and adjustments to be made to the equipment. More important, if the patient cannot tolerate a post-acute level of care, money has not been spent needlessly on equipment. Likewise, if the equipment thought to be the most desirable item at discharge turns out to be inadequate or less desirable for some reason and another item is required at a later date, money will not have been wasted. This scenario is especially true for patients requiring ventilators, several of which may be tried before the correct one is found. Also, sometimes the family finds, once the patient is home, that they cannot manage, and placement becomes necessary.

Because for some equipment long-term rental costs can easily exceed the purchase price, this factor must be considered when deciding whether to rent or buy. Ventilators are a good example. The purchase price of a ventilator, even with the cost of a service contract included, is far more advantageous than the rental cost. Most ventilators can be purchased for under $10,000 (the service contract is an additional $300 per month), whereas the monthly rental charges average $700 to $1000.

Service Contracts

If the equipment is serviced regularly, it can generally last for years. However, if it is purchased, routine maintenance may not be done. Thus, the prime drawback of purchase is that someone must assume the responsibility of paying for the routine maintenance and repairs that such equipment requires. When equipment is rented, the item continues to be the "property" of the equipment company, which is responsible for caring for it. However, when the item is purchased, these costs are then shifted to the new "owner." The only alternatives are to pay for the maintenance privately or arrange for it to be provided through a service contract.

A service contract basically covers the same services as those provided while the equipment was rented. Although a service contract can average several hundred dollars per month, these costs are cheaper than the cost of replacement or of deterioration of the patient's condition if the equipment fails. Unfortunately, this type of service is not routinely allowed by healthcare payors. Therefore, before purchase of equipment is considered, all factors must be taken into account.

Generally, when an item is rented, the rental price includes the routine maintenance required by the manufacturer and routine monitoring of treatment responses by the equipment company's professional nursing or respiratory therapy staff. Consequently, payment of a separate service contract is not required. Thus, before a ventilator is purchased, the case manager must be aware of the healthcare payor's policies for rental versus purchase. As stated earlier, if the ventilator is purchased, a monthly service contract must be considered, or, at minimum, a back-up ventilator must be readily available if the equipment fails or "routine" maintenance by the manufacturer is performed.

Equipment service contracts are almost a necessity for ventilators because the ventilator must be totally overhauled according to the manufacturer's specifications. As a rule, this is required for every 5000 to 8000 hours of use. During these times, the primary ventilator is sent out to be serviced and another is supplied in the interim. If a service contract is not maintained, the rental cost during the interim must be assumed by the healthcare payor.

Other Factors to Be Considered

If a non-network provider is used, case managers must not hesitate to negotiate discounted rates to ensure the overall cost effectiveness of the plan. Also, because of the costs associated with the need for equipment, case managers must be willing to "price shop" to ensure that the price is the best one available.

Sadly, the patient who is dependent on high-technology equipment may become the target of some opportunistic equipment companies. For this reason, all costs, the frequency of orders, and, more important, the amounts of equipment and related supplies must be closely monitored. Despite the fact that most DME items are available from the healthcare organization's network, this monitoring process should not be neglected.

Most DME companies provide free delivery, set-up, and teaching. Sometimes teaching is required while the patient is still an inpatient and discharge is imminent. In these situations, the company supplying the equipment to the patient should bring the equipment to the hospital so the patient or family can receive the actual teaching required there. In this way, the patient and family can be taught the needed procedures in the hospital and become familiar with the equipment. When this type of service is required, most healthcare payors do not reimburse the equipment company for this service; reimbursement starts at the time of discharge. In these cases, the company's professional staff or the home health agency must remain involved until the patient and family can demonstrate proficiency in all aspects of use of the equipment.

Equipment that must be customized (for instance, wheelchairs, seating pads, or trunk supports) requires outright purchase. However, until the special equipment arrives, similar equipment may have to be rented. This situation is always less than desirable because the interim equipment can cause unnecessary pressure sores or other problems that can be costly if procurement of the customized version is delayed for some reason. For this reason, the patient must be measured and the equipment ordered as soon as the need for this equipment is identified.

Some equipment requires modifications of the home and ramps. These modifications are rarely allowed by healthcare payors (the prime exception is workers' compensation). Consequently, the cost must be borne by the patient or family. When the family is unable to pay these costs, it may be wise to refer them to a fraternal organization. Volunteers from these organizations may be able to supply the labor, and the organization may be able to assist with covering the costs of any supplies used. Likewise, van lifts and modifications to vans or automobiles are not covered by healthcare payors (again, this is not true of workers' compensation). Costs then become the responsibility of the patient and family. However, depending on the patient and his or her motivation (and physical and mental abilities) to obtain gainful employment, the state department of rehabilitation or vocational rehabilitation may be a source of reimbursement.

Durable medical equipment and related supplies are commonly billed by using the Health-Care Financing Administration (HCFA) common procedural coding system (HCPCS). This is a set of codes used by Medicare and healthcare organizations for billing purposes because the codes are specific, among other things, for DME and ambulance services.

SUMMARY

Case managers must be familiar not only with the types of DME and those that fit the criterion of medical necessity, they must also be familiar with rental, lease purchase, and purchase options. Most equipment, if rented for any period of time, is more costly than outright purchase of such equipment. For this reason, many healthcare payors specify that if the rental price exceeds the purchase price, the equipment must be purchased.

Also, merely because a physician orders equipment does not mean that it is a benefit or that it is medically necessary. The case manager must know which items are medically necessary and which are for the patient's or the caregiver's convenience. Depending on the diagnosis, the medical necessity of the equipment, and its importance in preventing complications, some items that do not meet the medically necessary criterion may be approved through use of the extra contractual process. Unfortunately, the patient may have to do without some others. However, some so-called convenience items may be available through loan closets. Due to the many limitations and exclusions pertinent to DME, it behooves case managers to be familiar with alternative resources. If no such resources are found, the patient or family must be prepared to do without the items or assume the cost themselves.

Due to shorter stays in acute-care facilities and the discharge of patients who are more dependent on technology, the cost of needed durable equipment, if not watched closely, can be astronomical. More often than not, equipment should be purchased; however, before purchase occurs, a trial of rented equipment may be indicated. The keys to the final purchase are the service requirements of the equipment and provisions for patient monitoring. These are negotiated when the equipment is purchased if provisions are not already in place to have the service contract remain in force.

SELF-HELP DEVICES OR ADAPTIVE EQUIPMENT, OTHER TIPS FOR USE OF DURABLE MEDICAL EQUIPMENT, AND HOME MODIFICATIONS

Self-help devices and other factors related to the use of DME and home modifications are very important to the overall success of the case management plan. Because they may be excluded from the patient's healthcare coverage (workers' compensation is one exception), the patient or family may be required to assume a cost that is unplanned or for which there is "no money." This section also provides some helpful hints on how to make some of these items at home.

In all situations in which there is doubt, and before making any recommendations to the patient and family, always check with the attending physician about the feasibility of the alternative. Key resources that can be used for information or assistance in planning or designing self-help devices are the therapy teams (physical therapy, occupational therapy, and speech therapy) found in any rehabilitation unit, the local Easter Seals Society chapter, and the professional nursing or rehabilitation staffs of the local home health agency.

Clean Technique or Homemade Alternatives

Clean technique and homemade supplies are cost-effective alternatives to the high cost of sterile supplies once the patient is home and no longer requires the sterile technique and supplies used in the hospital. However, case managers must *always check with the physician first before implementing or suggesting this alternative to the family.*

Most homemade supplies cost less than 10 cents per item, whereas the same item, if purchased, can cost more than $1 to 2. For example, the savings achieved for a tracheostomy patient using clean technique for suctioning and care of the suction catheters versus sterile suction catheters can exceed $300 per month. The following sections highlight some examples of cost-effective homemade supplies or tips that are commonly taught by home health agency nurses and can be used in place of costly sterile ones if the attending physician agrees.

GENERAL TIPS

For patients confined to bed and without decubiti, corn starch spread on the lower sheet allows the patient to move about more easily and helps to prevent "sheet burn."

To assist in keeping urine smells to a minimum, full-strength white distilled vinegar can be used to wipe mattresses and plastic sheeting, tubing, and bags.

STERILIZATION OF WATER AND SUPPLIES

For disinfecting toilets and bedpans, the Centers for Disease Control (CDC) suggests using household bleach. Use a ratio of one part bleach to ten parts water.

In making any solution, the water, storage jars, and jar tops (metal screw type) can be sterilized by boiling the item or solution for 15 minutes.

Metal or glass containers or instruments should be used whenever possible (e.g., glass asepto syringes and baby food, mayonnaise, or peanut butter jars).

Two large "boiling pots" are necessary—one for water and one for receptacles or containers.

Once solutions have been sterilized, they should be stored in sterilized jars; other items can be stored in self-sealing plastic bags.

Hot soapy water and household bleach are two of the most commonly used disinfectants and are recommended by the CDC for disinfecting most items (such as those used for persons with tuberculosis or acquired immune deficiency syndrome [AIDS]).

HOMEMADE SOLUTIONS

In the following recipes, the salt, sugar, and soda dissolve better if the water is hot. All mixing and measuring must be done using sterilized containers or utensils.

Normal Saline:
1 teaspoon salt
1 quart boiling water (sterilized water)[3]
Mix well and keep in a sterilized closed
    container; replace every 24 hours.
Dakins Solution:
To make a 25% Dakins solution:
25 ml Clorox in 1000 ml H_2O or normal
    saline
To make a 50% Dakins solution:
50 ml Clorox in 1000 ml H_2O or normal
    saline[4]
Mix well and keep in sterilized closed
    container; replace every 24 hours.
Soda Solution:
1/2 cup baking soda
4 cups sterilized water
Mix well and keep in a sterilized container,
    store in the refrigerator, and replace every
    24 hours.
Acetic Acid Solution:
1/2 cup distilled clear vinegar
1 quart sterilized water[5]
Mix well and keep in sterilized container and
replace every 24 hours. The vinegar solution is
used to dissolve mineral deposits from urine
that often plug catheters, leg bags, inlets, and
valves of equipment. Leg and drainage bags
should be soaked approximately 8 hours in the
solution. Respiratory equipment should be
soaked for a few minutes, rinsed with clear
water, then drained and allowed to dry.

OTHER HOMEMADE SUPPLIES OR CARE

Egg Crate Mattress Care

If the patient has an egg crate mattress, it
can be washed in a bathtub with water and
detergent, rinsed thoroughly, and hung to dry.
Old egg crates can be cut into various sizes and
used as protectors for pressure points.

Brace Care

The leather lining of braces should be
cleaned with saddle soap or a leather cleaner
once a month. This increases the longevity of
the brace and helps to prevent the leather from
cracking.

Incontinent Pads

Incontinent pads can be made as follows:

- Several pillow cases
- One to two sheets of plastic cut to the size
  of the pillow case
- Several stacks of newspapers folded in half

Place plastic sheet in the pillowcase. Add about
a quarter- to a half-inch thickness of newspapers. When used, place the plastic nearest the
mattress. The plastic can be reused and wiped
clean with distilled white vinegar, and the pillow cases can be washed in hot soapy water.
The cost of these pads is minimal, whereas
purchased incontinent pads average more than
a dollar each.

Tracheostomy Care Kits

When clean technique is used, gloves are not
necessary; only good hand washing is required
prior to suctioning or caring for a tracheostomy.
Most of the supplies in a tracheostomy or
"trach" care kit can be obtained from local
tobacco or notion stores and can be made as
follows:

- Regular one-half inch hemming tape is available at notion stores and can be used in place
  of twill tape provided in disposable trach kits.
- Pipe cleaners or small brushes (available at
  local pipe or tobacco or variety stores) can
  be used to scrub the inner cannula.
- Gauze can be purchased in bulk from most
  pharmacies.

Tracheal catheters can be cleaned and reused
8 to 10 times before they become too stiff and
must be discarded. The catheters commonly
become cloudy after the second or third cleaning, but this does not affect their function. To
keep the catheters "clean," the patient or family
should store them in a plastic bag after each
use. Tracheal catheters are cleaned using the
following method:

- Flush the catheters with 2 tablespoons of
  hydrogen peroxide.
- Totally immerse them in a solution made of
  1/2 cup liquid dish detergent and 3 cups
  boiling water and soak overnight.
- Flush with 1/4 cup of boiling water.
- Wipe the outside of each catheter with a
  cotton ball saturated with isopropyl alcohol.
- Place in self-sealing plastic bag.

Urinary Catheter Care

Intermittent catheterization is a technique
used frequently for patients with a neurogenic
bladder or those who are continent between
catheterizations. Intermittent catheterization is
used only if the patient or family accepts the
procedure. In most cases, intermittent catheterization can be accomplished using clean technique. However, the final choice between clean

versus sterile catheterization technique is made by the physician and depends on the patient's particular circumstances.

With clean technique, urinary catheters can be used up to 7 days each if they are cleansed properly after each use. For cleaning catheters used in intermittent catheterization, the patient will require:

- Soap and hot water
- French rubber catheters (several)
- Receptacle in which to place urine (a toilet is OK)
- Self-sealing bags
- Clean towels and wash cloths
- Tube of water-soluble lubricant
- If the patient is female and is catheterizing herself, a mirror

Catheters are collected after each use in a towel, basin, or self-sealing bag for bulk cleaning. Collected catheters are washed with hot soapy water, rinsed in clear water, and stored in self-sealing plastic bags or clean towels. As with tracheostomy care, if clean technique is used, there is no need for gloves, only good hand washing.

Self-Help Devices

When a person is disabled, whether with a short-term or long-term disability, it often takes more time and effort than usual to accomplish daily tasks. It may also require unnecessary dependence on others or pose safety problems. Therefore, evaluation by a therapist for the use of self-help aids is as necessary as an evaluation for the use of any DME. In some cases, the simpler devices can be homemade, although the more technical ones cannot. Self-help aids or devices range from simple, large, or long-handled utensils to high-technology, breath-activated, or simple touch- or movement-generated electronic devices.

Despite the fact that commonly used self-help aids are readily available from most DME providers and specialized ones can be ordered, the costs of all of them must somehow be reimbursed. Therefore, decisions about coverage are made case by case and are based on medical necessity, not convenience. Unfortunately, reimbursement from healthcare payors is frequently limited to the standard models, and the patient and family must be prepared to assume the cost difference if deluxe items are preferred. Insurance coverage for self-help devices or aids is not common.

Case managers must keep in mind that the reason for obtaining self-help devices for the disabled or physically challenged is not for comfort but for promoting independence. Before self-help devices or aids are purchased, four major factors must be considered:

- Suitability
- Durability
- Ease of maintenance
- Ease of use

There are eight basic categories of self-help aids. These are:

- Bathroom
- Dressing and undressing
- Eating and drinking
- Personal hygiene and grooming
- Household or food preparation
- Communication
- Emergency response systems
- Mobility

Many of the following devices are not considered medically necessary and are excluded from healthcare payor coverage. Although many of these devices can be homemade, many others must be obtained from a DME company or a company specializing in self-help devices. In all cases, the key to evaluation is whether the device will allow the patient to function at his or her maximum potential.

DEVICES FOR DRESSING AND UNDRESSING

- Dressing sticks (two wooden dowels with cup hooks at the end that allow the person to pull on clothing)
- Twill tape loops sewn in waistbands (help in pulling on clothing)
- Buttonhook
- Zipper pull
- Stocking pull
- Long-handled shoe horn
- Velcro fasteners or seam closures to replace buttons or other closures
- Special adaptive clothing designed for the disabled (can either be made or purchased)

DEVICES THAT AID EATING AND DRINKING

- Special eating utensils (angled, swiveled, or long-handled or padded)
- Plate guards
- Dish with built-up sides and suction cups

- Special cups or glasses that are T-handled, two-handled, V-shaped, or have a weighted bottom
- Plastic clips or Velcro straps to secure eating utensils to the hand

PERSONAL HYGIENE AND GROOMING DEVICES

- Bedside commode
- Male or female urinal
- Bedpan (regular or fracture pan)
- Large, long, padded, or extended handles for toothbrushes, combs, hairbrushes, shaver or shower brushes
- Gooseneck or flexible tubing or special mounted mirrors

DEVICES THAT AID HOUSEHOLD OR FOOD PREPARATION TASKS

- Lap board
- Reacher (extension, claw, magnetic)
- Utility cart
- Baskets attached to walker or wheelchair
- Light switch extension
- Door knob adapters
- Pulley system
- Special handled or adapted knives, cutting boards, corner guards, or other food preparation devices
- Braille knobs
- Oven and food slide boards
- Oven sticks
- Special can and bottle openers
- Stove knob turners

COMMUNICATION DEVICES

Many communication devices are available through the local phone company. Families should be encouraged to explore this possibility whenever possible. For children under the age of 21 who are enrolled in school and eligible for Special Education, special communication devices may be available through the school district. However, in such cases the school district generally restricts use of any devices allowed to school hours. Other sources for communication devices are disease-specific organizations, speech and language centers, and the Title V Children's Medical Services program.

In all cases, the patient must be assessed to identify the appropriate device that allows him or her to communicate. Devices often include such items as:

- Telephone aids
- Flashing light or sound frequency system
- Amplifiers
- Electronic voices or viewers
- Communication boards
- Computers
- Braille watches, clocks, knobs, books, or writers
- Large-print books
- Talking books and devices
- Breath-activated systems

BATHROOM DEVICES

One of the first areas in the home requiring assessment for the use of self-help devices is the bathroom because safety factors must always be a concern. Some common bathroom aids are:

- Tub and shower handrails
- Bathtub seats and transfer benches
- Single-lever faucets
- Hand-held shower units
- Toilet frames or handrails
- Elevated toilet seats
- Hydraulic or mechanical bath lifts

EMERGENCY RESPONSE SYSTEM DEVICES

The emergency response system (ERS) is frequently used for frail elderly and disabled homebound people who are alone for any period of time. This system is an electronic telephone interception device that, when activated, secures the telephone line and routes the call to the local emergency room, where a preplanned emergency plan is activated. Many communities now offer this service. One of the best ways to locate information about this program is to call the local emergency room, state department of aging, or the local department on aging. The costs for a device of this type vary from program to program and in different communities, but for most systems the cost is very reasonable.

MOBILITY DEVICES

Mobility devices (see also the section on DME in the first part of this chapter) vary and depend on the extent of the patient's disability, the ability to move, the gait pattern, and the coordination, balance, transfer capability or strength, and endurance of the patient. Examples of mobility aids used for various levels of mobility and independence include:

- Wheeled walkers—used to conserve strength or promote independence.
- Platform walkers—used when both an arm and a leg are affected.
- Wheelchairs—used for persons with various levels of injury but primarily for those who are restricted in weight bearing or endurance.

For patients who are permanently confined to a wheelchair the chair must be custom-made because it must be not only the right weight for maneuverability but also the right height, width, and proportion to fit the patient's body measurements. Customized wheelchairs assist in preventing pressure areas and allow for proper body alignment. Special pads to prevent skin breakdown or pressure areas are a must for permanent wheelchair users. Quadriplegics and other neurologically impaired persons frequently require head or trunk supports as well as other supports, seating systems, or devices that allow them to sit with their bodies in proper alignment.

Patients who require a wheelchair intermittently frequently require chairs equipped with elevating leg rests and swing-away or removable arm rests. If they are to be as independent as possible, these patients often require additional equipment such as commodes or shower seats, slide boards or free-standing trapezes, or patient lifts if ease of transfer, toileting, and independence are goals.

For persons confined to bed a semi-electric bed with side rails and a trapeze allows independence; an alternating air mattress prevents pressure areas and skin breakdown; and a hydraulic or manual lift allows one-person transfer. Some patients confined to bed, such as those with a special cast or a spinal cord tumor, will require a reclining wheelchair because they are unable to achieve or tolerate an upright position.

To promote independence patients often require two different items intended for the same purpose. Dual equipment is usually not covered by healthcare payors. As a result, it may be necessary to obtain the "duplicate" item from a community agency or loan closet. Examples of situations in which dual equipment may be warranted include patients who can walk a short distance but are not yet totally independent. They also may lack the strength and endurance to walk any distance or stand for a period of time. Such patients may require both a wheel-

chair and a walker. Other examples of patients requiring dual equipment include those who may require both a bedside commode and a bedpan, or, in the case of a disabled student enrolled in school, an electric wheelchair may be needed in school, whereas at home the presence of carpet or other barriers makes the electric wheelchair inoperable, thus necessitating a regular wheelchair.

HOMEMADE SELF-HELP DEVICES

Many self-help aids can be made by converting ordinary household items to new uses. Sometimes the only modification required may be merely to increase the diameter of the part grasped because this decreases the force or effort required. Good examples of homemade self-help devices include the following:

- Wooden dowels to extend handles or make clothing pull sticks.
- Suction cups glued to the bottoms of items.
- Gooseneck or flexible tubing to create angles when necessary (e.g., mirrors with flexible or extended tubing when it is necessary to visualize oneself for self-care).
- Wood or metal to build up corners (e.g., to adapt plates or bowls with an edge to prevent food spillage when one has the use of only one hand or has muscle spasticity) or make corner guards.
- Bicycle grips, foam curlers, foam padding, or tape to build up handles.
- Three-inch foam ball with a hole in the center to hold pens, pencils, toothbrushes, eating utensils, hand-held safety razors, or other hand-held items.
- Bicycle baskets, trays, or cookie sheets with or without sides for carrying items.
- Terrycloth wrapped around water glasses to allow an easier grip and to prevent slipping.
- Tiered utility carts for carrying larger items.
- Velcro fasteners to replace zippers or buttons or to adapt openings or seams.
- Velcro straps to hold hand-held items.
- Pulleys and ropes.

Information about self-help devices can be obtained from occupational therapists or physical therapists. Information is also available from rehabilitation units, the local Easter Seals Society chapter, centers for independent living, the Blind Society, assistive device centers (often located at local colleges), and centers for deafness. In addition, patients or families should be encouraged to contact their local utility companies (electric, gas, and telephone) because they offer special programs and have many devices designed to aid the handicapped.

Architectural Barriers and Modifications

Architectural barriers in the patient's home make it difficult or impossible for the patient to function independently. They may also inhibit performance of necessary activities of daily living and prevent or inhibit the patient from entering or leaving the home, delaying social reintegration into the community, recreational activities, and employment. Unfortunately, many healthcare payors (with the exception of workers' compensation) and alternate funding programs exclude barrier modification or corrections from coverage. Consequently, the patient or family must pay for any expenses associated with these modifications.

Before the healthcare team can make recommendations for modification of barriers, they must know what barriers exist. They must also know whether the patient rents or owns the home. If the patient rents, landlord restrictions must be taken into account, and these often interfere with any recommendations. If the restrictions are too stringent, the patient may be required to relocate. In extreme cases, placement in a healthcare facility may be required until suitable housing can be located. Whenever barriers must be corrected, local building codes must be considered.

When assessing the patient and the patient's home for home care and the presence of potential barriers, the following factors must be evaluated:

- Accessibility to the outside and the driveway
- Ease of entrance and exit
- Accessibility to the bathroom, shower and tub, or toilet areas
- Accessibility to the bedroom
- Accessibility to the kitchen or eating areas
- Space available for high-tech equipment
- Width of halls and inside doors for maneuverability
- Presence of interior steps

RAMPS

It is often necessary to build ramps (either portable or stationary), widen doorways, or add safety railings to allow access to the home for people with mobility problems. The expenses associated with such home modifications or ramps, as stated earlier, are not allowable by most healthcare payors or alternate funding programs. The only exceptions are persons covered by workers' compensation, some vocational rehabilitation programs, and certain veterans. Case managers should encourage families who are unable to pay for making such modifications to contact fraternal organizations such as the Lions or Shriners to ascertain whether they can lend assistance.

Information about home modifications and home assessments as well as building plans for ramps are often available from agencies such as the centers for independent living, rehabilitation units, or the local chapter of the Easter Seal Society.

SUMMARY

Often self-help and mobility aids and necessary modifications to the home are excluded from the patient's healthcare coverage. Therefore, costs associated with procurement of these aids must be assumed by the patient or family. Many fraternal organizations or church or ethnic groups are willing to conduct fund raisers or assume responsibility for correcting barriers or making modifications to the home as a service project.

Regardless of the method of payment used, proper assessment of the need for self-help or mobility aids and correction of architectural barriers is an essential part of the process of providing continuity of care and maximizing the possibility of independent function.

The alternative and home-made supplies suggested in this section can potentially benefit many patients. However, before making any such recommendations or instituting any changes, all suggestions must be clarified and approved by the attending physician. The alternative supplies described here are especially helpful for patients and families who cannot afford the continued monthly out-of-pocket expense of purchased sterile supplies.

Sterile technique is the standard of care while patients are hospitalized, but once they are discharged, most home healthcare and infusion therapy agencies teach clean technique because it can be used safely in the home in most cases. Sterile technique is necessary primarily for the preparation of solutions and formulas, for the care of some wounds, for some intravenous administration of solutions or drugs, and for care of some skin sites.

Case managers should *never* suggest implementing clean technique until this has been approved by the attending physician.

PHARMACEUTICALS AND ENTERAL THERAPY

Pharmaceuticals

Despite the fact that most healthcare payors allow benefits for prescriptions and pharmaceuticals (Medicare is the one major exception), this does not mean that this benefit should go unwatched. This is true for all patients but expecially for case-managed patients. It is well known that most patients in case management have catastrophic and costly illnesses. Consequently, most of their drug costs are similarly high.

Due to the nature of the diagnoses in these high-risk patients, "routine" drug costs tend to be high, and in some the costs are exorbitant. Still others may be taking research drugs as part of a research program. Also, because of the diagnoses and the unusual drugs required, many drugs may not be available from the healthcare payor's pharmacy or infusion network. Thus it may be necessary to use a non-network provider, first seeking approval from the medical director and then negotiating an acceptable cost.

HEALTHCARE PAYOR REQUIREMENTS

Just because a drug is not included in the healthcare payor's formulary does not mean it is experimental. However, most healthcare payors (including Medicaid) maintain a list of the drugs allowed under their benefit structure. In most instances, not only must the drug be in the formulary, it must also be the generic equivalent of brand-name drugs; most healthcare payors will reimburse the cost of a trade-name drug only if documentation substantiates the medical need for this drug.

As a rule, healthcare payors exclude from benefit coverage all experimental or investigational services, and this includes any experimental, investigational, or "off label" pharmaceuticals. But many patients in case management caseloads, due to the nature of their disease, are participants in clinical trials and thus take drugs

that belong in these categories. For patients taking experimental drugs, laboratory tests to monitor the response to treatment are necessary. Unfortunately, like the drugs themselves, such tests may not be covered by the healthcare payor. Consequently, patients enrolled in clinical trials must be closely followed by the case manager to ensure that the costs are shifted appropriately and the patient is not required to assume these unexpected costs.

Medicare is one of the few healthcare payors that basically has no drug benefit. The few drugs Medicare does cover are pain medications for persons in a hospice program, immunosuppressive drugs following organ transplantation, some oral cancer drugs, and immunization for influenza. In essence, any person on Medicare is well advised to have Medicaid or a supplemental or Medigap policy or be enrolled in a managed care program that has a pharmacy benefit; otherwise, he or she should be prepared to pay for medications out of pocket. This lack of coverage for drugs is possibly the biggest void in the Medicare program. Case managers who have patients on Medicare must be acutely aware of this lack and must be ready to assist them in seeking alternative funds for payment of drug costs. Unfortunately, there is often no alternate funding available, and the expense must be paid by the patient or go without the drug. Over-the-counter (OTC) medications are rarely covered by healthcare payors, even with a prescription. Similarly, enteral therapy or formulas may not be covered either, because they are classified as OTC preparations. This is especially true if the formula is not administered by a pump and tube. Likewise, nutritional supplements, despite their importance, are rarely if ever covered. In addition to nonformulary drugs, over-the-counter drugs, and experimental drugs, other drugs excluded from coverage include drugs dispensed by a non-network pharmacy if the healthcare payor maintains a network; in these cases, if reimbursement is to occur, the drugs must be dispensed by the network pharmacy.

To help keep drug costs lower, many healthcare payors limit the number of pharmacies and infusion companies in their network or offer mail order pharmacy capabilities. This process decreases their costs by decreasing dispensing fees and improving compliance with their policies and procedures. The benefits to the patient include reduced out-of-pocket expenses. Also, with pharmaceuticals obtained from a mail order pharmacy, the cost is further reduced, and the patient has the added benefit and convenience of door-to-door delivery. If the patient is linked to a healthcare payor that does not maintain a pharmacy network, the case manager should encourage the family to explore procurement of drugs from a national mail order pharmaceutical company. Mail order pharmacies are a wonderful addition to any case management plan because they allow the patient and family more freedom for other tasks. As a result, case managers should use this resource whenever possible.

A word of caution about national pharmaceutical companies is in order. Because these companies are so popular, they are one of the resources referenced to patients and families by physicians, discharge planners, facility-based case managers, and especially large tertiary care centers and their staff when medications are ordered on discharge. Therefore, if the case manager's employer is a healthcare payor that requires the use of specific pharmacies, this information must be shared with the facility-based healthcare team at the time of admission. Likewise, case managers employed by the facility must always verify the pharmacy requirements of the healthcare payor. Otherwise, the patient and family may have to assume unnecessary costs because they will be linked to a pharmacy that will not be reimbursed by the healthcare payor.

FAMILIARITY WITH DRUGS

The fact that one drug has a variety of names causes confusion not only among nurses but also among other healthcare professionals and the general public as well. Nevertheless, it behooves case managers to be familiar with the common names of drugs, their uses, the standard of care for administration, and their costs. Such knowledge is necessary because drugs are often prescribed by either the chemical name, the trademark name, or the popular name given by the pharmaceutical company that manufactured it. To further complicate matters, if the same drug is manufactured by several different companies, each drug will have its own trade name. If in doubt, look it up.

Because of the many drug names and the complex actions of drugs, it is almost impossible to be familiar with every drug and its idiosyncrasies. However, the case manager is still responsible for being knowledgeable about the drugs prescribed for his or her patients. One of the most common sources of information about drug products is the Physicians Desk Reference

(PDR). This reference is an invaluable guide because it lists the conditions for which the drug has been approved; if a drug is not listed in PDR, it may be experimental for the condition, and this requires further investigation. It is imperative for case managers to have this reference source at their disposal. The PDR is an annual publication that offers specific details about drugs, such as composition, diseases for which use of the drug has been approved by the FDA, usual dosage, side effects, and contraindications. In addition, it is wise to maintain a notebook containing literature and resources on drugs, as well as phone numbers (e.g., Food and Drug Administration, infusion company pharmaceuticals) that may be useful when questions arise.

FOOD AND DRUG ADMINISTRATION

If questions do arise about a drug and whether it has been approved, the case manager may call the FDA's toll-free number directly for information about the drug in question. This agency not only approves drugs for general usage, it also approves other services, items, and devices, so it is an excellent resource for information on therapeutic interventions for clarification.

EXPERIMENTAL DRUGS

As a rule, the FDA requires drugs to go through three phases of development and trial to prove that they are reasonably safe and effective for treatment of a particular clinical condition. Until recently, these phases could take years, with phases one through three averaging 5 years. However, the AIDS epidemic changed some aspects of this process, and the FDA is now able to accelerate the drug approval process, making promising investigational drugs available earlier. If a drug is allowed to be released early, it is labeled an investigational new drug (IND).

Despite such early release for use in a specific condition, new drugs continue to undergo the process of clinical trials. The regulations ensure that careful controlled trials continue until the drug demonstrates effectiveness for the conditions for which it will be prescribed. Early release on the market does not mean that healthcare payors will automatically approve the drug, add it to their formularies, or assume responsibility for the costs.

Fortunately, if the drug in question is in the

investigational new drug category or in the last phases of a clinical trial (such as drugs intended for "compassionate use") or is used as an "off label" drug (see following paragraph), the healthcare payor may allow reimbursement for the drug. Reimbursement may be possible through several options, including outright approval, or special approval granted by the medical director, or use of the extra contractual process. The key to coverage is often merely the provision of sufficient information (especially cost savings data) that support and justify use of the drug.

Sometimes a drug has been approved by the FDA but its use may be required for a condition that was not included in the original FDA approval. Use of a drug under such circumstances is termed off label use. As with experimental drugs, some healthcare payors allow this and others do not. Healthcare payors that do allow such coverage follow the same process used for individual case review and coverage for experimental drugs when they review a request for off label use.

AVERAGE WHOLESALE PRICE

If network pharmacies or infusion companies are not available and a non-network pharmacy must be used, the case manager must be prepared to negotiate a discount to get the best price if drug costs are to be kept to a minimum. This process is required because there are vast differences between the billed charges and what is known as the average wholesale price (AWP). The average wholesale price is the price paid by the pharmacy for the drug obtained from the wholesaler or drug manufacturer. Pharmacies and infusion companies then add dispensing fees and profits that account for the vast differences in price. As a result, there is often room to negotiate discounts if the pharmacy or infusion company is willing. Also, because prices vary so widely, the case manager must compare prices before starting any negotiations. Such price comparison allows a baseline from which negotiations can start and ideally, a better overall final cost can be achieved.

DRUG UTILIZATION REVIEW

As stated earlier, drug therapy can be costly, especially when it is required over a long term or for a lifetime. For example, transplant patients are required to take cyclosporin, antire-

jection, or immunosuppressive drugs daily, for which costs average $1500 per month. Similarly, drugs for cancer and AIDS patients can easily cost $1500 per dose. Drugs for chronic pain can be just as costly. So monitoring drug usage is a must.

In addition to utilization review for medical and mental health conditions, many healthcare organizations have a drug utilization review program. These programs are designed to collect and analyze data and report the findings. Reports are than generated that show, at minimum:

- Overall drug utilization and costs.
- Areas benefiting from physician education.
- Patterns of drug utilization, costs, and physician dispensing practices.

The overall goal is to reduce costs and produce a program driven by a focus on quality.

Enteral Therapy Formulas

Because of the severity or nature of their illness or injury, many patients in case management require enteral therapy. Basically, enteral therapy consists of a liquid nutritional product administered into the gastrointestinal tract via a nasogastric, jejunostomy, or gastrostomy tube. Many healthcare payors allow enteral therapy as a benefit, but many others do not. Healthcare payors who do allow the therapy as a benefit do so if documentation supports its medical necessity. This therapy is medically necessary if the patient:

- Has an anatomic reason for an inability to swallow.
- Has a disease or pathologic lesion that prevents him from maintaining weight despite oral feedings.
- Requires the formula as the sole source of nutrition.

As a rule, enteral feedings that are excluded from coverage are those that are used as nutritional supplements to boost protein or caloric intake. This exclusion also covers formulas that are the mainstay of a dietary plan, but no pathology supports their use. Unfortunately, formulas are also frequently excluded because they are an over-the-counter item and because, regardless of the mode of administration or the formula's purpose, the general argument is that "the patient needs to eat and groceries are not a covered benefit."

When enteral therapy is needed, the case manager must attempt to seek approval for coverage through the extra contractual process or to procure the formulas from alternate funding sources (e.g., Medicaid, the Title V Children's Medical Services program, or the local Supplemental Food Program for Women's Infants and Children's [WIC] program). Coverage is necessary because far too often the costs of the formula may exceed the amount that the family, regardless of income, spends monthly for food.

COSTS AND PROCUREMENT

Because enteral therapy formulas can be costly, it may be necessary to negotiate discounts or per diem rates if the healthcare payor has agreed to pay for the formula and a non-network provider is used. As with pharmaceuticals, if the healthcare payor's network pharmacies or infusion companies can supply the formula, the patient may be required to use these providers. The only exception occurs when reimbursement for the formula is denied because it does not meet the criteria of medical necessity. In these cases, the patient and family have the right to use any provider they desire.

When the formula is not available in the healthcare payor's network and the patient receives the formula via a pump or by gravity flow, case managers must strive to ensure that payment for the formula and all related supplies is reimbursed using an all-inclusive rate. Such a rate will cover not only the formula but also all equipment and supplies and any nursing visits needed for direct care or teaching the family or caregiver how to administer the formula and use the equipment.

SERVICES REQUIRED

Patients receiving enteral therapy frequently require the skilled services of nurses from a home health agency or infusion therapy company. Such services are necessary until the patient and the family can demonstrate competence in administering the formula and changing the tube. The frequency and number of visits vary depending on the circumstances of the individual case. However, in most instances, this type of skilled nursing care is required only during the first 7 to 14 days; rarely are visits necessary beyond this time. If more visits are required, the actual notes pertinent to the need for skilled care must be reviewed

carefully, and continuation of coverage is determined on a case-by-case basis.

Other services that must be included in the case management plan include radiologic services, which are necessary to monitor tube placement. Depending on the patient's homebound status, a local company offering portable radiologic services may be required, contributing additional costs to the case management plan.

For babies and infants in whom the feeding tube is inserted and removed with each feeding, families or caregivers must be taught not only how to insert the tube but also how to recognize the signs and symptoms that the tube is placed inappropriately. In such cases, the skilled nursing visits from the home health agency or infusion company may be required (and are considered medically necessary) for a longer period of time than the initial 7 to 14 days typical of other cases.

Most gastrostomy feeding tubes or gastrostomy feeding buttons require little maintenance once the wound heals. Naturally, patient variables can affect the frequency of services. However, after the initial teaching of wound care and formula administration has been mastered, care may no longer be considered skilled. Care of such patients may then be classified as custodial. Also, because gastrostomy tubes are inserted directly into the stomach, little skilled care is actually required, even when the formula is administered through a pump. Because of these factors, gastrostomy tube feedings are rarely classified as skilled care, and rarely is this level of care reimbursable by healthcare payors.

The most common methods of enteral therapy administration are mechanical feeding pumps or feeding bags used with gravity flow. Despite the fact that most formulas are over-the-counter items, their bases vary—some have a powder base, whereas others are already prepared liquid products. Likewise, the formula bases vary for different and specific reasons and depending on the diagnosis. For instance, Pulmocare liquid is a lactose-free product that is frequently used for patients with respiratory problems, whereas TraumaCal liquid is frequently used for patients sustaining multiple injuries or burns. Infants and children with chronic diarrhea, malabsorption, cystic fibrosis, short gut syndrome, and other symptoms related to allergies or sensitivities to corn or cow's milk may require Soyalac, Isomil, or Alimentum. Although case managers are not involved with the actual writing of the order for the formula, they must be aware of and have contact with resources for procurement and nutritional counseling experts if families are to be linked with the most cost-effective supplier of the formulas.

In rare instances, formulas can be homemade. However, this is the least desirable method of procuring formulas and depends on the specific requirements of the case. If costs are an issue and access to alternate funding is nonexistent, the case manager may wish to explore this option with the attending physician. If this is possible, it is then critical to link the patient and family with a qualified dietitian who can calculate the nutritional needs accurately and assist the family in planning the right formula ingredients.

With few exceptions, administration of most enteral formulas can be accomplished using clean technique rather than sterile technique. Switching to this technique as soon as the patient is deemed medically stable by the attending physician is a method of achieving cost savings because this process decreases the costs associated with gloves and sterile water. Naturally, if a patient is confined to a facility, sterile technique is required, but these services are included in the overall daily rate.

SUMMARY

Although the patient's healthcare policy may cover the costs of drugs, if not carefully monitored, these costs can be exorbitant because often the patient's need for pharmaceutical products lasts for the long term or a lifetime. It therefore behooves case managers to include a method for monitoring medication usage and costs in the case management plan.

Because the cost of drugs can be exorbitant and vast differences in drug costs exist, case managers must make every effort to link patients to their healthcare payor's network pharmacies or negotiate discounts when the use of non-network pharmacies is necessary.

Because of the nature of their disease or injuries, many patients require enteral feedings. Although many healthcare payors allow reimbursement of enteral products, equipment, and supplies if the formula is administered by tube and there is documentation supporting its medical need, other payors do not. In contrast, formulas administered by mouth and those used primarily as a nutritional supplement may not be reimbursable by any healthcare payor.

Although many formulas are considered over-

the-counter products, they are also available from infusion companies; if they are, the family has a "one stop shop" for all their feeding supplies. Despite the fact that many formulas are OTC products, they are costly and vary in price, so if they are to be covered by the healthcare payor, the case manager must be prepared to negotiate a discounted rate or a per diem rate. When the patient is discharged home on a formula, an infusion company or home health agency is commonly required until the caregiver can demonstrate competence in administering the formula and changing the tube.

REFERENCES

1. United States Code Service 21 USCS (1997). Title §321. U.S. Administrative Public Health and Welfare Codes.
2. St. Anthony's Medicare Coverage Manual (1996). St. Anthony's Publishing, pp. 171–172.
3. Visiting Nurse Association (1996). Patient Education Manual–Sterile solution. Sacramento, CA, Visiting Nurse Association.
4. Visiting Nurse Association (1996). Op. cit., Dakins solution. Sacramento, CA, Visiting Nurse Association.
5. Visiting Nurse Association (1996). Op. cit., Acetic acid. Sacramento, CA, Visiting Nurse Association.

BIBLIOGRAPHY

Allman J (1996). Understanding of rehabilitation technology providers. Continuing Care 15(7):18–20.
Bertram GK, Katzung BG (1995). Basic and Clinical Pharmacology, 6th ed. Stamford, CT, Appleton- Lange.
Block SS (1991). Disinfection, Sterilization and Preservation, 4th ed. Philadelphia, Lea & Febiger.
Food and Drug Administration (1995). FDA Consumer from Test Tube to Patient: New Drug Development in the United States. Washington, D.C., U.S. Department of Health and Human Services, Publication No. FDA 95-3168.
Fisher JE (1991). Total Parenteral Nutrition, 2nd ed. Boston, Little, Brown.
Herfindal ET, et al (1992). Clinical Pharmacy and Therapeutics 5th ed. Baltimore, Williams & Wilkins.
The Homecare Case Management Source Book (1996). Malibu, CA, Miramar Communication Inc.
Lehne RA (1994). Pharmacology for Nursing Care, 2nd ed. Boston, Little, Brown.
Lesko M, et al (1993). What to Do When You Can't Afford Healthcare: An A–Z Sourcebook for the Entire Family. Kensington, MD, Information USA Inc.
MacLeod SM (1993). Pediatric Pharmacology and Therapeutics. St. Louis, Mosby-Year Book.
Pinnell N (1996). Nursing Pharmacology. Philadelphia, W.B. Saunders.
Resources for Persons with Disabilities and Chronic Conditions (1993). Lexington, MA, Resources for Rehabilitation.
Rice R (1995). Manual of Home Health Nursing Procedures. St. Louis, Mosby-Year Book, pp. 3–15.

Rombeau T, Coldwell MD (1993). Clinical Nutrition, Parenteral Nutrition, 3rd ed. Philadelphia, W.B. Saunders.

Shabino CL, et al (1986). Home Cleaning, Disinfection Procedure for Tracheal Suction Catheters, Pediatr Infect Dis 5(1):54-58.

Stanhope M, Knollmueller RN (1992). Handbook of Community and Home Health Nursing. St. Louis, Mosby-Year Book.

Williams SR (1997). Nutrition and Diet Therapy, 8th ed. St. Louis, Mosby–Year Book, pp. 447–478.

Chapter 10

Case Management in Specific Clinical Situations

COMMON HIGH-RISK CATASTROPHIC CASES

This chapter describes many of the most common diagnoses and situations found in patients in case management. There are no rules for the management of patients because every patient, family, and situation is unique. In addition, each case is affected by the patient's or family's coping ability or emotional stability, the intensity and severity of the illness or injury, the intensity and complexity of the care required, and the resources that are available or required to prevent rehospitalization or deterioration of the patient's condition. These variables affect all decisions made as well as the patient teaching required, the barriers to discharge, the overall case management plan, and the outcome. As stated earlier in the introduction to this book, the case manager's own organization and its policies, procedures, and criteria dictate the type and level of case management offered.

This section of the manual is designed to alert new case managers to the many factors involved in managing technologically dependent patients in their caseload. It is not the author's intention to paint a bleak picture but merely to offer an idea of the magnitude of the orders and issues that affect most cases. Usually the case manager is a welcome addition, and the family is delighted to have someone who can help them understand the issues involved and navigate the healthcare maze.

Case Management Plan

As stated earlier in this book (see Chapter 2), case management plans must be developed for specific patients and must include a composite of all data collected during the interview and assessment processes. The final plan is based on the following components:
• The treating physician's orders.
• The standards of care for the illness or injury outside the acute care facility.
• The patient's actual physical and psychological needs.
• The family's or caregiver's physical and psychological needs.
• The financial means or resources available to pay for the care.
• The availability of resources to meet the patient's level of care.

In all cases, the orders or services requested must be based on the patient's individual needs and must be specific to the patient or ordering physician. Standards of care for the community, region, or facility affect the success of any case that requires continuity of care. Because of the importance of standards of care, case managers must be familiar with the standards that affect healthcare providers and the healthcare delivery system. This familiarity must encompass not only local standards but regional and national standards as well, and recent legislation has also changed how health care payors must act on experimental issues. Without this knowledge, case management of all patients, but especially technologically dependent patients, is likely to be unsuccessful. Case managers should remember that what might have been done for one patient may not be necessary or appropriate for another! The same thing is true for hospital versus home care. What can be done in an acute care facility may not be possible in the post-acute healthcare arena. The case management plan, if developed and employed correctly, serves as a guide to obtaining access to care and linking patients to the necessary resources in a time-efficient manner as well as ensuring that resources are used effectively as the patient moves through the continuum of care.

In establishing the case management plan, it is essential to include short-term and long-term goals. Goals must be realistic and attainable for everyone involved and cannot be effective if input from the family is not allowed. The goals of the case management plan are greatly influenced by ethical dilemmas as well. Ethical issues and differences between the patient, family, providers, and payor, if not addressed and resolved or satisfied by a compromise, can result in failure of the plan. There will be times when the family's goals may differ from the goals thought to be important by the providers or payors. When these differences occur, crises and delays can be expected if a consensus cannot be reached about the relative importance of the goals.

To obtain the patient's and family's cooperation, the case manager must often help the family prioritize their goals, focusing on the ones that are most important or the ones that will result in the greatest improvement or have the greatest impact on the quality of life of everyone affected. As the assessment phase and the case management plan evolve, it is imperative for the case manager to not only identify resources to meet needs but also to point out any limitations or exclusions in the patient's healthcare benefits that could require application for the extracontractual or waiver process or application to an alternate funding program.

Because these processes are very detailed and time consuming, ample time must be allowed for events such as the health care payor's case manager to collect the pertinent justifying medical data and prepare the case for a coverage determination by the healthcare payor's medical and legal review processes for the extracontractual process or the family must be allowed the time to make application and receive a determination regarding acceptance for alternate funding (i.e., Medicaid).

Case managers who are unfamiliar with how the extra contractual process works must collaborate with their peers to become familiar with the process and the details required and to understand the importance of working as a team with the healthcare payor. This understanding is necessary because the extra contractual and waiver processes can serve as an excellent means of linking patients with appropriate levels of care, services, or items that would otherwise be lacking in the final case management plan because they are excluded or limited by the patient's own health benefit structure.

Multiple Diagnoses

Because many patients who are case management clients have multiple diagnoses and multiple needs, referrals are necessary to all resources specific for each diagnosis or issue. For example, if a patient with severe diabetes has an amputation and this amputation is further complicated by a stroke and cancer, referrals to community agencies for all three diagnoses are in order. In this case, the American Diabetes Association, the American Heart Association, and the American Cancer Society may be among the agencies utilized. Services from these agencies can range from information, education, and support groups to volunteers. In most cases the services obtained from these agencies will augment or enhance the patient's healthcare benefit coverage and the services reimbursed by the healthcare payor.

Head injuries may result in dual diagnoses (i.e., medical needs and psychiatric needs). When this occurs, the medical case manager and the mental health case manager must confer and determine which diagnosis is paramount. Likewise, they must decide which discipline, mental health or medical case management, is to assume responsibility for coordinating the resources necessary to manage the patient's care appropriately. Regardless of

which case manager assumes the role of the primary case manager, coordination of mental health and medical benefits, resources, and services must occur if both problems are to be treated. Far too often in patients with dual diagnoses, either role overlaps or role conflicts occur. Likewise, there is a potential for fragmentation and gaps in the care provided and in the establishment of resources available to aid the patient. These gaps and fragmentation of care can be avoided through close collaboration and excellent communication among all case managers involved. These two keys are essential if the patient is to meet the goals established by the healthcare team.

Home Care Versus Out-of-Home Placement

Healthcare professionals hear it said repeatedly that home is the best place for patients because they do better in their own surroundings and environment. However, at the present time, when patients are discharged sicker and sooner and require more complex care, home care can be very expensive, and, more important, it is not always appropriate for every patient. Therefore, when home care is contemplated, four basic factors must be considered. These factors can serve as guidelines in determining whether the patient can benefit from home care and whether the cost for such care is reasonable and acceptable to the healthcare payor and out-of-pocket expenses for the patient and family are manageable. The four factors are:

- The patient is ambulatory and can seek care provided by specific outpatient services, programs, or providers; if this is not true, it must be determined whether the patient meets the criteria for homebound care and whether the level of care can be adequately provided by home health care providers.
- The patient's medical, psychological, or psychosocial needs require continued care or supervision that can be provided in a home setting.
- The home environment is conducive to the treatment plan and to achieving the desired goals.
- The costs of the home care plan are comparable to or less than inpatient alternatives (e.g., continued hospitalization in an acute care facility, skilled nursing facility, subacute care facility, or rehabilitation unit), but despite the

reduced costs the quality of the care is essentially the same.

For many patients the costs of "basic" nursing care and equipment necessary for home care may exceed thousands of dollars per month. Not included in these costs are other charges (e.g., physician home visits, outpatient laboratory or radiologic services, pharmacy charges) for services that are necessary to meet the patient's needs. Thus, when evaluating all costs, home care can be far more expensive than placement. In other cases, numerous daily visits by professionals (e.g., nursing, physical therapy, speech therapy, occupational therapy, laboratory, radiologic services) requiring out-of-pocket copayments by the patient can make home care financially impossible for many patients. Consequently, out-of-home placement until the patient's condition is medically stable and can be managed more easily at home is usually the best plan.

Any number of examples could be cited to illustrate the foregoing statements; the following case is one of many possible ones. The patient in this case was a woman in her late thirties who suffered a major stroke. She was a single mother, her elderly parents lived out of state and were physically and emotionally unable to render the care she required (they were staying temporarily with her children), and her children (all teenagers) were in school. To further complicate matters, her insurance had very limited home healthcare benefits, the healthcare payor refused to consider the extra contractual process, which would have allowed 24-hour care in the home, and the patient and her family could not afford the cost of 24-hour care.

On the positive side, the children had an excellent loving relationship with their mother, and the patient's insurance did cover short-term rehabilitation, skilled nursing facility care, and short-term home healthcare. Despite the fact that the patient required total care, was aphasic, and had a major hemiplegia, the children wanted to bring their mother home. They would serve as her primary caregivers. The healthcare team developed a plan that made use of the skilled nursing care benefits in the patient's insurance package by carefully monitoring her care needs as she progressed through the continuum of care from one level to another. Each member of the team assumed the task of educating the children about the benefits of temporary placement in an acute care rehabilitation hospital and a skilled nursing facility before she came home. This plan not only allowed the patient to make the necessary gains

as she recovered, but also, and more important, it allowed the children to continue to learn the caregiver skills taught by the nursing and therapy staffs throughout each phase, ultimately resulting in the children becoming the caregivers. Implementation of this plan took hours of coordinated effort among all members of the healthcare team. It also took hours of counseling of the children by the social worker about the positive benefits of this arrangement. In the end, the children were able to complete their schooling, and the mother made the gains anticipated. By the time the patient was discharged, she was more independent, and the children were proficient in all aspects of her care and could serve as her caregivers without reservation.

Barriers to Discharge and Access to Care

Developing a case management plan for the discharge of a patient requiring complex care or one who depends on technological equipment requires considerable lead time (i.e., several days to weeks). This time frame is necessary for the patient and family to gain full acceptance of the plan, for any training to occur, and for all resources to be in place and ready to assume responsibility for the patient's care. For patients who are to be discharged home, the patient, family, and caregiver must be fully trained, and the home environment must be readied for the discharge. This itself can be a reason for delay, but it is not the only one. Costly delays can be encountered for any number of reasons, and although some of these are case specific, the following factors are often the primary culprits in the delays encountered in establishing a home plan:

- Inadequate home environment or, in some cases, no home.
- No family or caregiver.
- Family in-fighting, or family resistance to or noncompliance with the plan.
- Local physician unable or unwilling to accept responsibility for care.
- Local resources or agencies not available or unable to assume the required level of care.
- Transportation for follow-up appointments or services not available.
- Financial reserves inadequate, and patient is ineligible for alternate funding.
- Multiple psychological factors present in either the patient or the family.

- Patient, family, or caregiver nontrainable (i.e., language and cultural barriers, care is too repulsive or dexterity problems).
- Care too complex or beyond the standard of care for home care.
- Conservatorship for the patient required, and the process has not been started or completed.

In contrast, typical barriers to out-of-home placement include the following:

- Facilities not available or inadequate to manage the level of care required (this is especially true for patients who are children or for any patient who requires total care).
- Staffing inadequate in either number, type, or skill level (e.g., depending on state licensing laws, in many skilled nursing facilities a registered nurse [RN] is present only on the day shift, and licensed vocational or practical nurses [LVN or LPN] are available during the evening and night shifts, or the staff may not have the skill level and training to manage the patient).
- Facility available out-of-area, but this is unacceptable to family.
- Facility administrator unwilling to hire additional staff or to train existing staff.
- Financial resources of patient or family limited; they cannot afford the ongoing care if the patient's care needs are deemed "custodial," in which case, their healthcare coverage will terminate, and neither the patient nor the family is eligible for Medicaid.
- Total care required, and facility has a waiting list.
- Patient has infectious disease, and facility has no private room or cannot accept a patient with an infection.
- Patient's weight a problem (i.e., many facilities will not accept patients who weigh more than 200 to 250 pounds because this factor increases the probability of back injuries in their staff and increases workers' compensation claims).
- Intravenous therapy required, and staff is not certified to provide it.
- Delays in application for alternate funding encountered.
- Delays in conservatorship process encountered.
- Rates unacceptable to healthcare provider or healthcare payor, or healthcare payor must negotiate a reduced rate prior to transfer, or another facility must be found.

Although all such barriers vary with the individual case, if any barriers are encountered, the case manager frequently must make many daily calls to various facilities, whether local or regional, either to locate a suitable facility that can accept and render the care required or to ascertain the patient's status on the waiting list.

It is a well-known fact that healthcare professionals have an automatic tendency to blame barriers to discharge on the healthcare system in general. However, patient and family barriers are often encountered as well. These include such experiences and emotions as:

- Fear (e.g., fear of the unknown)
- Unrealistic priorities
- Insufficient motivation
- Previous unhappy experience with providers or resources
- Lack of knowledge of resources
- Lack of understanding of the problem (e.g., denial, emotions, language)
- Self-image
- Cultural or language factors
- Financial limitations
- Pride (e.g., too proud to apply for Medicaid because it is "welfare")

Communication

It must be kept in mind that families of patients who are catastrophically ill or injured are frequently under tremendous stress and often in a crisis situation, both initially and sometimes throughout the case; consequently, clear communication with such families may be difficult. As stated earlier, the success of case management involves clear, open, and honest communication with all participants—the patient, the family, and the healthcare team. Just as important is the fact that such communication must be conducted at a level that facilitates understanding by all parties. This is a critical link. Success also involves old-fashioned teamwork in which the case manager, regardless of his or her employer, becomes an integral part of the team. A successful case manager also acts and approaches the family or healthcare team in a proactive manner rather than a reactive one.

The power of communication with all parties—patient, family, physician, and healthcare team—cannot be overstated or underestimated. The actual frequency of communication depends on the individual case. However, it should always be frequent enough to ensure an actual sharing of information and an awareness by all case managers of the latest details of the case. In return, the patient, family, and healthcare team must also be kept informed about the progress of case planning as well as any delays encountered.

A good example of poor communication occurred in the following case. The patient in this case had a complicated postoperative course and eventually developed renal failure, which necessitated a kidney transplant. After the transplant he again had a stormy course, which resulted in multiple readmissions. Shortly after the last readmission, the case manager was notified that the patient had been terminated from his healthcare plan because his wife had lost her job and he had no coverage, not even through the Consolidated Omnibus Budget Reconciliation Act (COBRA). Because the employer had not supplied all the information about COBRA to the wife in a timely manner, the COBRA paperwork was subsequently submitted on the very last day on which the wife was eligible for filing it, and it appeared that retroactive coverage would not be possible because of the delays.

As a result, the healthcare payor could not authorize home care or infusion therapy because the patient appeared to be ineligible on the data base. To complicate the issue, the infusion company and the home healthcare agency were reluctant to accept the case because the only viable healthcare payor was Medicaid and they were not a Medicaid provider (but the only one in the immediate area), and despite the fact that the patient was eligible for Social Security's end-stage renal program and Medicare was to pay retroactively, the providers would not consider accepting the case. After many phone calls between the healthcare payor, the employer, the home healthcare agency, and the transplant team, it was discovered that the social worker knew of the wife's impending dismissal and was aware of the potential need to extend COBRA coverage, but she had not told the healthcare payor about it, nor had the wife during any conversation with her. In this case, the case manager could have worked with the employer and the patient to ensure a smooth transition of benefit coverage, whereas instead the transition was stormy, some frantic phone calls were placed, and the patient and his wife suffered a number of fears needlessly before a satisfactory end was finally reached.

Psychological Factors

Communication, both verbal and nonverbal, is also important in ensuring that any psycho-

logical factors or stressors associated with the case are recognized. The patient and family must be allowed to express their feelings. Depending on their responses, linkage to peer support or professional counseling may be necessary. Whenever possible, the patient and family should be informed of some of the actual and potential stressors they can expect to encounter and the mechanisms that can be used to alleviate them. This information allows them to recognize the stressors as they occur and to make appropriate arrangements to deal effectively with them. The best way to ensure that this occurs is to address these problems in the case management plan.

The ability to cope is affected by many factors, some of which are related to past experiences in dealing with crisis situations, the emotional well-being of the patient and family, the ability to cope in general, and the actual situation or circumstance causing the stress or crisis. Although stressors are not limited to the following situations, these factors and emotions are commonly encountered by case managers:

- Feelings of frustration are present because the patient and family believe that they are receiving conflicting answers or are not receiving the "true story" (i.e., they may have difficulty in communicating with or in obtaining access to the medical staff).
- Tempers are on edge; denial is the primary coping patter
- Feelings of hostility emerge owing to the unfairness of the situation or because the patient and family cannot accept the changes that have occurred in bodily functions or in body image (loss of the ideal or "normal" image of self or loved one).
- Emotions are so high that they only hear what they want to hear (i.e., they may have selective hearing).
- Exhaustion results from countless sleepless nights, improper nutrition, hurried hygiene, and worry; personal needs are forgotten.
- Feelings of disbelief are present; they cannot believe the situation is happening to them or that the condition might not improve.
- Feelings of overwhelming guilt occur; the impact of the responsibility they must face may or may not have set in.
- Fears of the unknown are always present; the impact of finances, bills, and care responsibilities may or may not have set in, and although it is often not spoken, the fact that death is a real possibility is in the background.

As the patient's condition changes or becomes chronic, it is common to see many or all of the foregoing reactions as well as feelings of frustration with the "system." Also, as the condition becomes chronic, other stressors occur related to problems such as lack of help, respite, or financial assistance; loneliness; isolation; and exhaustion. All of these are common reactions in families of patients with long-term problems. To assist in identifying any stressors and to prevent social isolation or escalation of the situation, it is imperative to link the patient and family with disease-specific support groups or agencies or professionally trained counselors. In these groups they can learn not only how to cope, they can also learn first-hand from their peers how to navigate the healthcare system.

An example of a case illustrating some of the foregoing reactions occurred many years ago. In this case, a baby was born several months prematurely and was hospitalized in a regional neonatal center. This case was not opened to case management because the child was progressing as anticipated, the family had been linked to the appropriate alternate funding programs, and there was no indication that the child would suffer long-term complications. On discharge, low-flow oxygen, an apnea monitor, and a daily visit for the first week by a nurse from the local home healthcare agency were ordered (all of which had been arranged by the hospital discharge planner). In addition, the parents had received adequate teaching and discharge instructions. All indications seemed to point to a normal discharge—correct? Wrong.

Approximately a week after the baby was discharged, the authorization request line for the health maintenance organization received a frantic call from the mother, who said that her child "was dying." The call was transferred to the case management department. During this conversation it was discovered that the baby was not accepting any nourishment, was losing weight, and was clearly at risk of hospitalization. It was also discovered that

- The mother had slept very little since the child had arrived home; she had been told by the residents and interns that "she needed to watch her baby because the baby could die," so she literally stayed near the baby all the time, watching it day and night.
- The mother (aged 18) and the father (aged 19) had been fighting for several days because she was inattentive to his needs, but paid attention only to the child.
- The mother and father had not had sex since before the child's birth.

- The mother had quit her job and had relocated to be near the regional center and the child; consequently, their income was greatly reduced, and they could not meet their monthly expenses.
- Because the mother had formerly paid the bills, this duty had long been neglected; several bills were now past due, and collection agencies were calling.
- The mother confessed that she did not feel comfortable holding the baby because the baby was not the "perfect" child she had dreamed of.
- Because of the long hospitalization, visits by a home health agency nurse had been approved, but these visits never occurred because the mother refused to allow the initial visit. Why? Her mother and mother-in-law had insisted that she forego this service because she needed to "bond" with the child (unfortunately, the home health agency never alerted anyone to this fact).

As these and other issues surfaced, it became apparent that this family needed help. The physician was called to see if an immediate appointment could be arranged to allow the baby to be examined. This was possible. In the return phone call to the mother, it was agreed that the case managers, one from the healthcare payor and the other from the local regional center, would meet the mother at the physician's office where a plan could be formulated. The following case management plan resulted:

- Using combined benefits of the extra contractual process and services from the regional center, 2 days of nursing care for 16 hours a day were approved, followed by 5 days of nursing care for 8 hours per day from the home health agency. This care allowed time for teaching the mother feeding techniques as well as observation of the child as the mother slept.
- The physician changed the baby's formula, and the parents were linked with the local Women's Infants' and Children's (WIC) nutrition program, which provided assistance in procuring the formula.
- The parents were linked with a local support group where they could learn care techniques and gain support from other parents of children requiring special care.
- The parents were linked with a marriage and family counselor to help them solidify their relationship.
- The parents were linked to the local consumer credit counseling services, which of-

fered assistance in dealing with their creditors and drew up a schedule for repayments that could protect their credit history.

In this case, despite the fact that the healthcare team thought that the needs of the baby and family had been met on discharge, they were not. This lack of recognition, combined with other stressors and misinterpretation (or selective hearing) by the parents of what was said, almost led to disastrous consequences. In this case, the final case management plan was essentially designed to provide caregiver respite and opportunities for the parents to learn caregiving techniques.

Teaching

Due to the complexity of care required by most case-managed patients, teaching and mastery of all care techniques, troubleshooting of problems, and correction of problems are the most vital of all the processes needed in planning for a move to an alternate level of care. Teaching is even more vital if the alternate level of care is to be the patient's home. Occasionally, patients being discharged to a post-acute care facility will require care that is so complex that the proposed post-acute care facility staff may require training in the specific details of the patient's care before the transfer is allowed. Although training the family concentrates on direct, "hands-on" care, it is not limited to this type of training. Sometimes teaching in the early stages of an illness may center on such issues as gaining an understanding of the specific diagnosis. It may also include such issues as gaining access to and use of resources, making lifestyle changes, planning the diet, and making decisions.

Case managers and all healthcare professionals must keep in mind that patients and caregivers must become as familiar with care techniques as healthcare professionals. Unlike professionals, who may be in the home for a relatively short period of time during the day or week, the family or caregiver often assumes responsibility for care for the greater part of a 24-hour day 7 days a week. More important, patients and families are expected to learn in a relatively short period of time what it may have taken the healthcare professional weeks or years to master.

Naturally, the substance of teaching varies in each case, but for all patients it must be started as soon as possible. Every patient who is capable of self-care must be taught this care or allowed the opportunity to learn it. With all patients, active participation in their own care must not be limited merely to their physical ability to perform the actual tasks. Self-care must encompass not only any physical care but also the chance to contribute actively to the choices and decisions necessary for care. Physical self-care for many patients is not always possible. However, the ability to contribute and make informed decisions helps patients to:

• Reduce their fears and anxieties about the unknown.
• Alleviate passive dependence on others.
• Encourage motivation and compliance.

If self-care is to be effective, it must be a collaborative effort between the patient and the teacher. The teacher must allow ample time for the performance of tasks and not become impatient if they cannot be completed in a reasonable time frame. Likewise, the creativity involved in performing a task must not be thwarted if the patient's method accomplishes the same result. Choices about how to accomplish the care are individual. Such choices are not the teacher's decision but the patient's because the patient must live with the consequences.

The key to teaching is that *every* body system must be assessed thoroughly, and all physical needs must be identified. From this needs assessment checklist, a plan for teaching can be developed. Possibly one of the best means of assessing each body system is to use a predeveloped questionnaire or checklist that can be modified to meet individual teaching needs. However, if in the course of asking questions other issues surface that may have an impact on the final plan, notes must be added to the checklist to ensure that these issues are captured and addressed in the plan. Because proper teaching is so critical for home care, many case management organizations have developed assessment forms for the use of their staffs. If such a form is not available, one can be developed using the guidelines listed below. If properly developed, this assessment checklist serves as the data base for the teaching program. Assessments for teaching must cover the following body systems, all care required for each system, and the corresponding teaching required to perform the care. The checklist also covers who will be taught and who will serve as the teacher (or teachers):

• Respiratory system
• Skin

- Gastrointestinal system
- Genitourinary system
- Nervous system
- Musculoskeletal system
- Cardiovascular system
- Mental capabilities
- Mobility and functional capabilities
- Communication abilities
- Emotional capabilities

Once the assessment has been completed and the areas of care or needs have been identified, a teaching plan can be developed. The final teaching plan must cover such areas as:

- Signs and symptoms of problems and when to call for help.
- Potential equipment needs and the training necessary to operate the equipment.
- Training required to ensure that all caregivers are proficient in all aspects of care, use of equipment, and troubleshooting techniques, as well as such minor details as proper storage and location of the equipment and supplies.
- Potential medical supplies needed—how many, when and where to order, and where and how to store.
- The medication regimen—dosages, times, storage, instructions, side effects, and contraindications.
- Nutritional and fluid needs for the patient's activity level as well as other nutritionally related issues that may include such details as:
  - Swallowing and feeding exercises
  - Formula preparation
  - Feeding tube maintenance and equipment
  - Identification of self-help feeding devices
  - Aspiration techniques
  - Signs and symptoms of dehydration or fluid overload
  - Feeding tube malfunction or malposition and troubleshooting; for infants, the actual reinsertion of the tube with each feeding
  - Proper positioning to prevent aspiration or choking
  - Radiologic services to verify tube placement (most often such services use portable equipment and are able to come to the patient)
- Oral hygiene and dental care:
  - How to brush and floss another's teeth or perform oral hygiene
  - Importance of scheduling frequent dental appointments (especially for persons who have an aversion to mouth care, an aversion

that is very common in children who are or have been ventilator dependent)
- Bladder program:
  - Application, cleaning, and emptying of drainage devices
  - Insertion and cleaning of catheters
  - Signs and symptoms of bladder infections
  - Signs and symptoms of urinary retention
  - Application of diapers
  - Importance of skin care
  - Signs and symptoms of vaginal infections
  - Sexual functioning and alternatives
  - Obtainment of urinary supplies
- Bowel program:
  - Signs and symptoms of constipation, how to prevent it, and how to treat it
  - How to administer an enema, insert a suppository, check for a fecal impaction
  - Diarrhea and how to treat it
  - Importance of skin care
  - Positioning the patient on a bedpan
- Autonomic dysreflexia:
  - What it is
  - Signs and symptoms and how to recognize it
  - Treatment
- Communication and speech needs:
  - Ordering or development and use of speech devices and communication systems or techniques
  - How to use devices or communication systems
- Seizures:
  - What to do when one occurs
  - Airway maintenance
  - Patient protection and use of devices such as helmets and pillows
- Muscle spasms:
  - Body repositioning
  - What to do when they occur
- Temperature regulation and measurement:
  - How to measure temperature and read a thermometer
  - Emergency measures for handling an elevated temperature
- Range of motion, repositioning, and techniques for preventing:
  - Footdrop
  - Contractures
  - Muscle spasms and spasticity
  - Skin breakdown
- Body mechanics for the caregiver.
- Application, removal, and care of antiembolic stockings, splints, braces, orthotics, or shoes.
- Patient lifting, manually or with a hydraulic lift.

- Patient transfers to and from bed, chair, car, and bathroom.
- Mobility and turning schedule for bedbound patients.
- Use of wheelchair and any other mobility device.
- Prevention and treatment of skin breakdown and decubitus.
- Foot and nail care.
- Use of pillows, foam pads, and padding.
- Use of special mattresses and beds.
- Wound care techniques, including clean versus sterile technique, irrigation techniques, preparation, procurement, and storage of solutions, procurement and storage of dressings, and signs and symptoms of wound breakdown and the need to seek further medical care.
- Signs and symptoms of heart failure, including:
  - Blood pressure measurements
  - Respiratory and pulse measurements
- How to take routine vital signs.

Any or all of these items can pertain to any patient. However, one of the main areas requiring teaching is encountered in patients requiring respiratory care. With these patients teaching must cover not only the signs and symptoms of respiratory failure but also frequently the following specialized areas:

- Signs and symptoms of respiratory infections.
- Use, care, and cleaning of all respiratory equipment.
- Oxygen administration, safety issues pertaining to oxygen, electrical use and electrical safety hazards.
- Nebulizer use, including administration of medications.
- Apnea monitor use, if applicable.
- Clean versus sterile technique.
- If the patient is ventilator dependent, all aspects of ventilator care must be taught, including information about the ventilator equipment, its parts, settings, function, dials, alarms, and how it all works; changing the circuits; storing and changing the batteries; how to assemble and reassemble all parts after cleaning; what to do if the ventilator malfunctions; and how to troubleshoot any problematic areas.
- Chest percussion and postural drainage.
- Auscultation for breath sounds.
- Nasal, oral, and tracheal suctioning techniques.
- Use, care, and cleaning of suction equipment and supplies.

- Tracheostomy care and maintenance, and troubleshooting emergency situations in patients with a tracheostomy (e.g., how to maintain the airway if the tracheostomy tube comes out); changing the tracheostomy tube; caring for the stoma; how to inflate the tracheostomy tube cuff and auscultate for cuff leaks and the importance of doing this.
- Hand bagging techniques (i.e., using an Ambu bag to breathe for the patient).
- How to maintain the patient's ventilation if an emergency occurs.
- How to remove a mucus plug.
- Cleaning, maintenance, storage, and ordering of all supplies and equipment.
- What to do in the event of a power outage.
- Signs and symptoms of respiratory distress and when to call the physician.
- Cardiopulmonary resuscitation.

As can be seen, the general teaching checklist is extensive. Add to this any other teaching the family may require (such as care of the patient with diabetes or a transplant or wound care), and the list becomes even more extensive. Not only must the family or caregiver be trained in all aspects of the care required, they must also know basic information about body mechanics and infection control and how to protect themselves when lifting or moving the patient or handling waste or soiled linens or dressings. Teaching of such information is necessary because in many cases the caregiver will be alone, and if injuries or infections are to be prevented, training in basic care and preventive techniques is imperative.

Once the teaching needs have been identified, the teachers of each task must be assigned and an actual teaching schedule agreed on by the caregiver, the patient, and the teacher. Because not all teaching can be done on the day shift, teachers must be found on all shifts. This ensures that the teaching schedule is maintained and kept within the time parameters established, thus minimizing delays in discharge.

One of the best ways to identify who will be responsible for teaching each task is to have a predischarge conference at which as many team members as possible are present. At this time, teaching duties can be assigned, and one team member can also be given the responsibility of serving as the primary teaching coordinator. Team conferences such as this should be attended by the patient, the family, and all health-care team members who have the day-to-day responsibility for care. These conferences must also include all post-acute care healthcare professionals who will be responsible for continued teaching, monitoring of the teaching-learning cycle, and the ongoing care on discharge.

TEACHING TOOLS

Teaching tools vary, but in most cases training consists of basic "hands-on" care. In some cases, teaching can be accomplished by using audiovisual materials and written literature. Depending on the facility, teaching can be further augmented by a home care manual. This manual not only enforces any teaching accomplished, but, more important, it serves as a reference tool once the caregiver is on his own.

Both patients and families benefit greatly when teaching is started long before discharge. Early teaching and actual practice of the physical care techniques required alleviate some of their concerns. The benefits are further enhanced if the family is allowed to troubleshoot problems and issues with professionals nearby. One of the very best ways to validate the fact that teaching has been successful is to allow the patient a trial weekend pass (or several) before the actual discharge occurs.

TRIAL PASSES

A trial pass (generally 48 hours) is critically important in the care of any technologically dependent patient because it allows an opportunity to identify any areas that may require additional teaching. For a trial pass to work as intended, it must be remembered that all equipment, supplies, and staffing must be in place just as they would be if the patient were actually being discharged.

Although it cannot be done with every patient and depends on the rules and regulations of the facility or healthcare payor, one mechanism that may be used when a pass is allowed is to simulate and actually plan for a real discharge (depending, of course, on the approval of the attending physician). In this case, prior to the transfer home for the "trial pass," the family makes all the arrangements with the business office just as if a discharge were to occur. A team member on each shift is identified who will assume responsibility for communication with the family during the pass. The family is given instructions in how and who to report to during the pass. If the pass is successful, this information is relayed to the business office, and the official discharge occurs at the end of

the trial pass. The patient is readmitted only if problems arise or when additional training needs are identified. Use of such a plan can potentially save hundreds of dollars in unnecessary ambulance fees, not to mention the stress and anxiety of readmission. Why readmit the patient, only to discharge him or her home again, if success was the outcome the first time?

TEACHING THE PATIENT AND FAMILY TO BE THE CASE MANAGER

It is vital to teach any patient and family in case management how to be their own case managers because most such patients have lifelong needs. Families and patients must know how and when to obtain access to outside resources. This process is essential if the patient's care is to remain of high quality and the patient is to move appropriately through the continuum of care when the professional case manager is no longer there to help. To ensure the continuity of care, six basic requirements must be satisfied in the process of training the family to manage their own case. These requirements are:

1. Identification and early referral to case management must take place, and all case managers must be introduced early to the patient, family, and healthcare team. Early referral allows time to build trust, rapport, and confidence. Also, the patient and family have someone to guide them through difficult situations in which they can learn firsthand how to manage their case.

2. Planning any case requires open, frequent, honest, and personal communication with all involved. As stated repeatedly in this manual, good communication is critical to prevent misinterpretation, duplication, fragmentation, omissions, and discrepancies in care. Good communication also ensures that the case management plan meets the patient's needs and that it is implemented in a timely and effective manner when the patient exhibits readiness for discharge. It also allows the patient and family to express their ideas and input, strengthens their confidence, and helps them to build their own communication skills in preparation for their assumption of the case manager role.

3. Crisis intervention mechanisms should be included in the case management plan to ensure that crisis atmospheres (which are common with case-managed patients) are alleviated. The use of a social worker or clini-

cal psychologist is an excellent resource that can assist in this area. Personal experience validates that some of the best discharges and case management plans are those in which the social worker and case manager work hand in hand with the patient and family, the case manager assisting them in establishing ties with community resources and the social worker helping them learn to cope. Provision of these mechanisms reassures the family and patient that they will not be abandoned in a crisis. More important, they are given a written guide or a list of resource personnel who can assist them when they are on their own and working through the crisis themselves.

4. A keen awareness on the part of the case manager to all available community, regional, and national resources and the patient's entitlement to their use builds the trust and confidence of the patient and family. This awareness is the pivotal element in case management and determines the success or failure of the case management plan because referrals are not limited to individual healthcare providers but frequently encompass a broad array of medical healthcare resources as well as social, financial, or other supportive formal and informal services or resources. Referrals may be made for direct care skills, counseling, meals, attendant care, respite care, support groups, transportation, or out-of-area placement. If the patient and family are involved in the decision-making and provider selection process and are given tips on how to access resources, they gain the confidence they need when they must do it on their own.

5. Teaching of the patient and family is necessary, not only the physical care techniques required but also how to access resources and exercise their appeal rights. Patients and family must know how to refuse to take a simple "no" from community resources and how to insist on receiving all denials formally in writing. This allows them to file a formal appeal and exercise their rights to services to which the patient may be entitled.

6. Patients and families must know when and how to obtain access to a professional case manager or other support system if their own attempts at case management or gaining access to care and resources fail.

POST-DISCHARGE TEACHING NEEDS

In many cases teaching continues even after discharge. In all cases, a mechanism for evaluat-

ing the teaching plan must be developed to ensure that monitoring of the plan continues throughout the duration of the care. It is important to identify a person who can assume a position after discharge similar to that of the inpatient teaching team coordinator; someone must be responsible for performing ongoing assessments of teaching-learning needs and for identifying areas that require further teaching.

A post-discharge teaching plan is essential to ensure that what was taught prior to discharge was relevant and that the family is not encountering problems or not reporting them. It is common for the team not to hear from a patient or family if things are going smoothly. In other cases, families do not call at all because they believe that their questions may be judged wrongly. Fortunately, others do call when unexpected problems arise or when they need reassurance.

On the proactive side, if case management continues after discharge by the same case manager and a good relationship and trust has been established between both parties, the patient or family often confides in the case manager realistically about the problems or limitations they encounter. In these cases, issues can be dealt with and the educational plans revised immediately. Such communication in itself allows an excellent opportunity for continual monitoring of the teaching-learning process.

For some patients (e.g., respiratory or infusion therapy patients), much of the post-discharge teaching is continued by the respiratory therapist or the nurses affiliated with either the durable medical equipment company or the infusion therapy company. As a rule, this teaching and any patient assessments, adjustments to the equipment or therapy, and reporting of responses to treatment to the physician are free when these professional disciplines are used because these services are included in the cost of the rental of the equipment or the overall nursing program established for the infusion therapy.

Fortunately, for many case-managed patients, a home health agency is involved after discharge owing to the patient's need for skilled care. Such agencies and their staffs are in a perfect position to serve as the person responsible for monitoring the teaching-learning process on an ongoing basis. If a home health agency is not involved and case management ceases at the time of discharge, one excellent means of monitoring the teaching-learning process is to establish a call-back system. Either a discharge planning team member or the facility-based case manager can be assigned this duty. Such a system allows an informal evaluation of the situation by a healthcare professional and offers a way to identify problems and find solutions before the problem leads to disastrous consequences. More important, it covers all patients, and nothing is left to chance.

In all cases, ongoing teaching-learning assessments are necessary to ensure that additional teaching occurs when issues are identified. Additional teaching is necessary when new caregivers are found, new equipment is required, changes in procedures occur and new skills are required, or changes in the level of care or condition occur.

Implementation, Monitoring, and Changes in the Case Management Plan

As stated earlier in this manual (see Chapter 2), the development, implementation, frequency of monitoring, and changes in the actual case management plan vary with the individual case. In most cases, referrals are generated early enough to allow time for planning the case without becoming involved in a crisis discharge atmosphere. Unfortunately, in others, in which for whatever reason the referral was delayed, a crisis atmosphere surrounding the discharge may surface. In such cases, the discharge and implementation of service often occur almost simultaneously with the referral. In these cases, of course, there is not only inadequate time to plan for appropriate linkage of the patient and family to the necessary resources, there is also inadequate time for teaching the patient and family if it is required and, equally as important, communication with the patient and family about issues and expectations.

Early referrals provide the benefit of adequate planning for locating appropriate resources and for smoothly implementing the plan. By all means, if a last-minute referral reveals that the discharge is not safe, the case manager must be prepared to substantiate opposition to the discharge either through documentation or discussion with the attending physician, the utilization reviewer, or other members of the healthcare team. The intensity and complexity of care required affect the frequency of monitoring as well as the type of monitoring technique used (by telephone versus on-site visits) and vary with the patient and case. The importance of performing reassessments on a regular basis cannot be overstated.

Likewise, the frequency of reassessments depends on such factors as medical or physical changes in the status of the patient (improvement, deterioration, or failure to change) or in his or her level of function; changes in the psychosocial status of the patient (e.g., loss of income, marital discord and separation, other crisis or stressors); and evolving educational needs (e.g., changes in the treatment plan, which necessitates a new teaching plan and then a new regimen of teaching or monitoring).

Equipment and Supplies

Although the actual equipment and supplies ordered vary with the patient, disease or injury, and level of impairment, many case-managed patients require an inordinate amount of expensive equipment and supplies. Factors affecting the amount of supplies and types of equipment ordered include the frequency of the patient's physical need for the item; the patient's mobility status; the distance between the patient and the supplier; and the presence of inclement weather conditions. Although most case-managed patients require voluminous amounts of supplies and duplicate items, many patients also require battery chargers and back-up batteries or battery-operated equipment. In areas where power outages are frequent, a portable generator is mandatory.

Not only do case-managed patients require expensive equipment, they also consume voluminous amounts of supplies. In most cases, supplies are ordered in 30- to 60-day increments. However, if the patient resides in a remote or rural area or in an area where accessibility is an issue, supplies can be ordered less frequently, such as quarterly or semi-annually. In all cases, proper storage (e.g., site, temperature) of all items must be considered and addressed in the case management plan.

For patients with respiratory disease, as much consideration must go into the selection of airways and accessories needed for ventilation as of the ventilatory device itself. This decision alone requires close communication with the healthcare team throughout the case but especially as the time for discharge approaches. Communication is necessary to ensure that the proper respiratory equipment and supplies are available and have been approved prior to the actual day of discharge and that the patient and family or caregiver have had adequate training in their use. Many respiratory patients, like other technologically dependent patients, require huge amounts of supplies. Additionally, much of their equipment must be ordered in duplicate because they require both a stationary ventilator and a portable battery-operated version.

The portability of equipment for all patients is vital if the patient is to be mobile and is to resume some sort of normal life. This "duplicate" equipment, however, can pose a problem if the healthcare payor will reimburse the provider for only one piece of like or similar equipment within a specified period of time. When this situation occurs, loan closets must be explored to find the alternate equipment, or approval through the extra contractual process must be sought.

In all cases, decisions about selection of equipment must be based on its suitability for the patient's home care needs, lifestyle, and home environment. Early identification of equipment needs well in advance of discharge is critically important to ensure a successful outcome because some equipment may have to be specifically made or adapted for the patient. This requires time. If not enough time is allowed, costly delays can ensue because the patient cannot be discharged until the equipment is available. In other cases, the discharge may occur, but loaned equipment may have to be supplemented in the interim. This latter method is the least desirable because it may hinder the patient's functional abilities.

HOME EVALUATION

For most technologically dependent patients, a home evaluation is necessary before the equipment is actually ordered and delivered and the patient is discharged. This is necessary to ensure that the home can accommodate the equipment and supplies physically, structurally, and electrically. Unfortunately, in many instances an actual home visit by the healthcare team is not always possible. If a home visit is impossible, it is wise to ask the family to measure and draw a replica of the space to be used. If this drawing indicates that the space is unacceptable, a visit by a local home health agency or even a local building inspector may be necessary. The physical dimensions are not the only factors that must be considered. It is important to ask the following questions:

- Is the house strong enough structurally to handle the weight of the equipment?

- Can the electrical panel accommodate the peak amperage required by all of the equipment? Note: All equipment must be assessed and the total amperage noted because most homes require extra electrical panels or circuits if they are to accommodate the equipment.
- Can the patient maneuver around the house? All doorways and hallways must be measured, and any barriers found must be corrected.
- Can the patient enter and leave the home safely, or are ramps or other accommodations necessary?
- Are the heating and cooling systems adequate to maintain temperature control because most technologically dependent patients have problems with body temperature regulation. Also, because of the heat generated by continuously operating equipment, adequate ventilation and air circulation is necessary.
- Where are supplies to be stored? Is there adequate space?
- Does the home provide hot water?
- Is there enough space to designate one area as clean and another as intended to hold dirty or used supplies?
- Physically, where will the patient spend most of his or her day? If a large portion of the day is to be spent in bed, then consideration must be given to relocating the patient area to the activity center of the home (i.e., the living room or family room).
- In all cases, the bathroom must be assessed for its ability to accommodate and contribute to personal care and toiletry activities.

If barriers are identified, corrections must be made as soon as possible. Other than workers' compensation, few healthcare payors reimburse the patient to correct barriers or modify the home for any of the foregoing reasons. This is an expense the family must incur. If the family cannot afford the necessary corrections, they should be encouraged to solicit assistance from a community volunteer or church group or a fraternal organization. Many such organizations are willing to make these repairs or corrections as a "service project."

Provider or Vendor Selection

The importance of appropriate provider selection cannot be underestimated because it plays an essential role in creating a successful plan. This topic is covered in more detail in Chapter 3. Ideally, selection of the provider should be started as early as possible. Early selection has several advantages: (1) if the organization's network is inadequate and is unable to accommodate the level of care required, there is enough time to locate another provider; (2) the provider's staff, the ones who will actually provide the care, have time to build a relationship with the patient and family, and any necessary staff training can be accomplished before the patient is discharged; and (3) the equipment can be delivered early, and the patient or family can practice with it and become familiar with the actual equipment that will be used on discharge.

Care of the Caregiver

Long-term care is the most common reason for caregiver burnout. As stated earlier, although some families are resilient and are able to cope, others are not. Many family structures may be stressed to the point of abandonment, frequent arguments, abuse, or divorce. For these reasons and others, care of the caregiver and family is as important as care of the patient. If the caregiver system fails, the consequences may be deterioration in the patient's condition or costly rehospitalization. If the caregiver system goes, so often goes the case management plan. The end result is long-term institutionalization. Therefore, respite care and appropriate training of the caregiver (or caregivers) are imperative.

Social isolation is a reality for many technologically dependent patients and their families. This is frequently due to such situations as the following:

- The patient and family live apart.
- The burden of care is overwhelming, the family or caregiver is physically and emotionally exhausted, and an outing "is not worth the effort."
- Moving all the equipment and supplies for an outing is too tiresome and overwhelming.
- The family's car or mode of transportation is inadequate to accommodate the patient and all the equipment. In some cases, there is no car because the patient and family rely on public transportation.
- Family members and friends may react negatively or be repulsed by the physical condition of the patient and some of the care needs that must be done.
- Families and patients are embarrassed about the patient's disabilities or appearance.

- After paying for medical expenses that are not covered by the healthcare payor, the patient and family cannot afford other expenditures even if they are for fun and offer a means to "get away."

The foregoing list is by no means all-inclusive, but it does give some idea of why, if arrangements are not included in the case management plan for socialization and respite, social isolation and caregiver burnout can occur. To encourage socialization, the case manager should at minimum urge patients and families to join disease-specific support groups when they are available. Disease-specific organizations and support groups are an invaluable resource for patients. In these groups the patient and family can learn first-hand how to solve problems and can share ideas. The powers and abilities of these groups should not be underestimated.

Examples of High Risk Flags

The following diagnoses are the ones most often used to flag cases for referral to case management (Table 10-1). As with all aspects of case management, diagnoses not on this list are not exempt—any case that poses a risk should be referred. Similarly, although a diagnosis may be listed as one causing automatic referral, once all the data in a particular case have been collected and assessed, it may be evident that the patient does not require case management.

Alternate Funding

Because of the many disabling conditions associated with the foregoing diagnoses and the possible lifelong consequences and continual need for healthcare services, it is imperative to evaluate such patients continuously or, when possible, link them with appropriate alternate funding resources. Why is this necessary? Because such resources can either assist with the payment for healthcare services or add needed income. Case managers must develop a schedule and include it in the case management plan whereby the financial status of the patient or family is assessed regularly. Such assessments are necessary because at any given time during the illness or recovery period the patient's healthcare coverage may terminate. Assessments are also needed when a request for ser-

TABLE 10–1
COMMON DIAGNOSES IN CASE MANAGEMENT PATIENTS

Cardiovascular and Thoracic Disorders[1, 2]

Cardiac arrest
Cardiac tamponade
Cardiomyopathy
Congenital anomalies of the cardiac or thoracic system
Congestive heart failure (severe)
Endocarditis
Gangrene
Heart failure
Heart transplantation, heart-lung transplantation, or
    rejection

Malignant hypertension
Mesenteric infarction
Myocardial infarction or complications
Myocarditis
Neoplasms of the cardiovascular or thoracic system
Pericarditis
Pulmonary hypertension (severe)
Stasis ulcers (severe, complicated)
Thrombophlebitis, phlebitis
Vascular disease (severe)

Connective Tissue Disorders[3, 4]

Progressive systemic sclerosis (scleroderma)
Rheumatoid arthritis
Severe osteoarthritis (multiple sites or complications)

Spondylitis and ankylosing spondylitis or spondylolisthesis
Systemic lupus erythematosus

Alimentary Tract, Hepatic, and Biliary System Disorders[5, 6]

Biliary atresia
Cirrhosis
Congenital cystic disease of liver
Esophageal varices
Gallbladder cancer
Hepatic coma, encephalopathy
Hepatic decompensation (severe)
Hepatic or portal vein thrombosis
Hepatitis (primarily B and C)
Hepatomegaly

LeVeen peritoneal shunt
Liver abscess
Liver cancer
Liver laceration (major)
Liver transplants or rejection
Pancreatic abscess
Pancreatic cancer
Pancreatitis
Portal hypertension

Disorders Associated with High-Risk Pregnancy[7–9]

Age under 15 or over 35
HIV+, AIDS
Early, threatened labor
Excessive vomiting
Fetal abnormality (known or suspected) affecting
    management of mother or unborn fetus
Hemorrhage in early pregnancy
History of or antepartum hemorrhage, abruptio placentae,
    placenta previa, fetal deaths, or previous neonatal
    history of sudden infant death

Hypertension complicating pregnancy
Infectious disease during pregnancy
Multiple gestation (known)
Maternal diabetes
Other placental or fetal problems affecting management of
    mother
Pulmonary or other emboli
Toxemia
Venous complications

Musculoskeletal System Disorders[3, 4]

Complicated fractures (traction, spica casts)
Complications of reattached limbs
Congenital muscular or skeletal anomalies
Crushing injuries
Multiple fractures
Muscular dystrophy

Osteomyelitis (complicated or with repeated admissions)
Severe decubitus, gangrene
Spinal cord injuries
Traumatic amputation

Metabolic and Endocrine Disorders[10, 11]

Congenital anomalies of metabolic or endocrine system
Diabetes insipidus
Diabetes mellitus (with complications or frequent
    admissions)

Hyperthyroidism—toxic
Neoplasms of endocrine system
Pancreas transplant
Parathyroid disorders with complications or tumors

Neonatal Disorders or Congenital Anomalies[12, 13]

HIV+, AIDS
Amyotonia congenita (Oppenheim's, Werdnig-Hoffman)
Atresia of bladder, esophagus, duodenum, liver, rectum, or
    anus
Birth trauma
Bronchopulmonary dysplasia (BPD or RDS)
Cerebral palsy
Chromosomal disorders
Cleft palate, cleft lip
Conjoined twins
Cystic fibrosis

Exstrophy of abdominal organs
Hirschsprung's disease
Intrauterine hypoxia or birth asphyxia
Malformation of central nervous system
Malformation of heart or vascular system
Malformation of urinary system
Malformation of respiratory system
Microcephaly
Myelomeningocele
Multiple anomalies
Prematurity (severe complications)

TABLE 10–1
COMMON DIAGNOSES IN CASE MANAGEMENT PATIENTS *Continued*

Neurologic Disorders[14]

Abscess (intracranial or intraspinal)
AIDS with neurologic complications
Amyotrophic lateral sclerosis (ALS)
Anoxic brain damage
Brain or other central nervous system (CNS) neoplasms
Cerebral palsy
Cerebrovascular accidents
Congenital neurologic anomalies (common)
Convulsive disorders (severe)
Guillain-Barré syndrome
Head or intracranial injuries
Hereditary degenerative disorders such as:
• Friedreich's ataxia

• Huntington's chorea
• Myasthenia gravis
• Tay-Sachs disease
• Wilson's disease

Multiple sclerosis
Paralysis, quadriplegia, or paresis
Parkinson's disease (severe)
Poliomyelitis
Subarachnoid hemorrhage, or other cranial bleeding
Spinal cord injuries or tumors
Tuberculosis of neurologic system

Respiratory Disorders[15, 16]

AIDS (fungal pneumonia, *Pneumocystis carinii, Candida,* and cytomegalovirus infections)
Apnea
Asphyxia with complications
Asthma (severe)
Bronchopulmonary dysplasia
Chest trauma or flail chest
Chronic tracheostomy with complications
Congenital anomalies of respiratory system
Chronic obstructive pulmonary disease (primarily end-stage or frequent admissions)
Crushing injuries to chest
Cystic fibrosis
Empyema
Laryngectomy

Legionnaires' disease
Lung abscess
Lung injury
Lung transplants or rejections
Major neurologic disease with respiratory complications
Neoplasms of respiratory system
Pneumonia with complications
Pneumonia, staphylococcal
Pulmonary emboli
Pulmonary fibrosis
Respiratory failure (RDS)
Systemic fungal infections (coccidiomycosis)
Tracheostomy (complications or new)
Tuberculosis with complications
Ventilator dependency

Renal or Urinary System Disorders[17, 18]

Complications of implants, grafts, or external stoma
Glomerulonephritis (acute or chronic)
Renal abscess
Renal artery sclerosis
Renal artery thrombosis and fistulas
Renal failure (acute or chronic)

Renal or bladder neoplasms
Renal or bladder rupture or trauma
Renal hypertension
Renal transplants or rejections
Stricture or trauma to ureters or urethra

Other High-Risk Disorders[19, 20]

Blood disorders (severe with complications):

• Anemia
• Hemophilia
• Leukemia
• Sickle cell anemia

HIV+, AIDS
Amputation with complications
Anorexia nervosa
Bone marrow transplants
Burns
Crush injuries
End-stage malignancies
Esophageal trauma, tumors
Failure to thrive
Fistulas (with complications)

Flail chest
Gangrene
Gunshot wounds
Intestinal malabsorption disorders
Lye or poison ingestion
Multiple trauma
Nutritional or vitamin deficiencies (severe—intractable nausea, vomiting, or intractable diarrhea)
Obesity with complications
Peritonitis
Radical neck dissection for malignancy
Septicemia
Short bowel syndrome
Stab wounds (if complications)
Ulcerative colitis (if complications)
Wound infections (multiple sites or complications)

vices is denied or when services are excluded or limited by the patient's healthcare benefit coverage.

Because of the importance of linkage to financial resources, case managers must maintain current knowledge of the commonly used alternate funding programs in the immediate vicinity of their offices and also in regions where the majority of their patients receive care. These programs undergo changes that result from budgetary constraints as well as from changes made in the laws or federal or state administrative codes that govern the programs. Each of the primary alternate funding programs is discussed in greater detail in Chapter 4. To remain knowledgeable about the resources available, case managers should keep current data relating to, at minimum, the referral processes, the basic eligibility criteria, and the appeal processes required by the major funding programs available to patients.

Because of variations in the programs, their eligibility requirements, and the manner in which eligibility is linked to services, it is wise to refer patients to such programs as soon as they are identified as possible candidates. Delays in the eligibility referral and screening processes are common. These delays are frequently due to such barriers as the following: (1) resistance by the patient or family, who must be counseled that alternate funding programs are not "welfare" but additional insurance; (2) the need to secure all the paperwork and receipts that may be required to establish financial need; (3) the agency's investigational process that is required to screen clients for eligibility; and (4) the agency's backlog in processing new requests. In addition to income programs, typical alternate funding programs to which patients may be referred are listed in Table 10-2.

Although many patients may be eligible for several programs at once, other patients, because of higher financial reserves, income, or assets will not qualify despite a demonstrated need for the program. In this latter category are those patients and families who have too much to qualify yet too little to pay for the services and care required. It is in these cases that the case manager must be as creative and innovative as possible if a plan that will meet the patient's needs is to be established. Sadly, in some cases, despite all efforts, no solution can be found. Less frequently, other sources of coverage may be found in the following situations:

- Regardless of age, if the patient has end-stage renal disease, referral must be made to Social Security's End-Stage Renal Disease program.

TABLE 10–2
ALTERNATE FUNDING

Adults	Children
Medicaid	Medicaid
Supplemental Security Income (SSI)	Supplemental Security Income (SSI)
Social Security Disability Insurance (SSDI)	Title V Children's Medical Services programs
Single parents with children: Aid to Families with Dependent Children (AFDC)	State agency responsible for administering services for the developmentally disabled
Veterans or retired from the military: veterans' benefits or CHAMPUS coverage	Dependent child of a person on active duty in any military service: Program for the Handicapped (PFTH)
Dependent spouse of a person on active duty in any military service: Program for the Handicapped (PFTH)	Dependent child of a person eligible for Social Security: any Social Security benefits to which he or she may be entitled.

- In some rare cases in which the patient may be undergoing an experimental or investigational procedure or service, he or she may be eligible for coverage of a portion of the care and services through a research grant. However, to be eligible, the patient must have the specific diagnosis for which the study is designed. Also, the research may be limited to patients in specific national university tertiary care centers.
- Another source of possible assistance, particularly when the patient's healthcare coverage limits or excludes some benefits, are funds available from some fraternal organizations. These organizations are often willing to assist with services ranging from payment for the services to assistance by volunteers when specific needs have been identified.
- For active duty military dependents, retirees, or their dependents, an excellent resource that may be explored for assistance when funding is limited or excluded by the Civilian Health and Medical Program of the Uniformed Services (CHAMPUS) now called TRICARE or the patient's other healthcare benefit package, is the Armed Forces family service agency programs. Information about the availability of such assistance can be obtained by calling a TRICARE health care finder or the nearest military treatment facility's health benefits advisor (HBA) or managed care or patient administration personnel. Also, depending on his or her specific needs, the patient may be eligible for some of the

CHAMPUS waiver programs for home care (i.e., home health care demonstration or the expanded home health care–case management demonstration project). Also, any patient needing specialized services such as a transplant may be eligible to have the procedure performed in any of the military centers of excellence (e.g., Wilford Hall Medical Center, Brooke Army Medical Center, Walter Reed Medical Center).

• If the patient is a veteran, contact with the nearest Veterans Administration Office or the local or regional Veterans Clinic or medical clinic can help the case manager determine whether the patient is eligible for any services that will be paid by the Veterans Administration.

Alternate Levels of Care

Many levels of post-acute care services are used by case-managed patients. Unfortunately, not all communities offer all levels of care, and it is common to encounter waiting lists for persons in need of complex skilled care. Consequently, out-of-area placement is necessary in many situations. Regardless of the setting of the alternate post-acute care used, the patient's progress must be closely monitored as the patient moves from one level of care to another. Monitoring is necessary to ensure that the patient is making progress toward the established goals, is receiving the care required to meet his or her needs, and is moving appropriately through the continuum of care. The following alternate levels of care are those most commonly used by the majority of patients:

• Subacute care facilities
• Acute rehabilitation care facilities
• Skilled nursing care facilities
• Home, with home health agency care for intermittent or hourly private duty skilled nursing care

Other facilities that may be required, depending on the diagnosis, include:

• Cardiac or respiratory rehabilitation units
• Inpatient or outpatient pain management units
• Outpatient therapy (physical, occupational, or speech therapy) facilities
• Post-acute care rehabilitation facilities for persons with a brain injury
• Intermediate care facilities for patients with

either less intense medical needs or developmental delay
• Mental health facilities, including psychiatric outpatient treatment facilities, residential treatment centers, substance abuse programs, and, in extreme cases, state hospitals

For frail elderly people, persons with a psychiatric disorder, or those with a mild or moderate developmental delay, the following types of facilities should be explored before the more restrictive ones are used:

• Adult day care centers
• Residential or board and care facilities
• Community care homes

Although a subacute care facility, rehabilitation facility, or skilled nursing facility may be appropriate for a child with special needs, these facilities may not be readily available. Consequently, many children are discharged home with any combination of complex needs and requirements for care and resources. Fortunately, some communities do offer facilities that specialize in pediatric skilled care, and some have day care centers that specialize in providing services to children with special needs. In addition, many communities have specialized care homes that are licensed to provide varying levels of care. For some of the most severely disabled children the only option for placement may be a state facility that provides long-term care.

Facilities designed to treat children and adolescents with a mental illness are likewise not available in all communities. Although many children and adolescents can benefit from outpatient programs, many require placement in a residential treatment center, community care home, or, sometimes, a state school or state hospital. If the child does require placement in any of these facilities, close coordination with the case manager from the agency responsible for mental health, the Department of Mental Retardation, or the Department of Education is vital to ensure that the child is placed appropriately. In most cases, these levels of care are not reimbursed by healthcare payors.

Other Community Resources

Due to the complexity of care required by case-managed patients and the fact that not all care may be covered by healthcare payors, case managers must be very knowledgeable about all community resources, whether local, regional, or national, that can be used to augment and enhance the proposed case management plan. Many patients may be eligible for services from several agencies. In all cases, the family should be encouraged to make contact with any agencies that can offer the assistance or information required.

Many disease-specific (e.g., American Cancer Society, United Cerebral Palsy Association), church (e.g., Catholic Social Services, Lutheran Social Services, Jewish Social Services), and ethnic agencies offer an entire array of services. Many disease-specific agencies are operational not only locally but also nationally; their national offices can be accessed by a toll-free telephone number. Services provided by such disease-specific agencies include at minimum information and referral, literature, educational classes, and support groups.

The power of the support received by patients and their families from these support groups cannot be overstated. Whenever possible, patients and families should be linked to the agencies designed to respond to the needs of patients with a particular disease. In addition to disease-specific, church, or ethnic agencies, the following community resources are commonly used by many patients:

- County choreworker or homemaker service agencies
- County public health clinics and services
- Emergency response systems
- Easter Seals Society
- Fraternal organizations
- Handicapped sports and recreation associations
- Handicapped transportation services (generally offered by local transportation authorities)
- Independent living centers
- Meals programs (delivered to homes or congregate sites)
- Legal advice, either from the local legal center for the disabled and elderly or a private attorney
- Library services
- Medical Alert identification bracelets
- Department of Rehabilitation or vocational rehabilitation services

For the visually or hearing impaired, referrals may be necessary to a center for deafness or blindness as well as to obtain assistance with such services as:

- Guide dogs for the blind
- Lions' eye and tissue bank

For children with special needs, referrals may be necessary to obtain such services as:

- Women, Infants and Children's nutrition program (WIC)
- Services offered by the Department of Education and Special Education
- Special Olympics or any of the agencies designed to provide handicapped recreational activities
- Special children's foundations (e.g., Make a Wish Foundation) for special projects or to fulfill a child's wish

Many communities offer art and play therapy as well as other programs designed to help children who have a terminal illness. Availability of these services can be ascertained by calling the local American Cancer Society or the nearest regional cancer center that specializes in pediatric cancer care.

For high-risk pregnant women referrals may be necessary to:

- County public health clinics for high-risk mothers and infants, or AIDS clinics
- Title V Children's Medical Services programs for genetic screening
- Planned Parenthood
- Women, Infants and Children's nutrition (WIC) program

For organ transplant candidates, case managers should link the patient to the nearest local organ procurement agency for any assistance or guidance that may be required, in addition to referring him or her to disease-specific groups and transplant centers.

Persons living alone may benefit from "friendly visitor" or "telephone visitor" programs offered by the local department on aging. These agencies are designed to serve seniors. Information about such programs can be obtained from the department on aging. This is an invaluable resource for information about any of its programs in the area that serve the senior population. Another excellent program is the emergency response system, which consists of a device worn by the patient that, when activated during a time of medical need, links the patient electronically to the nearest emergency room, which then mobilizes according to a prearranged emergency plan.

Certainly the community resources listed in this section are not all-inclusive. Each community offers a unique combination of resources. What is the best source for locating information about resources when a community resource directory is not available? The answer is the

TABLE 10–3
SERVICES TYPICALLY NEEDED AT DISCHARGE

Cardiovascular and Thoracic Disorders

Activities of daily living (retraining)
Antiembolic stockings
Cardiac rehabilitation
Counseling (role reversal, lifestyle changes, depression)
Energy conservation and mobility techniques

Job retraining
Nutritional counseling for weight control or reduction or fluid retention
Pain management
Wound care

Alimentary Tract, Hepatic, and Biliary System Disorders

Activities of daily living (retraining)
Counseling (body image, sexual function, lifestyle, depression)
Energy conservation and mobility techniques
Nutritional counseling for dietary and fluid restoration

Edema monitoring
Total parenteral nutrition
Gastric suctioning
Ostomy care and supplies

Connective Tissue Disorders

Activities of daily living (retraining)
Counseling (body image, sexual function, lifestyle, depression)
Energy conservation and mobility techniques
Gold therapy
High-dose steroids

Inter-articular joint injections
Job retraining
Pain control
Pool or water therapy
Nutritional counseling for weight control or reduction

High-Risk Pregnancy

Antiembolic stockings
Bedrest
Blood pressure monitoring
Counseling (frustration, lifestyle changes, altered sex life, depression)

Edema monitoring
Fetal monitoring
Nutritional counseling for weight control
Terbutaline therapy

Musculoskeletal Disorders

Antiembolic stockings
Energy conservation and mobility techniques
Hyperbaric oxygen
Muscle or nerve stimulation

Nutritional counseling for weight control or reduction
Pain control
Pool or water therapy
Wound care

Metabolic and Endocrine Disorders

Vitamin B_{12} injections
Diabetic education
Glucose monitoring
Insulin regimen

Nutritional counseling for dietary planning and weight control
Pain management
Wound care

Neonatal Problems or Congenital Anomalies

Specific to the diagnosis or anomalies

Renal or Urinary System Disorders

Blood pressure monitoring
Counseling (lifestyle changes, role reversal, sexuality)
Nutritional counseling for dietary and fluid restrictions

Pain management
Ostomy care and supplies

End-Stage Renal Disease

Blood pressure monitoring
Counseling for coping, role reversal
Dialysis shunt care

Energy conservation
Nutritional counseling
Possible self-dialysis

Neurologic Disorders

Antiembolic stockings
Activities of daily living (retraining)
Cognitive retraining
Counseling (role reversal, coping)
Job retraining

Mobility training and energy conservation
Pain management
Rehabilitation
Wound care

Respiratory Disease

Antiembolic stockings
Activities of daily living (retraining)
Counseling (role reversal, coping)
Energy conservation and mobility techniques

Job retraining
Nebulizer treatments
Respiratory rehabilitation

TABLE 10–4
TYPICAL EQUIPMENT NEEDS IN CASE MANAGEMENT

Cardiovascular and Thoracic Disorders

Antiembolic stockings
Adaptive clothing
Blood pressure cuff and stethoscope
Electric carts
Electrocardiogram supplies
Feeding pumps (portable and stationary) and supplies
Respiratory monitor and supplies
Infusion therapy, equipment, and all medications and supplies
Oxygen (stationary and portable) and supplies

Prosthetic devices
Ramps
Self-help devices (for feeding, dressing)
Suction equipment (portable and stationary) and supplies
Wedge pillow and other pillows or devices for positioning and support
Weight scale
Wound care supplies

High-Risk Pregnancy

Blood pressure cuff and stethoscope
Glucose monitor

Infusion pump, solutions, supplies, and medications
Home uterine monitor and supplies

Alimentary Tract, Hepatic, and Biliary System Disorders

Blood pressure cuff and stethoscope
Dressings, irrigation solution, and supplies
50-cc syringes (rectal neomycin)
Gastric suction or similar devices and supplies
Glucose monitor and supplies
Humidifier or cold mist
Infusion therapy equipment and all supplies (portable and stationary), medications, formulas, and solutions

Ostomy supplies
Oxygen (portable and stationary) and supplies
Scales (weight)
Tape measure
Wound care supplies, when applicable

Connective Tissue Disorders

Adaptive clothing
Adaptive eating, cooking, and writing utensils
Other activities of daily living and self-help devices

Ramps
Rails for shower, commode, or hallways
Splints and other orthotics

Metabolic and Endocrine Disorders

Assistive and self-care devices
Button infusor if insulin is required more than four times per day

Glucose monitor
Infusion pump and supplies (portable and stationary)
Regular or blind insulin syringes and supplies

Neonatal Problems or Congenital Anomalies

Stationary units and battery operated back-up units or monitors for all electronic equipment
Feeding pumps and supplies
Oxygen and supplies

Tracheostomy suctioning equipment and supplies
Infusion therapy supplies, solutions, and equipment
Ostomy supplies (common with neonates)
Suction equipment (stationary and portable)

Musculoskeletal Disorders

Adaptive clothing
Alternating air mattress and pump
Antiembolic stockings
Bedpan (regular or fracture) or toilet and bars and elevated toilet seats
Call system if confined to bed
Infusion pumps (stationary and portable), supplies, solutions, and medications
Pillows for patient lift, body support, and positioning

Ramps
Slide board
Traction unit (Bucks, pin, pelvic)
Wedge pillow and other pillows or devices for positioning and support
Trapeze (free-standing or bed)
Wheelchair (regular with removable arm rests, elevating leg rests, or reclining)
Wound care

Renal or Urinary System Disorders

Blood pressure cuff, stethoscope
Hemodialysis or ambulatory dialysis equipment and sterile supplies and solutions

Infusion pumps, solutions, supplies, and medications
Ostomy supplies
Weight scale

TABLE 10–4
TYPICAL EQUIPMENT NEEDS IN CASE MANAGEMENT *Continued*

Neurologic Disorders

Adaptive clothing
Adaptive feeding equipment
Adaptive activity of daily living devices
Alternating or special mattress
Antiembolic stockings
Call system
Catheter supplies (if self-catheterizing, mirror)
Communication devices
Decubitus supplies
Electric mobility carts
Elevated toilet seat or toilet rails
Feeding equipment and supplies (stationary and portable)
Foot board
Grab bars for toilet, shower, or hallway
Incontinent pads
Infusion equipment, solutions, supplies, and medications
Orthotics
Patient lift

Patient restraints
Prism glasses
Protective head gear
Ramps
Seating systems and supports (customized)
Slide board
Special cushions (often customized)
Splints, braces
Suction equipment and supplies (stationary and portable)
Trapeze (free-standing or bed)
Trunk supports
Walker (platform or regular)
Wedge pillow and other pillows or devices for positioning and support
Wheelchair (regular, reclining, specially made, removable arm and leg rests)

Respiratory Disease

Antiembolic stockings
Alternating air mattress or pump
Communication aids or call system
Dressing and supplies
Electric mobility carts
Feeding pump and supplies
Grab bars for toilet or shower or hallway
Humidifier or vaporizers
Infusion pump (for antibiotics or pain) (stationary and portable) solutions, supplies, and medications
In-home respiratory (apnea) monitor

Oxygen equipment (stationary and portable) and supplies
Percussors
Pump-driven or hand-held ultrasonic or intermittent positive pressure (IPPB) nebulizer
Sterile tracheostomy tube (extra) and other tracheostomy supplies
Suction equipment and supplies (stationary and portable)
Wedge pillow and other pillows or devices for positioning and support
Ventilator and all supplies

Other High-Risk Diagnoses

Dressings, solutions, other supplies for wound care (on occasion, continuous intermittent suction machine)

Feeding equipment (stationary and portable) and supplies
Infusion therapy (stationary and portable) equipment, supplies

---

yellow pages of the telephone book and eventually the case manager's own Rolodex file (see also Appendix in this manual).

Services Required for Discharge

The following services are frequently ordered by the treating physician for post-acute care on discharge. They may be ordered in any combination and in various frequencies. The final orders, of course, vary with the actual diagnosis and the patient's medical need. However, the following services are ordered most commonly:

• Home health agency services for intermittent or private duty (hourly) skilled nursing care

and skilled rehabilitation or therapy services or psychological counseling
• Social worker services
• Infusion services
• Durable medical equipment and medical supplies
• Laboratory or radiologic services that are portable and serve the homebound; if patient is not homebound, a linkage to outpatient services is ordered
• Transportation for follow-up appointments and any outpatient services, if patient is not homebound
• Detailed medication regimen and a pharmaceutical provider

In addition, orders such as those listed in Table 10–3 are also common.

Equipment Needs

The equipment ordered for each patient depends on the diagnosis and the patient's specific medical needs and functional abilities. The most frequently ordered equipment items for most patients include:

- Hospital beds, bedrails, and trapezes
- Commodes or bedpans
- Shower and bathroom devices
- Mobility devices

In addition, orders for the following items as listed in Table 10–4 are often seen.

☙ S U M M A R Y

The purpose of this section is to introduce the new case manager to the multitude of issues and problems that may be present in the various cases in his or her caseload. Most patients require voluminous amounts of equipment and supplies. Whereas some patients may require only an occasional laboratory or radiologic study, others require a multitude of such studies. Similarly, whereas one patient may require the use of a home health agency nurse for intermittent visits, another may require hourly care for extended periods of time (e.g., hourly or 24-hour care). So the services provided for one patient may not be possible or feasible for another.

In all cases, teaching of the patient and family is of critical importance. Teaching and a means of monitoring the teaching-learning process throughout the duration of the case must be incorporated into the case management plan. In most cases, teaching is started while the patient is still hospitalized, but it continues after the patient comes home. During this process, the family and patient must have a professional to oversee its effectiveness. More important, this professional must remain involved until the patient or family, or both, are proficient in all aspects of care.

Case management plans must be developed for specific patients, and all aspects of care of the patient and caregiver must be included.

CASE MANAGEMENT OF THE PATIENT WITH AIDS

Resource Authorities

Although home care and post-acute care for persons with acquired immunodeficiency syn-

drome (AIDS) have come a long way over the years, persons with AIDS present their own set of problems and challenges for the case manager. Treatment methods and resources for treating this disease vary greatly from community to community. However, larger cities such as San Francisco, New York, and Miami are leaders in the provision of care and treatment options for AIDS patients. Because they frequently use research, foundation, and other grant money for the evaluation of experimental and conventional treatments, they are willing to share information if it is needed. Case managers should not hesitate to call a specific department in a larger city directly when questions arise. Valuable other resources are the Centers for Disease Control and Prevention (CDC) and the federal Food and Drug Administration (FDA). Both of these agencies are invaluable if questions about treatments arise and the case manager requires assistance or information.

The Pros and Cons of Case Management

The literature supports the fact that in most cases, patients who are positive for the human immunodeficiency virus (HIV+) remain asymptomatic for years. Consequently, many of these patients are not included in a case manager's caseload until they develop AIDS. However, this consequence varies with the organization because many healthcare organizations require any HIV+ or AIDS patient to be included in the cases followed by case management.

Such automatic inclusion of all HIV+ and AIDS patients into case management caseloads can create problems. On the one hand, if the patient is being treated and the treatments are progressing as planned and if the patient has been educated about the potential resources available and he or she is working, one must really question what effect case management can have. During these early stages of the disease the patient generally receives specific diagnostic tests at regular intervals, and, depending on the CD4 and T-lymphocyte count and the viral load present, the patient may or may not be taking anti-HIV drug therapy. Many of these patients are employed, and, other than handling periodic requests for testing or medication, the case manager is not managing anything and has no impact on the disease course because the patient is receiving "normal" treatments.

On the other hand, if early intervention does

occur, it should be instituted for educational purposes. Early intervention can be a means of detecting problematic areas such as noncompliance and developing strategies for correcting them. For instance, early intervention allows an opportunity to address risk management techniques (e.g., safe sex, the importance of taking medications, the reasons for having tests done at the intervals outlined by the attending physician, and so forth). It also offers an opportunity to direct the patient to an accredited person who can provide counseling (i.e., an AIDS health educator).

However, if the disease is progressing as anticipated and the patient and significant other are linked to the appropriate resources, one must really question what there is to manage and whether case management can have an impact. In such cases, the case manager and the patient can remain in contact, and the case manager can be available for assistance if the need arises. This process allows the case manager to assist other AIDS patients who really need the services offered by case management. However, the choices here depend on the policies of the healthcare organization.

Unfortunately, the mere inclusion of this category of patients without specific guidelines to what is to be accomplished often only encumbers the case manager needlessly. It also raises doubt in the minds of HIV + patients, especially if they are included in the caseload of a healthcare payor's case management team. They fear that their employer will be apprised of their diagnosis, and the ultimate consequences for them may be job termination.

Due to the magnitude of the disease and the many other diseases and physical manifestations associated with the AIDS diagnoses, AIDS is the disease with which possibly the greatest number of case managers may be involved. When several case managers are involved, communication between all of them is critical to avoid duplication and fragmentation of care and the occurrence of a crisis atmosphere.

Also, it is important to educate HIV + and asymptomatic AIDS patients about the need to maintain regularly scheduled evaluations by their own physician or clinic. This is necessary to monitor the progress of the disease and to detect episodes of deterioration at their immediate onset.

Specialists

Because of the magnitude of the disease process and the fact that many patients have nu-merous medical and psychological problems, it is common to encounter many specialists and requests for a multitude of tests. It is also wise in cases such as these to work with the healthcare payor to have the patient linked to a specialist as his or her primary care physician because the traditional family practice physician may not be up-to-date on the latest treatment options. For instance, the specialists commonly used for referrals and treatment of AIDS are:

- Pulmonologists—for pulmonary manifestations
- Infectious disease specialists—for viral, fungal, or bacterial infections
- Gastroenterologists—for gastrointestinal manifestations such as small bowel and colon lesions and cytomegalovirus (CMV) cholangiopathies
- Ophthalmologists—for ocular and retinal manifestations
- Nutritionists—for nutritional guidelines, prevention of wasting syndrome, and evaluation of caloric needs
- Social workers or psychologists—for counseling for lifestyle changes, anxiety, and depression
- Pharmacists—for complex medication regimens
- Neurologists—for neurologic manifestations and dementia
- Cardiologists—for cardiac and pericardial disease
- Endocrinologists—for endocrine dysfunction secondary to opportunistic infections, malignancies, or drug toxicity
- Oncologists—for Kaposi's sarcoma or non-Hodgkin's B-cell lymphoma
- Obstetricians and perinatologists—for management of pregnancy and advanced gynecologic problems or monitoring of asymptomatic pregnant mothers

Major Barriers and Problems

Any healthcare professional working with AIDS patients can attest to the fact that AIDS is a disease that has possibly the largest number of complications and associated medical conditions. It is for this reason that the specialists listed above may be required in any combination and at any frequency throughout the course of the disease. These patients also have a multitude of psychological problems that can surface at any point in the course of the disease.

In all cases, it is imperative to link patients with appropriate counseling or support groups as soon as these problems are identified. Case management plans must ensure that resources for all these contingencies are included.

Barriers to care are often the biggest stumbling block for any AIDS patient followed by case management. Despite all the publicity about the disease, one of the most stubborn barriers to access to care continues to be fear and the stigma attached to the disease. Other barriers include the following:

- Lack of a home. If a home is available, it must have inside plumbing and hot water (the temperature of the water must be hot enough to require the use of gloves).
- Lack of local agencies willing to provide care.
- Lack of residential housing where the patient either can live or can use as a place for terminal care.
- Lack of financial ability to pay for medications or care. Most medications for these patients are extremely expensive, and often the patient is taking several medications.
- Lack of volunteers for grocery shopping or food preparation.
- Lack of a caregiver, or a high turnover rate or burnout of caregivers. In many cases, the volunteer caregiver (who may be the "lover") also has AIDS and may be as sick as the patient; or the patient has lost friends to the disease or has been deserted by all his or her friends; or the community has no volunteers.
- Fear of exposure to the disease and lack of willingness to accept education or knowledgeable information.
- Lack of parent or peer counseling or support groups.
- Lack of coordination between agencies and joint development of case management plans, leading to fragmentation or duplication of care.
- Lack of care facilities at all levels. (In some smaller towns, even acute care hospitals are reluctant to accept these patients, but the major problem is finding skilled nursing facilities, extended care facilities, and adequate board and care facilities or other home settings.)
- Difficulty of placing children born to AIDS-infected mothers; these children are offered for adoption or placed in foster homes.
- Lack of transportation to and from outpatient clinics and treatment facilities or for purchasing medications or grocery shopping.

- Unnecessarily expensive professional staffing required by many healthcare payor plans, which remains at the registered nurse (RN) and licensed vocational or practical nurse (LVN or LPN) level, whereas in fact home health agencies can frequently accomplish the care required through the use of home health aides and intermittent skilled nursing.
- Lack of clinics and outpatient sites in some smaller communities to provide care (e.g., chemotherapy, respiratory treatments, transfusions, and dialysis).
- Lack of coverage of experimental drugs and treatment options by other than research, foundation, or grant money because most healthcare payor plans do not cover experimental drugs or treatments.
- Lack of public education, tutors, or special education classes for children infected with the virus.

Equipment Needs

Because of the many physical manifestations of AIDS and the deterioration of body systems that is associated with the course of this disease, the following equipment and supplies are commonly ordered as the condition progresses. In all cases, patients must be continuously assessed for their level of functional ability and independence. Depending on the patient's physical abilities, consideration must be given to ordering both the stationary and the portable versions of many items if the patient is to remain as independent as possible. Typical equipment and supplies ordered include:

- Oxygen or other inhalation therapy unit and supplies
- Semi-electric hospital bed
- Wheelchair, walker, or canes (wheelchairs are common because often the patient lacks enough strength to walk)
- Shower chair, bath bench, shower or tub rails
- Bedside commode or toilet rails
- Intravenous solutions, equipment, medications, and associated supplies, including a sharps disposable container
- Feeding equipment and supplies
- Dressings and supplies for wound care
- Household bleach (the Centers for Disease Control and Prevention [CDC] recommends a 1:10 dilution of bleach [1 part bleach to 10 parts water] for use as a disinfectant or clean-

ing agent and full-strength bleach when disposing of excretions or body fluids in the toilet)
- Ziplock bags (for disposable waste)
- Reusable and sterilizable containers
- Gloves (only necessary when handling body fluid secretions)

Alternate Funding

Sources of alternate funding should have been explored long before the AIDS patient reaches the final stages of the disease. However, if this has not occurred, referrals to any of the following programs may be appropriate (see Chapter 4 for more details on these resources):

- Title V Children's Health Services program
- State agency responsible for handling developmental disabilities
- Medicaid
- Medicaid AIDS waiver
- Supplemental Security Income (SSI) and Medicaid
- Social Security Disability Insurance (SSDI) and eventually Medicare
- Ryan White funding

Also, for patients taking experimental drugs or treatments, case managers must be familiar with the healthcare payor's policy or position on experimental, investigational, or evolving technologic advances because they are frequently excluded from coverage. If a patient is taking experimental drugs or treatments, these must be monitored to ensure that any costs excluded by the healthcare payor are not shifted inappropriately to the patient.

Case managers must be familiar with their state's Title V Children's Medical Services program and its requirements for referrals for children with AIDS. Unfortunately, not every state's Title V program accepts such referrals or offers services to children with AIDS. In addition, it may be necessary to refer a child to a Special Education program because the child may not be able to participate in the regular educational program or setting. Depending on the child's disabilities, another program that may offer help is the state agency responsible for providing services to children with developmental disabilities.

Case managers must also know whether the community in which the patient resides is eligible for Ryan White funding. Ryan White funding is made available in many communities by the Ryan White Comprehensive AIDS Resources Emergency Act of 1990. This act provides emergency financial assistance to communities that are disproportionately affected by the AIDS epidemic. These communities are allowed monies to provide whatever essential services are necessary to maintain the patient.

In addition, this act established HIV care grants and demonstration grants. These grants are used for research and services for pediatric patients; for services aimed at early intervention; and for partner notification and development of guidelines for intentional infection. Case managers unfamiliar with this act and the resources within their state can contact the state's Health and Human Services department for information about the program.

Common Community Agencies

As mentioned previously, many patients with AIDS have a multitude of problems, some of which may not be covered by the healthcare payor because of limitations in or lack of coverage. When this occurs, AIDS patients are referred to many community agencies, including the following:

- AIDS Foundation
- American Cancer Society and Hospice
- Counseling for lifestyle changes and death and dying
- County health officer or public health clinics and nurses
- County in-home supportive services and homemaker programs
- Handicapped transportation
- Hemophilia Foundation
- Home health agencies or private duty registry
- Housing specific for providing AIDS services
- Outpatient clinics and laboratories
- Planned Parenthood
- Portable laboratories and radiologic capabilities, when patient is homebound
- Volunteer caregiver groups

Despite the fact that the patient may be eligible for referral to multiple agencies, it is wise to monitor the plan and the resources used continuously to ensure that services are not duplicated. When multiple agencies are involved, fragmentation of care and duplication of services can be a major problem because communication between healthcare professionals is often lacking. This lack of a very basic simple skill often contributes to the creation of a crisis atmosphere. Care should therefore be exercised to limit the agency numbers to a minimum and to encourage open and frequent communication. One excellent method of keeping crises to a minimum and maintaining open communication is for case managers to collaborate with each other, establish the case management plan jointly, and elect one person to act as the primary case manager.

Services Required for Discharge

As with referrals to community resources, patients with terminal AIDS frequently require many skilled and professional services. The attending physician commonly orders such providers and services as:

- Home health agency nursing services for:
  - Provision of actual skilled care
  - Drawing of blood for laboratory tests
  - Teaching family or caregiver all aspects of care
  - Monitoring and reporting response to treatment to physician
  - Teaching clean versus sterile technique and disinfection
  - Teaching disposal of waste products, supplies, or dressings, and, if applicable, compliance with infection control measures
  - Teaching signs and symptoms and when to call the physician
  - Teaching emergency care techniques (e.g., airway maintenance, suctioning) when applicable.
  - Teaching the importance of following the medication regimen, side effects, and contraindications
  - Coordination with other agencies
- Home health aides for provision of all personal care
- Social worker or psychologist services for counseling and linkage to other community resources providing psychological support not only for the patient but also for the family or significant other
- Rehabilitation therapy services such as physical therapy and occupational therapy for:
  - Conserving energy and maintaining endurance
  - Assisting mobility and transfers

- Using assistive devices
- Bed mobility (i.e., teaching the caregiver how to reposition or move the patient in bed)

In addition, it is common to see orders for such services as:

- Infusion therapy, when applicable, for:
  - Actual teaching of intravenous therapy techniques and administration of solutions or medications and all emergency techniques
  - Restarts and assistance with troubleshooting problematic areas
- Laboratory services for such tests or measurements as:
  - Frequent blood counts
  - Viral load
  - CD4 cell counts (T4 lymphocyte counts [total and percent])
  - Absolute T-cell values
  - Cultures (blood, stool, urine, and skin)
  - Western blot test
  - Antibody titers (enzyme-linked immunosorbent assay [ELISA])
  - Serum albumin
  - Serum globulin
  - Serum cholesterol
  - Erythrocyte sedimentation rate (ESR)
  - Platelet counts
  - Coagulation profiles
  - Calcium and phosphorus levels
  - Serum electrolytes
- Serologic tests for:
  - Cytomegalovirus (CMV)
  - Coccidioidomycosis
  - Histoplasmosis
  - Toxoplasmosis
  - *Chlamydia* pneumonia
- Other tests for:
  - Blood gases
  - Frequent chest x-rays
  - Urinalysis
  - Spinal taps
  - Sputum cultures
  - Skin tests
  - Kidney and liver function tests
  - Bone marrow biopsies
  - Gallium lung scans
  - Computerized scanning
  - Magnetic resonance imaging
  - Lumbar puncture
  - Tissue biopsies
  - Electrocardiograms
- Durable medical equipment company for:
  - Delivery of all equipment and supplies

- Respiratory teaching and monitoring
- Physician for:
  - Follow-up, monitoring, and changes to the treatment plan
- Other:
  - Frequent blood transfusions and linkage to the appropriate agency or facility for administration of blood
  - Multiple drug therapies and combinations and a pharmaceutical provider for these drugs

Anticipated Teaching

As with all patients, education of the AIDs patient or family and caregiver is critical. The professional home health agency or infusion therapy nurse must stay involved with the teaching until the patient, family, or caregiver is proficient in all aspects of care. When applicable, teaching must cover such areas as:

- Importance of hand washing and use of lotion after hand washing to prevent dry and cracking skin
- Use of gloves and protective garments
- Waste disposal and general care of the environment, personal items, eating utensils, linens, and so forth
- Instructions for pregnant caregiver, if applicable
- Wound and skin care or other specialized care
- Repositioning and mobility
- Feeding, nutrition, and hydration
- Bowel and bladder care and use and maintenance of all supplies
- Intravenous therapy and associated care
- General physical signs and symptoms and when to call the physician or seek professional attention
- Medication administration, signs, symptoms, contraindications, and where to dispose of sharps container
- Disinfection versus clean technique for waste and commonly used care items
- Understanding of the disease process and compliance with treatment
- Coping with the effects of the illness, isolation, psychosocial changes, physical limitations, body changes, and the importance of linkage to support groups or professional counseling
- Use of community resources
- Energy conservation

Common Diagnoses Associated with AIDS

The patient with AIDS has a multiplicity of other diagnoses and physical manifestations. When a patient has several diseases and problems it is imperative for each to be addressed in the case management plan with recommendations for care and treatment. Failure to do so can result in costly delays or deterioration in the patient's condition and in unnecessary rehospitalization. Some of the many diagnoses that may occur include hepatomegaly or splenomegaly, coccidioidomycosis, toxoplasmosis, coccidiosis, cytomegaly, isosporiasis, leukoplakia (gingiva, lip, or mouth), agranulocytosis, lymphadenopathy, mycobacteriosis, *Pneumocystis* pneumonia, reticulosarcoma, thrombocytopenia, hypoliposis, lymphadenitis, histoplasmosis, *Nocardia* infections, opportunistic mycoses, multifocal leukoencephalopathy, tuberculosis, Kaposi's sarcoma, Burkitt's tumor or lymphoma, immunoblastic sarcoma, primary lymphoma of the brain, strongyloidosis, *Salmonella* infections, and hematologic toxicity.

Common Physical Manifestations

The list of physical manifestations associated with AIDS is also lengthy. While some of these are minor manifestations, others are serious and must be dealt with by proper case planning to ensure that quality of care is maintained. Typical problems include dementia (organic or presenile) or confusion; headache; body wasting; premature graying or baldness; handwriting deterioration; insomnia; nausea and vomiting; volume depletion; sore throat; chronic vaginitis; blood disorders; weight loss, cachexia, or other nutritional disorders or deficiencies; diarrhea or gastroenteritis (infectious or noninfectious); mouth or skin lesions, oral candidiasis, thrush or macules or papules on the hard palate; persistent fever; herpes zoster, herpes simplex, or other chronic nonhealing viral or fungal skin disease; rashes, dermatomycosis, dermatophytosis, impetigo, psoriasis, or skin discolorations; arthritis (pyogenic or infective); dyspnea; fatigue or exercise intolerance; anemia (aplastic, hemolytic); enlarged or swollen lymph nodes; candidiasis of the lung, nails, skin, or vagina; pneumonia (hospital acquired or viral); septicemia; viral, fungal, or staphylococcal infections; depression; incontinence; blindness or diminished eyesight; neurologic involvement such as meningitis, encephalitis, memory loss, loss of concentration, behavioral changes, apathy, motor abnormalities, agitation, labile mood, delusions, hallucinations, mutism, quadriparesis or paraparesis, seizures, tremors, discoordination, poor balance, hyperreflexia, hypertonia, sensory neuropathy, painful dysesthesias or paresthesias, neurogenic bladder, ataxia, malaise, irritability or diplopia or photophobia; and, in small children or infants, one might see lack of ability to reach expected developmental milestones or failure to thrive.

Typical Drugs

Patients with AIDS may be taking any number of medications in large daily quantities. In addition to other medications, whether oral, intravenous, or via other routes of administration, HIV+ and AIDS patients commonly take any combination of the drugs in the following list. Because of the AIDS epidemic, the FDA has relaxed some of the criteria or time frames that were formerly required for drug testing. New drugs are therefore being approved and marketed more quickly than in the past. The following list of drugs includes those that are in use as of this writing.

- Retrovir
- Pentamidine
- ddI (dideoxyinosine)
- ddC (dideoxycytidine)
- d4T
- Saquinavir
- Hivid
- Neupogen
- Epogen
- Diflucan (fluconazole)
- Videx
- Trimethol sulfa
- Intravenous ganciclovir
- Dapsone
- Pyrimethamine
- Amphotericin B
- Clarithromycin or Biaxin
- Megace
- Bactrim or Septra
- Foscarnat
- Acyclovir

Many HIV+ and AIDS patients are intravenous drug users, and when this fact is known, these patients often cannot be discharged until the treatment course and intravenous access have been discontinued. If this occurs, placement in a skilled nursing facility or subacute care facility that offers intravenous therapy is necessary.

As stated earlier, the AIDS epidemic was the stimulus that created changes in the speed with which drugs became available on the market. Thus, many drugs now being taken by HIV+ and AIDS patients may be under FDA investigation and are considered investigational or experimental in nature. When this occurs, care must be taken to make certain that all drugs authorized are FDA approved because many healthcare payor plans will not cover the cost of experimental or investigational drugs or any treatments associated with monitoring the drugs' effectiveness. If the patient is not linked appropriately to research funding or if approval is not obtained from his or her healthcare plan for the drugs, the costs often become the responsibility of the patient.

Fortunately, many healthcare payors do reimburse if the drug is classified as an investigational new drug (IND). However, this process varies with the healthcare payor, and if a drug is approved, sufficient medical information and cost benefit analysis must be supplied at the time the request for authorization is submitted. If a medication is unfamiliar, research must be undertaken to validate that the drug is FDA approved. One of the simplest ways to do this is to call the FDA or the nearest medical center that provides care for AIDS patients. They can be located by calling the toll-free directory assistance service.

Terminal Care

Terminal care methods vary from physician to physician. While many physicians prescribe any combination of treatments until death occurs, others take a more palliative approach and order only care that alleviates pain and discomfort. Regardless of the method used, for patients who require terminal care, referrals to a local home health agency or hospice agency are frequently necessary. These agencies provide not only skilled nursing care or custodial care but also the assistance and support required by the caregiver or the family during the dying process.

Because many AIDS patients in the end stages of their disease have no home and no family or caregiver and are living on a limited income, many communities offer the services of congregate housing and care for these patients. Although their services vary, many of these homes offer care and services to persons who need a place to live; others continue to allow the patient to reside there and provide terminal care. Case managers unfamiliar with these services can locate information regarding such projects by calling (1) the nearest AIDS foundation; (2) physicians who specialize in AIDS care; (3) another case manager or discharge planner; (4) the closest tertiary center's clinical nurse specialist who specializes in AIDS care; and (5) the state Health Department or office handling AIDS patients.

🔖 S U M M A R Y

Persons with AIDS are often among the most challenging for a case manager because they frequently have little income, no home, and their family and friends have deserted them. Although many healthcare organizations offering case management automatically include the AIDS diagnoses in the caseloads that must be followed by case management, case managers should be careful to follow only those patients who truly require assistance.

Because AIDS patients frequently have several diagnoses, referrals to many specialists as well as to numerous community agencies are common. All patients and caregivers must be informed of community resources and alternate funding programs to which they might be entitled.

CASE MANAGEMENT OF CANCER AND HOSPICE PATIENTS

The Pros and Cons of Case Management

Cancer can occur at any age and in any tissue or organ, and regardless of the type of organization offering case management services, a significant number of cancer patients is usually found in most case management caseloads. Case management involvement can occur at any stage of the disease. However, because survival rates are increasing, cancer, like many other diseases, is now considered a chronic disease for many patients. With this in mind, many case management organizations have shifted their efforts from providing terminal care case management to early education. The purpose of most early intervention efforts is to educate the patient and family about the disease and the options for treatment and to offer information on local or national resources.

However, case variables and the type of case management offered by the healthcare organization (e.g., facility-based case management, community-based, or healthcare payor) dictate whether early involvement is appropriate. The following factors also are common indications for earlier intervention:

- There is evidence that quality of care issues are present.
- Poor discharge planning has occurred, with evidence of fragmentation or duplication of services.
- There is evidence of frequent emergency room use or related readmissions.
- Patient and family education about community resources and alternate funding is necessary.
- There are requests for experimental or investigational procedures or drugs.
- Extensive surgical treatment or treatment rendered in a tertiary care center is present, and the treatments or lengths of stays appear to be longer or more complex than is usual and customary.
- There is evidence that this could be a high-dollar case.
- There is evidence that the treatment course will be long or that the patient will require frequent admissions.
- A bone marrow transplant will probably be required.
- There is evidence that the treatment course is not appropriate or underutilization of treatment is identified, and the patient must be moved to a center of excellence or tertiary care center that specializes in cancer care.

Common Treatment Modalities

Although cancer is not limited to the following, the most common forms of cancer are:

- Leukemias
- Lymphomas
- Solid tumors

- Adenocarcinomas
- Sarcomas
- Retinoblastomas
- Neuroblastomas
- Malignant melanomas

Throughout the course of treatment, the focus of the treating team will be on the tumor and any metastases, the type of treatment (surgery, chemotherapy, or radiation therapy) or combination of treatments that will be necessary, and the site where the treatments will be rendered. In the early stages of cancer, hospital case managers or discharge planners, the healthcare payor's case manager, the home health agency's nurses, and the physician's office staff are invaluable resources for the patient and family. For instance, they are helpful in establishing the resources necessary for outpatient care, coordinating admissions, and educating the patient and family about their healthcare benefits, community resources, and alternate funding programs to which they are entitled.

Centers of Excellence or Tertiary Care Centers

Historically, most treatments have been administered in the clinical setting of acute care hospitals. With the advent of shorter lengths of stays and proliferating outpatient services, many treatments are now available in the home or in various outpatient settings. However, caution must be exercised when cancer patients are discharged to ensure that any post-acute care the patient requires can be administered safely and efficiently in an outpatient setting or at home. This is necessary because some treatments, according to the standards of care for the condition or treatment modality, cannot be given safely in anything other than an acute care setting. Also, owing to the complexities of new treatment modalities (e.g., experimental procedures), many cancer patients now receive their care in centers of excellence or tertiary care centers.

Any cancer patient who is hospitalized in a tertiary care center must be evaluated for the feasibility of case management. This is necessary not only because these patients are sicker but also because their medical costs (as well as their out-of-pocket costs) at a tertiary center can be exorbitant. The increase in cost results not only from the types and frequency of the care given but also from the fact that many such centers will not contract with healthcare payors. Many centers are also not willing to negotiate discounts or consider other forms of reduced rates for reimbursement. Thus, the costs of the services must be paid. Out-of-pocket expenses can be high because many patients must drive long distances or even relocate temporarily to be near the treating facility.

In tertiary centers costs can average several thousand dollars per day because charges are based on the full fee-for-service rate, and if services and costs are not monitored closely, the patient's healthcare benefits can be quickly eroded. Although cost is a concern, the actual treatment program is a matter of concern also. This is due to the fact that many of these tertiary care centers are teaching centers, and complex cancer cases make excellent subjects for teaching. Medical students, however, are not attuned to the business world of medical finances. Consequently, lengths of stay must be closely monitored to ensure that the patient is moved to a lower level of care or back to the local community as soon as it is medically possible to do so. Such monitoring not only saves healthcare costs but, more important, it ensures that the patient's healthcare benefits are preserved for use at a later time.

Experimental or Investigational Services

When cancer patients are hospitalized in tertiary care centers, the case manager must be keenly aware of treatments that are experimental or investigational as opposed to those that are recognized as the standard of care. Many tertiary care centers and teaching facilities are affiliated with clinical drug or treatment trials or studies, and, as stated earlier, experimental and investigational treatments (as well as any associated treatments, testing, or services) are often not reimbursable by healthcare payors.

When cancer treatments or drugs are identified as experimental, the case manager must ensure that the healthcare payor has issued, in writing, the appropriate coverage determination for the treatment in question. Without a prior authorization, reimbursement may be denied. If close attention is not paid to this detail, the patient and family may be burdened with unexpected financial obligations.

Although a coverage determination for an experimental or investigational service or item varies with the healthcare plan, many healthcare payors do pay for such services or drugs.

This is especially true for drugs classified as investigational new drugs (INDs) and for drugs in the later phases of their clinical trials and for which favorable results are emerging from the studies. It is also true for drugs used for conditions classified as "off-label use." In these cases, reimbursement occurs if prior approval has been issued by the healthcare payor.

A good example of a procedure that is still in the experimental stages and remains under close scrutiny and for which coverage varies from plan to plan is autologous bone marrow transplantation (ABMT). This treatment in most cases has not been recognized by most authorizing bodies as efficacious for the disease under treatment and may not be covered by the healthcare payor. If reimbursement is to occur, the procedure must be authorized before the beginning of the treatment by the healthcare payor.

If the transplant or procedure is denied by the healthcare payor, legal action against the healthcare payor frequently ensues. These cases become very labor intensive for all case managers involved. To prevent such occurrences, it is imperative for all case managers involved to collaborate on the work required. For instance, if the case manager is associated with a facility, his or her job may be to collect all pertinent data for the healthcare payor that point to medical efficacy. In contrast, the healthcare payor's case manager may collect all pertinent data and possibly perform a cost analysis, preparing all this information for medical or legal review and the final coverage determination.

To verify whether a treatment or drug is experimental or investigational, two of the case manager's best resources are the Food and Drug Administration (FDA) and the National Cancer Institute (NCI). Case managers should include the current phone numbers of these agencies in their phone directories. These agencies are most helpful not only in answering questions and defining the status of the treatment or drug in question but also in sending literature and directing the caller to centers of excellence that are participating in specific trials, when information of this type is necessary.

Of course, until the patient is actually entered into a study and the experimental services are started, healthcare benefit coverage for all services is, in most cases, allowed. However, it is common to find that, once the patient is enrolled in the study, all services related to the subject under investigation are excluded from healthcare coverage. Similarly, for patients participating in drug studies, all healthcare services required by the patient are covered by the healthcare payor with the exception of the drug treatment itself and related laboratory or radiologic studies ordered to monitor its clinical effectiveness.

How is a case manager to know when a treatment or drug is experimental or investigational? Basically, one's awareness is heightened when medical information raises doubt about it or points to the fact that the treatment or drug is other than a standard of care or is not recognized as such by the medical profession. If doubt arises, one of the best ways to clarify the status of the issue is to review a copy of the consent form the patient is asked to sign (or did sign). Providers by law are required to inform patients about the treatment they are to receive and whether the treatment is a standard of care or experimental (California has a Human Experimentation Act that further emphasizes this requirement).

Any facility or physician that enrolls patients in clinical trials must inform the patient of its status, and the patient must sign a statement that he or she has been informed of this fact and is aware of his participation in a clinical trial. The consent form clearly states that the patient understands that the treatment is experimental and grants consent to participate in the trial.

Complex Treatments

In addition to the few patients who are entered in clinical trials, many cancer patients in case management caseloads require complex treatment modalities that in themselves necessitate frequent hospitalizations. Unfortunately, many of these are chemotherapy treatments that cannot be administered safely in an outpatient or home setting. If a hospital stay is necessary, it is often for a short term, 2 to 3 days.

These short stays are necessary not only for the chemotherapy treatments themselves but also for any follow-up laboratory and radiologic studies or monitoring by nurses and physicians. Also, because of the toxic nature of the treatments, frequent changes in physician orders and treatment planning are commonly encountered. In addition, many patients require frequent administration of blood or blood products and control of pain, nausea, and hydration throughout the duration of the treatment. Case management plans are therefore often in flux and require frequent changes and close communication with everyone involved.

Certainly, among the many drugs used in cancer management, many are recognized as safe to administer in a home or outpatient setting when they are given by themselves. If given in combination with others, the patients frequently are hospitalized, as stated earlier, for a short-term admission. If in doubt about the setting to be used for administration of the drug, one of the best resources for information is the pharmacist at an infusion company.

Services Required for Discharge

Side effects of radiation therapy or chemotherapy vary with the treatment course. However, the physician's orders are directed toward detecting and correctly treating such side effects as nausea, vomiting, diarrhea, chills, fever, lethargy, fatigue, cystitis, mucosal ulcerations, skin rashes, hyperpigmentation, hot flashes, decreased libido, leukopenia, and anemia. Some of the more serious side effects may result in hospitalization of the patient; these include such conditions as renal, liver, or cardiac toxicity, hyperglycemia, deep vein thrombosis, pulmonary fibrosis, bone marrow suppression, cerebellar and conjunctival toxicities, and peripheral neuropathies. As the orders are changed to correct the side effects, the case management plan must be readjusted as well. Likewise, services must be implemented to correspond with the patient's needs or the changes made by the physician's orders.

Because of the many side effects and toxicities that occur, any combination of laboratory and radiologic studies as well as hospitalization may be necessary throughout the treatment course. The treatments ordered to correct these effects vary with the symptom or sign and the physician, and the case management plan may have to be changed many times to correspond to these changes. Important to the plan are provisions for teaching the patient and family about the side effects and what corrective actions to take as well as when to call the physician for treatment or guidance.

One common side effect of cancer treatments is low blood counts, which sometimes results in the need for blood transfusions. Consequently, case managers see frequent orders for blood transfusions and drugs such as Epogen or Neupogen. Although many home health agencies and infusion companies can now safely administer blood and blood products in the home, this is not a recognized service that is provided by all such agencies.

Case managers must therefore be familiar with the agencies in their communities that provide services to cancer patients and know which treatment modalities the agencies can and cannot administer. If certain treatments cannot be performed in the home, arrangements must be made with the nearest hospital or outpatient facility to perform them. In such cases, it may also be necessary to arrange transportation for the patient to the facility.

As stated earlier, the side effects of chemotherapy are numerous, and when they occur the patient must be watched closely by the professional team. Monitoring is a service that is frequently provided by the home health agency or infusion company nurses. This service includes close monitoring of vital signs paying close attention to the appearance of pain, skin and mouth conditions, bowel and bladder function, and hydration and nutritional intake, and alerting the physician when problems are identified so that changes can be made to the treatment plan. As the physician's treatment plan or orders are adjusted, the case management plan must be adjusted accordingly. This is necessary to ensure that the plan is kept current and that appropriate resources and agencies are identified in order to reach the stated goals.

The actual frequency of home health agency visits depends on the requirements of the individual case, but the nurse should visit at least one to two times to perform assessments and any related teaching. The home health agency must stay involved with the patient until all aspects of the required care are mastered by the patient, family member, or caregiver. The frequency of review and extensions for actual coverage of skilled home care visits varies with the individual case.

Pain Management

Many cancer patients take high doses of pain medications. These medications are commonly administered orally, intravenously, intramuscularly, intrathecally, subcutaneously, or via special surgically implanted pumps. Pain in cancer patients is possibly the most undertreated condition in the medical arena. Sadly, the lives of many patients are totally uprooted because of pain; even worse is the fact that many patients must live in excruciating pain or die an agonizing death because attention to pain management was neglected. Surprisingly enough, many healthcare professionals are ignorant of the importance of pain management in these patients.

Not all excruciating pain occurs among the dying. It can occur at any time during the disease process, and when identified, it must be dealt with appropriately. Case managers must pay careful attention to this detail and make every effort to seek solutions that allow these patients to live and die as free of pain as possible.

One of the best resources for consultation and recommendations on pain management is the hospice team and its pharmacist or medical director. If there is no hospice team in the patient's general area, the case manager may wish to consult with a pharmacist or his or her own organization's medical director for advice or recommendations. Another excellent source for consultation is a pharmacist from an infusion therapy company. When a formal hospice agency is not involved in the case, the case manager must often assume the role of advocate, interacting with the patient's physician and family and relaying the recommendations of the person consulted.

Patients in extreme pain must take a pain medication in doses that are high enough to allow them to function in a reasonable manner without pain. Unfortunately, many lay people (and yes, some professionals) ignorantly view such dosages as a mechanism for addiction! It is not. In these cases, special attention must be paid to educating the patient and family about the benefits of such a treatment program.

Equipment Needs

Although equipment needs vary from patient to patient, the most common items required by terminally ill cancer patients may be a hospital bed, bedrails, and a bedpan. Depending on their mobility status and level of consciousness, others may require a wheelchair or walker and possibly a commode. Those with respiratory or secretion problems may require oxygen or suction equipment and supplies. Others who are in severe pain and are receiving medication administered other than orally may require some form of infusion device and the necessary and sundry supplies needed for its administration. Similarly, patients who are unable to eat orally may require a feeding pump and its related supplies.

One of the most important and common needs of terminally ill patients who are confined to bed is incontinent supplies and pillows. These are necessary if the patient is to be kept clean, dry, and properly positioned. Unfortunately, because these items are rarely reimbursed by healthcare payors, either the family must pay privately for these items or they must secure them through the local American Cancer Society or other loan closets.

Community Resources

The American Cancer Society is one agency the case manager must be familiar with because it is not only a service agency, it is also dedicated to research. This agency is possibly one of the most important ones used by cancer patients.

Most American Cancer Society agencies offer a full array of services, but services vary from community to community. However, this agency commonly provides such services as support groups, durable medical equipment from its loan closets, bandages and other dressings, incontinent pads, one-on-one volunteer visitors for specific diagnoses (i.e., Reach to Recovery) or for caregiver respite, information on local resources such as hospice agencies, and transportation for patients to and from the treatment facility (if the patient is ambulatory and can ride in a private car). Other community agencies commonly used for cancer patients are:

- Handicapped transportation
- Homemaker and chore worker services
- Telephone reassurance programs or volunteer visitor programs
- Child care services, if applicable
- Fraternal organizations, if applicable
- Church, ethnic, or social service agencies
- Special education or tutoring programs for children

Barriers to Discharge and Access to Care

The two most frequent barriers to home care for cancer patients are lack of a primary caregiver and treatment that is too complex to be administered outside the acute care setting. Other barriers associated with access to care for cancer patients include:

- Patient requires custodial care (often the patient requires total care, but skilled care is not needed), but the healthcare payor will not pay for it and the family does not have the financial resources to pay privately for help.

- Care needs are of such intensity, complexity, or frequency that the skilled nursing facility or home care agency cannot manage the level of care.
- Patient is confused, noisy, or combative.
- Facility is full and there is a waiting list.
- Patient is a child or young adult, and the staff are unfamiliar with the care needed for this age group.

Alternate Funding

When working with cancer patients it is very important for the case manager to encourage the patient and family to explore the benefits offered by any "cancer" or other income (short-term or long-term disability) policies they may have. Many of these policies can assist with payment of the terminal needs of the patient. This is especially true when care is denied or is not a benefit of the primary healthcare policy and the patient must pay privately for this level of care.

Likewise, alternate funding programs must be explored because they can assist with either income or copayments, cost charges, and deductibles. Because many patients with cancer do not have other supplemental insurance policies, the family must then be encouraged to explore such financial options as:

- Unemployment benefits and state disability benefits, if available
- Medicaid
- Title V Childrens' Medical Services program
- Supplemental Security Income (SSI)
- Social Security Disability Insurance (SSDI)

While many of these programs are income programs, Medicaid and the Title V Children's Medical Services programs are not; these programs may be available to assist with reimbursement of medical services that are limited or excluded from the patient's primary healthcare policy. Medicaid and the Title V Childrens' Medical Services programs vary in eligibility requirements and the treatment benefits allowed. Therefore, it is imperative for case managers to be very familiar with their state's requirements for eligibility and with the benefits allowed.

If income is needed, SSI, SSDI, unemployment benefits, or state disability income may be programs that can be explored by the pa-

tient and family. Unfortunately, SSI is for low-income persons who have no assets, and not everyone who applies is eligible; persons who are eligible for this program are also eligible for Medicaid. The SSDI program is for persons who have been deemed totally and permanently disabled. Unfortunately, because of the requirements needed to qualify and the processing time required, many patients die before they become eligible for benefits (income). However, this should not discourage the family from applying as soon as the need is identified. This is especially true since patients with cancer are living longer and care is now chronic instead of terminal, and some form of income is required for basic survival when a person is unable to work. As stated in the section on Social Security (see Chapter 4), if a patient remains on SSDI for 24 months, he or she is entitled to Medicare to assist with payment of medical costs.

Hospice

Unfortunately, not all communities offer the services of hospice through a formal program. While hospice services are not limited to persons with cancer, the name has historically been equated with cancer, and it is included in this chapter for that reason. When a community does offer hospice care, these agencies are a wonderful asset to any plan. The purpose of any hospice program is to provide the support and palliative care (relief of pain and uncomfortable symptoms) needed by patients in the final stages of their disease. It also allows these patients to live as fully and comfortably as possible.

Hospice services can be provided by either grassroots organizations that rely strictly on volunteers to formal programs, either Medicare certified or not, which generally provide their services for reimbursement but can if necessary render the services free of charge.

TYPES OF HOSPICE PROGRAMS

Formal hospice programs can be broken down into the following types:

- Hospital-based
- Home health agency
- Independent community agencies

All three types offer a coordinated interdisciplinary team approach in which the focus is on the patient and the family. These programs provide any combination of medical, psychosocial, and spiritual support as required. The goal of hospice is to allow the patient to remain at home with family and friends as long as possible.

Although hospital and home health agency hospices can provide all services, including periodic inpatient care as needed for short-term care or respite, this may not be the case for the independent community hospices. Independent community hospices must frequently augment their services by subcontracting with home health agencies for some of the skilled nursing services required by patients. This statement does not imply that these agencies do not have merit, but only that two or more agencies may be involved as the hospice provider.

Although most hospice care is administered in the home environment, it can also be provided to persons living in a skilled nursing facility. Because of the nature of the disease and the unpredictability of the outcome, some patients may require occasional short-term admissions for pain control, for other physical needs, or for respite of the caregiver. The final case management plans must contain provisions for such occurrences.

ADMISSION CRITERIA

Hospice care is usually available to terminally ill patients who are no longer receiving curative treatment for their disease. Most patients are accepted into a hospice program if their life expectancy is less than 6 months and if the treatments received are palliative rather than curative in nature. In addition, some hospices require the patient or family to allow the physician to write a "do not resuscitate" (DNR) order. In such cases, the patient or family agrees to this directive, and a signed statement to this effect is maintained in the chart.

Most referrals to hospice care are generated by healthcare professionals. However, referrals are accepted from any source. Timeliness of the referral is important because there are times when the hospice provider may have a waiting list and cannot accept the patient. If this occurs, it may be necessary to establish a mock hospice team until the formal hospice agency can accept the patient. In these situations, the patient is linked to a home health agency for any skilled care required. The personal care needs of the patient and respite for the caregiver are provided by volunteers recruited from

the community or church. Bereavement counseling is offered through local churches and their pastoral services or the home health agency's social worker.

Once accepted or "admitted" into a formal hospice program, families generally become very involved with the patient's care. In most cases the patient's primary caregiver is a family member or several family members, and support is given by either volunteers or the professionals on the hospice team. Occasionally the hospice agency accepts a patient who lacks an identified primary caregiver, but these instances are rare because toward the very end of the patient's life, the level of care may increase. This increase in care requires hourly skilled nursing care or admission into a skilled nursing facility if no caregiver is available on a 24-hour basis.

MEDICARE CERTIFICATION

There are many types of hospices nationwide. However, for reimbursement purposes, many healthcare payors require hospices to be certified by Medicare. Basically, such certification means that these hospices meet minimum standards for care. However, if the only hospice in the area is not Medicare certified, this factor should not prevent the case manager from establishing the patient with hospice. In these cases, the case manager may be required to seek approval for use of this agency through the extra contractual process, showing the cost advantages for use of the agency versus continued inpatient care.

If use of the extra contractual process is not possible, creativity may be called for in using any benefits available from the patient's healthcare coverage or finding and using free community service agencies. In such cases, the patient's healthcare benefits (e.g., home health care, durable medical equipment, and pharmaceuticals) are augmented by volunteer services offered by church, ethnic, or other community groups for the respite and emotional support of the family. If the case manager is unfamiliar with the patient's community resources, one of the best sources of information is the American Cancer Society.

Medicare divides its hospice care into benefit periods. To be eligible for hospice benefits, the patient must have Medicare Part A. The benefit format allows patients to be accepted for care and coverage for an initial 90-day period, followed by another 90-day period if services continue to be required. Additionally, another 30-day extension can be granted, and this is followed by a final extension for an indefinite period if the patient continues to demonstrate need. For patients without Medicare, if the patient's healthcare policy allows hospice as a benefit, many healthcare payors follow Medicare's guidelines in regard to benefit periods. All patients entering a hospice program must file an election form stating that they understand that care is palliative rather than curative.

SERVICES PROVIDED

In general, formal hospice programs provide their services at an all-inclusive per diem rate if the care specified is reasonable and necessary for palliative management of the terminal illness. As a rule, the following services are covered under this per diem rate:

- Nursing services (either direct services or services performed under the supervision of the registered nurse)
- Physical therapy, occupational therapy, or speech therapy
- Medical social worker services
- Counseling services (pastoral, bereavement, or other)
- Dietary services
- Physician services
- Short-term inpatient care (including respite and procedures necessary for pain control and acute and chronic symptom management)
- Continuous home care (up to 8 hours or more per day, if necessary during short periods of crisis)
- Medical appliances and supplies
- Outpatient drugs and biologic preparations for pain relief and management of symptoms

Rarely does the hospice agency supply 24-hour nursing care except for short-term respite care or during crisis situations. If the family cannot manage to provide the care themselves, consideration should be given to admitting the patient to a skilled nursing facility. Unfortunately, two of the most common barriers to placement in such a facility are: (1) the facility cannot admit the patient for whatever reason, and (2) the family or patient refuses admission.

The Patient on Chemotherapy

Many cancer patients need chemotherapy, which can be administered safely at home; thus

the need for acute hospitalization or post-acute care hospitalization is reduced or eliminated. The feasibility of home-administered chemotherapy depends on the chemotherapeutic agent used and the standards required for administration of the drug. As with any patients receiving long-term intravenous therapy, a central line may be inserted prior to discharge, or the patient may be admitted or scheduled for the procedure in an outpatient setting. However, the actual mode of access depends on the individual case.

Although many chemotherapeutic agents can be administered at home, many others cannot. In these situations, the patient must be readmitted for short-term stays for the actual administration of the drug, blood work, and monitoring by the healthcare team. These admissions will be scheduled at regular intervals every month or every few weeks.

READINESS FOR DISCHARGE

Readiness for discharge depends on the individual case and on the disease. However, the following criteria are often helpful in determining whether a cancer patient can be discharged on chemotherapy:

- The outpatient treatment course is financially feasible.
- The patient is clinically stable.
- The patient is taking a nonexperimental chemotherapeutic agent, and the drug is appropriate for home use.
- The patient has tolerated the initial course of chemotherapeutic agent without problems.
- The patient and family accept home care.
- The patient and family or caregiver can be taught all techniques required.
- The patient has an established venous access that is adequate (a central line is best).
- The patient's home has an adequate physical layout and a clean environment.
- The necessary medical resources are available.

SERVICES REQUIRED FOR DISCHARGE

Patients who require the administration of chemotherapy in the home when discharged frequently need the following services:

- Home health agency or infusion therapy provider with 24-hour capabilities for skilled care involving:

- Monitoring, assessment, and reporting of responses to physician.
- Teaching of all aspects of care and emergency precautions or situations plus monitoring the teaching–learning cycle until the patient or family is proficient in care.
- Drawing blood for laboratory tests.
- Actual provision of skilled care until the patient, family, or caregiver demonstrates proficiency in all aspects of care.
- Restarts or troubleshooting of problems.
- Registered pharmacist or infusion supplier with 24-hour availability for:
  - Preparation of chemotherapy solutions, delivery of supplies, intravenous therapy pump, equipment, and solutions.
  - Troubleshooting and equipment maintenance and operation.
  - Review of changes in drug or frequency of administration with physician.
  - Review of medication regimen and recommendations to the healthcare team if adverse reactions are encountered or other pharmaceuticals are needed (e.g., pain control, bowel regimen, antiemetic use).
- Physician for:
  - Follow-up, monitoring, and changes to the treatment plan.
- Durable medical equipment company for:
  - Delivery of other durable medical equipment and supplies if applicable.
- Laboratory or radiologic services for:
  - Appropriate outpatient laboratory tests or panels, or radiologic services (offered either in an outpatient setting or via a portable unit dispatched to the patient's home).
- Other services:
  - Counseling or peer support groups to help the patient and family in coping with the illness and possible death.
  - Home health aides for assistance with any personal care (depending on the patient's disability).

ANTICIPATED TEACHING

If the patient or family is to assume responsibility for the administration of chemotherapy, teaching is imperative. Teaching for patients who need chemotherapy must encompass at least the following areas:

1. Understanding of the disease.
2. Knowledge of the drug (action, side effects or toxic reactions, dose).
3. Care of intravenous catheter and venous access site.
4. Safe handling and storage of drug and disposal of waste products.
5. Signs and symptoms of complications or problems.
6. Nutritional needs, hydration and antiemetic use, pain control, and bowel elimination regimen.
7. Procurement of supplies.
8. Troubleshooting of equipment and intravenous line when problems arise.

Additional topics include:

- Availability of community agencies or resources.
- Coping with the illness, psychosocial changes and limitations, physical changes, and death.

EQUIPMENT NEEDS

The actual durable medical equipment required by the patient undergoing chemotherapy depends on the diagnosis and on the intensity and severity of the disease. However, at minimum, chemotherapy patients require:

- Infusion therapy equipment, solutions, heparin, and supplies (including chemotherapy spill kits and waste containers).
- Dressings for site care.

COMPLICATIONS

Most complications resulting from infusion services for chemotherapy in cancer patients are preventable if meticulous attention is paid to techniques, if observation and monitoring are performed, and if corrective actions are implementd when problems are identified. When complications do occur they are frequently associated with such causes as:

- Infiltrations
- Phlebitis
- Infection
- Sepsis
- Dislodgment, kinking, or occlusion of the tubing or catheter
- Untoward effects of the agent (nausea and vomiting, hair loss, decreased blood counts)
- Thrombosis
- Difficulty in maintaining venous access if a central line is not used
- Major event separation (central line) of tubing and catheter during tubing changes, causing air embolism
- Pneumothorax, hemothorax (although these are rare)

BARRIERS TO DISCHARGE AND ACCESS TO CARE

With all technology-dependent patients, and chemotherapy patients are not exempt from this category, barriers to discharge and access to care are common. In most cases, the barriers associated with the discharge to home of a cancer patient include the following situations:

- The caregiver or family is not available or is unteachable (two factors that often affect a person's capacity to learn include vision and manual dexterity).
- Community resources are not available.
- The patient and family are not accepting of home care.
- The chemotherapeutic agent is not appropriate for home administration (too complex or dangerous).
- The home environment is unsanitary.

SUMMARY

Case management of cancer patients occurs at various stages of the patient's illness. Due to the fact that many cancers now require chronic care, case management is best done in the early stages of the illness. It is during this phase that education often plays the biggest role.

Cancer care is costly, and for those patients in tertiary care centers, the case manager must pay particular attention to the need to move the patient to another level of care as soon as he or she shows readiness for such a move.

Although most chemotherapy treatments are recognized as standards of care, some are not. The case manager must research drugs or treatments that are not familiar to ensure that such treatments will be reimbursed by the healthcare payor. Also, while many treatments are known to be safe for home care or outpatient administration, many are not. In such cases, cancer patients may require frequent short-term stays in the hospital while these treatments are administered. If this is the case, the case management plan must address this need.

Hospice is a wonderful addition to any case management plan, and case managers must know which agencies in their area are available to assist with this function. Unfortunately, situations will occur when a hospice agency is not available, yet the family desires to take the patient home for terminal care. In these cases, a mock hospice plan can be developed utilizing any healthcare payor benefits for the skilled care required and community volunteers to assist the caregiver with the nonskilled needs or to provide respite.

CASE MANAGEMENT OF THE END-STAGE RENAL DISEASE PATIENT

The numbers of patients with chronic renal failure or end-stage renal disease in case management caseloads can be significant. These patients have a multitude of medical, psychological, and socioeconomic needs that are costly not only in actual expenditures but also, and more important, in the quality of life of both the patient and the family.

The causes of end-stage renal disease in chronic renal failure patients can be many and varied and range from diabetes, congenital anomalies, sepsis, trauma, burns, or drug intoxication to specific diseases, especially those related to cardiac or respiratory failure, metabolic disorders, and older age. While many patients in this category must undergo dialysis for the remainder of their lives, many others are candidates for transplantation, and still others die awaiting a transplant.

Patients with end-stage renal disease in chronic renal failure often present a greater challenge to case managers than other cases because community resources available to manage this category of patients are frequently nonexistent. This void places an additional burden on the patient and family because they must be referred to services that may be out of the area and must assume the extra costs associated with travel to those agencies. To further complicate the situation, many patients are unable to work owing to their disease and disability. Thus, until they qualify for Social Security benefits or welfare, loss of the breadwinner of the family or of additional income adds further to an already stressful situation.

Treatment Modalities

During the past decade, the healthcare delivery system has developed different treatment modalities for the end-stage renal disease patient. These new modalities assist the patient and family in adjusting to the medical condition, the rigors of the treatments, and the situation in general. For instance, years ago, the arduous process of hemodialysis was the only mode of dialysis available, and it was offered only from a facility-based unit. The patient had to travel to the facility several times a week for the dialysis treatment, which was necessarily partner-assisted. This type of treatment caused any number of insurmountable problems, including unemployment and added costs for transportation, and fostered a dependent personality. The problems resulted from the fact that dialysis became the patient's "life." These treatments greatly affected the patient's lifestyle and ability to function normally and independently.

With the advent of technologically complex care administered in outpatient and home settings, all this has changed. We now see end-stage renal disease patients undergoing various types of dialysis, many of which allow the patient to maintain a fairly active and normal lifestyle. Other than hemodialysis, the common dialysis modalities in use include:

- Continuous ambulatory peritoneal dialysis (CAPD)
- Intermittent peritoneal dialysis (IPD)
- Continuous cycling peritoneal dialysis (CCPD)
- Equilibrium dialysis (EPD), which is frequently used only in an inpatient setting for nonambulatory patients

In addition to a more active lifestyle, each of these modes offers different methods of dialysis, different time schedules, and different complexities of care as well as a choice between partner-assisted dialysis and totally self-administered dialysis.

These choices are certainly a contrast with the days of hemodialysis. These new modalities not only offer the patient an opportunity to choose the type of treatment he or she prefers, they can also help the patient overcome some of the psychological characteristics typical of the disease and the treatments. Choice of dialysis not only affects the psychological well-being of the patient, it also affects his or her ability to work and his financial reserves. Additionally, it affects the amount of community resources that may otherwise have been required to augment the case management plan or the healthcare benefits available.

Regardless of the mode of dialysis selected, all patients require some form of extracorporeal or peritoneal long-term access. This long-term access is established either by creating a subcutaneous arteriovenous (AV) fistula shunt or by implanting a peritoneal catheter.

The most common reasons for inpatient care involve the initial placement of the dialysis access, complications related to the patient's other medical conditions, or problems associated with the AV shunt or peritoneal catheter. Otherwise, most care for patients on dialysis occurs in an outpatient setting or at home.

Treatment Team

All treatment planning and monitoring of responses to treatment in the patient with end-stage renal disease are provided by a multidisciplinary nephrology team approach. This nephrology team is composed primarily of healthcare professionals that may include such specialists as a nephrologist, psychiatrist, facility-based case manager or discharge planner, social worker, specially trained nursing personnel, and a nutritionist. Many teams also include members of the surgical transplant team, since many patients in this disease category are candidates for renal transplantation. Other members of the treatment team must include any non-facility-based case managers who will be involved with the care or coordination of resources when the patient is discharged (e.g., healthcare payor case manager, home health agency case manager).

As with all transplant patients, if the patient lives in a remote area, the local physician, who will be following the transplant team's treatment recommendations, must be considered a member of the team despite the fact that he or she is only in contact with the team by phone. Such an arrangement ensures the existence of open lines of communication to facilitate the ongoing regular treatment and monitoring the patient requires. The transplant patient's care after discharge is local, and he or she is seen by the transplant team only at the intervals scheduled or requested by them.

Medical Management of Patients on Dialysis

Many end-stage renal disease patients are diabetics or have other diseases that require medical management at the frequency directed by their attending physicians. However, in addition, patients on dialysis must pay meticulous attention to their dietary needs, fluid restrictions, and medications, and case management plans must address these needs. Diets must be specially prepared because these patients have numerous dietary requirements (e.g., special protein, sodium, potassium, and phosphorus requirements) as well as restrictions on fluid. Therefore, linkage with a dietitian who can assist the patient with dietary planning is critical. An additional resource for dietary planning, as well as for other needs, is the literature available from such organizations as the National Kidney Foundation and the American Diabetes Association.

In addition, the case management plan must consider any medications taken for the patient's other medical conditions. The medication regimen for a person on dialysis typically consists of multivitamins, B-complex vitamins, folic acid, vitamin C, ferrous sulfate, anabolic steroids, and oral phosphate. For patients on peritoneal dialysis, laxatives or stool softeners are included in this regimen. Also, because many dialysis patients are anemic, many receive medications such as Epogen or blood transfusions. If blood transfusions are required, they are frequently administered in an outpatient setting or at the local blood bank. In some communities, the home health agency or infusion agency staff is trained and qualified to administer blood to homebound patients. However, this latter capability varies with the particular agency.

Despite the fact that the physician may order a medication or item and the patient has a "written prescription" (like the prescriptions for many of the medications listed above), many over-the-counter (OTC) medications or items are not reimbursed by healthcare payors. This lack of reimbursement imposes an additional financial impact on the patient's already strained budget. For other medications that are reimbursed and are classified as "maintenance" drugs, linking the patient with a mail order pharmacy, if allowed by the healthcare payor and acceptable to the patient, is an alternative measure that can greatly decrease out-of-pocket expenses for prescription medications. Typically, mail order pharmacies offer two important features to their patrons—door-to-door delivery and reduced rates.

To monitor the effects of treatments, patients are subjected to a great number of laboratory tests and radiologic studies. Although most of the patient's laboratory tests are done in an outpatient setting, sometimes the patient may be confined to home. If this is the case, the case management plan must include provisions for linking the patient with laboratory or radiologic providers who offer "portable" services to the homebound. The laboratory tests or radiologic studies typically ordered vary with the individual case. However, the following laboratory tests and radiologic studies are ordered fairly regularly for persons with chronic renal failure or end-stage renal disease:

- Urinalysis
- Renal function studies
- Serum creatinine testing
- Blood urea nitrogen (BUN)
- Creatinine testing
- Radiologic studies
- Intravenous urography
- Cystograms or renal sonograms
- Ultrasound (pelvic or renal)
- Computed tomography (CT)
- Angiography
- Venography
- Magnetic resonance imaging (MRI)
- Renal biopsy

Psychological Impact

Aside from the medical factors associated with chronic renal failure or end-stage renal disease, the psychological stressors associated with this disease make the patient and family constantly vulnerable to crises. It is common to see the following psychological stressors and emotional reactions: anxiety, depression, fear of death and the unknown, loss of independence, role reversal, resentment, loss of income or greatly reduced financial resources, loss of and changes to body image and function, denial, guilt, hostility, and ambivalence or marital discord.

Anger at the whole situation is common on the part of both the patient and the family. Whereas the patient may direct his or her anger at the treating team, the family's or dialysis partner's anger may interfere with his or her ability to function or cope or to offer the emotional support the patient needs. With this in mind, the case management plan should include provisions or action plans to link the patient and family to support groups or professional counseling.

Complications

Patients with chronic renal failure and end-stage renal disease are susceptible to any number of complications, which range from clotting of the AV shunt or peritoneal dialysis catheter; fever; nausea, vomiting, weight loss, and anorexia; malaise or lassitude; dyspnea; cardiovascular arrhythmias; pericarditis; stroke, air embolus; pericardial tamponade; hemorrhage (e.g., gastrointestinal, intracranial, retroperitoneal, or intraocular); metabolic disturbances (e.g., hyperkalemia and hypokalemia, hypercalcemia, hypermagnesemia); hypotension or hypertension; pruritus; seizures; muscle cramps or twitching; restlessness; insomnia; decreased mental status, confusion, or dementia; and full-blown psychiatric disorders such as schizophrenia and manic depression.

Many of these complications require unexpected inpatient acute care. Therefore, lengths of stay are unpredictable. They are based solely on the intensity and severity of the complication and the resulting care required. Nevertheless, the final case management plan must contain provisions for addressing these issues.

Alternate Funding

The most important alternate funding program for patients with chronic renal failure or end-stage renal disease is Social Security; these patients should be referred to this program as soon as possible because persons with this disease who are on dialysis or in need of an immediate transplant may be covered by a special program offered by Social Security. This program is designed to assist with the costs associated with dialysis and transplantation if the patient (or, in the case of a child, the parent) qualifies for Social Security (call the local Social Security office for more details; see also the section on Social Security in Chapter 4). Basically, to be eligible for this program, the patient must have been on dialysis for 3 months or have entered a transplant center for the actual transplant before Medicare coverage can begin. In the interim, and for the first 30 months after the patient begins to receive Medicare, the person's employer-paid or other health insurance is primary. After 30 months, Medicare becomes primary, and any other healthcare coverage is secondary. Medicare coverage continues until 36 months after a successful transplant. Medicare can be reinstituted any time after this period if rejection occurs and the patient requires another transplant.

A major expense associated with transplantation is the cost of immunosuppressants. As a rule, these drugs can cost an average of $1500 per month and even if covered by a healthcare payer, out-of-pocket copayments can add additional expenses to an already strained budget. Because of these costs, it is often necessary to explore the patient's potential eligibility for Medicaid or other alternate funding sources. Alternate funding programs that may be explored are:

- Title V Children's Health Services program (if 21 years old or younger)
- Supplemental Security Income (SSI) and Medicaid
- Research funds (if the transplant is experimental)

Community Resources

Although most end-stage renal disease patients receive dialysis from an outpatient facility (either facility-based or free-standing) or use a self-administered program at home, a few require placement in a skilled nursing facility, and transportation must be arranged to and from the dialysis unit. If placement is required, not all skilled nursing facilities accept this category of patient. The most frequent reason is lack of coverage by the healthcare payor because many of these patients, due to their general debilitated condition, may require merely "custodial" care rather than skilled care. In contrast, many others require very complex skilled care in addition to dialysis. In these cases, the nondialysis treatments may require more nursing hours with their consequent expenditures, for which the skilled nursing facility's administrator is willing to assume responsibility.

Another reason for difficulty in placing such patients in skilled nursing facilities lies in the fact that many skilled nursing facilities simply cannot manage the dietary requirements, nor are they willing to assume responsibility for transporting the patient to the dialysis center for the treatment. Unfortunately, the patient must then often be placed out of the area, established with a dialysis center, and arrangements made for transportation for dialysis.

Regardless of where the patient is placed or lives, possibly the greatest need is the need for transportation. Most healthcare payors will not reimburse for "nonmedical"-related transportation. Also, because of automobile and workers' compensation liability coverage, many community agencies that do offer transportation require the patient to be ambulatory and be able to get in and out of a car without assistance. So, unless the patient is fairly self-sufficient, this mode of transportation is limited as well.

Locating transportation can be an arduous process because it may be necessary to contact multiple agencies. If an agency cannot be located, a schedule for volunteer drivers may be needed if the patient can depend on family and friends. In other cases, the patient may require transportation in a wheelchair car or another form of nonmedical-related "ambulance" service. Unfortunately, this mode of transportation may or may not be reimbursed by the healthcare payor. Consequently, costs must be assumed by the patient or by Medicaid, if the patient qualifies for Medicaid and the state Medicaid program allows this form of transportation.

Since the patient is usually followed by a nephrology, transplant, or dialysis team, there is often little reason for home health agency care. If a home health agency is required, it is frequently used to assist with any skilled care needs related to other conditions, or for teaching or other skilled care needs related to the mode of dialysis. If a home health agency is needed for skilled care, the nurse must remain involved with the case until the patient or family is proficient in the care required.

If the chronic renal failure or end-stage renal disease patient is discharged to home, other community agencies or resources that may be useful in the final case management plan may include:

• American Kidney Foundation
• American Diabetes Association
• Support groups
• Church, ethnic, or community social service agencies (used mainly for transportation, support groups, or assistance with shopping or personal care, when applicable)
• Disease-specific agencies (those related to the underlying cause of the renal failure)
• Handicapped transportation services
• Chore worker or homemaker services
• Organ procurement transplant center
• Emergency response system
• Hospital or independent dietitian
• Medical-alert identification bracelet
• Outpatient laboratories or radiologic or imaging centers or, if the patient is homebound, centers that offer portable services

Equipment Needs

Although the patient with a newly transplanted kidney requires little if any equipment, patients in need of dialysis require a voluminous amount of monthly supplies and solutions in addition to their dialysis equipment. The best sources of such equipment and supplies are national vendors who specialize in dialysis equipment and related solutions and supplies and door-to-door delivery. However, before establishing a patient with a national vendor, the case manager must always verify with the healthcare payor the provider of choice. Otherwise the patient may be financially liable for the equipment and supplies until transferred to a vendor that will be reimbursed by the healthcare payor.

In addition to dialysis equipment and supplies, these patients must be assessed for any other equipment that may be required for other specific diseases or debilitating conditions. In most cases, this equipment will be available from a local durable medical equipment vendor.

Anticipated Teaching

As with all patients, if the patient administers his or her own dialysis, teaching is critical (see also the later section in this chapter on transplants and the teaching recommendations for these patients). At minimum, the patient or dialysis partner must be taught:

• The importance of meticulous attention to diet and fluid restriction
• The importance of recognizing signs and symptoms
• Compliance with the dialysis regimen
• The importance of paying meticulous attention to administration of dialysis
• All necessary care associated with self-administered dialysis
• All aspects of care related to other medical conditions

Barriers to Discharge or Access to Care

Barriers to discharge are common for this category of patients. The greatest challenge for a case manager in working with end-stage renal disease patients is the lack of resources to support the needs associated with dialysis (e.g., limited or nonexistent dialysis centers in the patient's general vicinity or community, and transportation to the dialysis center). Other barriers include the following:

- There is no home, or the home lacks running water or telephone service.
- Local community resources to support dialysis needs are limited or nonexistent.
- The home environment is unsanitary.
- There is no family or caregiver (sometimes one may be available but is unable to assume responsibility for care).
- There is no transportation.
- The local physician is not available or is unwilling to accept responsibility for care.

SUMMARY

Patients with chronic renal failure or end-stage renal disease generally have other medical conditions that must be addressed as well as their need for dialysis and control of their kidney disease. Due to the advent of new treatment modalities, many patients can now administer dialysis to themselves at home, thus maintaining a somewhat normal lifestyle. Unfortunately, for those patients who must receive their care from an outpatient center, two of the most stubborn barriers to gaining access to this care are a lack of local facilities that offer this type of care and transportation of the patient to the outpatient facility.

This category of patients has multiple stressors related to their disease and the necessary lifestyle changes. Therefore, the patient's active participation in choosing his or her preferred mode of dialysis and linkage to support groups or professional counseling are critical.

CASE MANAGEMENT OF THE CHRONICALLY ILL OR DISABLED CHILD OR THE CHILD WITH SPECIAL NEEDS

Demographics and Overview

National statistics indicate that approximately 10% of all births have a catastrophic outcome—either death of the infant or a severe birth defect. Add to this the number of children who develop a severe illness or sustain a catastrophic injury, and the numbers can be astronomical. These numbers certainly exert a substantial effect on our healthcare resources and the dollars spent on healthcare, but no price can be placed on the quality of life that the child and his or her parents must frequently endure.

Because children with special needs have a multitude of diagnoses, conditions, malformations, and injuries, the variations seen in the capabilities and needs of families and the services offered to them are just as diverse. This section attempts to outline some of the many issues involved in managing pediatric patients. However, it is virtually impossible to outline everything because each case has its own set of variables. Pediatric case management plans must be very individualized and case specific. Consequently, because of the intense and complex care associated with pediatric cases and the fact that resources for this category of patients tend to be sparse, the amount of energy and effort needed by the case manager to coordinate and implement the final plan is tremendous.

Not only does illness in this category of patients require an inordinate amount of healthcare resources, more important, it takes a heavy toll on the family, both emotionally and financially. Unlike adults, who might develop or sustain a catastrophic illness or injury but live a few years longer, children with a chronic illness or injury are dependent on their families or the healthcare "system" for a lifetime. Consequently, families must be prepared for the difficulties ahead and must be taught how to navigate the healthcare system to take care of their child and of themselves as well.

Although chronically ill or disabled children have special needs, so do their parents, especially the mothers or caregivers. As such, caregivers must be watched closely, and arrangements must be made to ensure that timely respite is available and caregiver burnout prevented. The best solution is to establish respite care whenever possible. This respite may be available through volunteers (it must be remembered that if the child is technologically dependent, volunteer caregivers must be trained in whatever skilled care techniques are required to allow the primary caregiver respite), day care centers that specialize in caring for sick children, short-term foster home placement, or skilled nursing facility admission.

Unfortunately, respite care is often excluded from healthcare benefit coverage or is unavailable in some communities. It is therefore helpful for case managers to become familiar with respite alternatives, to know how to seek respite via the extra contractual process, and to discover what respite services are available from the state agency responsible for developmental disabilities. Familiarity with this latter agency is very important because many children requiring care have developmental disabilities. If the child is a client of this agency, respite services may be available. If for some reason the child is not eligible and respite care is required, the case manager may be required to seek approval for this level of care through the extra contractual process if it is available. If not, other community resources (e.g., church groups) must be explored to discover volunteers, who must then be trained.

Community Resources and Alternate Funding Programs

Families are expected to be able to navigate the healthcare system and to be knowledgeable about the resources available to help them, yet many healthcare professionals are unaware of which community resources and alternate funding programs can serve sick children and their parents. This ignorance on the part of both parents and professionals is one of the main reasons for denial of services—lack of timely referral. For instance, each state has a Title V Children's Medical Services program that can provide medical coverage for a chronically ill or disabled child if the child meets certain eligibility criteria. The eligibility criteria and medical treatment reimbursement capabilities vary from state to state, but this should not deter case managers from making referrals if the child appears to have an appropriate diagnosis. In most states, the earlier the referral is made, the more time is available to complete the eligibility process and determine the benefits.

Additionally, any child with a developmental delay may qualify for services from the state agency responsible for serving persons with developmental disabilities. It is common for children to be eligible for both programs. Whereas the Title V Children's Medical Services program is designed to assist children with special needs, the agency for developmental disabilities is intended to help clients with developmental disabilities who are at risk of long-term care. This agency's primary purpose is to keep the person from being institutionalized. However, if a person does require institutionalization, this organization is often the pivotal point for entry, assisting families with all the arrangements necessary for placement.

Each state is required by federal mandate to provide a free and public education to every child from birth to age 21 even if the child has a medical condition that interferes with his or her schooling. Under the Individuals with Disabilities Education Act (formerly Public Law 94-142), schools are required basically to provide whatever care and services are needed to ensure that the child will receive a free public education. Once the child has applied for Special Education, the school district must develop an individual educational plan (IEP), which specifies which services will be provided by the school district (this includes instruction in special schools such as those for the deaf and blind). States vary in the level of services they provide, but case managers must be knowledgeable about what services are available in their state for children needing special access to education.

As stated repeatedly in this manual, the case manager must be familiar with the alternate funding programs available to help patients because many of these programs can be used to augment healthcare payor benefits that are excluded or limited from the patient's insurance policy. These programs are not only of critical importance in enhancing benefits, but also, if the patient is denied care from the healthcare payor (for example, if the needed services are not a benefit or if the patient has exhausted his benefits), reimbursement may be available from the alternate funding source if the patient meets the eligibility criteria.

Other alternate funding programs that may be explored by families include:

- Medicaid
- Supplemental Security Income (SSI)
- Medicaid waiver programs, if applicable
- Medicare for the disabled person under age 65 if the child is a dependent of a parent who is already on Social Security Disability Insurance (SSDI)
- Social Security's End-Stage Renal Disease program, if applicable
- Ryan White funding for children with AIDS, if applicable

As with all alternate funding, the foregoing programs are frequently overlooked or access to them fails owing to inappropriate timing of the referral. Most often they are overlooked because it is thought that the healthcare payor will cover all expenses. Unfortunately, another reason they are overlooked is that they are viewed as a form of "welfare" or as a program "for the elderly" and thus not applicable for younger patients. Another reason for delayed referrals is that when families attempt to gain access to these programs themselves, they may receive an initial refusal at the time of inquiry and, due either to stress or to lack of knowledge of the healthcare "system," they go no further. In these cases, despite the fact that the child may have been eligible, the family has not received an official denial of services, and thus they cannot exercise their right to appeal. Should the child be referred properly at a later date, it may be too late to be eligible for services they may have been eligible for all along.

With this in mind, case managers must make sure that they are very knowledgeable about the referral and appeal processes for the alternate funding and public entitlement programs in their state. Families must be encouraged to follow through on any referral made and to exercise their right of appeal if services are denied. Despite the fact that the appeal process is labor intensive and another source of frustration for the family, families do win, but often success occurs only with the encouragement or intervention of a healthcare professional as the family pursues the appeal.

Other Resources

Although no one likes to speak of the subject, death is a real possibility for many chronically ill children or children with special needs. When death is expected, linkage with a hospice or other support services must not be overlooked. Many communities offer programs that are specifically designed for terminally ill children. In addition to typical skilled nursing care and hospice services, these programs use play and art therapy and other techniques that allow children to express their emotions and thoughts about death. For children who die in a tertiary care center miles from home, case managers should be familiar with resources that can be used to assist families with any costs associated with bringing the body home, if the family cannot assume this expense themselves.

When a chronically ill child or a child with special needs requires frequent or extended hospitalization, families should be informed of the fact that many tertiary care centers can arrange for local housing at a reduced rate. The purpose of this housing is to help families avert costly hotel or motel bills. More important, it is used to provide a home-like setting during the remainder of the treatment. Possibly the most famous of these programs are the Ronald McDonald Houses associated with large tertiary care centers that specialize in technologically complex pediatric care. Regardless of the name, these housing resources offer a home-like environment for families at nominal to no cost while the child is hospitalized or receiving outpatient treatment. Information on such housing arrangements can often be obtained from the social worker or case manager at the tertiary care center.

Another community service that is not well known is assistance with some transportation costs. Although funds for this service vary from state to state, if the child is eligible for treatment and services from the state's Title V Children's Medical Services program and the family cannot afford the costs associated with transportation, this program may be able to assume a portion of the costs. Other agencies that may be used for this purpose are the American Red Cross, American Cancer Society, United Cerebral Palsy Association, Easter Seals Society, and other volunteer groups. If the child is eligible for the Civilian Health and Medical Program of the Uniformed Services (CHAMPUS), now called TRICARE, and his or her care has been approved under the Program for the Handicapped (PFTH), funds for mileage costs (at a greatly reduced rate) associated with transportation of the child to and from the treatments may be available.

One frequently overlooked resource is the use of facilities operated by such organizations as the Shriners and Saint Jude's. Such facilities are designed to provide free care to technologically dependent children or those who require specialized care and treatment. For instance, the Shriners is known for its orthopedic and burn care, and Saint Jude's cancer and respiratory services for children are well known.

Because pediatric resources are limited, case managers must be very familiar with the resources that are available in their immediate area. Likewise, they must be familiar with national children's resources or facilities that accommodate children with special needs. One of the best ways to stay abreast is to maintain regular contact with other pediatric case managers. Programs and situations that affect children with special needs and are constantly changing include the following:

- Alternate funding sources, public entitlement programs, and the charges for each.
- Legislation or budgetary cuts that affect the availability of resources and patient rights and entitlements to them.
- The various appeal processes.

- Waiting lists for specialized services or for public programs (e.g, Medicaid, Title V Children's Medical Services programs, conservatorship, skilled nursing facilities).
- Changing capabilities of frequently used agencies, especially those relating to staffing and levels of expertise.

Children with special needs may need any number or combination of community resources. Although many of these resources are disease specific, some are "vendors" for the local Title V Children's Medical Services program or the agency responsible for administering services to the developmentally disabled. When a child is eligible for benefits from both the healthcare payor and the alternate funding or entitlement program, coordination with these vendors is critical even if the child's healthcare payor is the primary payor and requires use of its own network providers.

Approval of such providers is critical because use of the same agency by all payors of services has several advantages. For instance, it allows an opportunity for open and frequent communication, and permits less fragmentation and duplication of care; it helps to keep confusion to a minimum, and allows the family some control over the numbers of persons going in and out of the home. Unfortunately, in many cases such approval and coordination of agency use is limited to the extra contractual process. In others it may not be possible at all if the extra contractual process is disallowed or denied or the healthcare payor has stringent rules about the use of only its own contracted or network providers.

Genetic Services

Because so many disorders have a genetic component, most states offer some variation of genetic services and testing. These services are frequently provided by the state's Title V Children's Medical Services program. As with all state agency services, the types and amount of testing offered vary from state to state. Genetic counseling services provide families with an understanding of the problem and the disease and offer information about the future risk of recurrence.

Genetic counseling services include any tests necessary to confirm the carrier status of prospective parents or to detect actual fetal defects in pregnant women. Tests commonly associated with detection of a defect include:

- Amniocentesis
- Chorionic villus sampling (CVS)
- Ultrasonography (US)
- Maternal serum alpha-fetoprotein screening (MSAFP)
- Percutaneous umbilical blood sampling (PUBS)
- Chromosomal studies
- Southern blot
- Other carrier disease-specific screening tests

Genetic diseases frequently seen in case managers' caseloads include such conditions as:

- Down's syndrome and trisomy 21
- Tay-Sachs disease
- Friedreich's ataxia
- Sickle cell anemia
- Thalassemia
- Muscular dystrophy
- Hemophilia
- Hunter's syndrome
- Lesch-Nyhan syndrome
- Cystic fibrosis
- Huntington's disease
- Retinoblastoma
- Wilms' tumor

Developmental Delays

Because any of these genetic disorders can have catastrophic outcomes, many children born with birth defects or genetically linked diseases will qualify for developmental disability services, many of which are mandated by the Developmentally Disabled Act of 1984. Under this act, states must provide services that contribute to the "habilitation" of developmentally disabled persons. The term developmentally disabled is generally defined as a severe chronic disability that:

- Is attributable to a mental or physical impairment or a combination of both.
- Becomes manifest before the person attains the age of 22.
- Is expected to continue indefinitely.
- Results in a substantial limitation of function.
- Results in a need for specialized services for an extended period of time or for a lifetime.

In addition to the genetic diseases listed earlier, developmental delays can be caused by such conditions as:

- Stroke in a young child.
- Anoxia or other causes of brain damage.
- Traumatic brain damage.

- Severe orthopedic or neurologic trauma that leaves the child with severe developmental delay or paralysis.
- Severe cardiac or respiratory condition.
- Cerebral palsy.
- Severe mental retardation.

Any of these conditions can cause a condition severe enough to qualify the child for services. The key is to refer the child as soon as the condition is identified and let the agency determine whether the child meets the criteria established for eligibility. Delays in the referral process are frequently the main cause of denial of reimbursement for services and care. It is unfortunate that many medical professionals do not understand that the above diagnoses often cause developmental disabilities; instead, they associate the services provided by this agency with patients labeled "handicapped" or "retarded." Thus, the primary reason for delays in services or noneligibility for services is the timing of the actual referral.

Although most states serve these children through the state agency responsible for administering services for those with developmental disabilities (e.g., Department of Mental Retardation, Department of Developmental Services), California has vendored these duties to agencies called regional centers. At present there are 21 such centers statewide, and California is the only state that offers this separation of duties. However, the services provided by these regional centers are no different from those provided by other states.

Because institutionalization in a state hospital is viewed as the avenue of last resort, the state agencies responsible for handling services for the developmentally disabled "vendor" the necessary care and services to providers to prevent such institutionalization. Although the frequency and types of services provided vary from state to state, vendors typically are home health agencies, durable medical equipment companies, child day care centers, hourly private care or homemakers' service agencies, skilled nursing facilities, or other licensed facilities that are capable of rendering the level of care required. All these services are intended to assist the caregiver with housekeeping and child care chores or to offer respite. If respite is required, the home care hours may be increased. If not, temporary arrangements for foster care or out-of-home placement in a skilled nursing facility may be made.

If the disabled person is an adult and is referred to the developmental agency before the age of 22, services may continue past this age and range from long-term board and care and vocational services and training to placement in a skilled nursing facility.

Skilled Nursing Facility Care

Placement in a skilled nursing facility is one of the largest voids in pediatric case management. Finding a skilled nursing facility that is willing and able to accept patients under the age of 50 is difficult and is almost impossible if the patient is a child. Case managers must therefore become familiar with all levels of skilled nursing care, whether provided by local, regional, or national facilities, that are capable of meeting the needs of children with special needs.

How are such facilities found? Often the process involves calling the state agency responsible for licensing and certifying skilled nursing facilities. Sometimes this information can be found by networking with peers or by calling community resource agencies that are specifically designed to handle pediatric services. Unfortunately, many facilities that can offer the needed care will be located out of the area, adding additional burdens and strains on the family and the child. When out-of-area or out-of-home placement is necessary, the case manager must work closely with the family, keeping communication open, honest, and proactive. The emphasis must be on the quality of care that will be afforded the child.

Equipment Needs

Many children with special needs require not only specialized high-technology "skilled" care, they also require specialized high-technology equipment. Of course, the need for equipment varies with the individual and the specific disease involved, but in most cases the equipment must be ordered specially and custom-fitted specifically for the child. Also, because of the child's continued growth, regular replacement of many items will be necessary, and a routine monitoring schedule should therefore be built into the final case management plan.

When ordering pediatric equipment it is important to use durable medical equipment companies that specialize in providing and fitting equipment for children. Many of the technicians working with these companies have undergone specialized training pertinent to measuring and making the equipment. Also, these companies are frequently vendors for alternate funding programs such as the Title V Children's Medical Services program or the state agency responsible for developmental disabilities. As stated earlier, it is important to make every attempt to coordinate the provision of services and use the durable medical equipment companies that are vendors of the alternate funding programs designed to assist persons under the age of at least 21 if Title V programs are involved and beyond this age for other agencies. This coordination decreases the risk of nonreimbursement if the healthcare payor declines to pay for the service or provides inadequate reimbursement to cover the total costs of the equipment, which will be an expense the family either cannot afford or is not prepared to assume.

Home Health Agency Services

As with durable medical equipment companies, case managers should try to ensure that home health agency care is likewise coordinated using vendors or home health agencies approved by alternate funding programs whenever possible. Unfortunately, as stated earlier in this manual, many healthcare payors insist that the providers used belong to their own network. If this is the case, the case manager may find it necessary to use the extra contractual process, explaining the advantages of use of other providers to ensure the overall success of the case.

If it is possible to use a provider that is also a vendor for an alternate funding program for which the child is eligible, it is important to develop the case management plan jointly with the case managers for these programs and the home health agency. Joint planning is important because it prevents the following unfortunate consequences:

• Fragmentation or duplication of services.
• Too many case managers, all acting on similar issues.
• Multiple calls to the physician by all case managers about the same problem.
• Families not knowing which case manager to call.
• Lack of communication between all caregivers and all parties.

FREQUENCY OF SERVICES

When a pediatric or adolescent patient requires home care, the actual number of hours or frequency of services provided by the agency varies from case to case because, although some technology-dependent children and their parents can manage with intermittent home health agency care, these instances are rare. Frequently, nursing care is required on an hourly basis, the average amount of time ranging from 8 to 16 hours per day. Due to the complex care required, many patients require round-the-clock nursing care for an indefinite period of time.

Since many healthcare benefit packages place limits on home care, coordination of this benefit with the alternate funding programs for the exact number of hours required is critical. This is especially true if the quality of care is to be maintained and unnecessary hospitalizations avoided. However, before home care is recommended or implemented, approval must be obtained from the healthcare payor, especially if benefit coverage is limited to providers within the healthcare payor's network. If linkage to home care is made without this approval and payment for the services is denied, the family could experience unexpected outlays of money that may not be reimbursed until the child can be linked with a network provider approved by the healthcare payor.

Communication

The key to pediatric case management as in all case management is communication. Not only must case managers communicate with the family, it is vitally important that they communicate with the healthcare team as well. Case variables dictate the frequency of communication that is recommended.

Case managers must pay close attention to communication not only of the details of the child's physical care needs but also of the elements of what is being communicated and how it is communicated. Frequently these elements revolve around the parents' coping skills and level of maturity and whether or not they understand what is being said to them by the healthcare team.

Communication with the parents must be open, honest, and frequent and must be phrased in language they can understand. Case managers must always keep in mind that parents and families are under tremendous stress at this time, and that receiving too much information at one time can be so overwhelming that they may fail to absorb most of it. Information that might seem clear and simple to healthcare professionals can be very confusing to parents and families. When it is apparent that the parents are confused, the case manager must explain the details in a manner that allows them to be absorbed. The timing of all communications, even for basic information, must be matched to the parents' emotional readiness if they are to understand the relevance of the information. If the patient and family are not familiar with the English language, interpreters are necessary. In such cases, not only is a general interpreter required but also one who is familiar with medical terminology. If such an interpreter cannot be found, much information can be misinterpreted, and the result can be costly in terms of the quality of care.

Naturally, parents differ widely in their ability to know how to ask for information. In some cases, the parents know when and how to ask questions. Other parents are too intimidated to express themselves or ask questions, or they think the questions will be considered "dumb." In such situations, the case manager may need to help the parents formulate questions or actually be present when the questions are asked. In other situations, the case manager must assume the role of an advocate until the family is able to assume this responsibility themselves.

Anticipated Teaching

Because community resources in the pediatric post-acute care arena are sparse, many children with special needs are discharged home. When this occurs, it is necessary to ensure that the family and caregivers are fully trained in all areas of the child's care. In addition, when they live in a remote location and have limited access to community resources, the parents must fully understand the child's illness and know what to do in an emergency. In addition, they must be able to operate and clean all necessary equipment, be able to troubleshoot their own problems and know when to seek help, and demonstrate proficiency in all areas of care. This proficiency includes a knowledge of what to do when the equipment fails, all relevant medical issues, and how to administer cardiopulmonary resuscitation when necessary.

A child with a chronic illness or injury often has special needs for the remainder of his or her life. Consequently, the family must be taught how to be the case manager for the child. In this capacity, they must know:

- What community resources are available and whether the child is entitled to these resources and programs.
- How to navigate the system and barter for services.
- How to file a formal appeal when services are denied.
- What services can be provided by special education programs and other alternate funding programs and how the process works.
- When and how to obtain access to a professional case manager when difficulties are encountered.

The teaching required for the family of a child with special needs is, in many cases, an ongoing task. For all such teaching, both the child and the family must be assessed for their level and style of learning. Although the case manager in most cases is not responsible for the actual teaching, it is wise for the case manager to monitor the teaching process. Suggestions for the use of charts, pictures, dolls, or actual equipment may be necessary if teaching or learning difficulties are noticed. Some outcomes of this teaching may be for the parent to be able to:

- Verbalize why the child is using the equipment or requires the care.
- Verbalize an understanding of the modifications in lifestyle or routines necessary to care for the sick or dying child.
- Demonstrate proficiency in:
  - All care techniques.
  - Appropriate use of equipment and supplies.
  - Troubleshooting problems.
  - Making tubing changes, when appropriate.
  - Cleaning procedures for all equipment.
  - Administration of medications, side effects, and contraindications.
- Verbalize signs and symptoms and when to call for help, and, when applicable, demonstrate proficiency in cardiopulmonary resuscitation.
- Identify resources for maintenance of equipment or procurement of supplies.
- Identify resources for home care and respite services.
- Identify resources for emergencies and disasters.

- Identify emergency back-up plan during power failures or equipment breakdown.
- Identify other resources, support services, and sources of alternate funding.

Just as critical as establishment of a teaching plan is the need to monitor the teaching–learning cycle. This simple task is necessary not only to ensure that all aspects of care are taught but also to evaluate the patient's needs and to ensure that changes are made in the case management plan when changes in the treatment plan are made by the physician. Monitoring of the teaching–learning cycle should be included in all case management plans, not just those relating to children with special needs.

Stresses and Emotional Responses

When children with special needs require services lifelong, multiple stressors are commonly present not only in the parents but also in the child. When stressors are identified, families should be encouraged to seek support either from professionals or from peer support groups. Therefore, the case management plan must include a mechanism for assessment and an action plan that links the patient and family with the appropriate resources. Common stressors associated with caring for chronically ill children or children with special needs include the following emotions or situations:

- Feelings of loss of independence owing to the significant burden of care required and the lack of resources for the care of sick children and respite care of the caregiver.
- Resentment due to lost opportunities and lost income (i.e., mothers especially are in this category because they have had to give up their careers to assume the caregiver role).
- If a sibling, feelings of possible neglect because the sick or injured child requires all the attention; siblings often act out their feelings, and behavior problems are common.
- Social isolation imposed by the 24-hour demands of care and lack of financial reserves for other than the expenses required for the sick child's care.
- Anger about such things as the time commitment needed or the burdens the child now places on the family.
- Unrealistic expectations for the child's recovery.

- Shock, guilt, or grief for the loss of a normal child or family.
- Denial that the child has special needs, which forces the child to perform beyond his or her capacity, or, alternatively, results in a tendency to seek treatment from all sources whether or not they are realistic.
- Financial burdens due to limited or excluded healthcare benefits or to the fact that benefit coverage is limited to acute skilled care rather than long-term or custodial care.
- Limited or nonexistent community resources designed to assist children with special needs.
- Marital discord, separation, desertion, or divorce due to the stresses imposed by care.
- Lack of bonding between the parent and the child with special needs, leading to such outcomes as failure to thrive, abuse, and abandonment.

Although some families have no resilience, others have an abundant supply of this quality. Families without resilience frequently require professional counseling if they are to meet the demands of their duties. When this need is identified, the appropriate resources must be coordinated and implemented immediately. If support and counseling are unavailable or inadequate from free community resources and the person has mental health benefit coverage, coordination with the healthcare payor's mental health review staff is necessary.

Regardless of the parents' abilities, the emotional demands of providing care for these children can be overwhelming. Therefore, linkage of the parents with support groups is a valuable community resource. Here parents can learn first-hand from others how to cope, how to navigate the "system," and how to bypass bureaucratic obstacles. These support groups often serve as an extended family and may become the only "social outings" the family allows themselves.

Probably the saddest result of the stress and pressure that occur in these cases is seen when parents of children with special needs abuse the child. As stated previously in this manual, there are varying forms of abuse, and careful observation is needed to detect not only the obvious signs of abuse but the nonvisual signs as well. State laws mandate the reporting of suspected abuse, so it behooves case managers to know the requirements for reporting abuse in their state. Professional counseling or support groups must be provided for families or caregivers found to be abusive as soon as any form of abuse is identified. Abusers need to know that anger at the unfairness of their situation is a common feeling but that it is possible to express anger in ways that will not harm others. In other situations, the child may have to be removed from the abusive atmosphere and placed in another home or facility.

Emotional Support for the Child

Children may require counseling and support just as much as their parents. When stressors for children are identified, the parents must be encouraged to seek assistance as soon as possible. Stressors for chronically ill children or children with special needs are frequently related to a number of the hurtful experiences in their lives; among them are:

• Pain and discomfort
• Frequent hospitalizations and outpatient treatments
• Possible restricted growth and development, disfigurement, or deformity, causing decreased self-esteem
• Restricted activity and an inability to be involved with their peers
• Taunting, mocking, or harassment by others
• Parental abuse
• Social isolation
• Lack of educational development
• Many psychiatric conditions, including anxiety and depression as the most common

Of course, not all children and their families have these experiences or endure these situations or conditions as every family is different. Some families are able to cope and sustain themselves, but others will succumb to the pressures and demands created by the chronically ill or disabled child.

Barriers to Discharge or Access to Care

Many of the foregoing problems could be dealt with if healthcare benefit coverage and community resources were available. Lack of community resources is the biggest hurdle to obtaining care for families of children with special needs. Some families need help, whereas others just need to "get away" for awhile and experience some "normalcy" in their lives. Barriers typical for children with special needs include the following:

• Providers or facilities that specialize in or are trained in pediatric care are limited or are found only in the larger cities.
• There is a lack of understanding by the general public (this includes healthcare workers) of pediatric diagnoses and needs, or the family's frustrations in dealing with a system that cannot meet the child's needs.
• The programs, services, and alternate funding agencies (e.g., Special Education or the Title V Children's Medical Services program) are inconsistent in quality and vary from state to state and from county to county, and, more important, families face endless bureaucratic obstacles in gaining access to them.
• Poor coordination and lack of joint development of the case management plan among providers, agencies, and the healthcare payor's case manager lead to fragmentation, duplication, and sometimes denial of services.
• Heavy caseloads, due to the sheer number of children with special needs, limit the ability of the case manager to work individually with patients and their families.
• Programs may be staffed by poorly or inadequately trained personnel who are insensitive to the needs of families.
• Respite care is lacking.

Because there are so many case variables, case managers must be creative as they establish case management plans. This creativity is needed to make use of any combination of services from the various agencies and programs to create a "package" that meets the needs of the child. The importance of networking with other case managers who specialize in pediatric case management cannot be overstated; this simple task is extremely helpful as one sets about researching community resources and creating an individualized case management plan for the child.

Case Management of Neonatal Patients

Because neonates frequently make up a large portion of a case manager's caseload, a separate section is included under Children with Special Needs. Neonatal births often result in high dollar expenditures for the healthcare payor and the family as well. Thus, this category of patients must be automatically included among the referral flags used by healthcare organizations that provide neonatal services. The high costs associated with neonatal births are attributable to such factors as the anomalies of the baby, the complexity of the care required, the fact that these babies are cared for in regional centers that specialize in neonatal care, and the length of time it takes to stabilize the child for discharge, to name a few.

Not only do neonates consume enormous amounts of healthcare resources while they are hospitalized, similar consumption may continue after they are discharged. As a result, case management of neonates may be more labor intensive than other cases followed. Because few post-acute care facilities are available for neonates, many neonates who would otherwise be placed in a facility are discharged home. Training of the caregiver or healthcare professionals who will be providing the care must therefore be started as soon as possible to avoid delays in discharge. The training required is related to the intensity of services needed, the complexity of the care, and the severity of the illness. It also depends on the maturity and capabilities of the parents.

Adding to the difficulties of establishing services for a neonate is the fact that the area in which the parents live frequently lacks the resources necessary to manage the child. This factor in itself can be the primary culprit that precludes an earlier discharge.

READINESS FOR DISCHARGE

The criteria used to gauge the neonate's readiness for discharge depend on the individual case as well as the particular neonatal center. However, for most neonates, readiness for discharge is related to such factors as:

- Ability to control the head
- Ability to maintain body temperature in an open environment
- Increased weight gain, or weight stabilization on the feeding regimen used
- Follow-up care by physician available
- Maintenance schedule for medications and feedings established; adjustments not required daily or weekly
- Home evaluation or assessment completed by public health nurse or home health agency nurse
- Teaching of parent, caregiver, or professional and any back-up caregivers adequate; or family has successfully completed a 12-hour trial

period of full care if they are to be the primary caregiver for any period of time
- Follow-up care by medical resources or other healthcare agencies available

ALTERNATE FUNDING

Any neonatal baby should have been referred long before discharge to any alternate funding program to which he or she is entitled. If the referral has not been made before discharge, it may be too late by the time of discharge to obtain any assistance.

Alternate funding programs to which a child may be entitled for services include the Title V Children's Medical Services program (however, not all Title V Children's Medical Services programs cover acute care or neonatal care, so the case manager must be very familiar with what services are available in his or her state), Special Education, and the state agency responsible for services to the developmentally disabled. The latter two agencies are very important because many neonates require infant stimulation programs and other developmental services if they are to progress and develop appropriately and keep up with their peers. Also, as stated earlier, many of these babies have severe neurologic disorders that qualify them for developmental disability services. For further information, see the sections in Chapter 4 corresponding to these three programs.

SERVICES REQUIRED FOR DISCHARGE

The actual services required on discharge are no different for a neonate than for any other patient and depend on the individual case. However, the following services are commonly ordered:

- Skilled nursing care from a home health agency that offers 24-hour availability for:
  - Monitoring and reporting problems, including progress or regression, to the physician
  - Provision of actual skilled care (nursing care can range from intermittent skilled nursing care to hourly private duty nursing and depends on the diagnosis and level of care required as well as many other variables)
  - Teaching of all techniques to the family or caregiver until everyone is proficient in all aspects of the child's care
  - Drawing of blood samples for laboratory tests

- Laboratory services (24-hour on-call availability) for:
  - Hematocrit and reticulocyte counts weekly
  - Electrolytes weekly
  - Nutrition and antibiotic levels, if applicable
  - Theophylline levels
  - Blood gases
  - Caffeine levels
- Registered pharmacist or, when applicable, an infusion supplier (24-hour on-call availability) for:
  - Home delivery of premixed medications, intravenous solutions, and supplies or formulas
  - Troubleshooting of infusion equipment problems
  - Review of medications and solutions with the physician
- Durable medical equipment company (24-hour availability) for:
  - Home delivery of durable medical equipment and supplies and teaching of equipment operation, if applicable
  - Troubleshooting equipment problems
- Physician for:
  - Follow-up, monitoring, and changes to the treatment plan
- Others for:
  - Respite or back-up caregiver support
  - Identification of parent support groups

ANTICIPATED TEACHING

Many neonates have a variety of medical conditions or anomalies, and varying degrees of intensity and complexity of care are required. Consequently, it is imperative to start teaching as soon as possible. At minimum, teaching of parents or caregivers of a neonate must include the following to be ready for discharge:

- Cardiopulmonary resuscitation or other emergency procedures (as indicated by diagnosis)
- Feeding techniques (including tube insertion), if applicable
- Weight control
- Signs and symptoms of fluid overload, infection, dehydration, and medication reactions
- When to call the physician or seek professional help
- All aspects of the specialized care required (for example, many neonates have one or more of the following conditions: a tracheostomy, a ventilator for breathing, or an ostomy, or they require total parenteral nutrition or tube feedings on discharge. The family or caregiver and sometimes the professional nursing staff must be trained in all techniques needed for care prior to discharge. Also, teaching must continue until the family and any back-up caregivers are proficient in the care)
- How to administer medications
- Airway maintenance and knowledge
- How to read infant "cues" of stress as opposed to illness
- How to make or purchase supplies
- Clean versus sterile technique
- Proper storage of solutions
- Methods of coping with the impact of the illness and necessary changes in lifestyle
- Use of community resources

EQUIPMENT NEEDS

The actual equipment and supplies needed vary depending on the diagnosis and actual procedures or treatments proscribed. However, in most cases, neonates require the following equipment and related supplies:

- Stationary as well as battery-operated equipment (this includes a battery charger) to allow mobility for the child and a normal lifestyle
- Liquid oxygen system and supplies
- Apnea or oximetry monitors
- Feeding equipment and supplies
- Ostomy supplies
- For a ventilator-dependent child—all equipment and supplies
- For a tracheostomy-dependent child—all equipment and supplies

COMPLICATIONS

Most complications leading to rehospitalization or problems are preventable by paying meticulous attention to details, maintaining close observation and monitoring, and implementing corrective actions when problems are identified. Typical complications associated with the ongoing care of a neonate are:

- Infections
- Complications with catheters
- Shunt malformations, when applicable
- Severe diarrhea or constipation
- Wound site complications, when applicable
- Fluid overload
- Failure to thrive (dehydration, inability to nipple, suck, swallow, or obtain enough calories)
- Caregiver burnout

BARRIERS TO DISCHARGE AND ACCESS TO CARE

Although barriers vary with the patient and are related to the intensity and severity of the illness or the complexity of care required, common barriers to the discharge and access to care of a neonate include the following:

- A home or other care resource is not available.
- Home conditions are inadequate, such as lack of heat, water, and cleanliness.
- Age or maturity of parents is inadequate, or their ability to comprehend or learn is limited.
- Closest healthcare resources are too far, or resources are unavailable.
- Known abusive situation or environment is present.
- Transportation is not available.
- Physician is not available or unwilling to assume responsibility for care.
- Telephone access is not available.

SUMMARY

It is literally impossible in a book of this type to list each test and service a child with special needs may require on discharge. This section merely outlines some of the considerations that must go into planning for the care of a technologically dependent child or a child with special needs. It also outlines some of the basic resources one may wish to explore when establishing the care and resources required by either the child or the family.

One of the most common barriers, outside of a lack of providers that specialize in pediatrics, is the prevalence of untimely referrals to alternate funding programs, such as the state Title V Children's Medical Services program or the state agency responsible for offering services intended for those who are developmentally disabled. When this occurs, the child may be denied access to programs for which he is eligible in the time of greatest need.

The chronically ill or injured child often becomes the chronically ill or injured adult. As a result, services and care may be needed for the person's entire life. Therefore, it is important to train families to be their own case managers and teach them how to negotiate the "system," calling on the professional case manager only when they encounter obstacles.

CASE MANAGEMENT OF THE DIABETIC PATIENT

Diabetes mellitus (DM) and its complications are possibly one of the most frequent underlying causes of problems seen in patients in case management caseloads. No age, sex, or specific population is exempt. Not only is diabetes costly in terms of health care dollars, it is also costly in terms of the quality of life many diabetic patients must endure.

Types of Diabetes

Although diabetes has two major classifications—type 1 DM (insulin-dependent diabetes mellitus) and type 2 DM (noninsulin-dependent diabetes mellitus)—it is type 1 with its assorted and systemic complications that can lead to end-stage diseases. Thus, these patients are the ones most frequently seen in case management. But type 2 diabetes is the most prevalent type, and these diabetics are not exempt from complications such as cataracts, glaucoma, and neuropathies.

Other Medical Disorders

Healthcare professionals are witness to the fact that people with diabetes are often afflicted with an array of other debilitating medical conditions, for most of which the underlying culprit is DM itself. Other than gestational diabetes, which occurs during pregnancy and in patients with pancreatic cancer, type 1 DM frequently starts before the age of 30. Due to its early onset, diabetes thus makes these patients more susceptible to a variety of other expensive conditions such as retinopathy, neuropathy, nephropathy, and foot and lower extremity ulcers, infections, or amputations. Many of these complications lead to other, more serious conditions such as neurologic disabilities, chronic renal failure, end-stage renal disease, blindness, and sexual dysfunction. It is due to these complications and the complex treatments required that many diabetic patients require hospitalization and other related healthcare services, leading to their inclusion in case management caseloads.

Unfortunately, because of the cost of care, many case management organizations concentrate their efforts on type 1 diabetics or those in the end stages of the disease. As a result, they may offer limited or no benefits other than medication coverage for a type 2 diabetic on oral medication. For example, many do not cover diabetic educational classes for prevention and control of the disease at the time of the initial diagnosis or in the early stages of the disease when the patient exhibits a readiness for learning. Thus, complications that could have been prevented are not addressed until it is too late.

However, many complications of diabetes can be prevented if the patient is proactively involved in his or her care planning in the early stages of the disease or from the onset of the diagnosis. Prevention especially depends on aggressive and intensive hyperglycemia control. This control can be accomplished by carefully monitoring the glucose level, making adjustments in the insulin dose, administering accurate doses of insulin, making allowances in dietary and insulin schedules for variations in activity levels, and paying meticulous attention to skin and foot care.

Insulin

The type of insulin used and the frequency and mode of administration vary with the individual and the details of the specific case. Although past methods of insulin administration were limited to subcutaneous injections using any combination of insulin types, strengths, and frequencies, recent studies have proved that patients often achieve the best results if they have four shots of insulin per day—one shot of regular insulin with each meal and one of NPH insulin at bedtime. With the advent of newer technology, certain categories of type 1 diabetics are candidates for more innovative insulin injection devices such as continuous subcutaneous insulin infusion pumps or button infusors. The button infusor is a small device inserted under the skin and is useful for persons who must take four or more injections per day. The subcutaneous infusor is a small external device worn by the patient that administers subcutaneous injections of insulin at predetermined times throughout the day via a small needle inserted into the patient's abdominal wall.

Equipment and Medical Supplies

Equipment needs vary depending on the body systems affected by the diabetes. How-

ever, all type 1 diabetics require at minimum a glucose monitor, lancets, and related supplies plus insulin, syringes, alcohol, and all supplies needed for administration. Additionally, diabetic children require urinary ketone testing supplies, and patients who are candidates for an insulin infusor need the infusor, insulin, and all related supplies.

Laboratory Tests

All testing depends on the intensity and complexity of the disease and the patient's other medical conditions. In addition to glucose testing, performed by the patient, type 1 diabetic patients typically require the following tests, which are performed at varying frequencies:

- Blood urea nitrogen test at least once per year.
- Chemistry panels as deemed appropriate by the attending physician.
- Serum creatinine studies at least once per year.
- If wounds are present, frequent wound cultures and other laboratory studies to monitor the responses to antibiotic therapy.
- Ophthalmologic examination at least once per year.

Other Services

Many new type 1 diabetics require short-term outpatient clinic or skilled home health agency services after they are diagnosed. This is necessary to ensure that the teaching–learning cycle continues until the patient can, at minimum, administer his or her own insulin injections, accomplish the glucose testing regimen, understand the side effects of insulin and the disease, and know when to seek professional help. In some cases the home health agency nurses may become involved during their visits to the patient for other medical conditions or complications, such as wound care and infusion therapy.

Similarly, for a blind insulin-dependent diabetic, a home health agency is frequently necessary to train the family or caregiver in insulin administration and all facets of glucose monitoring. Blind diabetics who live alone can often self-administer their own insulin if they have access to prefilled syringes that are filled by either the home health agency or a pharmacy. If the patient is blind and has not been previously exposed to courses in independent living, independent living centers or the society for the blind are excellent resources for referral. From these sources the patient can obtain information about his or her options and education to aid independent functioning. In all cases the home health agency must be allowed to follow the diabetic patient until both the patient and the family are proficient in administering the required care.

Because many diabetic patients have neuropathies, chronic pain for them is a reality. Although diabetics with neuropathy will not respond to a pain management program, studies have proved that they often respond to certain medications designed to increase perfusion to the nerves. In such situations, case managers must make every effort to ensure that the case management plan provides for an evaluation by a neurologist or pain management specialist. Once this evaluation has been completed, the plan must include provisions for initiating any pain management techniques recommended and monitoring the patient's responses.

In addition to the American Diabetes Association and its local chapters, other community agencies that may become involved with diabetic patients are many and varied; their involvement depends on case variables. However, the following agencies are often helpful for diabetic patients:

- Assistive device centers
- Blind society and services such as Braille libraries, readers for the blind and other blind services, training, and schools
- Church, ethnic, or community social service agencies for volunteers and drivers and respite care
- Support groups
- Choreworker or homemaker services for shopping, personal care, and housekeeping
- Diabetes educational classes
- Department of Education and Special Education or information on blind schools if the child is under the age of 21
- Department of Rehabilitation and vocational rehabilitation services
- Handicapped transportation services
- Independent living centers
- Utility company for special mechanical modifications for appliances
- Organ procurement program, if the patient is a transplant candidate

Alternate Funding

Depending on the extent of their disability and the complications of the disease, many diabetics maintain a fairly active lifestyle. Thus, they continue to be gainfully employed and retain their healthcare coverage. It is only when complications occur or the disease reaches the end stages that unemployment or a reduced income and loss of healthcare coverage force the patient to rely on alternate funding sources. Alternate funding programs that the family should be encouraged to explore include:

- Medicaid
- Social Security Disability Insurance (SSDI)
- Medicare for the blind and disabled under the age of 65
- Social Security's End-Stage Renal Disease (ESRD) program
- Supplemental Security Income (SSI)

Families of children under the age of 21 should be encouraged to apply for services that may be available from the local Title V Children's Medical Services program. Depending on the child's disabilities, they may also need to apply for services available from the state agency responsible for providing developmental disability services or the Department of Education.

Because many patients with diabetes are candidates for transplantation (kidney, kidney–pancreas, or islet or segmental pancreas transplantation), other sources of coverage that can assist with payment for the transplant may be required. For instance, while most of the transplants just mentioned are recognized as the standard for care, there is a chance that one or more may be considered experimental and thus may be excluded from reimbursement by the healthcare payor or alternate funding source.

When this occurs, the case manager must help the patient and family locate a program that will allow the transplant to occur. This may mean finding a tertiary care center that may be performing the transplant in question under a research grant. However, the primary means of funding a transplant when reimbursement is denied by the healthcare payor is private donations or the fund-raising efforts of a local fraternal organization.

Psychological Impact

As with any long-term illness or injury, the psychological impact of dealing with a chronic debilitating condition takes a toll. Diabetic patients are not exempt and display an array of psychological responses to their illness and its accompanying problems. Reactions and emotions such as the following are common:

- Anxiety
- Depression
- Fear of death and the unknown
- Loss of independence and role reversal
- Loss of income and financial resources
- Loss of body image and physical changes, especially after amputation
- Denial
- Manipulative personality due to chronic pain and dependency
- Guilt
- Hostility

With this in mind, case managers must include in the case management plans efforts to ensure that the patient and the family are knowledgeable about the appropriate resources, such as support groups or professional counseling, that can help when needs are identified.

Anticipated Teaching

The primary focus of teaching diabetics about their disease is to emphasize the importance of keeping the patient's hyperglycemia under control and preventing latent complications. All type 1 diabetics require monitoring and instruction in insulin administration techniques and signs and symptoms of hyperglycemia or hypoglycemia. Although dietary restrictions are no longer endorsed by the American Diabetes Association, dietary teaching is required to manage the patient's weight and to make adjustments in insulin and dietary intake according to varying levels of activity. Therefore, patients must be linked to educational classes as early as possible.

One of the best methods of diabetic education is formal educational classes, many of which are offered through outpatient programs at local hospitals. Unfortunately, not all healthcare payors reimburse for this level of service because it is classified as educational as opposed to "medically necessary." When such a denial is encountered, the case manager must make every attempt to obtain approval, which may include use of the extra contractual process.

If all attempts to enroll the patient in a formal educational class fail, educational literature can be obtained from the American Diabetes Association. Similarly, many community hospitals, the

local chapter of the American Diabetes Association, and even some healthcare payors offer "informal" classes or distribute information. Some of these classes are free. For programs for which a fee is charged and no reimbursement is available from the healthcare payor, the costs must be assumed by the patient using out-of-pocket funds, or, if he or she is eligible for Medicaid, by Medicaid. Medicaid reimbursement for this type of service varies from state to state; some states do not allow it.

Education about diabetes is necessary to ensure that the patient or family at minimum:

- Understands the disease process.
- Can demonstrate proficiency in administration of his or her insulin regimen, if applicable.
- Understands the importance of recognizing signs and symptoms of problems and knows when to seek immediate medical care.
- Understands the importance of paying meticulous attention to foot care.
- Understands the importance of monitoring activity levels and dietary requirements.

Education sessions may also cover such areas as:

- Wound care.
- Administration of intravenous antibiotics, total parenteral nutrition (TPN), or other intravenous drugs and solutions.
- Use of the insulin pump.

In these cases, the "teacher" must stay involved until the patient or family is proficient in all aspects of care and knows how to troubleshoot problems, recognizes the signs and symptoms of problems, and knows when to call for help.

Barriers to Discharge or Access to Care

The most stubborn barrier to care for diabetic patients occurs in the early stages of the disease. It is then that patients can benefit most from a formal educational program. Yet, as stated earlier, educational programs are frequently excluded from the patient's healthcare plan. Also, because many diabetic patients are not involved in planning their own care and treatment regimen, their commitment to the rigors of any program established is weak or absent. Barriers to discharge or access to care are encountered most frequently in the end stages of the disease when the patient has multiple and complex medical needs. These barriers include the following factors:

- No local community resources are available to meet the needs of the patient.
- There is no family or caregiver.
- Transportation is lacking.
- The patient is unable to qualify for Medicaid financially but does not have enough money to pay privately for services.
- Personality disruptions cause adversarial relationships, and the local physician is then unwilling to accept responsibility for care.
- The care level required is too intense for skilled nursing facility admission.
- Despite multiple chronic conditions leading to "total care or dependence," the patient is classified as requiring custodial care only, and the services required are not reimbursable by the healthcare payor.

Certainly the list of barriers is not limited to these. Each diabetic patient has his or her own set of variables that affect the presence of barriers in obtaining access to care.

SUMMARY

Type 1 diabetic patients frequently have other serious medical complications that further increase their inability to function. Unfortunately, one of the most serious voids in healthcare coverage is the lack of reimbursement for education needed by the patient in how to manage his or her disease.

Depending on their condition, many diabetics are candidates for transplantation, and while most transplants are recognized as a standard of care, many are not. When this situation occurs, the case manager must be prepared to assist the patient and family in seeking alternative routes of reimbursement. Because of their disabilities, many type 1 diabetics are eligible for Social Security and other alternate funding programs.

A critical factor in fostering the patient's motivation and compliance with his or her medical care is active patient participation in planning his or her own treatment regimen. Commitment to and compliance with the medical regimen can also be gained by early education, which fosters an understanding of the disease and the best methods of caring for themselves.

CASE MANAGEMENT OF THE GERIATRIC PATIENT

Demographics

As our population continues to age and live longer, case management faces the possibility of gaining a whole new focus and role as care shifts from a system of reimbursement for acute care to one of chronic or maintenance care. The healthcare system in general is now treating an older clientele who frequently have one or more chronic health conditions. These conditions are complicated by a host of psychosocial and environmental factors, many of which require some supervised care, which allow the patient to maintain some level of independence, unlike the situation in facility-based care.

Any case manager whose caseload includes many elderly patients must be knowledgeable about Social Security, Medicare, Railroad Retirement, or other retirement plans in which the patient did not contribute to Social Security. Likewise, he or she must possess a knowledge of any Medicare risk programs in the area, Medicaid, Supplemental Security Income (SSI), and other state and local community agencies that provide services to a geriatric clientele. Such knowledge is necessary to ensure that linkage with programs to which the patient is entitled occurs appropriately.

Referrals

Case managers involved with the elderly often find that their involvement results from many factors. As with all patients followed by case management, the high-risk diagnoses or flags mentioned in the preceding sections serve as the most common reasons for referral. However, case variables such as age, prior medical history, level of care required, resource availability, family involvement and interest, and who pays for the case manager's services are some of the most common variables that contribute to the final decision to open the case.

The majority of elderly patients require "maintenance" or "custodial" care, and this level of care is not covered by Medicare or most insurance policies (the only exceptions are some private custodial care policies and Medicaid). In all cases of case management for geriatric patients, it is important for case managers to explore the area of financial assets and liabilities with the patient and family. This exploration is necessary to determine whether the patient can possibly qualify for Medicaid or SSI when funds are limited or nonexistent. Because many patients require custodial care and the patient and family must pay privately for these services, families must be informed about the potential cost outlays and the possible alternate funding programs for which the patient might be eligible once the familiy's financial reserves are depleted.

The search for resources to meet any patient's needs, through either private or public programs, creates its own set of problems. However, planning care for the elderly is further hindered by the lack of community and caregiver resources. Unfortunately, as the population ages, case managers can expect to see further limits on more and more resources, further restrictions in admission requirements, and outright termination of services. These limits are the result of greater demands placed on services, budgetary restrictions, and cuts or elimination of programs.

Assessments

Before conducting the initial interview and assessment, the case manager, with the patient's or conservator's permission, must collect as much pertinent medical, social, and cultural information as possible. This information may include:

- Present and past medical history, including past and present physical, mental, and functional limitations.
- Family history and dynamics.
- Socioeconomic history.
- Emotional and psychosocial history and evidence of memory.
- History of alcohol, smoking, and drug use.
- Family or caregiver availability and abilities and limitations.
- Resources used in the past.
- Patient and family financial status and insurance policies.

Demographic information about the patient can come from a variety of sources, but the four most common are:

- Questionnaires
- Medical records
- Consultation with physician or other healthcare professionals
- Visual and interactive assessments of the patient

As with all patients, assessment of the geriatric patient must be thorough and comprehensive if the final case management plan is to be valuable and based on individual data.

Interviews

As much information as possible must be gathered before the initial interview. Whenever possible, it is wise to interview the geriatric patient in the patient's own home environment. However, as stated earlier in this manual, such on-site assessment and interview capability depends on the policies of the case manager's healthcare organization.

A home visit is ideal because it does not place additional financial burdens on the patient and family for transportation or a caregiver. Likewise, distractions or disorientation of the patient are reduced because the patient is in his or her own familiar environment. If at all possible, as many family members as possible, including the caregiver, should be present for the interview. This is desirable because they can then be interviewed collectively or individually. Case variables determine which method of abstracting the relevant data to be used in the final case management plan is best or most appropriate. The initial assessment interview must be of reasonable length, possibly no longer than 2 hours. Certainly additional phone contacts or other visits can be scheduled if more information is required. The home visit allows an opportunity to view or evaluate:

- How the patient moves about in his or her own surroundings and conducts his or her activities of daily living.
- The need for any mobility aids or other adaptive equipment.
- Any structural barriers (both interior and exterior) that, if not corrected, might affect the final plan.
- The patient's and family's cultural or religious beliefs, customs, or practices.
- The actual home conditions and environment and its compatibility with the patient's needs and the distances to the nearest resources and sites of medical care.
- Interactions between the patient and family (they are likely to be more relaxed in their own home environment and therefore interact or respond more freely).

- All medications and their storage.
- Food and its storage and preparation area.
- Accessibility to and from the home.

Geriatric Case Management Plans

Although case managers like to state that their case management plans are "individualized," most such plans are actually generalized for the specific illness or injury, and case variables are then added to "individualize" each plan. Because of our aging population, the problems associated with chronic health conditions, the fact that chronic health conditions can be "catastrophic" and expensive, and the fact that in the future most costs associated with provision of care for the elderly will be borne by the patient and not Medicare or insurance policies, case management plans for the elderly must really be as comprehensive and individual as possible. Additionally, they must cover the entire spectrum of care anticipated for the patient as he or she progresses or fails to progress.

The specific nature of the plan is especially necessary because case managers are often involved only long enough to establish the plan and close the case. Therefore, geriatric case management plans must be developed to serve as a long-term guide for the patient and family. To execute this type of planning requires time and individual consideration. For instance, time is required to locate resources, since much of the care required is custodial in nature and not skilled. Because care is custodial, it is rarely covered by insurances. Consequently, a limited fixed income is the most common barrier to obtaining access to care and resources.

In most cases, an array of resources is necessary if the patient's needs are to be met in the least restrictive environment. Contrary to popular belief, most patients can and should remain at home. Placement should be considered a last resort. Thus, the case management plan must limit alternative placement recommendations to those that require the fewest restrictions as the patient moves through the continuum of care.

Because the case manager may not be involved in the case for an extended period of time, the plan must contain provisions whereby it can be revised by the family or significant other as the patient's condition changes. In addition, it must provide methods for reestablish-ing case management services by the patient or family should the need arise. More important, the plan must be developed to serve as a long-term guide for the family, listing the possible conditions that may trigger evaluation of which resources or alternative care sites are appropriate for the next step. It is wise to include approximate costs for each level of care along with recommendations for financial avenues or options that may be explored by the family. Like all plans, the geriatric case management plan involves mutual agreements about problems and goals, identification of resources, and alternatives. The final plan must address such issues as:

- The patient's and caregiver's needs, including physical, functional, social, educational, spiritual, and cultural needs.
- Financial abilities and alternate funding sources of assistance.
- The level of care and resources that meet the patient's needs or allow him or her to function at the maximum level of independence.
- Provision for the health and safety of both the patient and the caregiver.
- The informal community resources that can be used to support or augment any formal healthcare provider benefits.
- Problems and recommendations for nonmedical issues, such as nutrition (e.g., home-delivered meals, self-preparation of meals, congregate sites), transportation, architectural renovations of the home, assistive devices, and durable medical equipment.
- Alternative arrangements, such as facility care, if the home plan turns out to be not feasible or ceases to be the level of care required.
- Alternative arrangements for skilled care and administration of such care as well as respite for the caregiver.

Nutrition and Use of Medications

Two major areas that must be included in the final case management plan are nutritional needs and medication usage. These are two of the most common causes of problems seen in the elderly. Although problems in both areas may be related to the specific factors listed in the following sections, one major underlying cause of these problems is lack of money. Most elderly people, even healthy people, are living on very fixed incomes, which may or may not meet their everyday expenses. In the case of the elderly sick person, the additional costs of medications or unexpected outlays for special diets create a financial deficit that forces the patient to make a choice between basic necessities and the need for treatment of the medical condition. In any event, details of these two important aspects must be included in the final case management plan.

NUTRITIONAL CONCERNS

It is a well-known fact that nutritional needs are affected not only by the normal physiological changes associated with aging but by psychosocial and environmental factors as well. Some of the factors that affect nutrition and can explain why the elderly person may not eat properly include the following:

- Cultural preferences
- Religious observances
- Behavioral patterns, depression, and grief
- Special dietary needs
- Decreased vision
- Decreased taste and therefore decreased food appeal
- Lack of motivation to eat alone or "cook for one"
- Inability to shop owing to mobility problems or lack of transportation
- Limited financial ability to purchase food, especially food needed for a special diet
- Limited or nonexistent food preparation area, limited food storage area, or lack of cooking or eating utensils
- Limited geographic area served by the local home-delivered meal program
- Limited or nonexistent congregate meal sites
- Dental problems
- Reduced or limited activity

Some of the problems caused by nutritional needs in the elderly can be illustrated by the following example. In this case, the elderly gentleman lived alone in one of the downtown hotels. Despite the fact that he really was a candidate for placement, he flatly refused to be discharged anywhere else than to his room. Therefore, arrangements were made for the necessary equipment, home health agency services, and delivery of his meals. Unfortunately, during the assessment interview, questioning never elicited whether or not he had eating utensils. His meals were delivered, but he couldn't eat them until the home health agency nurse discovered that he lacked utensils and

provided them for him. Needless to say, after this experience, this simple question was added to the discharge questionnaire used for patients being discharged home, especially to a hotel.

MEDICATIONS—THE MAIN CULPRIT

The use of medications by the elderly is another major problem area, which must be carefully assessed and addressed in the final case management plan. In addition to noncompliance in taking medications for whatever reason (e.g., lack of funds to pay for the drugs, forgetfulness), older patients are also at risk of adverse reactions to their medications. These reactions may result from changes due to the normal processes of aging or from the fact that the patient may be taking multiple medications for various medical conditions. For instance, changes due to aging frequently occur in the processes related to digestion, elimination, and absorption and metabolism of drugs. Also, the patient's level of physical activity or inactivity or the actual diagnosis affects the response to medications. Similarly, the mere use of multiple medications for various medical conditions makes the elderly, who often have several diagnoses, highly susceptible to a variety of problems related to medication usage and compliance.

The reasons for noncompliance with medication use can be many and varied. Among them are the following:

- Limited finances
- Complexity of the drug regimen
- Inaccessibility of a pharmacy
- Inability to open containers
- Fear of drug dependency or desire to avoid unpleasant side effects
- Failure to discard outdated or discontinued medications
- "Pill sharing"
- Conflicts with religious or cultural beliefs
- Depression and feelings of hopelessness or despair
- Inadequate eyesight
- Inadequate supervision
- Forgetfulness or confusion
- Failure to report use of over-the-counter drugs

Case managers must assess all prescription as well as over-the-counter drugs used. This is best accomplished by using detailed questioning techniques or a questionnaire or better yet, a home visit where all can be visualized. The keys to managing medication use in the elderly are to take a detailed drug history and then to establish a means of ensuring that the patient is monitored for drug use and drug reactions as well as for compliance with any regimen established by the physician.

Monitoring and compliance with drug regimens is an important element of care for the elderly, and provisions for such must be included in all geriatric case management plans. Monitoring can usually be accomplished by soliciting the assistance of family members or friends. Not only the patient but also the families and caregivers must be educated about the importance of medications and schedules. One of the best ways to remind patients with memory deficits to take their medications is through the use of calendars or written reminders of times and frequencies of doses, including which pills to take and how many to take. Also, many visiting nursing agencies will establish a medication regimen by prefilling syringes or containers with drugs and posting reminders of when the drugs must be taken.

Family Involvement

Families caring for an older parent are just as overwhelmed and confused as families caring for a child with special needs. However, there is one major difference, and this is one of finances. While most younger patients have healthcare coverage for most of their medical needs, the elderly often do not. This financial deficit occurs because most elderly people need custodial care rather than skilled care, and custodial care is not covered by most healthcare payors. Consequently, the financial worries add to an already strained situation.

Families of the elderly need to be linked with support groups and services just as much as families of younger patients. Such support groups strengthen families and allow them to cope better with their situation. They also often help to relieve any guilt felt by families as they struggle with their decisions about care for their elderly parents or relatives. Often adult children promise their parents that they will never place them in a nursing home, yet, due to the demands of care and a lack of resources, this promise in many cases must be broken.

The involvement of the family is essential. Their level of involvement plays a key role in determining the relevancy and success of the case management plan. Unfortunately, achiev-

ing this involvement is not always any easy task. The full cooperation of the family in the development of the case management plan depends on several factors, three of which are very common. First are their feelings about the patient in general; second are their reactions to the illness or injury; and third is the fact that they may not reside in the same community as their elderly parent. Therefore, educating the family about the specific details of the disease and the available resources is one of the best mechanisms for alleviating their fears.

In discussions with the family, the case manager must use a proactive approach to alleviate the stigma of Medicaid and "nursing home" placement. It is important always to make every effort to describe Medicaid as "insurance" and to portray "nursing homes" not as a step in the final process of dying but as institutions where the quality of care can be maintained. Naturally, the case manager's ability to overcome such fears depends on the family. However, if their behavior remains adamant or their reluctance to accept information continues, the case manager may be required to close the case if alternatives cannot be found that satisfy their needs and demands.

Community Resources

LEVELS OF CARE

If facility-based care is included in the case management plan as an alternative, the patient, family, and caregiver must be made aware of all the various levels of care within the patient's given community. Case managers must also keep in mind that just because a patient is elderly does not mean that he or she automatically requires a skilled nursing facility or its equivalent. Care for the elderly, or any patient for that matter, must be found in the least restrictive environment that can meet their needs. If out-of-home placement is required, facilities that may be explored include:

- Senior housing (assisted or independent)
- Residential care home
- Community board and care home
- Intermediate care facility
- Skilled nursing facility (also frequently referred to as a nursing home by lay persons), locked psychiatric facility, or Alzheimer's facility
- State institution (this is rare and should be the very last resort)

Among these, the most costly are skilled nursing facilities and state hospitals. Care in these facilities ranges from skilled nursing care to custodial care. Although some patients in skilled nursing facilities can be cared for at home, the costs associated with the care or supervision required are often far higher than the daily or monthly rates charged by a facility. Skilled nursing facilities are the largest provider of long-term institutional custodial care. Staffing in these facilities consists of professional nursing and rehabilitation staff as well as nursing aides. Care in most skilled nursing facilities costs an average of $4000 per month or more. State hospital costs are even higher.

For patients who require an intermediate care facility, board and care facility, or residential care home, admission is frequently based on the patient's ability to ambulate and function normally, bowel and bladder control, actual physical care needs, medication requirements, and the facility's licensure. Much of the care provided at facilities of this type is rendered by unskilled aides or nonlicensed staff. The average costs vary significantly for all levels of care and from region to region.

Likewise, costs for home care vary greatly depending on the patient's actual care needs. Unfortunately, in some cases home care is far more costly than facility-based care if one adds all the costs—hiring help, meal preparation or delivery, equipment, and medications. Also, case managers must keep in mind while drawing up the case management plan that facility-based care usually provides the maximum benefits required to meet the patient's care needs while maintaining the quality of care and the patient's safety. Families must be informed of all alternatives and allowed to make their own choices about home care versus facility-based care.

Although not listed in the foregoing paragraph as a facility, adult day care centers are a wonderful resource for any adult who might need care or socialization during part of a day or week or while their caregiver works. Adult day care centers generally operate from Monday through Friday and belong to one of two types, the medical model, in which some skilled nursing services are available along with socialization, and the social model, in which services are primarily designed to meet the social needs of the elderly. Many centers offer transportation to and from the facility. Charges for this type of service vary, but generally they are based on a sliding scale pegged to the patient's or family's income.

OTHER COMMUNITY AGENCIES ASSOCIATED WITH THE ELDERLY

Besides home health agency services, attendant care services, durable medical equipment services, adult day care, and skilled nursing facility care, the resources that can augment any case management plan for geriatric patients frequently include the following:

- Meal programs, whether home-delivered or at congregate sites
- Friendly visitor programs
- Telephone reassurance programs
- In-home supportive services (usually housekeeping or chore worker services provided either through community programs or through private pay resources)
- Emergency response system
- Handicapped transportation services
- Church, ethnic, or social service agencies
- Senior housing units
- Legal services for the elderly and disabled
- Library services (e.g., home delivery of books for the visually impaired)
- Respite services
- Disease-specific agencies for support groups or literature

Certainly this list is not limited to these resources because each community varies in the types of services provided. Also, accessibility to some services is directly linked to the patient's financial assets and ability to pay.

Alternate Funding

Because most elderly people are receiving Social Security and Medicare, the most common alternate funding sources are:

- Medicaid
- Supplemental Security Income (SSI)
- Private health policies (e.g., cancer, custodial care, nursing home)
- Agencies with a sliding scale
- Medicare Part B, for those who have not previously applied

Other Issues Affecting the Elderly

While he or she is involved with the geriatric patient, the case manager is in a prime position to detect such unfortunate occurrences as neglect or abuse. The geriatric person living at home is a prime target for abuse and is also at risk for the most prevalent form of elder abuse—neglect. Case managers have not only an ethical obligation to report suspected abuse or neglect, in many states they are legally obligated to report any suspected abuse or neglect to the nearest adult protective services agency. Although in many states such reporting is mandatory, in other states it is voluntary. In any case, the case manager is well advised to learn the county or state reporting requirements for the state in which the client resides.

Just as important is a basic knowledge of what kinds of activities constitute abuse. Most groups on aging identify the following activities as forms of abuse:

- Active neglect—intentional failure to provide care by denying food, medicine, or personal hygiene.
- Passive neglect—unintentional failure to fulfill caregiver duties.
- Psychological abuse—infliction of mental anguish by insulting, demeaning, ignoring, making threatening remarks, or isolating the patient.
- Financial abuse—illegal or unethical exploitation of a person's funds, property, or assets.
- Physical abuse—intentional infliction of pain or injury.

Obvious signs of neglect or abuse include:

- Bruising, lacerations, or skin sores.
- Frequent broken bones.
- Unmet medical needs.
- Excessive clutter or filth.
- Few or no social contacts.
- Feces or urine not properly disposed of.
- Rotting or molding food in refrigerator or on counters.
- Reported use of frequent emergency room services for anxiety attacks, difficulty in breathing.
- Claims history of multiple emergency room services at various emergency rooms or urgent care centers.

Other signs that may be recognizable by an alert case manager include:

- Depression or depressive behavior
- Withdrawn behavior or extreme passivity
- Anxiety
- Hostility
- Excessive weight loss
- Physical injuries
- Recent impoverishment

When any of the foregoing signs are discovered, referral to the appropriate agency must be undertaken immediately. It is then the responsibility of the agency to conduct an investigation of the reported issues.

Dealing with geriatric patients raises another issue—that of the patient's or family's wishes for resuscitation or continuation of treatments. To support his or her wishes, the patient may write a Living Will or request that a do not resuscitate (DNR) order be drawn up. If the patient has been declared incompetent, his or her appointed conservator is responsible for doing this for the patient. All case managers must be familiar with the laws and regulations pertaining to these two documents because the mere presence or existence of these documents may not be a sufficient guarantee that they will be honored when or if they are needed. If a Living Will or DNR order is known to exist and is valid, this information must be included in the final case management plan.

Dealing with the elderly presents another issue that is not often found in performing case management for other age groups. This concerns what to do if patients cannot speak for themselves or are not competent to make informed decisions, which are made for them by a third party—the conservator or family. This presence of this situation intensifies the need for the case manager to consider all consequences and available alternatives. Subsequently, all actions must be documented. This documentation is necessary to substantiate the ethical soundness of the case manager's actions if situations arise at a later date that challenge the final plan.

In situations like this, when the patient is incompetent but has not been declared such and no conservator or guardian has been established, the case manager must be familiar with the laws and regulations pertaining to establishing the conservatorship process in the area where the patient lives, the time frame required for this process, and which agencies or professionals are responsible for implementing it. In many states the conservatorship process, due to backlogs, can take several months from the time of application to assignment of a temporary conservator. When this occurs, frequently nothing can be done but wait until the final conservator is appointed. This situation has a significant impact on the case management plan because often the patient cannot be moved nor can money be accessed to establish care at an alternate site until the conservatorship process is completed.

Barriers to Discharge or Access to Care

Possibly the most common barrier to obtaining access to resources and services for the elderly is financial limitations. Many elderly are living on limited or fixed incomes that barely cover the basic essentials of daily living. Consequently, if out-of-pocket expenses are necessary for medical care or services (especially because many services are classified as custodial rather than skilled), the person must make a choice. Unfortunately, this choice is often to do without the medical care or the medications required. Other barriers commonly seen in case management of the elderly include:

- Lack of availability of resources (e.g., level of care or location of resources)
- Lack of transportation
- Lack of availability of caregivers
- Resistance to stigma associated with "nursing home" placement or application for Medicaid
- Reluctance to accept care or services or make a change in residence or lifestyle
- Borderline incompetence and refusal of care or services
- Limited fixed income

❧ S U M M A R Y

Improper or inadequate case management planning for the elderly can lead to increased adverse conditions, readmissions, or admission to an inappropriate level of care. If the case management plan is not specific and the patient, family, or caregiver is not educated about the availability of community resources, patients will inappropriately use the emergency room when a minor problem arises. Also, because resources are often limited for this category of patients, case managers must familiarize themselves with the community resources that serve the elderly. The goal of any case management plan must be to maintain or enhance the patient's level of function and allow him or her to function in the least restrictive environment.

Despite the fact that the elderly patient often needs help and assistance, this level of care is rarely considered skilled. In reality, it is nothing more than maintenance or custodial care or assistance with the activities of daily living. Unfortunately, custodial or maintenance care is not reimbursable by the elderly person's primary healthcare payor—Medicare. Therefore, geriatric case management planning involves finding appropriate resources that are cost effective and financially affordable by the patient.

Because the elderly are often vulnerable to exploitation or abuse, case managers who work with geriatric clients must constantly be attuned to the signs and symptoms of abuse and neglect.

CASE MANAGEMENT OF THE MENTALLY ILL PATIENT

Overview

Because mental health is a specialty in itself, mental health case management (like pediatric and geriatric case management) should be performed by persons who specialize in the field. However, in reality, many case management organizations do not have separate mental health and medical case management programs. Therefore, this section is included as a means of assisting case managers who must assume a dual role. It also aims to educate case managers about the complexities associated with mental health case management.

Although medical case management has been around for years, mental health case management as it is known today has been slower to evolve. However, as the venue of providing mental healthcare continues to change and treatment modalities change from traditional inpatient care, physician office visits, and group therapy to other forms of outpatient care, so must the focus of mental health case management. Long gone are the days when "mental health case management" consisted merely of monitoring and limiting days of service through the utilization review or retrospective review processes. The same thing is true of the social worker versions of case management, which merely linked mentally ill persons with basic resources.

Why has nursing case management taken so long to arrive in the mental health arena? The answers are many and varied; possibly the most obvious reasons are:

1. For the most part, healthcare payors have provided very few if any mental health bene-

fits, and once the person exhausted his or her "lifetime" benefits, care was shifted to the public payor—Medicaid. Medicaid was either unwilling or unable to invest the necessary resources to really care for the person.

2. Insurance reimbursement methods provided little incentive for the provider to consider cost-effective alternatives or other forms of reimbursement.

3. Like their counterparts in the medical-surgical arena, mental health providers have been reluctant to change from their traditional methods of providing care because the "new" ways were not consistent with their practice patterns, philosophies, or professional experiences.

4. Although deinstitutionalization occurred in the 1970s, alternatives to inpatient care have not materialized.

Also, during the past decade, new challenges to the mental health system have emphasized the facts that we have more persons in need of mental healthcare and that access to care has not always been ideal. When patients need care, "someone" has to be able to advocate and assist these patients in gaining access to the services to which they are entitled.

Some other reasons for the change seen in mental healthcare include:

- The erosion of family and social support systems.
- Fragmentation and lack of resources due to budgetary cuts for many community programs or resources.
- Destigmatization of mental illness, which allows more persons to recognize and accept mental healthcare.
- The increased complexities and stressors of life and society in general, which have led to increased mental health symptoms and chemical dependency.

Because of the complex nature of mental illness and the fact that many patients are chronically disabled (either by the nature of the dysfunction or because they have not been able to gain access to treatment), case managers assigned to mental health must be specialists in their field. They must also possess a broad knowledge of:

- Diagnosis and treatment modalities specific for mental health disorders.
- Services and providers that can best serve the patient given the limited or nonexistent healthcare coverage.

- Patient rights and confidentiality laws (e.g., federal Privacy Act and the Comprehensive Alcohol Abuse Prevention, Treatment and Rehabilitation Act).

Case managers must be keenly aware of the requirements imposed by these acts, since mental health information pertinent to the patient is closely regulated by these acts. In addition, case managers must possess a knowledge of the acts that are specific and pertinent to the release of information and the type of information protected by these acts.

Diagnostic Flags

As in medical case management, lengthy admissions and diagnostic flags are not always the criteria one uses to classify a mentally ill patient for case management. Certainly flags are useful, but in cases appropriate for mental health case management the diagnoses and need for services are intertwined with other influences such as age, behavior patterns, family dynamics, past medical or mental health history, adequacy of the original treatment plan, compliance with the treatment plan, standards of care, availability of resources, and financial capabilities or alternate funding programs available. Despite these variables, the following diagnoses are frequently associated with mental health case management:

- Adolescent adjustment reactions
- Manic depressive bipolar disorders
- Schizophrenia
- Sexual abuse
- Chemical dependency
- Major depression
- Dual diagnoses
- Multipersonality disorder

The symptoms commonly associated with these diagnoses are also intertwined with case variables, and these symptoms may be the reason for a referral. Common symptoms that add to mental health case variables may include:

- Inability to perform from day to day in any capacity or role or to conduct the normal activities of daily living
- Disruptive behavior and agitation
- Immobilizing symptoms
- Emotional states of agitation
- Anxiety and panic reactions
- Impulsive or overaggressive behavior
- Impaired sense of reality caused by hallucinations, delusions, or paranoia

- Severe, incapacitating depressive episodes that leave the patient nonfunctional or suicidal
- Self-destructive behavior
- Homicidal tendencies
- Inability to interact with others
- Defiant behavior
- Explosive behavior

Mental Health Care Professionals and Programs

Treatment of the symptoms or diagnoses is provided by any combination of providers and programs. Typically, the healthcare professionals, programs, and services associated with mental healthcare include:

- Psychiatrists
- Psychologists
- Psychiatric nurses
- Social workers
- Marriage and family counselors
- Certified chemical dependency counselors
- Acute inpatient psychiatric facilities
- Long-term state facilities
- Partial hospitalization programs
- Residential treatment centers (adolescent and children)
- Outpatient programs
- Individual counseling and psychotherapy services
- Group psychotherapy
- Family therapy
- Pharmacologic therapy
- Psychoanalysis
- Diagnostic evaluation and testing
- Home health agency care
- Substance abuse programs, inpatient and outpatient
- Medication management programs

Some mental health and substance abuse programs are designed to treat both adults and children. However, in most cases, child and adult services and programs are provided by separate professional entities. Therefore, case managers must be knowledgeable about all treatment modalities, levels of care, and the types of patients served by the various programs.

As stated in the later section in this manual on brain-injured patients, "dual diagnoses" often complicate the recovery period. Dual diagnoses in these cases take careful coordination of care if both the medical and psychiatric con-

ditions are to be treated. However, with mental health patients dual psychiatric diagnoses may be a reality. As a result, mental health benefits can swiftly be eroded. Consequently, mental health case managers must often apply for the extra contractual process if the patient is to receive the necessary treatment. In these cases, careful use of benefits coordinated with community resources is also critical. If benefits are coordinated with other resources and there is more than one case manager, development of a joint case management plan is critical if fragmentation, duplication, and gaps in care are to be avoided and access to care maintained.

Communication

As reiterated throughout this manual, communication with any case-managed patient is of critical importance, and this is also true of mental health patients. Certainly, open, honest, and frequent communication should be conducted with the patient, but because of the patient's mental status or perception of reality, this may not always be possible. In such cases, communication is often conducted with the family or conservator instead.

Because diagnoses and related illnesses are closely protected by laws, the case manager must use extreme caution in relaying and conveying information. Also, if the patient has not signed a consent form or if a court-appointed conservator has not been established, communication may be held to a minimum or directed to a specific contact. Inability to communicate information greatly hinders development of the case management plan and establishment of the patient with the necessary resources and treatment modalities.

Case Management Plan

Development of the mental health case management plan differs very little from development of plans for medical cases. Consequently, the same seven steps needed for development and monitoring of a case management plan are followed:

- Assessment and collection of pertinent medical data
- Organization of the data for planning
- Coordination and referral
- Negotiation of discounts or reduced rates when non-network providers are used

- Initial and ongoing counseling and education
- Implementation of plan
- Reassessment and development of plan during periods of crisis or chronicity or throughout the time the case is open to case management

As with any patient under case management, the ultimate goals of mental health case management are to:

- Ensure that care is appropriate.
- Provide care at the appropriate level.
- Ensure that services and providers selected are effective in rendering treatment and that deterioration or rehospitalization is prevented.
- Ensure that care is provided in the most cost-effective environment to obtain optimal cost savings.

Mental health case management uses virtually the same implementation techniques as those used in medical case management, the goals of which are to:

- Help the patient gain access to appropriate resources for diagnosis and treatment.
- Assist the patient and family in obtaining access to community resources that can augment their mental health benefits.
- Monitor the patient's progress and make recommendations for alternate treatment modalities.
- Assist the family in applying for conservatorship, when applicable.
- Advise the family how to gain access to the support they require to cope with the situation.

Because many mental health conditions are chronic, many of these processes will be required sporadically throughout the patient's lifetime. Also, as in medical case management, there is no "cookbook" to follow. Whereas some of the techniques listed above may be required only once, others may be repeated throughout the case. As in medical case management, these processes occur in no sequential order. Nor is there any set number of services or providers that may be involved in the case at any given time.

Families dealing with the mental illness of a parent, spouse, or child react no differently than families dealing with a medical illness in the family. When psychological problems or feelings of being overwhelmed surface or are identified, they must be dealt with and the family linked to support groups or professional counseling. Because of the multiple problems associated with mental illness and the fact that most such conditions are chronic, it is common to see entire families in therapy. Reactions such as the following are common:

- Feelings of frustration with the system.
- Exhaustion due to sleepless nights of worry or fright and fear of the unknown if the patient is abusive or violent.
- Anger over drained financial resources due to lack of reimbursement, benefit limits, or exclusions by the healthcare payor.
- Anger and frustration with the insufficient numbers of agencies or facilities that can adequately manage the patient.
- Anger over why the situation is happening to them.

The key to the success of a mental health case management plan is the level of trust the patient has in his or her case manager. Trust increases the commitment of the patient and family to the final plan. Depending on the severity of the dysfunction, the mental health case manager often assumes the role of advocate to ensure the provision of appropriate care, especially medication management.

Medication Management

It is a well-known fact that a primary culprit in the exacerbation of any illness is the management of medication usage regardless of the patient's condition or the diagnosis. Although management of medications is important for all patients, it is imperative for mental health patients because this is often the thread that keeps these patients out of the more expensive facilities. Medication management not only allows patients better control and use of their mental health benefits, it also decreases the risk that their benefits will be prematurely exhausted by preventing frequent and costly inpatient admissions or treatments.

As most healthcare professionals know, mental health benefits are severely limited by healthcare payors and benefit packages. Until recently, with the passage of the Mental Health Parity Act, many healthcare payors placed day or dollar limits or a yearly or lifetime maximum on benefits; others exclude specific diagnostic categories such as learning disorders, eating disorders, attention deficit hyperactivity disorder (ADDH), and autism from benefit coverage. Other healthcare payors simply limit coverage to inpatient care and offer minimal coverage for outpatient benefits or treatments, while still others limit care to a select panel of providers or professionals. Under the new Mental Health Parity Act dollar limits can no longer occur and mental health inpatient care must be comparable to any medical benefits allowed by the healthcare payor.

Alternate Funding and Community Resources

Due to the chronicity associated with mental illness, case managers must work closely with the patient and family or conservator to make sure that they apply for any alternate funding programs to which the patient may be entitled. These programs include:

- Supplemental Security Income (SSI)
- Medicaid
- Social Security Disability Insurance (SSDI) and Medicare
- General assistance (GA) and food stamps if the patient is unemployed
- State unemployment or disability income (SDI), if applicable
- Special Education if the patient is 21 years of age or younger and is still enrolled in school
- Title V Children's Medical Services program (some states offer assistance with treatment for mental illness)
- State agency responsible for providing services for developmental disabilities
- State agency responsible for mental health services

To ensure that the mental health case management and physician's treatment plan is complete and that the patient receives the maximum benefits allowable, linkage with community resources may be necessary. Such agencies can be used to augment healthcare benefits that are limited or exhausted. Agencies that case managers may want to explore when they are developing mental health case management plans include:

- Crisis intervention programs
- Abuse and domestic violence programs
- Infant and foster care shelter programs
- Family service agencies
- Ethnic, church, or other support groups or other community service agencies
- State and county departments of mental health
- County department of social services
- Volunteers of America, Salvation Army, and similar programs
- Veterans Administration programs (for veterans only)

Typical Providers

ACUTE CARE PSYCHIATRIC HOSPITALS

Like medical and geriatric patients, not all mentally ill patients require inpatient care, and patients should be placed in the least restrictive environment possible consistent with their care and safety. However, patients showing acute symptoms or who are suicidal may require admission to an acute care psychiatric hospital.

Acute care psychiatric admissions provide a multidisciplinary approach that allows daily visits by a psychiatrist and skilled nursing care and observation. Inpatient admissions also allow the entire multidisciplinary team to conduct assessments and implement therapy designed to stabilize the acutely ill patient. Depending on the patient's diagnosis, an inpatient program offers one-on-one intervention or constant observation, seclusion, or restraints; pharmacotherapy and skilled observation of responses to drugs and other treatments; skilled interventions including any other tests or therapy necessary, including electroshock therapy (ECT); and any combination of individual, group, or family psychotherapy sessions as deemed necessary.

PARTIAL HOSPITAL PROGRAMS

During the past decade, partial hospitalization programs have surfaced as a cost-effective alternative to inpatient care. In a partial hospital program the patient is exposed to the same multidisciplinary team and provided with all the services normally associated with inpatient care. However, these patients are allowed to return home in the evenings and on weekends to maintain some normalcy in their lives. In addition to decreasing costs, these programs have helped to decrease the stigma associated with mental illness. Thus, they have allowed patients to maintain more intact relationships with peers, family, and coworkers. More important, these programs increase self-esteem because the patient can continue to work.

Many healthcare payors use the partial program in place of inpatient care, thus extending the mental health benefits they provide. In these situations, one inpatient day is frequently exchanged for two partial days of treatment. Partial programs vary from half-day to full-day programs, and this often includes evening and weekend programs as well.

Partial programs are important for patients who require a step-down unit because they allow such people to bridge the transition from hospital to home in incremental moves. Additionally, the programs are useful for persons who require continued care and consistent support to maintain the clinical stability they achieved while in the acute care setting. They are also useful for people who are unable to maintain stability even when receiving other types of outpatient services.

RESIDENTIAL TREATMENT CENTERS

Residential treatment centers (RTCs) provide 24-hour care for adolescents or children who have a psychiatric illness that is too severe to be effectively treated in a less restrictive level of care. They are also intended for any child who cannot be treated at home within the family unit even with the help offered by other outpatient services. Patients entering a residential treatment center must be medically and psychiatrically stable and capable of participating in the program. To remain in the program, the patient must show clinical improvement, and the family must actively participate in the program as well. Such progress allows the patient to be discharged to a less restrictive level of care and eventually reintegrated into the family unit. The therapeutic program offered by residential treatment centers includes at least the following components:

- A multidisciplinary team approach
- Active family involvement
- Twenty-four hour nursing assessments and skilled nursing care
- Individual, group, and family psychotherapy

In addition, some of these programs provide other therapies, prevocational and vocational training, and regular or Special Education classes.

OUTPATIENT PROGRAMS

Outpatient programs are probably the most common mode of therapy used to treat mental illness today. These programs are typically provided in the privacy of the therapist's office. However, some group and family sessions are conducted in outpatient facilities. Outpatient programs are designed to treat both acute and chronic illnesses. They consist of the following treatment modalities in any combination:

- Individual counseling and psychotherapy
- Group psychotherapy
- Family psychotherapy
- Pharmacotherapy
- Diagnostic evaluations and psychological testing
- Home health agency care

HOME HEALTH AGENCY SERVICES

Traditionally, home health agency care has centered on care of medical-surgical patients; mentally ill patients have not had access to this level of care. However, as care has shifted from inpatient to outpatient care, home health services for people with mental illness have evolved. As with any other patient, mental health clients receiving home health agency care must meet the same criteria for "homebound" or "skilled" nursing care for the agency to provide the care and receive reimbursement. Unfortunately, not all home health agencies provide this kind of care. If they do, case managers must ensure that it is provided by licensed personnel who actively practice in the mental health field. Case managers assigned to serving mentally ill patients must familiarize themselves with the home health agencies in their area that provide this service.

STATE HOSPITALS

State hospital placement is rare but is occasionally necessary for patients who are so severely impaired mentally that traditional mental healthcare is of no avail. Although state hospital placement can be voluntary, entrance in most cases occurs through a court order and the conservatorship process. Because of the complex requirements for state placement, all case managers working with mental health patients must be very familiar with their state's laws and the requirements for entrance to such hospitals.

State hospital care is rarely reimbursed by healthcare payors because most patients require custodial care. Also, by the time state hospital placement occurs, any mental health benefits that were available have been exhausted. Therefore, the most common source of payment for state hospital care is Medicaid.

Substance Abuse Programs

When treatment for substance abuse or chemical dependency is desired or recommended, benefits are often payable only under the mental health benefit structure. This is unfortunate because many healthcare payors thus use stringent guidelines for the type and length of program they will approve. Similarly, as with other mental health benefits offered, many apply the same stringent day, dollar, or lifetime limits to the chemical dependency or substance abuse programs they offer. Some healthcare payors offer "substance abuse programs" that cover nothing more than a 3-day detoxification regimen; the case manager must then assist patients who want treatment to gain access to free services in the community, or the patient must assume the costs of such treatment himself. Nevertheless, if treatment is allowed, the programs offered can be divided into the following categories:

- Detoxification programs (both inpatient and outpatient)
- Inpatient rehabilitation programs
- Structured outpatient programs
- Day treatment programs
- Individual or group outpatient programs

In most cases, chemical dependency programs are offered in an outpatient setting. The actual treatment given depends on many factors relating to the patient's chemical dependency and the characteristics displayed by the patient. Chemically dependent patients typically:

- Have used the substance over a prolonged period of time.
- Frequently are high or intoxicated and are unable to fulfill their obligations and duties.
- Have a marked tolerance for the drug or substance and show characteristic withdrawal symptoms when the substance is stopped or reduced.
- Show manipulative or abusive behavior that seriously impairs their social, family, occupational, and educational function.

Inpatient admissions for a substance abuse patient, if necessary, frequently result from:

- An unstable medical condition that was exacerbated by or resulted from the substance abuse behavior, withdrawal, or impending withdrawal.
- An unstable psychiatric condition that places the patient at risk of injury to himself or others.

- A life-threatening episode that resulted from drug or alcohol intoxication and overdose.

When admitted as an inpatient, the substance abuse patient remains hospitalized until he or she is medically stable and the substance abuse problem can be managed at a lower level of care such as a day treatment program. Most chemical dependency programs last for 4 weeks, and often the actual treatment program can be a combination of inpatient and outpatient care. Both inpatient and outpatient programs offer a multidisciplinary team approach, the team being composed of mental health professionals who specialize in chemical dependency.

Day and evening treatment programs are designed to serve patients who cannot maintain abstinence during the transition phase back to the community. These programs allow the person to continue to work while he or she receives treatment after the normal work day. In a day program, the patient receives treatment during the day hours and returns home at night. These programs are like partial programs only the focus is on substance abuse. The primary difference between the two programs is the time spent (per day or week) in the program.

Regardless of the setting, chemical dependency programs offer the following minimum components:

- Individualized treatment planning
- Assessments of patient's psychological, physiological, and psychosocial function
- Substance abuse counseling
- Skilled nursing care (but not in the social model)
- Weekly individual, group, or family psychotherapy sessions
- Treatment planning for aftercare and arrangements for such services as half-way houses, group homes, or other community support services that help the patient remain sober
- Relapse prevention planning
- Active participation in Alcoholics or Narcotics Anonymous programs

Programs designed for children have the same components but also include psychoeducation classes.

✂ SUMMARY

This section offers a brief overview of some of the many programs available for mental health care if the patient's individual healthcare benefit package offers mental health coverage. Unfortunately, mental health benefits are often severely limited. This, combined with the fact that many mental health conditions are chronic, means that any healthcare benefits allowed by the healthcare payor are often exhausted quickly. Eventually, many patients fall through the cracks because they have no money for treatments or medications. Thus, case management for this category of patients is necessary if the quality of care is to be maintained and the patient allowed to receive the care he or she requires.

CASE MANAGEMENT OF THE NEUROLOGICALLY IMPAIRED PATIENT

Regardless of the case manager's employer, neurologically impaired patients comprise a large portion of any case management caseload. The most frequently encountered neurologic impairments can be divided into four groups: high-risk neurologic conditions (e.g., stroke), Alzheimer's disease, acquired or traumatic brain injury, and spinal cord injuries. Neurologic conditions that come to mind first are spinal cord injury and traumatic brain injury. However, case management is not limited to these diagnoses. Any patient who has a significant neurologic impairment that affects his or her quality of life, influences the healthcare organization's costs, or requires coordination with community resources and alternate funding programs must be evaluated for case management.

The extent and type of case management offered by an organization affects the case manager's level of involvement with the patient. For example, if the case manager is from a facility, he or she may be involved only while the patient is hospitalized, whereas the non-facility-based case manager may remain involved indefinitely. As has been stated previously, regardless of which organization employs the case manager, if more than one case manager is involved in a case, all must work together cohesively if goals are to be reached, resources readied for discharge or the next level of care, costs contained, and the quality of care maintained.

General Neurologic Conditions

CASE PLANNING

If the case manager is other than a facility-based case manager, he or she must make every effort to become an integral part of the neurology or rehabilitation team as soon as possible. This is necessary to become knowledgeable about all case details because this case manager may be the one who will be involved with the patient over the long term.

From a clinical standpoint, early involvement allows the case manager to know first-hand when the patient is ready for transfer, to make recommendations if the patient requires a more specialized level of care, and to arrange approval for the next level of care when the patient demonstrates readiness for it. Early intervention allows the case manager, when applicable, to act as an advocate for the family, assist them with questions and answers, keep them informed about the patient's condition, and request their input into the case management plan.

Throughout the patient's hospital stay, the team, through their treatment plan, will be identifying and defining the patient's cognitive, psychosocial, physical, and medical needs, including short- and long-term goals, much of which must be included in the data collected for the final case management plan. It is much better for the case manager to obtain this information first-hand, since the final case management plan is based on the patient's pre-injury history as well as the recommendations of the treating team and the physician's orders.

TYPICAL NEUROLOGIC DIAGNOSES

Case management flags for neurologic diagnoses vary with the organization, and the following list is only an example; however, these diseases indicate the types of conditions that should be evaluated for their case management potential:

- Anoxic brain damage
- Neurologic congenital anomaly
- Cerebral palsy
- Amyotrophic lateral sclerosis
- Spinal cord and brain neoplasm
- Spinal cord or traumatic brain injury
- Cerebral vascular accident
- Muscular dystrophy
- Multiple sclerosis
- Severe parkinsonian disorder
- Chorea
- Dystonia
- Alzheimer's disease
- Guillain-Barré syndrome
- Myasthenia gravis

- Duchenne's dystrophy
- Aneurysms

Each of these neurologic disorders has its own set of symptoms, related remedies, treatment modalities, and case variables. What might be right for one disorder may not work for another. Although many neurologic disorders can start with mild symptoms and never become any worse, others may become progressively worse. Others are severe from the outset.

Many patients with mild symptoms may not be candidates for case management, especially if the treatment course is progressing as anticipated. However, they should be assessed anyway. Often these patients and their families may not require any services, but others may need information about community resources, dietary counseling, and other health-related classes pertinent to their disorder.

In contrast, patients with severe symptoms or those in the end stages of disease must be assessed for possible case management because many of them have multiple skilled nursing needs. Although many patients can be sent home, others may benefit from either a short-term inpatient or an outpatient rehabilitation program. Many of these patients will require some form of "rehabilitation" on an ongoing daily basis over an extended period of time. The key to encouraging patients to reach their maximum level of functional independence is to refer them to therapy and a rehabilitation program as soon as possible.

REHABILITATION

Although rehabilitation is discussed in more detail in the section on rehabilitation in Chapter 11, it merits a separate section here as well because it is a vital component of successful treatment and renewed quality of life in all neurologically damaged patients. Every patient with a neurologic illness or injury must be afforded the opportunity for rehabilitation, and the initial assessments must be done as early as possible.

In most cases, the rehabilitation team assesses the patient within 72 hours of the occurrence of neurologic trauma or brain injury or the reason for admission. Despite the fact that the patient may be in the intensive care unit, formal rehabilitation and assessment must be started as soon as possible. However, for formal rehabilitation to be effective, the patient must be medically and surgically stable and able to

benefit from a bedside program. Even patients in coma must be started on a formal rehabilitation program, which consists of splinting, bed positioning, and progressive stimulation. Therefore, in all patients with a neurologic illness or injury, at least the following areas are assessed:

- Bed positioning
- Range of motion
- Splinting
- Skin care
- Bowel and bladder management
- Nutrition management
- Respiratory management (often the most important problem for patients in coma)

As in all cases involving rehabilitation, the most appropriate indicators of progress are the patient's functional abilities. Some tools that are widely used to measure these abilities include the disability rating scale, the functional assessment measure, the functional independence measure, the Rancho Los Amigos cognitive functioning scale, and the Glasgow coma-outcome scale. These assessment tools assist the treating team in determining the type of rehabilitation services the patient requires. For instance, patients who have reached a level VI or VII on the Rancho Los Amigos scale are considered cognitively capable of discharge and ready for an outpatient or post-acute care program.

For patients with other neurologic disorders, the key to discharge is the patient's capacity to participate in rehabilitation. This ability is frequently measured not only in the scope and depth of their functional abilities and deficits but also in their ability to tolerate a minimum of 3 hours of therapy per day.

Rehabilitation is best accomplished by a multidisciplinary team directed by a physician who specializes in physical medicine and rehabilitation. This physician is referred to as a physiatrist. The acute rehabilitation multidisciplinary team often comprises professionals from the following healthcare disciplines:

- Nursing
- Nutrition
- Occupational therapy
- Speech pathology
- Physical therapy
- Discharge planning or facility-based case management
- Pharmacy
- Recreational therapy
- Social work

- Specialist in durable medical equipment or prosthetic specialist
- Other appropriate specialists (e.g., cognitive retrainer, vocational rehabilitation specialist)

Although the patient with a neurologic disorder may have had a "rehabilitation" assessment shortly after he or she was admitted, another extensive evaluation is usually performed by the rehabilitation team before the patient is admitted to the acute rehabilitation unit. This evaluation consists of assessment for cognitive, physical, behavioral, and psychosocial functional levels. Based on this evaluation, an interdisciplinary treatment plan is developed that encompasses all aspects of the patient's physical, functional, psychological, and cognitive care. This plan includes at minimum the following elements:

- Medical, physical, and nursing management
- Nutritional management
- Rehabilitation therapy modalities
- Neuropsychological management
- Psychosocial counseling
- Educational plan
- Vocational rehabilitation plan

Family members must be encouraged to participate actively at all levels in the rehabilitation program. They can participate in actual therapy sessions and case conferences, and they can ask specific questions of the rehabilitation team.

Once the patient is moved to the rehabilitation unit, continued progress in such things as activities of daily living, cognition, social and vocational skills, and functional abilities must be documented by the rehabilitation team. This charted documentation assists the case manager in making recommendations or arrangements for the most appropriate post-acute care rehabilitation program at discharge.

Length of stay in the acute rehabilitation unit varies greatly and depends on the patient's medical needs and rehabilitation potential. Generally speaking, the length of stay varies from several weeks to several months, and therefore close communication between the rehabilitation team and the healthcare payor's case manager is absolutely critical. Such communication is necessary to ensure that premature denials of coverage are not issued, and benefit coverage continues until the patient is ready for discharge to the next level of care.

If the patient is to be discharged to his or her home, a weekend pass is often ordered before discharge. This "pass" allows the patient and the team an opportunity to test the skills learned and identify further areas that require correction before final discharge is ordered. Passes are useful in preparing the patient for reentry to the community, and in some cases more than one pass may be required before the patient is deemed ready for final discharge. Unfortunately, not all healthcare payors recognize these passes as medically necessary, nor will they reimburse the rehabilitation facility during the patient's absence. In these cases, the family must pay the facility privately if the case manager cannot convince the healthcare payor to reimburse or cover this event.

EXTENDING COVERAGE

The patient's readiness for discharge is gauged by evaluation of the following points in case conferences or therapy or chart reviews: (1) the patient is making progress; (2) the patient has not yet reached his or her maximum functional potential as outlined in the original goals; (3) the patient is learning a home therapy program, if applicable; and (4) there are other skilled or custodial needs that require case planning attention.

The patient must be motivated to participate in therapy, whether it is physical therapy, occupational therapy, or speech therapy. This fact is evident by the patient's cooperation with the exercises themselves, and, after discharge, by compliance with appointments or involvement in a home therapy program.

Many patients, despite the fact that they remain in a severely impaired state, may be classified as chronic or custodial. This classification is the hardest for patients and families to accept because it often means that the healthcare payor will exclude benefits or terminate coverage. Even when the patient is so classified, it is critical for all his or her needs to be evaluated and plans made to provide all the physical care required; any training required by the caregiver should be addressed as well, and resources must be identified in the case management plan.

POST-ACUTE CARE COSTS

Many patients with a neurologic illness or injury who are not candidates for an acute rehabilitation unit may be candidates for admission to a subacute care facility. Here they can continue to receive therapy while their other skilled care needs are met. Costs of subacute care vary significantly. However, if a contracted or negotiated rate is possible, the final costs can amount to an average of approximately $500 to $700 per day. In contrast, costs at a skilled nursing facility are less than half this amount, and consequently, many healthcare payors tend to consider this the least costly alternative. As stated elsewhere in this manual, quality of care and benefit outcomes should be the driving force behind case management alternatives when it comes to choosing levels of care, not costs.

The lengths of stay in both skilled nursing facilities and subacute care facilities vary. For instance, most patients in a subacute or extended care facility are admitted for short-term care until they show readiness for discharge to a skilled nursing facility or home. In contrast, some patients with severe neurologic impairments require placement in a skilled nursing facility for long-term or lifelong care.

ALTERNATE FUNDING

Although it is common to associate neurologic disorders with older patients, and one automatically thinks of stroke and brain tumors, this is not always true. Many patients with the severest neurologic disorders are children. These families should be encouraged to apply for any program benefits allowed by the local school district and its Special Education program, the local Title V Children's Medical Services program, and the state agency responsible for providing services to the developmentally disabled.

Other important alternate funding programs that may be worth exploring for all patients (including children) are Medicaid, SSI, and SSDI. Some important provisions of these three programs are as follows:

1. If the patient is eligible for Medicaid, Medicaid coverage starts immediately, and this coverage can assist with out-of-pocket medical expenses. Keep in mind that Medicaid is always a secondary payor even when healthcare benefits are limited.
2. Patients eligible for Supplemental Security Income (SSI) are also eligible for Medicaid. In addition to income, therefore, persons in this category have some healthcare coverage through the Medicaid program. In some instances, SSI recipients may also be eligible for homemaker-type services or chore-worker services. However, this benefit varies from state to state and from county to county.

3. Persons eligible for Social Security Disability Insurance (SSDI) are entitled to monthly Social Security checks. If the person remains on SSDI for 24 months, he or she automatically receives Medicare Part A insurance and has the option to enroll in Medicare Part B. Every effort should be made to encourage patients to enroll in Part B because this portion covers physicians' charges and outpatient care. Also, many healthcare payors require the patient to have Part B to be entitled to healthcare payor benefits.

Many persons qualify for all programs. Unfortunately, it is the person with low income or limited assets who often falls into the "gray" area when it comes to eligibility for Title V Children's Medical Services or Medicaid. Such patients often have too little to pay for the necessary services yet too many assets (primarily income) to qualify. If in doubt, the case manager should make the referral and let the experts at the various agencies determine the patient's eligibility.

Any patient with a spinal cord injury or severe neurologic impairment who has the potential and motivation to seek gainful employment should be encouraged to work with the rehabilitation team's vocational specialist or the state Department of Vocational Rehabilitation. Such cooperative effort is necessary for admission into a training program or sheltered workshop where the person can be retrained for possible employment if unable to resume his or her previous occupation.

As with all patients in case management, all insurance policies must be explored (e.g., motor vehicle insurance and other healthcare insurance policies) to determine the possibility of coordination of benefits. This is especially true if the neurologic injury was the result of an automobile accident or if it happened on another person's property. All third-party liability (TPL) cases (and this includes victims of violent crimes) must be explored to determine the ability of the third party to assume all or part of the costs. Additionally, patients and families must be encouraged to explore all benefits payable from unemployment and disability income plans, workers' compensation benefits, or any other possible source for income or healthcare coverage.

TYPICAL POST-ACUTE CARE SERVICES

Many patients with a neurologic illness or injury have a variety of physical and mental needs. Families or caregivers must be taught all aspects of their care if the patient is to be discharged home. Depending on the level of care and the intensity or severity of the condition, arrangements must be made for respite care and support groups for the patient and his or her immediate caregivers.

Skilled Nursing Facility Rehabilitation

Although most patients suffering from neurologic disorders can be cared for at home, a small percentage of patients with very severe impairments require placement. Most often such patients are placed in skilled nursing facilities owing to the severity of the disorder and the level of care required. Unfortunately, in many instances, such patients may have to be placed for the long term. Long-term skilled nursing facility placement is not a benefit provided by most healthcare payors. Thus, either families pay privately or care is reimbursed by Medicaid. Sadder still, many children with very severe conditions have to be institutionalized in state hospitals because there are few resources available to handle long-term placement of severely disturbed children.

If reimbursement for care in a skilled nursing facility is to occur, the facility must have the capacity to administer and continue any therapy or "rehabilitation" that was started prior to admission. This is the key factor regardless of whether the patient is discharged to a skilled nursing facility or a subacute care facility. It is even more important when the goal is to move the patient eventually to an acute rehabilitation unit or home.

Unfortunately, not all skilled nursing facilities offer a full range of rehabilitation therapies or the interdisciplinary composition of the rehabilitation team. Commonly, the skilled nursing facility's therapy program depends on its commitment to rehabilitation and how therapists are employed. For instance, while one facility may directly employ licensed therapists and offer therapy at least twice daily, another facility may contract for therapy services. In this facility, therapy is provided once daily, or, in some cases, the duty may be delegated to a therapy aide when the "therapy program" is developed by the therapist.

It is therefore necessary to do research and evaluate which facilities have the appropriate capabilities to manage the needs of neurologically impaired patients; then the patients' progress must be monitored to ensure that the goals are met. For patients placed in a skilled nursing facility in anticipation of a move to a rehabilitation unit at a later date, monitoring is essential to be sure that progress is being made at the expected rate. If it is not, and the therapy is found to be less intense than that promised by the facility's admission personnel, a move to another skilled nursing facility may be necessary. If such a situation should occur, the case manager must be prepared to initiate the necessary changes while informing and educating the patient and family of the reasons.

Home Care

For patients with neurologic impairments who are discharged home but still need continued rehabilitation from an outpatient facility, the case manager must make every effort to find outpatient rehabilitation facilities in which the program is staffed by a multidisciplinary rehabilitation team. In most cases, these units are associated with acute rehabilitation hospitals. These treatments are scheduled daily or intermittently and concentrate on continued cognitive or physical rehabilitation. Costs for outpatient therapy vary. Unless an all-inclusive rate can be agreed on, average costs range from $100 to $175 per hour per therapy session or professional discipline.

Occasionally the neurologically impaired patient is discharged home but requires some variation of skilled nursing care. If this happens, the family must be taught all aspects of the required care. Like therapy, the costs for home care vary, and without an all-inclusive rate, most home health agency visits range from $100 to $150 per visit. If hourly skilled nursing care is required, costs may average $100 per hour.

Equipment and Supplies

Possibly the greatest need of patients with a neurologic disorder is equipment, and in many instances, this equipment must be specialized and fitted specifically to the patient's body size, posture, and deformity. In addition, seating pads and pressure point pads are not a luxury, they are essential; the costs are minimal compared to the costs that can occur if complications, especially decubitus ulcers, develop.

Many neurologically impaired patients, especially those with spinal cord injuries, are confined to a wheelchair. Wheelchairs can vary from fully electric ones operated by breath-activated devices to extremely lightweight models. Because of the cost of wheelchairs (e.g.,

$500 for a standard wheelchair to $25,000 for a fully electric model), many healthcare payors (with the exception of workers' compensation) limit coverage to the most utilitarian model suitable for the condition and exclude deluxe models. If the patient or family insists on a deluxe model, they may be required to pay any difference in cost between the amount reimbursed for the utilitarian model and the actual cost of the model ordered.

Occasionally, some patients require two wheelchairs, or what may be classified by the healthcare payor as a "duplicate purpose" item. In addition, children require frequent changes in their chair or seating systems or even a new chair as they grow. Two good examples of the need for dual purpose items may be cited: (1) For independence at school a young child may require an electric wheelchair, whereas at home, because of the presence of carpet and other internal or exterior barriers, a manual wheelchair is required. (2) A patient may be able to ambulate only a very short distance, for which some type of mobility device is required, such as a walker; however, owing to limited strength and endurance, the patient may also require a wheelchair for most of his or her mobility needs.

Equipment needs and related supplies vary greatly from patient to patient. However, neurologically impaired patients commonly require such items as:

- Stationary and portable
  - Suction devices
  - Oxygen devices
  - Ventilators
  - Infusion devices for intravenous therapies, parenteral nutrition, or feeding formulas
- Batteries and battery-charging units
- Urinary supplies
- Semi-electric hospital beds or special beds (e.g., air-fluidized beds, body float mattresses)
- Commodes or raised toilet seats, toilet rails
- Shower benches, shower or bath hand-held devices or long-handled devices and shower rails
- Multiple assistive and adaptive devices that allow self-care and feeding
- Braces, splints, casts, and hand or wrist orthotics
- Lap trays
- Seating and positioning systems
- Special wheelchair control devices
- Special tires for the wheelchair
- Grab bars, trapezes (free-standing or attached to the bed)

- Patient hydraulic lift systems
- Slide boards
- Orthotics for proper support or positioning of limbs
- Abdominal binders
- Specialized seating pads

Equipment and services that are often excluded from benefit coverage by many healthcare payors (the only exception being workers' compensation) include:

- Communication devices
- Environmental control devices
- Ramps and home modifications or structural or electrical corrections
- Specialized vans and modifications to motor vehicles (e.g., hand controls, wheelchair lifts)

When equipment or necessary modifications are excluded or not allowed even through use of the extra contractual process, the case manager may wish to explore with the family the feasibility of obtaining assistance from a fraternal organization (e.g., Lions, Shriners, Elks). These organizations hold fund raisers that may assist with the financial costs of medical services or items that are excluded or limited. Similarly, these organizations are wonderful sources of volunteers who can help with the labor costs associated with building ramps and correcting structural or environmental barriers.

Anticipated Teaching

Educational needs required to meet the needs of neurologically impaired persons depend on the intensity and severity of the condition and the intensity and complexity of the care. In all cases, all aspects of skilled care must be mastered by the patient, family, or caregiver before the patient is discharged from either the hospital or the home health agency. Key areas requiring teaching include, at minimum:

- Suctioning and airway maintenance
- Proper positioning and skin care to prevent skin breakdown and contractures
- Proper bowel and bladder care, including removal of fecal impactions, enema administration, and catheterizations, when applicable
- Proper transfer techniques or body mechanics for both the caregiver and the patient
- Proper range of motion exercises
- Proper feeding techniques
- Medications—administration, side effects, contraindications
- Pain control
- Proper use and care of all equipment

COMMUNITY RESOURCES

Community resources vary depending on the actual disease or neurologic disorder and the patient's age. However, the most frequently used community resources for patients with neurologic impairments are:

- Easter Seals Society
- Disease-specific organizations (e.g., American Heart Association [stroke patients], Muscular Dystrophy Association, and Brain Injury Association)
- Handicapped transportation services
- Emergency response systems
- Congregate or home-delivered meal programs
- Friendly visitor programs or volunteer telephone reassurance programs
- Providers of portable radiologic and laboratory services, if patient is homebound
- Independent living centers or assistive device centers
- Adult day health or adult day centers
- Church, ethnic, or other social service agencies for volunteers, transportation

BARRIERS TO DISCHARGE AND ACCESS TO CARE

Barriers to discharge and access to care for the neurologically impaired patient are common because many of these patients require total care, yet the care required is custodial. Consequently, two of the most persistent barriers are inadequate funds to meet the long-term needs of the patient and the unavailability of a caregiver. Barriers vary from patient to patient, but among the most common are the following:

- Unavailability of agencies or caregivers that can provide the necessary care and support.
- Unavailability of durable medical equipment companies that can provide the equipment.
- Delays in ordering specialized equipment, causing delays in patient discharge.
- Absence of local parent and peer support groups.
- Lack of coordination between agencies, with subsequent fragmentation of care.
- Insufficient transportation to and from outpatient facilities and treatment facilities.
- Insufficient numbers of professionals trained in pediatric neurologic care or other skilled care.
- Inadequate numbers of care facilities that can accept a total care patient, a patient with Alzheimer's disease, or a child with a severe neurologic handicap.

- Backlogs in public entitlement programs or delays in the application process if the patient needs a conservator.
- Inadequate home conditions (e.g., lack of heat, water, or cleanliness or presence of structural barriers).
- Abusive home situations.
- Unavailability of respite care for caregiver relief.

Alzheimer's Disease

The end stage of Alzheimer's disease presents its own challenges, especially when it comes to care and placement. Referral for case management may come at any stage of the disease; however, for case management to be most effective, patients should be referred as early in the disease process as possible.

It is in these early stages that families can be advised about resources and a plan can be devised that can serve as a guide as the disease progresses and more services are required. This early intervention also allows the family to make financial plans and to research resources for care, respite, or the psychological support that may be required as the disease progresses. As is true of resources for neurologically impaired children, resources for the Alzheimer's disease patient are sorely inadequate (especially facilities for care and respite care). In addition, many Alzheimer's disease patients need custodial care, which is not reimbursable by the healthcare payor. Thus, funding and the costs of care are a real issue. As a rule, many of these patients require placement, but because care consists of custodial care and supervision in a protective (often locked) facility, reimbursement from the healthcare payor is excluded from coverage. Reimbursement for care must then be sought from private funds or from Medicaid. Case managers working with Alzheimer's disease patients should encourage the family to explore pertinent community resources in addition to Medicaid and Supplemental Security Income (SSI).

If difficulties in placement are encountered, it is usually because of lengthy waiting lists and inability to qualify for alternate funding such as Medicaid. If a facility is found, it may be out of the area, causing hardship on the family, especially the elderly spouse. Like location of a facility, respite care is just as difficult to find; often it is either unavailable or, if available, the spouse lacks the financial resources to pay for it. Unfortunately, these factors are the major reasons for caregiver burnout. Thus, case management is just as important during the end stages as it is at the time of diagnosis because the caregiver may be as much or more in need of help as the patient. It is during the end stages of the disease that a case manager may be able or required to help the family in gaining access to appropriate resources.

Acquired Brain Injury or Traumatic Brain Injury

Healthcare journals validate the fact that advances in emergency care and acute medical-surgical treatment modalities are increasing the numbers of "survivors" of acquired brain injury (ABI) or traumatic brain injury (TBI). Brain injuries now represent a significant portion of healthcare expenditures by private healthcare payors and alternate funding programs (e.g., Medicaid) as well as out-of-pocket expenses by patients. Not only are the costs of treatment significant, brain injury is also an area of explosive growth in terms of:

- The quality of life endured by many "survivors" and their families
- Patient numbers
- The variety of treatment modalities and services (both inpatient and outpatient)
- Healthcare dollar spending

The segment of the population most affected by brain injuries is the young, who for the most part were relatively healthy before the accident. When this young age is combined with the advances in technology taking place in medicine and healthcare, the result is an increased number of survivors. Although most traumatic brain injuries are associated with motor vehicle accidents, they can result from any trauma to the brain, such as gunshot wounds, sports injuries, falls, child abuse (e.g., shaken baby syndrome), assaults, and so forth.

Not only is the care of brain-injured patients costly in terms of the actual money spent for care, the quality-of-life "costs" for the patient and the family cannot be calculated; many "survivors" are left with significant cognitive, motor, sensory, social, and vocational deficits as well as a so-called decreased quality of life.

The brunt of these costs must be assumed by the patient's family or the taxpayers because many healthcare payors, with the exception of workers' compensation, exclude or severely limit the amounts they pay for rehabilitation benefits. Many more exclude post-acute care rehabilitation programs for patients with brain trauma because these programs, which focus on "education" and retraining, frequently do not fit the typical "medical" model.

Although many of the costs associated with acute care are paid by healthcare payors, in children and young adults with brain trauma or brain damage referrals must be made to the local Title V Children's Medical Services program, the state agency responsible for providing developmentally disabled services, and the Department of Education as soon as these children are identified. These referrals for potential assistance are necessary to ensure that payment for long periods of rehabilitation services continues without disruption. For adults, referrals to alternate funding programs such as Medicaid should be encouraged as soon as financial needs are identified. Unfortunately, Medicaid has limited or nonexistent coverage for acute care rehabilitation services. Thus, because many patients have long-term needs, the family must be trained in as many aspects of therapy and treatment disciplines as possible to ensure the goals for the patient can be reached even when funding is limited or nonexistent.

INITIAL TREATMENT

As in all trauma cases, trained emergency personnel treat and maintain life support, if necessary, for the brain-injured person while they are en route to the emergency room. The more severely brain injured patients are taken directly to a regional trauma center if one is available. If such a center is not available, the patient must be taken to the nearest emergency room and then transferred as soon as he or she has been evaluated and stabilized.

Persons who suffer the least severe brain injuries often are discharged directly from the emergency room after evaluation. In contrast, moderately to severely injured patients are admitted, generally to an intensive care unit. These patients often have also sustained other traumatic injuries. These injuries include, for example, trauma to the internal organs, fractures, facial injuries, lacerations, nerve damage, or spinal cord injury, all of which further complicate the situation. Consequently, any trauma patient, especially one with a severe head injury, should be admitted or transferred to a regional trauma center as soon as possible.

Most trauma centers have the capability to

perform a thorough evaluation, which consists of consultations with specialists from neurology, neurosurgery, orthopedics, cardiology, dentistry, plastic surgery and other appropriate disciplines. Of prime importance is the trauma center's radiologic and diagnostic expertise, not to mention its capabilities in surgery, intracranial pressure monitoring, neurologic intensive care, and physical rehabilitation medicine.

Ideally, any brain trauma patient should be referred to case management as soon as possible after the injury. One of the primary purposes of case management during these early stages is to ensure that the patient is at the most appropriate level of care. If the patient is not at the appropriate level, he or she must be so identified and moved as soon as medically feasible. Most patients with traumatic brain injuries or acquired brain injuries are sent to an acute care rehabilitation unit when: (1) they are medically and surgically stable, and (2) they can benefit cognitively (generally when at level IV on the Rancho Los Amigos scale) from an intense rehabilitation program.

COGNITIVE THERAPY

Cognitive therapy is an essential component of effective brain injury rehabilitation. This therapy involves improving the patient's memory, judgment, and ability to concentrate. It also involves retraining in the ability to perform the simple tasks we all take for granted such as safety awareness, balancing a checkbook, buying groceries, riding a bike, driving, and so forth.

Unfortunately, cognitive therapy is not always covered by all healthcare payors (the prime exception being workers' compensation). Although cognitive therapy may be covered if it is part of the entire rehabilitation process, in other instances it may not be reimbursed if it is a "stand alone" therapy. Consequently, the healthcare payor's case manager is an invaluable member of the team. He or she can state whether cognitive therapy is a benefit and can alert the team if it is not; similarly, he or she can say whether the extra contractual process can be used for the coverage required. This sharing of information is critical for planning. Collaboration also allows time for case managers to locate alternative resources if reimbursement is not allowed.

ADMISSION CRITERIA FOR REHABILITATION

Although the normal standard for admission into an acute physical medicine and rehabilita-

tion program is 3 hours of therapy per day, 5 days a week, many brain-injured patients, including stroke patients and those with any other neurovascular disorder causing brain damage, may not be medically or cognitively ready for therapy at this level of intensity. Although some patients are able to meet the criterion of 3 hours of therapy, others are only stable enough to benefit from two to three 15- to 30-minute sessions per day.

The more severely brain injured patients are generally transferred to an acute rehabilitation program, whereas those in coma or those who are cognitively not ready for an acute program may be transferred to a facility-based subacute care facility or a skilled nursing facility where they can continue to receive the appropriate treatments. Here again, depending on the patient's healthcare coverage for rehabilitation, some patients have coverage, and others do not.

Patients whose rehabilitation treatments are covered by a healthcare payor must, in most cases, continue to demonstrate progress; this classifies them as receiving "skilled" care. If progress is not made, coverage by the healthcare payor terminates because they are then reclassified as receiving "custodial" care. In these cases, if the patient cannot be discharged, the family must pay privately for the care or seek eligibility for Medicaid.

Inadequate coverage threatens the successful accomplishment of the goals established by the team. As a result, the family must be taught how to administer the therapy at home to prevent the patient from sliding backward and losing the gains made while enrolled in a formal acute rehabilitation program.

When evaluating a patient for his or her readiness to progress to the next level of care, the patient's overall cognitive abilities must be taken into account. Also, whereas some patients may progress and are able to tolerate each level as they reach it, others may require a trial period of rehabilitation at the new level; sometimes it may be necessary to extend the trial period an additional 3 to 4 weeks or longer to ascertain the appropriateness of the program. This process is necessary because many brain-injured patients make very slow but steady gains, often punctuated by periods of plateaus in which no progress is made. Consequently, their progress in rehabilitation is not as predictable as that of patients with other neurologic disorders.

POST-ACUTE CARE

As stated earlier, while most inpatient acute rehabilitation and outpatient "traditional medical model" rehabilitation programs are usually covered by healthcare payors, many post-acute care rehabilitation programs are not. For this reason, case managers may have to seek approval for (or act as the patient's advocate for) this portion of the rehabilitation program via the extra contractual process. This is especially true if the patient shows potential improvement in functional gains.

Owing to the unpredictability of brain injury and its effects on the patient's progress and recovery, the case manager must work closely with the family, helping them plan realistically (e.g., financially; for learning how to provide the care; for possible role reversal, and so forth) throughout the duration of the case. Families must be prepared for both the emotional and financial consequences associated with placement of the patient in a skilled nursing facility; many such patients will be reclassified as requiring custodial care if they show no change or potential for change in either cognitive or functional abilities.

Services frequently used for brain-injured patients may be provided at home, in an outpatient center, transitional living center, or board and care home. Augmenting these might be services or training provided through Special Education or vocational training programs, supportive employment, sheltered workshops, and day care programs. These services generally fall into the category of "custodial" care or "educational" program and are not covered by most healthcare policies.

Of course, the behavioral, cognitive, and physical deficits of the brain-damaged patient must be the deciding factors in choosing the appropriate level of care and services. However, if financial coverage is not available, other factors must be considered as well; the "best" case management plan can then be developed in light of these new circumstances. This "best" plan may be developed by considering other resources the patient may be presently utilizing, or it might consist merely of a list of resources that the family can research for care options.

Fortunately, the majority of patients with moderate brain injury and good recovery potential are discharged home and continue their therapy using an outpatient program, whether this therapy is administered in an outpatient setting or in the patient's home. Typically, these patients require a combination of skilled rehabilitation services.

For instance, whereas one patient may require continued cognitive therapy along with physical therapy, occupational therapy, and speech therapy, another may require cognitive therapy, continued psychological services, and possibly vocational rehabilitation with no physical, occupational, or speech therapy. Still another patient may need only physical therapy, occupational therapy, or speech therapy. The actual level of services required depends on the nature and severity of the brain injury and the patient's response to the treatments. The scope of services is often dependent on the healthcare payor and the actual coverage of rehabilitation benefits.

For patients with behavioral, memory, or judgment deficits, or those who cannot tolerate the intensity of an acute rehabilitation program, or those who continue to make very slow progress (i.e., due either to complex medical conditions such as a tracheostomy or skin or decubitus care, or to a Rancho Los Amigos rating below level IV), placement in a skilled nursing facility or subacute or extended care facility may be necessary. These patients will remain institutionalized until (1) the complexity of their care needs decreases, (2) they can withstand the intensity of a rehabilitation program, or (3) they reach a plateau and are reclassified as needing custodial care.

Nonmedical Models

For brain-damaged patients discharged to a post-acute care rehabilitation facility, therapy is frequently provided in a "nontraditional and nonmedical model." This level of rehabilitation is frequently described as "transitional living rehabilitation" or as a "community reentry program." Despite the fact that these programs are classified as "nonmedical," they are actually far from being nonmedical.

The primary difference between the medical and nonmedical models is in their licensure. Also, because the emphasis in these nonmedical models is on a "home therapy milieu," these programs are typically located in the community and offered in a home or apartment setting instead of in an institution. Consequently, facilities of this type are frequently licensed by board and care regulations rather than by those used to license facilities.

The programs presented and the staff responsible for providing the therapy are far from nonmedical. Most of these "nonmedical" post-acute care brain injury programs offer a closely supervised and active therapeutic program that operates 5 to 7 days a week. The program emphasizes retraining the individual to a point where he or she reaches a functional level of independence cognitively and behaviorally or is no longer "at risk." Staffing includes:

- Neuropsychologists
- Occupational therapists
- Speech therapists
- Physical therapists (who may or may not be present depending on the physical needs of the patients)
- Program case manager
- Program medical director
- Recreational therapists
- Vocational specialists
- Cognitive trainers
- Nursing personnel
- Other appropriate specialists

Because of the popularity of the post-acute rehabilitation facility as a mode of treatment, it is often possible to negotiate an all-inclusive per diem rate that is favorable to all concerned. These rates and the ability to negotiate vary significantly from program to program. However, if rate negotiation is possible, an average daily or all-inclusive rate of $300 to $700 is often feasible. Average length of stays also varies; however, stays ranging from 3 to 6 months are common, depending on the severity of the patient's brain injury.

Since the level of care for transitional living rehabilitation is not standardized or monitored by state licensure agencies, case managers must monitor patients closely during this phase to ensure that they are making progress and that discharge occurs when appropriate.

TERMINATION OF BENEFITS

Patients with brain damage who are entering transitional living rehabilitation or community reentry programs commonly experience termination of healthcare coverage because many healthcare payors exclude this level of care. Not only is coverage denied for continued care, the extra contractual process is also denied. If this occurs, the case is frequently terminated from case management by the healthcare payor's case manager. When termination of benefits occurs, either the family must assume the role of the case manager or coordination of the patient's case is assumed by the transitional or community reentry team's case manager.

Unfortunately, if insurance benefits are terminated, treatment is often likewise ended because few families can afford the costs of these programs by themselves. The final outcome of the case usually hinges on the financial ability

of the family. If the family can afford to pay privately for this care, treatment can continue; however, if they can't, or if the patient's care is reimbursed by Medicaid, this level of rehabilitation care is probably not covered.

Consequently, many of these patients whose insurance benefits have terminated are vulnerable to "life on the streets" or institutionalization. It is therefore imperative to work closely with the family during all stages of rehabilitation to ensure that the family is trained to assume the care required and that they have applied for or are aware of the alternate funding programs to which the patient may be entitled. Additionally, they must be trained to assume the role of case manager at any given time.

OTHER LEVELS OF CARE AND TRAINING SITES

Once the patient has reached the goals established for the transitional or post-acute care level, he or she may receive services at other levels of care such as:

- Home-based rehabilitation (i.e., patient is sent home and the rehabilitation team comes to the home versus the patient going to an outpatient rehabilitation center)
- Day treatment programs
- Day training programs
- Sheltered workshops
- Supportive work programs
- Supportive living centers

Day Treatment Programs

Day treatment programs provide a broad range of services and continue the cognitive and behavioral therapies that enable the brain-damaged patient to function and perform the activities of daily living. These programs are provided either by acute rehabilitation units, certified skilled nursing facilities, or transitional community reentry programs. In some areas, similar programs are provided by local chapters of the Easter Seal Society; however, the capabilities of Easter Seals chapters vary from county to county and from state to state.

As a rule, the patient participates in these programs 4 to 8 hours per day on a regularly planned basis. Costs of the program vary, but the average for this type of program ranges from $350 to $600 per day. Care in day treatment programs is frequently reimbursed by healthcare payors because therapy is provided by typical "medical model" clinicians.

Day Training Programs

Day training programs are similar to day treatment programs, but the focus is on patients whose functional and cognitive deficits are not severe enough to require a day treatment program but are sufficiently incapacitating to hinder patients from participating in a sheltered workshop.

Day training programs are frequently offered by such groups as the Salvation Army, Purple Heart, or the local Easter Seals Society chapter. The goals of such programs are designed to return the patient to some form of gainful employment. Entry into the program is coordinated by the rehabilitation team's vocational specialist, who in turn works closely with the state Department of Vocational Rehabilitation and its staff. This level of care is paid for through assumed private funds, workers' compensation, or the state's vocational rehabilitation program if the patient has the potential to return to work; it is not reimbursed by the healthcare payor.

Sheltered Workshops

Sheltered workshops provide services and experiences to persons who have progressed to a point where they are able to resume some form of economic independence. These programs focus on such areas as prevocational skills, task orientation, appropriate work behaviors, fine motor skills and coordination, and preparation of the person to perform occupational tasks at an acceptable level.

The programs are provided by such groups as the Salvation Army and Purple Heart. Like day training programs, sheltered workshop programs are coordinated by the rehabilitation team's vocational specialist or the counselor at the state Department of Vocational Rehabilitation if the patient has the potential for gainful employment. This level of care is reimbursed through use of private funds, workers' compensation, or state funds. Healthcare payors do not reimburse services provided at this level of care.

Supported Work Programs

In supported work programs the person is returned to the work environment, generally at or above minimum wage. Training, supervision, and supportive services are provided by the rehabilitation agency (e.g., Salvation Army, Purple Heart) that assumed responsibility for the person's training in the sheltered workshop.

Once a person has reached this stage, he or she is rarely involved with the rigors of medical rehabilitation, and the healthcare payor is not responsible for any reimbursement of costs.

Home Care

Home is the ultimate goal for the brain-injured patient. However, the details of each individual case will determine whether this goal can be met or realized. Case variables also dictate the level of care and the intensity of services that can be arranged at home. Persons who are homebound and continue to need skilled nursing care or skilled services can certainly qualify for any of the skilled nursing services or therapies offered by home health agencies if the patient's healthcare policy covers home care. Depending on their functional abilities, many patients are discharged home and continue to receive therapy in an outpatient program, since they are not "homebound." In contrast, homebound patients continue to receive therapy at home until they are deemed candidates for an outpatient facility.

If the patient cannot be cared for at home and does not meet the criteria for an outpatient level of care, placement in a supportive living or board and care home designed to provide services to brain-injured persons may be appropriate. There are two categories of such facilities—intensive supportive and supervised living facility. In intensive supportive facilities the patient may live in an apartment or rooming house and have 24-hour on-call supervision and daily interaction with the rehabilitation team specialists. Those in a supervised living facility live in board and care homes. Here supervision and meals are provided, but essentially the person lives as independently as possible.

Spinal Cord Injury

Spinal cord injury (SCI) is one of the most common neurologic disorders found in many case managers' caseloads. Consequently, case managers must assess any patient with a SCI to determine the likelihood of opening the case. Case management may be necessary because once the patient with a SCI is stabilized and the treatment of any medical difficulties has been resolved, rehabilitation must start. The literature supports the fact that everything taught in the next 4 to 6 months has a significant impact on the patient's future quality of life. Thus, it is important to ensure that the patient is transferred to a rehabilitative facility as soon as possible and that the patient and family are prepared for this event. The most obvious person to arrange and oversee this process is a case manager, who can then follow the patient throughout his or her course of treatment.

GOALS

It must be kept in mind that patients with SCIs have experienced an instantaneous and devastating event that has changed their lives forever. In these patients, as in all others, resilience and coping abilities vary from patient to patient. Therefore, the goals established for the patient and the focus of treatment must be based on individual, realistic, and meaningful factors. In addition, the goals must address both the physical and mental needs of the patient and must be directed toward the patient's potential rather than dwelling on lost functions.

Spinal cord injured patients (and their families) undergo many dramatic emotional episodes and lifestyle changes. Consequently, they must have access not only to medical care but also to psychological support that can assist them in dealing with, at minimum, their emotional upheaval, changes in their socioeconomic status and their personal relationships, and sexual dysfunctions.

COMPLETE OR INCOMPLETE SPINAL CORD INJURY

Spinal cord injuries are described as complete or incomplete. Patients with incomplete injuries have motor or sensory function below the level of the injury and have various degrees of paralysis or numbness. Consequently, these patients have the best potential for recovery. In contrast, a person with a complete SCI has no voluntary muscle tone or sensation below the level of the injury, remains paralyzed, and has numerous functional limitations. Additional factors that limit functional outcomes in these patients include:

- Significant spasticity
- Inadequate range of motion, resulting in contractures
- Lack of patient acceptance of the injury
- Poor family or social support
- Poor environmental or living conditions
- Limited function or presence of disability preceding the injury
- Other complicating factors associated with

spinal cord injury (e.g., traumatic brain injury, stroke)
- Compromised mental health status

REHABILITATION

If the patient with a SCI is hospitalized in a community hospital that does not offer a comprehensive physical medicine and rehabilitation (PM&R) program, the case manager must advocate the patient be moved as quickly as possible to a site where this level of care can occur. The success of rehabilitation depends on the care and treatment received for the many problems that occur in a person with quadriplegia (may also be termed tetraplegia) or paraplegia. The outcome also depends on how quickly the patient is referred to rehabilitation. Complications not only are costly, they also impede the achievement of goals and can close the small window of opportunity that exists for successful rehabilitation.

Case managers must maintain a list of the various rehabilitation units in their region or state (and even some national units). This list should contain not only names and phone numbers but also pertinent information about the levels of SCI that can be handled by the various facilities. Not all facilities admit or can render care for patients with all levels of SCI (e.g., patients with high cervical fractures who are ventilator dependent).

Although the philosophies of rehabilitation differ at different facilities, the treatment teams at each facility must agree on a uniform approach that allows instructions to be presented to the patient in an intelligible manner. This allows goals to be met and ensures that the patient receives the maximum benefits of a teaching or learning program.

KEY PROFESSIONAL DISCIPLINES

As stated earlier in the section on rehabilitation (see Chapter 11), formal rehabilitation begins while the patient is still in the intensive care unit. It consists of range of motion exercises, bracing, splinting, and positioning to prevent contractures and skin breakdown. This level of rehabilitation is critical because patients with SCIs are potentially vulnerable to a variety of complications unique to their injury, and every precaution must be taken to prevent them. Therefore, nursing care of these patients is highly specialized. These nurses provide routine nursing care to meet the patient's medical needs, and they work closely with the patient, providing direct skilled care and teaching for such functions as:

- Skin integrity and care
- Bowel and bladder care
- Control of autonomic functions such as blood pressure and pulse

Two other key professionals in the life of a person with a SCI are the physical therapist and the occupational therapist. These therapists must perform comprehensive evaluations of the patient as soon as possible after the injury to ascertain the functional level of neurologic injury, establish long-term goals, and devise a treatment plan.

Although nursing care, physical therapy, and occupational therapy are critical, the patient with a SCI also frequently requires services from other rehabilitation team members as well as many other consultations and treatments. Consultations are often required with specialists in pulmonary medicine, urology, neurosurgery, orthopedic surgery, dentistry, internal medicine, plastic surgery, and other subspecialties. In addition, both the patient and the family need the emotional and psychological support given by social workers, clinical psychologists, and psychiatrists.

The occupational therapist and physical therapist play a pivotal role in the life of the spinal cord injured patient and in the rehabilitation process. Their evaluations cover seven major areas:

- Sensory testing
- Motor control
- Respiratory functions
- Joint range of motion
- Muscle tone
- Skin integrity
- Functional levels

The results of these evaluations allow the therapists to identify the patient's functional capabilities, and on this basis, the rehabilitation team can then develop a goal-directed plan. While the physical therapist concentrates on mobility, motion, gait, strength and endurance, and muscle tone, the occupational therapist works with the patient to develop motor skills and strengthen the upper extremities. The goal of therapy is to allow the patient to return to an optimal level of functioning with as much independence as possible.

Both therapists work jointly in selecting exercise equipment, adaptive equipment, and orthotic devices. All equipment, whether ordered by the physical therapist or the occupational therapist, is recommended on a case by case basis. Although it is important to order the equipment early enough to avoid delaying the discharge, it should not be ordered too prematurely because changes may occur in the patient's status.

EQUIPMENT AND SUPPLIES

The key to the success of rehabilitation and the integration of patient with a SCI into society is the selection of proper equipment. Equipment needs for a SCI patient are costly. Many items classified as "convenience" items for the majority of the healthcare payor's insured population are absolute necessities for a person with quadriplegia. Many items must be custom-fitted and made specifically for the patient with a particular level of injury and function. Thus, it is critically important for the case manager to argue on the patient's behalf for the appropriate equipment.

Such advocacy is necessary because periodically the extra contractual process may be required to gain approval of the desired equipment, especially if the items are classified as deluxe or convenience items. Proper equipment is the key to independence and prevention of costly complications such as decubitus ulcers and contractures. Consequently, case managers must be keenly aware of the healthcare payor's policy on coverage or how to request the process when durable medical equipment and supplies are required.

Because of the presence of limits and exclusions in many policies, the healthcare payor's case manager must be included as a member of the rehabilitation team as early as possible. This ensures accurate communication about any limitations or exclusions in the policy. More important, it encourages exploration of alternate funding programs, which may be used to help in alleviating the costs required for procurement of the anticipated equipment and services as well as income for general living expenses. Although workers' compensation has few exclusions, patients with SCIs must, like all patients, be evaluated for their potential eligibility for any alternate funding programs (e.g., Social Security Disability Insurance [SSDI]).

The appropriateness of the wheelchair and seating system selected for patients with a SCI cannot be overemphasized. Wheelchairs are not a frill—they are a medical necessity! Although standard wheelchairs (economy models) can cost from $500 to $750, an electric chair that has been custom-made for the patient averages $15,000, and as much as $25,000.

Not all SCI patients require an electric chair. However, many require a lightweight standard model with any number of "customized" modifications, which increases the average cost of the chair. These added charges naturally fall outside the limits of many healthcare payor benefits, since many payors stipulate that benefits are limited to the standard or economy model. The key in such situations is for the case manager to be willing to argue strongly for the patient and the type of equipment required. The case manager must remember that if patients with SCIs are allowed only a standard or economy wheelchair, complications and costly outcomes can be anticipated. Therefore, the case manager must be prepared to argue convincingly, outline costs and disadvantages to the healthcare payor, and plead the case of patients who need specialized equipment and appropriate services.

Likewise, if the patient is a child, the need for "replacement" equipment or parts as the child grows must be considered. In these cases, case managers must work closely with the rehabilitation team and a specialist from the durable medical equipment company to obtain a wheelchair that allows the child to grow. If the appropriate wheelchair is obtained, it can often be used for several years. In contrast, the seating system, which keeps the child properly aligned in the chair, must be replaced as often as the child experiences significant growth spurts. However, the cost of the seating system is nominal compared to the cost of a new wheelchair. If the patient's healthcare benefit coverage for such items is limited, the local Title V Children's Medical Services program, the state agency handling services for the developmentally disabled, or Medicaid may be able to assist with replacement costs.

When managing children with SCIs, it is critically important for case managers to become familiar with durable medical equipment companies that specialize in making customized pediatric equipment. These companies have specially trained personnel who are knowledgeable about measuring and fitting the equipment to the child appropriately and accurately. Unfortunately, not all durable medical equipment companies offer this specialized service.

Just as important as wheelchairs, cushions, and seating systems for the SCI patient is bathroom equipment. Prior to discharge it is advisable for the therapist to make a home visit to evaluate the bathroom and living quarters. If this is not possible, the family must submit a detailed sketch of the home that includes room dimensions and distances in the home. This serves as a guide in ordering the final equipment and allows the treating team to identify barriers that must be corrected before the patient is discharged.

COMMON PSYCHOLOGICAL REACTIONS

The patient who experiences any neurologic impairment (e.g., stroke, brain tumor, amputation) goes through several stages of psychological reactions and readjustments. However, these reactions are often magnified in patients with SCIs as they realize that they face a need to make major lifestyle changes and possibly a life of dependency on others. Consequently, case managers must be cognizant of the resources needed to address these psychological needs. These resources must be included in the case management plan as needs are identified.

Psychological support is critically important for the SCI patient, as much so as the services of nurses and therapists. Not only is this care needed initially, it can be needed during the long term as well. For example, it may be used initially to assist the patient in dealing with periods of confusion, disorientation, denial, depression, anxiety, and grief; as the chronic nature of the problem becomes evident, it may be used to help the patient (and family) deal with such problems as:

- Lifestyle changes
- Life rhythm disruptions (sleeping patterns, toilet habits, sexuality)
- Perception of illness or injury
- Body image and function
- Learning ability
- Emotional reactions (reduced self-esteem, coping ability, labile moods)
- Forced dependence and role reversal
- Continued anger and hostility
- Chemical abuse
- Verbal abuse, child abuse
- Marital discord
- Separation, desertion, and divorce
- Financial problems
- Potential risk of suicide

In the same vein, attitudes about sexuality must be dealt with because they play a vital role in achieving the long-term goals of successful rehabilitation and increased self-esteem. For instance, some male patients may wish to bank sperm, while females may have questions about pregnancy or birth control. All related topics and questions must be dealt with openly and honestly and at the time the question arises.

COMMON PHYSICAL MANIFESTATIONS

Case managers must also be very familiar with the physical problems that plague patients with SCIs. Although some of the following conditions surface while the patient is still hospitalized, most occur after discharge. If neglected or not recognized and treated expeditiously, costly outcomes ensue. Common problems associated with rehospitalization or complications of the SCI patient include:

- Urinary tract infections, calculi, and kidney failure
- Urinary and fecal incontinence
- Skin breakdown, pressure areas, and decubitus
- Constipation and impactions
- Spasticity
- Contractures
- Pain and sensation (with amputees, phantom pain)
- Difficulties in weight control
- Blood pressure and autonomic dysreflexia
- Heterotopic ossification
- Difficulties in temperature regulation
- Deep vein thrombosis
- Edema of the extremities
- Breathing and respiratory problems
- Muscle atrophy and wasting
- Dry, scaly skin
- Ingrown toenails
- Excessive flatus
- Scoliosis (improper trunk balance)
- Ataxia
- Drop foot
- Autonomic dysreflexia
- Reflex dystrophy syndrome (RSD)

In addition to teaching the patient how to recognize and manage problems, most SCI centers send the patient home with a "spinal cord" manual. This manual allows the patient to continue the learning-teaching cycle because both the patient and the caregiver can read and see how to manage any problems and can recognize when to seek professional care. These manuals include not only pictures and text but also community resource information and are a valuable asset.

DISCHARGE PREPARATION

From the time of admission onward, the treating team teaches the significant other or the caregiver all the related skills necessary to allow the SCI patient to be discharged. Unfortunately, one significant barrier to discharge is often the lack of a caregiver. If a caregiver is not available, the healthcare team faces a greater challenge in planning a discharge that will allow the patient to function in the least restrictive environment.

Despite the fact that the rehabilitation program for patients with SCIs lasts for several months, many patients still require outpatient therapy or home health agency follow-up for either continued therapy or nursing care. The actual admission and length of stay in the program depends on case variables. For instance, a patient in a Halo vest may be discharged from the rehabilitation unit with an outpatient program. When the Halo is removed approximately 12 weeks later, the patient must be readmitted to the rehabilitation program to continue his or her therapy (e.g., for balance training and mobility without the Halo).

Ventilator dependency or a traumatic or acquired brain injury further complicates the discharge planning process, and these conditions and their requirements for care must be considered during development and implementation of the case management plan.

SUMMARY

Neurologic disorders present their own special challenges to the medical case manager. Treatment programs vary in philosophy and in the level of brain or SCI they will accept. Most treatment programs last for many months, and are followed by an outpatient program that may also last for an extended period of time.

The SCI patient may be followed for life by, at minimum, a physiatrist and the outpatient rehabilitation clinic. In addition, he or she may be referred to any number of other specialists when complications arise. Because many of these patients have permanent disabilities and their care is chronic, their healthcare payor benefits are often exhausted. When this happens, patients must rely on some form of federal or state assistance.

Brain damage, regardless of etiology, can be one of the most challenging problems faced by case managers. This is particularly true as the patient moves from the traditional medical model of rehabilitation to nontraditional models that focus on retraining the individual to reach his or her maximum cognitive, behavioral, and functional potential.

Long-term deficits are problematic, and the case manager must work closely with the family to work out a permanent financial plan that will account for the anticipated ongoing needs and care. Rehabilitation of the patient with brain trauma or brain damage can be a slow process in which progress may not occur on a regular and predictable basis as in other forms of rehabilitation. Ultimately, regular assessments are a must, and the appropriate rehabilitation program must be matched to the needs identified.

CASE MANAGEMENT OF THE TRANSPLANT PATIENT

Types of Transplants

Transplants are often among the top ten diagnoses found in certain case managers' caseloads. Not only are the transplant procedures themselves costly, the patient's physical deterioration and medical care before the transplant can be, in some cases, just as expensive or more so. Not measurable are the changes in quality of life that the patient and family must endure. As medical technology has expanded, so has expertise in organ transplantation. Transplants of the following organs or tissues are now common:

- Heart
- Heart-lung
- Single or double lung
- Liver
- Liver segment
- Pancreas
- Pancreas segment
- Pancreatic islet cells
- Intestines
- Stomach and intestines
- Kidney
- Kidney-pancreas
- Bone marrow, autologous or allogeneic

Therefore, transplant candidates must be included in any referral criteria for case management and opened to case management as soon as possible.

Case Management Involvement

Once the patient has been identified as a candidate for transplantation, a referral to case management is in order. Early referral allows time to explore the patient's eligibility for healthcare benefits and an opportunity to meet the patient and family to establish rapport. With all transplant candidates, the actual level of involvement by the case manager depends on the organization's policies. However, a minimum of two case managers is commonly involved with the patient and family; one is the transplant center's case manager, and the other represents the healthcare payor.

During the inpatient stay for the actual transplant, the facility-based case manager is frequently more involved than the healthcare payor's case manager. However, this does not decrease the importance of collaboration between both case managers. Communication is necessary to ensure that the treatment course is progressing as anticipated, that healthcare payor benefits are communicated, and that as the discharge planning process approaches, referrals for post-acute care or procurement of pharmaceuticals or other medical service needs are directed to the appropriate providers. If the patient is linked to a healthcare payor that specifies which providers must be utilized, it is critical for this information to be relayed to the transplant team. Otherwise, the patient may be linked to the wrong providers and then held financially responsible for costs until the services can be transferred to the appropriate network provider.

Transplant Center Evaluation

Each transplant center requires specific medical information to perform the initial evaluation for candidacy for the transplant, and it may be necessary for the healthcare payor's case manager to assist in obtaining this information. Therefore, both case managers must work closely together to prevent delays. Such close collaboration is also needed to ensure that the patient is linked to the appropriate transplant center within the healthcare payor's network. Because most healthcare payors maintain a provider network that includes transplant centers, it is important for the transplant evaluation to occur at the transplant center that will be approved by the healthcare payor. (Also in the case of patients having insurance from Medicare or Medicaid, the facility selected must meet Medicare's or Medicaid's certification process and actually be certified by them.) If it is not, a denial for coverage may ensue if the transplant evaluation could have been done at the healthcare payor's network provider.

In all cases, basic patient demographic information must be shared, and this includes submission of copies of the patient's medical records. Despite the fact that specific laboratory tests may have been done before the request for the evaluation, the transplant team may request that all or some of the tests be repeated, since testing requirements often are specific to each transplant center. If additional tests are required, it is vital to coordinate these requests with the healthcare payor's case manager. If this is not done, and it turns out that the laboratory test or other tests were available or could have been done in the healthcare payor's network, a denial may ensue if all tests did not receive prior authorization.

Once the patient is accepted for an evaluation, the initial transplant evaluation includes, at minimum:

- A complete medical history and physical examination
- Routine laboratory testing and blood typing
- Blood serologies
- Pulmonary and cardiovascular tests
- Prothrombin tests
- Twenty-four hour urine protein and creatine clearance tests
- Radiologic studies
- Immunologic typing and testing
- Other organ-specific tests

In addition to an extensive medical work-up, the patient and family must undergo psychiatric testing to ensure that they can cope mentally with the stressors and demands of a transplant and can perform the necessary duties associated with follow-up care of the transplant. At the time of the initial evaluation, the patient and family are given specific information pertaining to the transplant as well as information about housing, transportation, and financial expectations. The most common reasons for denial of a transplant are:

- Age (although most centers do not directly restrict age)
- Presence of multisystem disease not correctable by a transplant
- Presence of recent infections
- Presence of acute peptic ulcers or liver disease

- Presence of malignant neoplasms (i.e., patients must be disease-free for varying periods of time, but this is not an across-the-board exclusion)
- History of alcohol or drug abuse
- Presence of irreversible brain damage

National Registries

When a patient is accepted as a candidate for a solid organ transplant, he or she is placed on the organ transplant list and his or her name is entered in a national registry called the United Network for Organ Sharing (UNOS). This organization is divided into 11 regions and is responsible, among other things, for maintaining a national list of all patients awaiting organ transplantation. Similarly, if the patient is a candidate for an unrelated allogeneic bone marrow transplant, the relevant data are submitted to the National Bone Marrow Donor Registry (NBMDR).

Once the patient is on the appropriate waiting list, the actual waiting time for transplantation will vary depending on the organ or tissue type required, the patient's medical condition, and the urgency of the need. Although the waiting time varies from center to center and there is no "average" waiting time, published data from the UNOS indicate that "waiting times can be as short as one year to five years depending on the type of transplant."[21] In reality, because of the limited supply of organs, many patients die awaiting a transplant.

Because the passage of time limits the viability of solid organs, patients who are "waiting" must wear a pager. This is necessary because once an organ is found, they have a relatively short time available in which to arrive at the transplant center. Depending on their medical condition and the circumstances, some patients actually relocate to be near the transplant center. It may be necessary for the case manager to link others with a free volunteer pilot association to arrange their flight to the center. In other cases, the patient must arrange for commercial air or land travel. If this is not possible, air ambulance transportation may be required, depending on medical urgency and the patient's medical condition.

After Care

Most transplant centers require the patient to receive immediate post-transplant care from the transplant center's outpatient clinic. These patients are seen daily or as often as required by the transplant team. Depending on the outcome of the procedure and the patient's medical course, some patients may require a home health agency or infusion services on discharge; responses to the treatment and the progress of the transplant are monitored by the transplant team. For these reasons, most transplant centers have arranged to provide discounted housing and transportation and use a specific home health agency or infusion agency.

Unfortunately, if after care requires the services of a home health agency, and these services are not included in the rate agreed on between the transplant center and the healthcare payor, a separate rate negotiation may be necessary. Otherwise, reimbursement problems or a denial of coverage can ensue. This is especially true when the patient's benefits are linked to a specific provider network. To prevent such events, close communication between the facility case manager and the healthcare payor's care manager is critical. This ensures claims will be paid and the family will not be responsible for the "non-network" provider's charges.

Providers

Medicare uses very stringent criteria to certify transplant centers, and consequently many healthcare payors adhere to the same guidelines in their coverage language. Thus, healthcare payors often specify that transplants are allowed only in those centers that are "Medicare certified." If the transplant is not done at such a facility, reimbursement may not be allowed. In such cases, the patient will be financially liable for the procedure if research funding is not available. Many healthcare payors make similar requirements of bone marrow transplant centers. These centers are required at minimum to be a member of the National Bone Marrow Donor Registry.

To ensure that all providers used are appropriate, the facility-based case manager must coordinate all details with the healthcare payor's case manager. Similarly, the healthcare payor's case manager must know which types of transplants are performed at the most frequently used centers and which post-acute care providers they may utilize. Just as important is a knowledge of the capabilities of other transplant centers, nationally and in other parts of the state. This information is necessary for pa-

tients whose condition and transplant type cannot be done at a network provider and a "non-network" center of excellence must then be found.

If the transplant procedure cannot be done at the network transplant center, the case manager must be prepared to request approval through the extra contractual review process or negotiate a reduced rate for the actual services to be rendered. For instance, liver transplantation is a benefit provided by most healthcare payors; however, not all liver transplant centers may be certified to perform the procedure for every diagnosis. Likewise, not all facilities are certified to perform pediatric transplants.

If the appropriate transplant center is not in the healthcare payor's network, the case managers in the case must collectively be prepared to guide the patient to the appropriate center, making the necessary arrangements for care and reimbursement. It is wise, therefore, for case managers to keep a current list of frequently used transplant centers in their reference files. At minimum, this list should include:

- The transplant medical director's name.
- The phone numbers of the center, financial coordinator, transplant coordinator, clinical nurse specialist, case manager, and social worker.
- Specific details of what medical and patient demographic information is required at the time of referral.
- Types of transplants performed and any information about the center's outcomes and transplant history.

Alternate Funding and Finances

Most transplant candidates are in the end stages of their medical condition or the disease underlying the reason for the transplant and are unable to work. Case managers involved with transplant patients must encourage patients and their families to explore and apply to all alternate funding programs to which the patient may be entitled.

In addition, transplant patients and families must be encouraged to explore all income sources and other healthcare benefit policies and unemployment benefits. For instance, if the patient has the appropriate work history with Social Security or is a spouse or dependent of a person on Social Security disability, the patient should be encouraged to apply for Social Security Disability Insurance (SSDI). Likewise, if the patient is 21 years old or younger, he or she may apply to the local county or state Title V Children's Medical Services program. These alternate funding programs, if the patient is deemed eligible, frequently can augment the patient's healthcare benefits or income when those benefits are limited or voids exist.

As explained in the section on Social Security in Chapter 4, the process of applying for SSDI takes several months. With the exception of patients in Social Security's End-Stage Renal Disease (ESRD) program, the patient must draw SSDI for 24 months before he or she is eligible for Medicare. Many patients die during this lengthy wait, and others die during the wait for the actual transplant. Even though the patient has applied for the program and has received income during the 24 months (if eligible), he or she will not have Medicare, nor will he or she receive income from Social Security during the initial 5-month eligibility determination period. However, Social Security has special rules for patients with end-stage renal disease, and benefits can begin after 3 months of dialysis or when a transplant is performed, whichever comes first.

The Title V Children's Medical Services program, on the other hand, does not provide any income. If the child meets the eligibility requirements for the state's program and if benefits are limited or excluded by the healthcare payor, the program may assist with payment for the needed services.

Most solid organ transplants are recognized as a standard of care. However, some transplants are deemed experimental. In such cases, the transplant is frequently excluded from healthcare benefit coverage, and this exclusion may apply to alternate funding coverage as well (i.e., Medicare, Medicaid, and Title V Children's Medical Services programs). Although limited in scope and very restrictive, research funds or grants may occasionally pay for transplants for patients who qualify. In these situations, patients and families must be encouraged to apply for this alternate funding source through the financial counselor at the transplant center.

Other resources that may be explored for reimbursement for an experimental transplant or transplants excluded by the patient's healthcare coverage are local fraternal organizations or church or ethnic service agencies. These organizations frequently provide monies raised from fund raisers and contributions for such purposes (either in part or in whole), and the family should be encouraged to apply for any services and funding that may be available from these sources.

Transportation

Depending on the patient's physical condition, the urgency of the transplant, and the distance to the transplant center, transportation needs at the time of the actual transplant must be considered. In most cases, patients are able to arrange for transportation via commercial or private means. However, if the patient's physical condition is critical, ground ambulance or air ambulance transportation may be in order.

Many communities have access to a volunteer pilot organization (e.g., Angels of Mercy) if the transplant center is more than 500 miles away and the patient has limited resources. These volunteer pilots operate a free nonambulance network 24 hours a day, 7 days a week. Regardless of the actual diagnosis, it is wise for case managers to be familiar with this invaluable transportation resource even for nontransplant patients. It is also important to maintain a list of current transportation phone numbers and to share these numbers with patients and their families.

Beneficiaries of the Civilian Health and Medical Program of the Uniformed Services (CHAMPUS), now called TRICARE, may be eligible for free transportation by the military's air medical evacuation system if an air ambulance is required. Information about this resource is available by calling any military treatment facility or Scott Air Force Base in Illinois.

Psychosocial Aspects of Transplantation

The psychosocial and emotional demands on both the patient and the family who are facing a potential or actual transplant can be a significant influence on the patient's health and well-being. Not only will role reversals and disruptions occur in family routines and duties, the financial stressors alone can be insurmountable. Consequently, case management planning must provide for these likely events because these stressors must be dealt with and the patient and family referred to counseling as the various needs are identified.

Financial pressures are exacerbated when (1) the illness involves the primary breadwinner, (2) the transplant contemplated is considered experimental or investigational and the medical efficacy of the procedure and outcomes have not been proved, (3) the patient is a child and the parent(s) must quit their job or take a leave of absence, or (4) the transplant must be performed out of the area, and the patient and family must be relocated or separated. In such cases, if the patient is the breadwinner and loses his or her job, the family's daily income vanishes and often their healthcare insurance as well. In such cases, the patient and family may not have sufficient financial resources or reserves to pay for continuing the insurance benefits, even through the provisions of the Consolidated Omnibus Reconciliation Act (CO-BRA).

Depending on their personal assets, many patients may qualify for Medicaid. Unfortunately, if the patient has any financial resources at all, he or she may be disqualified from Medicaid until these resources have been exhausted. Exhaustion of private assets brings additional stresses such as guilt about being on "welfare," divorce, or bankruptcy, further magnifying an already devastating situation.

Another source of pre- and post-transplant stressors is the presence of limited funds for procurement of medications. If the patient does not have sufficient financial resources to procure his own medications after the transplant, this factor must be considered when candidacy for transplantation is contemplated. This is especially true for patients who are eligible for Medicaid, because Medicaid funding for transplant medications is almost nonexistent.

Although the patient's medical needs frequently dominate every phase of the transplant, the linkage of the patient and family to psychological support services is vital. This support may be obtained from such sources as:

- Support groups (church groups, organ-specific groups, and other community disease-specific agencies)
- Psychiatrists
- Psychologists
- Family counselors
- Clinical social workers

Referral to psychological support is warranted when the following situations or emotions are identified:

- Unrealistic hope for a cure exists
- Denial
- Fear of the unknown and death
- Anxiety or depression, especially as the real-

ity of the illness and its overall impact is absorbed
- Guilt
- Role reversals and demands
- Sexual dysfunction
- Helplessness and frustration
- Changes in body image
- Changes in strength and endurance
- Dependency and lifestyle changes
- Protectiveness

As stated earlier, not all kinds of transplants are done at every transplant center. Therefore, another stressor often seen in transplant patients is separation anxiety. Not only does the patient now face a life-and-death situation, he or she also faces separation from the family. The separation also places additional strains on the family such as isolation and unexpected financial burdens. These stressors are magnified when the potential transplant candidate is a child because frequently one parent remains with the child while the other remains at home working or caring for the other children. Whenever the case manager identifies such stressors, he or she must make every attempt to provide the patient or family with some form of counseling, whether offered by a healthcare professional or a support group.

Experimental Transplants

When a transplant is one that is considered experimental, it is absolutely critical for all case managers to collaborate about the needs and details that arise. Thus, when a transplant referral comes to a healthcare payor's case manager from a transplant center and the requested transplant is not the usual and customary request for the diagnosis or is known to be experimental, special precautions must be taken. Many healthcare payors exclude experimental or investigational services or items from reimbursement, and the patient and family must fully understand the potential financial implications of such a transplant. Consequently, for transplants that are known to be experimental or that raise doubts, all case managers involved must work closely together to make sure that all the information and medical facts justifying the transplant are made known. If they are not, the transplant may be denied coverage when it might have been covered if all the facts had been presented at the time of the review and coverage determination.

If doubt is raised about the procedure, or if

the transplant is known to be experimental, what can case managers do? In addition to requesting the standard medical information about the evaluation or the transplant, the healthcare payor's case manager must query the referral source regarding the standard of care status of the actual transplant. Another way to accomplish the same thing is to request a copy of the consent form the patient will sign. If the transplant is known to be experimental, the patient must be informed of this fact and must acknowledge his or her awareness of it by signing the consent form. If the patient is not informed of participation in an "experiment," the facility performing the procedure can be subjected to significant monetary fines and other penalties.

If there is doubt about the transplant and its status the case manager or the healthcare payor's medical director must conduct research to find information from key national resource groups about the status of the transplant. In many cases, the organization's legal counsel must be consulted for guidance. Sources that can assist with verification of the status of the transplant include:

- Center for Health Care Technology (CHCT)
- National Institutes of Health (NIH)
- National Cancer Institute (NCI)
- Other major tertiary transplant centers throughout the country
- On-line computer information, if the software is available, through such programs as Medline, GratefulMed, and Scientific America

Although the research modalities used to evaluate whether a transplant is experimental vary with the healthcare payor or organization, the primary reason for research is to validate that the procedure is indeed experimental. In many cases this research is conducted when the request for the initial evaluation for the transplant is submitted. In other cases it is conducted when the patient is deemed a candidate for transplantation and it is known that the outcome procedure, the transplant, is experimental.

The actual approval or denial of the initial evaluation varies from payor to payor. For instance, some payors indicate that if the evaluation is approved, this approval will set up a "right of expectation" that the transplant will be covered, even though it is experimental and excluded from coverage. In contrast, other payors view the approval of the evaluation process as a second opinion. In either case, it is imperative for all case managers to be familiar with the requirements of the healthcare payors for the evaluation process. In all cases, both facility-based and healthcare payor case managers must work closely together to avoid delays in the approval process and to ensure that all information is submitted as expeditiously as possible.

Financial Arrangements

Because of potential limitations, voids, or exclusions in many healthcare policies, the case managers employed by the facility and the healthcare payor must work closely with the transplant patient and the family to ensure that financial resources are in place to cover all aspects of care. Although the actual transplant costs are covered by the healthcare payor, other financial obligations associated with the transplant may be excluded. Frequently these costs involve housing arrangements for pre- or post-transplantation monitoring or transportation to and from the transplant center. Because not all transplants are done at every transplant center, many transplant candidates must relocate temporarily and reside near the transplant center. This burden adds to an already strained budget because these expenditures are excluded from healthcare policy reimbursement.

As a rule, if the transplant is a covered benefit, expenses associated with the transplant are covered. These expenses include HLA and HLA-DNA (histocompatibility locus antigen and histocompatibility locus antigen-deoxyribonucleic acid) testing, which are necessary to determine whether the donor organ or tissue matches the recipient's. Healthcare payors vary in their policies on organ acquisition costs or testing. For example, many payors will not pay for any expenses related to the harvesting of the donor organ; and in the case of an allogeneic bone marrow transplant, tests of living related donors may be covered whereas tests of unrelated donors and donor searches are not. In other cases, the costs of donor harvesting are covered if they are billed by the recipient's hospital, not the donor's hospital. Other healthcare payors do not cover any donor charges.

Commonly, many plans exclude any charges related to services rendered to the donor prior to brain death; these are paid by the donor's insurance. In patients needing an allogeneic bone marrow transplant from an unrelated donor, much of the testing and search costs must be borne by the patient or family, and in many cases, they must rely on fraternal organizations and other groups that conduct fund raisers to assist with raising the money needed.

CHAMPUS Coverage for Allogeneic Bone Marrow Transplantation

If the patient who needs an allogeneic bone marrow transplant has no other insurance and his or her primary healthcare coverage is by the Civilian Health and Medical Program of the Uniformed Services (CHAMPUS [now TRI-CARE]), he or she must be referred or evaluated by the Wilford Hall Medical Center's transplant team in San Antonio, Texas. This referral or evaluation must be done prior to any evaluation or transplant procedure performed by a civilian transplant center. Referral to this center is necessary because before reimbursement can occur, a nonavailability statement (NAS) must be issued from Wilford Hall Medical Center. This nonavailability statement stipulates that the services required by the patient were not available from Wilford Hall Medical Center. The nonavailability statement then allows the patient to undergo the evaluation or have the transplant performed in a civilian transplant center. More important, it allows the transplant center to be paid.

A word to the wise—Wilford Hall Medical Center, like many military treatment facilities, is a state-of-the-art center of excellence. This facility matches or exceeds the standards set for any civilian center of excellence, and case managers should not underestimate its capabilities. If the patient has CHAMPUS (now TRI-CARE) coverage, the case manager should take a proactive role in advocating that the transplant occur at Wilford Hall Medical Center or the military transplant center designated. Not only will the transplant be performed in a state-of-the-art center, but also most services related to the transplant are free, including most outpatient care and medications.

Indications and Contraindications for Transplantation

The following list (although it is not all-inclusive) offers some guidelines to the indications and contraindications recommended for the various types of transplants. Each healthcare payor has its own list of acceptable conditions that it will allow for benefit coverage. It behooves case managers to be very familiar with this list and the processes required for approval or denial when requests are generated because not every transplant listed below is a standard of care for certain conditions. Nor have all been approved as efficacious by the approval bodies; thus, certain transplants continue to be tested in clinical trials and remain experimental (at this writing this is true for solid organs and bone marrow transplantation).

HEART TRANSPLANTATION

Indications[22, 23]

- Functional class III or IV (New York Heart Association classification) or heart conditions with poor 6-month prognosis for survival that are not amenable to other medical and surgical treatments
- Under age 50 years (occasional exceptions, especially younger patients or physiologically young patients may be considered; this is one indication that varies with the transplant center)
- Healthy except for end-stage cardiac disease
- Medically compliant; patient must be capable of following a complex medical regimen for the rest of his or her life after the transplant
- Emotionally and psychologically stable with a demonstrated realistic attitude to past and current illness
- End-stage cardiac disease individuals who have exhausted alternative medical and surgical treatments and have a current status of poor prognosis due to cardiac function (less than 25% chance of survival for 6 months; this often includes persons with cardiomyopathy and valvular disease)

Contraindications

- Systemic disease (e.g., severe peripheral cerebrovascular disease; insulin-dependent diabetes; cancer or any other condition associated with a shorter than normal expected lifespan; chronic obstructive pulmonary disease)
- Active systemic infection such as AIDS or HIV
- Pneumonia, recent or unresolved pulmonary infarction; any infiltrate on chest x-ray is a relative contraindication
- Severe pulmonary hypertension with a fixed pulmonary vascular resistance of over 6 to 8 Wood units
- Moderate to severe prerenal azotemia or hepatic abnormalities (acceptable if mild to moderate in severity and secondary to right heart failure)

- History of central nervous system disorder
- Morbid obesity
- History of alcohol or drug abuse, or mental illness considered to interfere with a disciplined medical regimen
- Renal dysfunction not explained by underlying heart disease and not deemed reversible
- Age older than 70 years
- Severe systemic hypertension requiring multidrug therapy for even moderate control (e.g., multidrug treatment to attain diastolic pressure of <105 mmHg)

HEART-LUNG TRANSPLANTATION[24, 25]

Indications

- Eisenmenger's syndrome
- Cystic fibrosis
- Primary pulmonary hypertension
- End-stage pulmonary or cardiopulmonary disease
- Life expectancy less than 1 year
- Age no more than 50 to 55 years (heart and lung, bilateral lung) or 60 to 65 years (single lung)

Contraindications

- Active infection or systemic illness
- Psychological disorder
- Active alcohol or drug dependence
- Life-limiting conditions such as renal or hepatic failure, malignancy
- Previous major thoracic surgery
- Lack of compliance with supportive medical regimens or lack of rehabilitation potential
- HIV+ or AIDS
- Morbid obesity
- Irreversible brain damage
- Insulin-dependent diabetes with neuropathy, retinopathy, or peripheral vascular disease

LUNG TRANSPLANTATION[26, 27]

Indications

- Chronic obstructive pulmonary disease (bronchiectasis, emphysema)
- Alpha-1-antitrypsin deficiency
- Primary pulmonary fibrosis
- Cystic fibrosis
- Primary pulmonary hypertension

Contraindications

- Insulin-dependent diabetes
- Active drug, alcohol, or cigarette dependence

- Active infection
- History of malignancy within the past 5 years
- Chronic pulmonary emboli
- Lupus erythematosus
- Primary pulmonary hypertension
- Myogenic respiratory disease
- Renal insufficiency
- Cor pulmonale with gross cardiomegaly
- HIV+ or AIDS

LIVER TRANSPLANTATION[28, 29]

Indications

- End-stage liver disease for which other available medical and surgical treatments have been exhausted
- Extrahepatic biliary atresia for which hepato-portoenterostomy has failed
- Chronic active hepatitis with progressive liver failure and a life expectancy of less than 6 months
- Primary and secondary biliary cirrhosis
- Hepatic vein thrombosis with progressive liver failure and ascites that has not responded to anticoagulants or portal decompression surgery
- Sclerosing cholangitis with chronic nonsupportive inflammation of the bile ducts with no history of multiple surgeries, extrahepatic duct disease, or the presence of biliary infections
- Presence of imminent death
- Inevitable irreversible damage to the central nervous system
- Deterioration of quality of life to unacceptable levels
- Primary hepatic malignancy confined to the liver but not amenable to resection
- Alcoholic liver disease in patients who develop evidence of progressive liver failure despite appropriate medical treatment and cessation of alcohol abuse
- Postnecrotic cirrhosis
- Budd-Chiari syndrome
- Wilson's disease
- Primary hepatoma
- Fulminant liver failure
- Alpha-1-antitrypsin deficiency
- Hemochromatosis

Contraindications

- Active systemic infection
- Encephalopathy with edema or irreversible brain damage
- Congenital anomalies that prevent surgery

- Primary hepatic malignancies extending beyond the margin of the liver
- Metastatic hepatobiliary malignancy
- Severe hypoxemia due to right-to-left intrapulmonary shunt
- Severe renal or cardiopulmonary disease (may require dual organ transplantation)
- HBsAg-positive donor and HBeAg-positive recipient
- Prior abdominal surgery, particularly in the right upper quadrant (relative contraindication)
- Lack of sufficient psychosocial stability to ensure compliance
- Active alcohol or drug abuse
- HIV+ or AIDS

SIMULTANEOUS KIDNEY AND PANCREATIC TRANSPLANTATION

Indications[30]

- End-stage renal disease
- Age younger than 50 years (generally 18 to 50 years)
- Glucose control problems (e.g., frequent hypoglycemia or hypoglycemia awareness)
- No disabling advanced diabetic neurovascular complications
- Type 1 diabetes mellitus
- Good understanding of the uncertain benefits of a successful pancreatic transplant beyond glycemic control

Contraindications

- Coronary artery disease manifested by poorly controlled angina, congestive heart failure, or ejection fraction <50%
- Peripheral vascular disease manifested by leg ulcers or previous amputation
- History of alcohol or drug abuse, or mental illness that would interfere with the recipient's ability to participate in a disciplined medical regimen
- Stenosed or occluded renal vein or arteries
- Congenital disorders such as hypoplasia, aplasia
- Hereditary disorders such as Alport's syndrome, polycystic kidney disease, pyelonephritis
- Renal cell carcinoma
- Multiple myeloma
- Wilms' tumor
- Hemolytic-uremic syndrome
- Thrombotic thrombocytopenic purpura
- HIV+ or AIDS

KIDNEY TRANSPLANTATION

Indications[31, 32]

- Diabetes mellitus
- Amyloidosis
- Henoch-Schönlein purpura
- Congenital kidney disorders
- Metabolic disorders
- Polycystic kidney disease
- Toxic nephropathies
- Obstructive uropathies
- Renal cancer, Wilms' tumor, or tuberous sclerosis
- Trauma and resultant renal vascular disease
- Irreversible acute renal failure
- Irreversible chronic renal failure
- Scleroderma
- Systemic lupus erythematosus (inactive)
- Macroglobulinemia

Contraindications

- Heart disease severe enough to create unacceptable risks during the surgical procedure or immediate postoperative period
- Age over 70 years; generally, persons over 70 years old or those who are intolerant of dialysis are considered on a case-by-case basis
- Malignant disease within the last 5 years and no recurrence within a minimum of 1 year
- Active alcohol abuse or other chemical abuse
- History of noncompliance or psychiatric disease of such magnitude that postoperative compliance will be jeopardized
- Irreversible brain damage
- Active liver disease
- HIV+ or AIDS
- Obesity over 150% of ideal body weight
- Active infection

BONE MARROW TRANSPLANTATION

Indications[33, 34]

- Malignant disorders
  - Acute lymphocytic leukemia
  - Acute nonlymphocytic leukemia
  - Chronic myelogenous leukemia
  - Preleukemia
  - Hairy cell leukemia
  - Chronic lymphocytic leukemia
  - Hodgkin's and non-Hodgkin's lymphoma
- Select solid tumors
- Nonmalignant disorders (acquired and congenital)
  - Aplastic anemia

- Severe combined immunodeficiency disorder
- Myelofibrosis
- Osteopetrosis
- Hematologic disorders
  - Wiskott-Aldrich syndrome
  - Fanconi's anemia
  - Diamond-Blackfan anemia
  - Cyclic neutropenia
  - Chediak-Higashi syndrome
  - Chronic granulomatous disease
  - Thalassemia
- Mucopolysaccharide storage diseases
- Lipid storage diseases
- Lysosomal storage diseases
- Bone marrow transplant recognized as standard therapy for the diagnosis

Contraindications

- Age over 55 years for allogeneic transplantation and age 65 for autologous transplantation
- Active systemic infection
- HIV+ or AIDS
- Psychological disorder
- Alcohol and drug dependence
- Life-threatening conditions such as cardiac, renal, or liver failure

INTESTINAL TRANSPLANTATION

Indications[35]

- Short bowel syndrome
- Crohn's disease
- Gardner's syndrome
- Radiation enteritis
- Superior mesenteric artery or vein thrombosis
- Trauma to intestinal vasculature
- Intestinal atresia
- Gastroschisis
- Volvulus
- Necrotizing enterocolitis (NEC)
- Microvillous atrophy
- Pseudo-obstruction

Contraindications

- Drug or alcohol dependence
- Life-threatening condition such as cardiac, renal, or liver failure
- HIV+ or AIDS
- Malignancy
- Active infection
- Extensive atherosclerosis
- Advanced neurologic dysfunction
- Severe cardiopulmonary insufficiency

Anticipated Teaching

Teaching varies with the organ transplanted and the transplant center. However, all case management plans must provide for teaching the transplant patient. At minimum, teaching of transplant patients before discharge must cover the following areas:

- Importance of compliance with follow-up laboratory testing, biopsies, and any specific instructions pertinent to the transplant and clinic visits
- Importance of compliance with taking immunosuppressants or antirejection medications
- Importance of not ignoring changes in condition or body cues and when to call physician. These signs generally include:
  - Signs and symptoms of rejection and prevention (and for bone marrow transplants, signs and symptoms of graft-versus-host disease [GVHD])
  - Signs and symptoms of infection and how to prevent infection (e.g., safe sex, gardening, travel, handling of pets, avoidance of persons with an illness)
  - Activity restrictions (especially lifting, strenuous exercises, and sexual limits)
  - Exercise recommendations
  - Dietary recommendations and restrictions and special diets
  - How and when to contact transplant personnel (routine and emergency)
  - Importance of follow-up both regularly and annually
  - Importance of maintaining general health (especially dental appointments and vaccinations)
- Medication regimen, side effects, and contraindications
- Mechanisms of coping with psychological effects of transplant and lifestyle changes; when and where to seek help
- All aspects of infusion, wound, or nasal gastric tube care or other skilled care needs

Discharge and After Care

As the transplant patient's condition stabilizes and the time for discharge approaches, arrangements are made to provide post-acute care either in the center's outpatient transplant clinic or by the patient's own attending physician in his or her local community. The actual arrangements depend on the outcome of the transplant and any complications that may be present, the transplant center's criteria for immediate postoperative care, the patient's place of residence and accessibility to medical care in his or her local community, and the referring physician's willingness to assume responsibility for the care.

Depending on the transplant, some patients are required to remain near the transplant center for 2 to 3 months after discharge for monitoring. For this reason, a home health agency is rarely used to monitor the actual transplant. However, a home health agency may be required for skilled care needs unrelated to the transplant.

All patients with transplants are at risk of rejection at any time. Consequently, they must take antirejection drugs indefinitely and require frequent blood studies, biopsies, and other tests to measure the toxicity of the drugs and the symptoms of rejection. All patients require, at minimum, annual follow-up examinations and tests by the transplant center. Thus, the after care of a transplant patient is costly, since the cost of antirejection drugs (immunosuppressives) alone can exceed $1500.00 per month.

READINESS FOR DISCHARGE (ALL TRANSPLANTS)

As the time for discharge approaches, the following criteria may assist in identifying which patients are ready for discharge. These criteria may include the following:

- Patient's condition is stable with no signs of deterioration.
- There is no fever or signs of sepsis or active rejection.
- Patient is not on intravenous antibiotics or intravenous immunosuppressive medications (occasionally a bone marrow transplant patient may go home while taking intravenous antibiotics, but this is rare).
- Patient understands the physical signs and symptoms of rejection (this includes graft-versus-host disease [GVHD] for bone marrow transplants), the medication regimen, including contraindications and side effects, and the importance of adhering to the schedule of post-transplant follow-up testing.
- Nutritional status is adequate, and any nausea and vomiting or diarrhea has been controlled.
- Caregiver is available to assist with routine tasks because many patients suffer from fatigue.

- Hematologic, platelet, and other laboratory studies are within the desired range.

Additional criteria may be applied to patients with specific transplants, as follows:

Kidney Transplants

- No dialysis is necessary.
- There are no signs of acute tubular necrosis (ATN).
- There are no signs of active rejection.

Liver Transplants

- Teaching of family or caregiver has been started or completed if the patient requires care related to:
  - Feeding tube or total parenteral nutrition line
  - T-tube
  - Dressing changes

Heart Transplants

- Patient understands the importance of frequent heart biopsies, since this is the prime means for detecting rejection.
- Patient understands the importance of salt-restricted diet.

Bone Marrow Transplants

- Platelet transfusions have been discontinued or decreased or can be performed on an outpatient basis.
- Patient is out of protective setting.
- Teaching of family or caregiver has been initiated or completed for care of:
  - Feeding method (total parenteral nutrition or enteral nutrition)
  - Infusion services, medications, and line care
- Patient understands importance of using sunscreen lotion.
- Patient understands importance of avoiding crowds and wearing masks in public (must be worn for several months after the transplant).
- Patient understands importance of avoiding persons with known viral or fungal diseases.
- Patient understands importance of recognizing GVHD (allogeneic transplant patients).
- Patient understands importance of recognizing signs and symptoms of other body dysfunctions or complications associated with long-term bone marrow transplantation.

SERVICES REQUIRED FOR DISCHARGE (ALL TRANSPLANTS)

Services required at discharge for transplant patients depend on any transplant complications that may be present and the center's requirements for immediate and ongoing monitoring. However, because most transplant patients must reside near the transplant center, the conditions that require continuous care or monitoring are generally accomplished by outpatient services offered by the transplant center. This is not true in all cases, however. The following services are commonly required:

- Many liver transplant patients require an extended care facility (ECF), subacute care facility, skilled nursing facility, or home health agency (HHA) for skilled nursing services such as dressing changes, T-tube care, or care of a feeding tube or total parenteral nutrition (TPN) line until the family, caregiver, or patient has mastered the required techniques.
- Bone marrow transplant patients, if discharged with a TPN line, nasal gastric (NG) tube, or enteral feedings, require a home health agency for care and continued teaching until the techniques have been mastered by the patient, family, or caregiver.
- Social worker or psychological counseling or support groups frequently continue after discharge to help the patient and family learn methods of coping with the disease and necessary lifestyle changes.
- In many cases, the newly transplanted patient is seen weekly at the transplant center for several weeks after the transplant for testing and evaluation to ensure that the organ is functioning well.
- If the transplant patient is discharged to his or her own community or lives a great distance from the transplant center and transportation costs are a problem, the patient's local attending physician is required to perform any necessary biopsies or order any laboratory studies, sending the slides and results of these tests to the transplant center for review and recommendations. If changes are made to the treatment regimen by the transplant physician, the local attending physician must implement these changes. Arrangements must be made by the patient to be seen at least monthly by the transplant team, or as often as specified by the team.
- If home health agency services are used, they are likely to be used not for care and monitoring of the transplant but for care or retraining of other body systems that deteriorated prior to the transplant, or for training or actual administration of infusion services, TPN, NG tube care, enteral feeding care, or wound care. The home health agency must stay involved until all care techniques have been mastered by the patient, family, or caregiver. The services most commonly required from a home health agency are:
  - Physical and occupational therapy for strength, mobility, and endurance.
  - Skilled nursing care for compliance with medication schedule, other identified specific skilled nursing needs, blood pressure monitoring, infusion services, wound care, or reenforcement of teaching or teaching diabetic care to new steroid-induced diabetics.

LABORATORY TESTING

All transplant patients are required to have laboratory tests performed once or twice weekly for 4 to 6 weeks after the transplant. Therefore, the case management plan must provide for this. The following list includes the tests most transplant patients require at any frequency after discharge:

- Blood urea nitrogen (BUN)
- Creatinine
- Blood glucose
- Complete blood count (CBC)
- Cyclosporin levels, either serum or whole blood
- Screening chemistry panel
- Platelet count
- Ultrasound and biopsies

In addition, liver transplant patients require:

- Liver enzymes and other tests to measure liver function and signs of rejection.

Kidney transplant patients require tests such as:

- Urinalysis and urine cultures and other tests specific for measuring kidney function and signs of rejection.

Bone marrow transplant patients require tests such as:

- Serologic studies and bone marrow biopsy to measure bone marrow function and graft-versus-host disease or rejection.

Heart transplant patients require tests such as:

- Heart biopsies, performed on a regular basis and at the frequency outlined by the transplant team. Frequency varies according to the needs of the patient. However, this test is the prime means of monitoring rejection. If the patient is in rejection, the frequency of biopsies will increase.

- Any other tests specific for measuring heart function and signs of rejection, including chest x-ray, cardiac catheterization, electrocardiograms.

Pancreas and intestinal transplant patients require tests such as:

- Ultrasound examinations and biopsies, as indicated.

EQUIPMENT COMMONLY ORDERED

Durable medical equipment for transplant patients is rarely needed. However, if it is required, the case management plan must identify what is required and where it will be obtained. If equipment is required, it is often needed for disabilities that occurred prior to the transplant or for postoperative complications. The actual equipment ordered is directly related to the need. In general, the equipment ordered will include the following:

All kidney-pancreas transplant patients require a glucose monitor and supplies if they were not purchased prior to the transplant.

Any transplant patient discharged home with intravenous or enteral feedings will require the appropriate supplies and solutions as well as dressings for care of the site.

Many liver transplant patients require dressings and related supplies for care of the abdominal wound.

MOST COMMON COMPLICATIONS

As preparations for discharge continue, the transplant team's teaching plan generally covers complications and how to deal with them. For all patients, the following areas should be addressed. Patients must know what to do when:

- Fever greater than 100.5°F or 38.5°C occurs.
- The nutritional status is altered or the patient is unable to keep food, fluids, or medications down.
- The hematologic status is altered, as evidenced by laboratory studies.
- There is an increase in the liver function study results.
- Pain and tenderness occur over the transplant site (not in bone marrow transplant patients).

- An infection occurs (colds, pneumonia, wound infection).
- Cyclosporin toxicity or antirejection drug(s) toxicity or reactions occur.
- Shingles or herpes occurs.

In addition, although teaching varies according to the organ transplanted, it must include what to do and who to call when complications occur. The following lists for each type of transplant describe the specific topics that must be covered.

Bone Marrow Transplantation

- Diarrhea of more than 1 liter in 24 hours
- Oral infections and candidiasis
- Skin pigmentation changes
- Dryness of mouth, eyes, vagina
- Soreness, redness, or blisters of fingers and toes due to chemotherapy toxicity
- Fungal infections

Kidney Transplantation

- Weight gain beyond desired limit (3 kilograms)
- Decreased urine output

Heart Transplantation

- Fluid overload
- Arrhythmias other than those commonly associated with a heart transplant
- Weight gain beyond desired limit

Lung Transplantation

- Fluid overload
- Weight gain beyond desired limit

Stomach-Intestine Transplantation

- Diarrhea
- Alterations in nutritional status and inability to retain fluids or food

BARRIERS TO DISCHARGE OR ACCESS TO CARE

Although barriers to discharge of a transplant patient vary with the particular patient, the following factors or situations are commonly seen. Also, postoperative complications and the complex care they require present additional barriers to locating appropriate resources. Typical barriers associated with the discharge of transplant patients include:

- Lack of a caregiver
- Limited or nonexistent access to resources

- Unavailability of local physician
- Inadequate home conditions (e.g., water, heat, cleanliness)
- No transportation for follow-up care or inadequate transportation
- Patient, caregiver, or family is not teachable

SUMMARY

Patients who are either candidates for or actual recipients of a transplant are typical of the categories of patients found in a case manager's caseload. Patients who need a transplant are highly charged and emotional because they know they will die if an organ cannot be found. Therefore, it behooves the case manager to be knowledgeable of resources and to take a proactive approach in assisting the patient and family in locating the most appropriate resources for care.

Although many factors affect these patients, two of the major ones are the high costs associated with treatment and a lack of income. These factors are caused by either services that are limited or excluded from the healthcare policy or high out-of-pocket copayments and deductibles. The impact is especially severe when the transplant recipient is the breadwinner for the family or is a child, in which case one of the parents must quit his or her job to take care of the child. Also, costs for care and drugs are a primary concern. Due to these factors, exploration of alternate sources of income or funding is imperative, and case managers must be very knowledgeable about such resources.

CASE MANAGEMENT OF RESPIRATORY DISEASE PATIENTS

Patients with respiratory diseases represent a large portion of any medical case management caseload regardless of the organization employing the case manager. As with so many medical diseases, no age, sex, or specific population is exempt.

Typical Diagnoses

Case management of persons with respiratory conditions can be instituted for many and varied reasons. In most cases it is necessary because these patients require a voluminous amount of equipment as well as complex and often skilled care, the caregiver requires teaching, or respite arrangements must be made for volunteers, who must be trained in skilled care. All of these are necessary if the caregiver is to assume responsibility for care.

Although a large percentage of patients are in the end stages of their disease, an almost equal percentage require acute care and have a multiplicity of complex skilled care needs; still others are in the very early stages of disease and require teaching and linkage to appropriate resources. Respiratory disease patients in medical case management caseloads commonly have such diagnoses as asthma, advanced chronic obstructive pulmonary disease (COPD), end-stage cardiac disease, emphysema, cor pulmonale, neoplasms, respiratory failure, hypoxemia, airway obstruction, and many conditions related to prematurity, congenital anomalies, trauma, and near death situations involving respiratory complications.

Although many of the foregoing diagnoses are related to prematurity, congenital anomalies, and other medical conditions, many others are related to environmental irritants, and most are attributable to years of smoking or inhalation of noxious irritants. As with many patients followed by case management, healthcare expenditures for respiratory conditions can be astronomical if they are not controlled. However, the cost in terms of human suffering and the person's or family's quality of life cannot be measured. Respiratory problems are also a major cause of disability and death in both the young and the old.

Respiratory Team

Although many respiratory disease patients are followed by their primary care physician or local general practitioner, others are followed by internists who specialize in pulmonology or are board-certified as pulmonologists. In addition to the physician, other members of the respiratory team include specially trained nurses, clinical nurse specialists, respiratory therapists, nutritionists, discharge planners, respiratory team case managers, physical therapists, occupational therapists, psychologists, and social workers.

As stated repeatedly in this manual, nonfacility-based case managers must make every attempt to become a member of the team as soon as possible. This is necessary for several reasons. One is to open communication to expedite the sharing and identification of problems and issues, since care will usually be necessary for the long term, and possibly for the life of the patient. Another reason is that discharge planning for this category of patients is frequently more arduous than for other patients because some community resources are limited or nonexistent.

This lack of community resources is particularly evident for those patients who require "total care" or have complex care needs. For instance, in the case of a patient requiring total care, assistance is often needed with all activities associated with daily living, but this type of care is not considered skilled but custodial. When care is deemed custodial by the healthcare payor, reimbursement for services may be nonexistent. For patients requiring complex care, the needs for care may be so complex that post-acute care providers are reluctant to accept responsibility for care because they do not have the staffing to manage this level of care. Also, patients with complex skilled care needs may require hourly care for weeks or months and then maintenance care for years. Again, this type of care may not be a benefit of the patient's individual healthcare coverage because many healthcare payors place day, hourly, or dollar limits on the home care portion of the policy.

Treatments Required

For all respiratory disease patients the aim of treatment is to correct the immediate respiratory crisis, maintain oxygenation, alleviate excessive breathing workload, maintain electrolyte and pH balances, control infections, maintain the airways, and keep secretions cleared (either via coughing or suctioning). Thus, the patient should be able to function at the maximum level allowed by the condition. These treatments are also a means of preventing complications and exacerbations.

Respiratory patients are likely to experience many inpatient admissions. Many of these admissions result from noncompliance with the treatments and medical regimen as well as from the patient's medical condition and complications. As a result, the physician may change the patient's treatment orders frequently. Some of the most common reasons for admission in-

clude secondary infections (e.g., *Klebsiella*, *Pseudomonas*, *Proteus* infections), sepsis, airway obstruction, respiratory failure or other multiple organ failure, ileus, tachycardia, pneumothorax, pulmonary emboli, edema of both lungs or lower extremities, and so forth. These complications result in additional variables in the case and frequently complicate existing barriers to placement or transfer to another level of care. In all cases, action plans for these crises must be included in the case management plan.

Although the actual respiratory condition dictates the mode, type, and frequency of the treatment, typical treatment orders often consist of low-flow oxygen therapy; ventilation with positive end-expiratory pressure (PEEP), continuous positive airway pressure (CPAP), and other methods of maximizing lung function; humidification; antibiotic therapy; and the use of cortisone, bronchodilators, diuretics, and other drug therapies (e.g., theophyllines, beta-adrenergic agents, anticholinergic agents, and anti-inflammatory agents). For hospitalized patients, short periods of oral or nasal endotracheal tube insertion for suctioning and clearing of secretions may be added to any other treatments the patient may be receiving.

In addition, orders are commonly given for some form of chest physical therapy for postural drainage, breathing exercises, and strength and endurance exercises. Likewise, many patients require tube feedings or TPN to meet their nutritional needs. Some treatments are administered only in an inpatient setting, but many others continue when the patient is discharged. Thus, depending on their technologic needs, a respiratory patient's home environment may resemble a small hospital unit.

Patient motivation is a major factor in patient selection for pulmonary rehabilitation, and patient selection is based on the severity of the respiratory diagnosis. Pulmonary rehabilitation programs are designed to teach the patient and family how to live within the constraints of the disease and disability. If a pulmonary rehabilitation program is considered essential for the success of the case, both in terms of quality of life and in overall cost savings, the case manager must make every effort to seek approval for it from the healthcare payor. Although healthcare payors are beginning to recognize the importance of pulmonary rehabilitation, many still do not include it in their coverage. If this program is denied coverage, approval should be sought via the extra contractual process.

Depending on the diagnosis and the other case variables, most nonventilator patients can be discharged home. When they are, equipment requirements can vary, but respiratory patients commonly require multiple items of equipment, supplies, and services. Requirements for the actual care of these patients depend on the diagnosis and treatment orders written by the attending physician.

If a home health agency is involved, coverage of these services by the healthcare payor is frequently limited to those services considered medically necessary and skilled. Even for these services, coverage may be limited to one to two intermittent skilled nursing visits. Teaching of skilled techniques, medication administration, or direct administration of skilled care may be allowed for the short term. Long-term hourly skilled care may be possible through use of the extra contractual process or alternate funding sources. The family must often make arrangements for this level of care through their own funds or volunteer caregivers, but in some cases placement may be the only alternative.

Ventilator-dependent patients require an inordinate amount of equipment and skilled nursing care. The greatest need is a caregiver who can be trained to administer all levels of the required care and services, including any required help with activities of daily living. To coordinate this level of care, much planning must be done by all case managers involved and the healthcare team before the actual discharge.

For patients in need of long-term ventilator support, case managers must be careful not to purchase the ventilator until the appropriate ventilator has been selected for the patient. Many healthcare payors do not allow reimbursement for duplicate items of equipment in a specified period of time. Before any decision is made about the feasibility of purchasing a ventilator, factors such as the potential for weaning and the scope of services allowed by renting the equipment must be considered.

On the surface, purchase often seems far more economical; however, it may not be when one considers all the relevant factors. For instance, when the equipment is rented, the rental costs include the services of a respiratory therapist, routine maintenance of the equipment, and replacement of the unit if it requires servicing by the manufacturer. When rental is converted to a purchase, these services cease. If a monthly service agreement that includes these services is not established, the healthcare payor or family must assume these costs. Despite their nominal monthly cost, many healthcare payors do not allow approval or reimbursement for service agreements. When such a

denial occurs, arrangements must be made to ensure that support services, monthly monitoring of the patient, adjustments to the equipment settings, and routine maintenance of the equipment continue. Therefore, as the case management plan is developed, these important elements must be considered and included in the plan.

Ventilator Weaning

While most ventilator-assisted patients can be weaned long before discharge, many others cannot. In some situations, those who cannot be weaned initially may be candidates for a ventilator weaning program. Ventilator weaning capabilities vary from patient to patient because techniques of weaning vary from facility to facility. Weaning readiness is based on many factors that typically include clinical findings such as continued evidence of improved lung function and the patient's ability to tolerate short periods off the ventilator. In most cases, weaning goes smoothly and is accomplished within a relatively short period of time. However, for some patients, this does not happen. For them, weaning is often a long and arduous process, and some remain ventilator dependent for the rest of their lives.

If attempts at weaning fail prior to discharge from the acute care facility, most candidates for ventilator weaning are admitted to a skilled nursing facility or care facility that specializes in ventilator weaning. Others, however, owing to case variables such as the intensity and complexity of their care or the refusal of the patient and family to accept placement, are discharged home.

If weaning attempts prove fruitless in patients admitted to a skilled nursing facility or care facility, these patients will be candidates for long-term care. This care can be given at home if the patient and family agree and caregivers can be found who can manage the care required. Others will require long-term placement in a skilled nursing facility that specializes in long-term ventilator care.

Psychological Factors

Like many patients with chronic and debilitating conditions, respiratory disease patients are not exempt from psychological problems or personality disorders. A whole array of psychological factors may surface, and typically, these patients can be very demanding, manipulative, angry, and hostile, venting their emotions at the treating team or family members.

Anxiety and depression are possibly the most common factors seen; the anxiety is due to hypoxia and a feeling of asphyxiation, and the depression is caused by the patient's changing lifestyle. Also, depending on the person's degree of debility, many respiratory disease patients are dependent on others, and this dependency intensifies their reactions and responses. Consequently, it is a major cause of marital discord. It is also a factor in the occasional difficulty experienced in gaining access to follow-up care and treatment by physicians and other healthcare providers. These professionals have had previous exposure to the patient and have elected not to resume responsibility for services in future episodes of need.

Consequently, for all respiratory disease patients and their families, appropriate resources should be identified in the case management plan, even when psychological factors are not obvious; at minimum, the patient and family should be apprised of available support groups should they elect to take advantage of this type of service. In most cases, such groups emphasize helping the patient and family overcome some of their fears, serving as a "social outlet," offering an opportunity to share experiences, and allowing an opportunity to learn how to navigate the healthcare delivery system and overcome obstacles associated with obtaining access to services in the long-term care system.

Testing

Most respiratory disease patients require frequent laboratory tests and radiologic studies to monitor the disease course and the responses to treatment. The case management plan must provide for these tests and the corresponding resources required (e.g., outpatient laboratory or radiologic services or portable services that come directly to the patient's home). The following tests or services are often ordered:

- Chest radiologic studies
- Sputum cultures
- Lung volume tests (i.e., total lung capacity, functional residual capacity, and residual volume)
- Arterial blood gases (ABGS)
- Pulse oximetry

- Serum electrolyte, pH, and other blood studies
- Bronchograms and other tests and procedures
- Computed tomography (CT) scans

Alternate Funding

Assessments and referrals to any alternate funding sources (especially if they provide income) are critical and are an absolute must in planning cases for the respiratory disease patients. Assessments for financial assistance must be done continuously and included in the case management plan. This is essential because respiratory patients often have major out-of-pocket expenditures for their care (e.g., some healthcare payors do not cover any durable medical equipment, others may impose large copayments, and most impose limits on home care and exclude such services as attendant care). Referrals are also necessary because many respiratory patients are unable to continue working. When this occurs, they not only experience a loss of income, they lose their healthcare coverage as well because they cannot afford to continue payments of the coverage even through the provisions allowed by the Consolidated Omnibus Reconciliation Act (CO-BRA). Because many respiratory disease patients are no longer able to work, they may be eligible for unemployment or state disability benefits, Medicaid, or Supplemental Security Income (SSI).

Many respiratory disease patients will qualify for Social Security Disability Insurance (SSDI) and eventually Medicare for the disabled under the age of 65. Because the application and approval process is lengthy, any patient identified as a possible candidate for SSDI must be referred as early as possible.

Similarly, all children with a respiratory diagnosis must be evaluated for possible referral to the local Title V Children's Medical Services program. Depending on the child's disabilities and needs, referral to the state agency responsible for developmental disabilities and the Department of Education may also be necessary. Because of differences in eligibility factors and treatment options for acute care versus chronic care, it is vital for case managers to be familiar with the policies and referral criteria for local and state agencies.

Because of their disease, many respiratory disease patients may become candidates for a lung or heart-lung transplant. Although in general these transplants are recognized as a standard of care for most such conditions, if the transplant is considered experimental for the patient's disorder, the case manager may have to seek extra contractual approval for it. If this fails, the patient and family must be given assistance in locating research funds and transplant centers that can perform the transplant. The same assistance is needed for patients who are taking investigational or experimental drugs while enrolled in a clinical trial. If research funds are not available for such treatment, the case manager may have to apply for approval using the extra contractual process or help the family locate a fraternal organization that can possibly help with payment for the necessary services (in whole or in part, depending on the organization and its fund-raising efforts).

Community Resources

Although most care for respiratory patients occurs at home, many patients, owing either to complications or noncompliance, require frequent inpatient admissions and treatments. When home care is not an option, placement in a skilled nursing facility or care facility that specializes in respiratory disorders is usually the alternative. As stated elsewhere in this manual, care in specialized facilities is generally short term and is designed to continue the treatment until the patient's condition has stabilized and he or she can be transferred to home or to a skilled nursing facility where long-term care can continue (however, the skilled nursing facility must be capable of providing the level of care needed). Because of their oxygen needs, many respiratory disease patients are not candidates for placement in a board and care home because fire and other local ordinances and licensure restrictions prohibit use of this level of care in these facilities.

Because of their skilled nursing care needs, many homebound patients qualify for home health agency services, which are reimbursed by the healthcare payor. Others need custodial care and assistance with the activities of daily living. In these cases, the patient or family must assume responsibility for payment for the services. It is these patients with custodial care needs that pose one of the greatest challenges to case managers. Not only do most of these patients have a limited or nonexistent income to pay for services, many also require assistance with every aspect of their lives. These patients are frequently classified as requiring "total care." Finding resources to assume responsibility for providing total care is difficult because, in most cases, the availability of such care is directly related to finances and the ability to pay.

Fortunately, many respiratory disease patients receive their care in an outpatient setting or at home. To augment the patient's healthcare benefits, the following community agencies are commonly involved with respiratory patients:

- American Lung Association
- Support groups
- Church, ethnic, and community social service agencies (mainly for volunteers and transportation)
- Handicapped transportation services
- Chore worker or homemaker services
- Organ procurement programs
- Pulmonary rehabilitation programs
- Emergency response systems
- Hospital or independent dietitians
- Laboratories and imaging centers that offer outpatient services, or, if the patient is homebound, portable services

Equipment Needs

The equipment needs of nonventilator-dependent respiratory disease patients vary depending on the patient's actual diagnosis and state of debility. However, the equipment required for many of these patients includes:

- Oxygen system (stationary, portable, and back-up E tank)
- Continuous positive airway pressure (CPAP) devices and all related supplies
- Apnea monitors
- Pulse oximeters
- Suctioning equipment (stationary and portable) and related supplies
- Feeding pumps (stationary and portable) and related supplies
- Infusion pumps (stationary and portable) and related supplies, solutions, and medications
- Wheelchairs, walkers, or other assistive mobility devices
- Bedside commodes or toilet rails and elevated toilet seat
- Other assistive devices that enable the patient to conserve energy

Anticipated Teaching

Teaching for the respiratory care required is imperative. At minimum, the case management plan must ensure that the patient and family receive instruction in the following topics:

- The respiratory disease process
- Airway maintenance and what to do in emergent situations
- Signs and symptoms of respiratory distress and when to seek medical attention
- All aspects of skilled care (e.g., suctioning, intravenous therapy, wound care)
- Basic knowledge about:
  - Equipment maintenance and routine cleaning
  - Position changes
  - Breathing exercises
  - General exercise to maintain strength and endurance
  - Dietary requirements and restrictions
  - Compliance with treatment regimens
- Postural drainage and chest percussion techniques
- Training in cardiopulmonary resuscitation
- Clean versus sterile technique

Barriers to Discharge or Access to Care

Although barriers vary with the individual, the following barriers to discharge are commonly associated with many patients with severe respiratory conditions:

- No home.
- Home structurally or electrically inadequate to handle the weight of the equipment and the amperage requirements.
- Caregiver unavailable or unable to manage the level of care required or understand instructions.
- Skilled nursing facility unable to manage the level of care required.
- Local community resources unable to accept responsibility for care, for example, (1) many respiratory disease agencies require that patients live within 45 to 60 minutes maximum of their agency, and inclement weather conditions or difficult terrain often rules out many patients; (2) a home health agency may be available but does not offer professional staff that can administer the respiratory care required or manage a ventilator-dependent person, especially if the patient is a child.

- Transportation to outpatient facilities or treatment unavailable.
- Location of patient's residence is remote or is in an area with frequent power outages.
- Family unwilling to accept placement or home care.
- Physician or other healthcare professionals unwilling to continue treatment or provide care due to personality disruptions or noncompliance with treatment regimens.
- Respite care services not available.
- Patient financially unable to qualify for Medicaid but lacks sufficient financial reserves to pay for care or assume out-of-pocket expenses.

The Ventilator-Dependent Patient

Many respiratory disease patients are ventilator dependent, and since this category of patients presents possibly the most difficulty in establishing care, it is included in this section. Case management planning for these patients is essential not only for all medical care and needs but also for identification of psychological factors and the corresponding resources needed to assist the patient and family in dealing with such issues. Counseling is often necessary because long-term hospitalized patients often experience separation anxiety and need assistance in coping with their new life. In other cases, both patients and families may require help in coping with the ventilator patient's "dependency."

The most critical needs for discharge planning include securing and training all caregivers and professionals, procuring equipment, and identifying and implementing all services and resources. In addition, the case management plan must include arrangements for emergency actions to be taken by local utility companies or paramedic intervention if emergencies occur. Consequently, the planning list for resources and resource implementation is lengthy.

READINESS FOR DISCHARGE

Readiness criteria for discharge of the ventilator-dependent patient vary depending on a host of individual details. However, in most cases, the following guidelines apply:

- The patient must be clinically stable.
- The airway must be secure and patent.

- The laboratory and radiologic data are within an acceptable range as determined by the treating physician.
- The patient's functional abilities are not markedly deteriorating.
- The patient, family, or caregiver can understand and implement the teaching required.
- The initial teaching program for the patient, family, caregiver, or professionals has been started or is near completion.
- The patient and family are emotionally and mentally stable and accepting of the transfer to home.
- The family is accepting of the impact and need for technologically complex care at home.
- A home is available and is environmentally safe and structurally sound enough to support the weight of the equipment; its wiring is suitable for the amperage the equipment requires; and there is telephone access.
- The necessary medical and emergency resources are available.
- The family has adequate financial resources to pay for the care that will be required.

SERVICES REQUIRED FOR DISCHARGE

As with readiness criteria, the services required at discharge for the ventilator-assisted patient vary with the details of the case. However, most ventilator-assisted patients require the following services:

- Skilled nursing care from a home health agency (24-hour availability) for:
  - Monitoring and reporting of problems and patient's status.
  - Teaching of clean versus sterile technique for suctioning and preparation of supplies.
  - Optimizing patient's ability to be as independent as possible.
  - Actual provision of all skilled care until family member or caregiver is able to assume the care either part-time (8 to 16 hours) or full-time (24 hours).
  - Education of the family or caregiver about all skilled and custodial care techniques, signs and symptoms, and administration of medications.
- Respiratory therapist (24-hour availability) from a durable medical equipment company or home health agency for:
  - Education of family or caregiver about respiratory techniques and the use and operation of all equipment.
  - Information about troubleshooting equip-

ment problems and making equipment adjustments.
  - Assessment and reporting of patient's response to treatment to physician.
- Durable medical equipment company (24-hour availability) for:
  - Actual delivery of all equipment, supplies, and replacements as necessary (note: Ventilators need routine servicing, and when this occurs a back-up ventilator must be readily available).
- Laboratory services (24-hour availability) for:
  - Blood gas determinations.
  - Other blood studies as ordered by physician.
- Physician for:
  - Follow-up, monitoring, and readjustment of orders.
- Others for:
  - Notification of emergency community services such as nearest paramedic service, telephone and power companies, and fire and police stations about the presence of a ventilator-dependent patient in their vicinity in the event of problems.
  - Alternate plans for care if problems occur; caregiver burnout or respite care needs or changes in the patient's or family's status (e.g., admission to a skilled nursing facility).
  - Arrangements with local power company for possible discounted rates.

ANTICIPATED TEACHING

As with all patients, although the actual details of the teaching vary with the individual patient, the case management plan for respiratory disease patients, particularly ventilator-dependent patients, must identify all teaching needs, the teachers, the people who will be taught, the relevant time frames for teaching, and any other resources that may be required. In most instances, teaching related to the care of ventilator-dependent patients must cover such areas as:

- Clean versus sterile technique. (Once home, and if the attending physician agrees, many "sterile" supplies and solutions can be "home-made" or substitutes can be used if the patient can be switched from sterile to clean techniques. This change can potentially save considerable money but can only be done if the attending physician concurs and the family or caregiver can be trained.)
- Signs and symptoms of respiratory distress or

other medical problems and when to seek professional help.

- Ventilator and other equipment operation, care, and cleaning; troubleshooting of equipment problems.
- Safety issues (e.g., electrical or power failure, equipment or oxygen failure, dislodgment of tubes, maintenance of patent airway).
- Actual skilled care, which must continue until the caregiver is proficient in all aspects of care (e.g., changing tracheostomy tubes, airway maintenance, feeding techniques if nutrition is other than oral, suctioning).
- Medication administration, side effects, and contraindications.
- Use of community resources, including respite care.
- Methods of coping with illness and long-term ventilator care, the impact of illness and technologically complex care on the family, lifestyle changes, limitations.
- Physical therapy for chest therapy (i.e., chest precussion), postural drainage, general exercises for mobility, independence, and conservation of strength, and body mechanics for the caregiver.
- Understanding of the disease process.
- Cardiopulmonary resuscitation and other emergency measures (e.g., replacement of tracheostomy tube and airway maintenance).

EQUIPMENT NEEDS

The equipment needed for ventilator-assisted patients is voluminous. Not only must these patients have basic durable medical equipment, they also need many pieces of respiratory related equipment. While much of the equipment can be rented, some of it must be purchased outright, especially the supplies necessary for operating the equipment. Also, outright purchase of equipment does not include the disposables and other soft goods required. Thus, these items are required monthly for the entire time the equipment is in use. Plans for the resources that will be used to procure the equipment must be included in the case management plan. The following equipment and supplies are commonly ordered for these patients:

- Call system (tap bell or call system)
- Bedside commode or bedpan
- Hospital bed, bedrails, and trapeze (sometimes a patient lift may also be required)
- Humidifier
- Shower chair

- Walker or wheelchair (depending on the patient's needs, the wheelchair may be specially adapted to carry the ventilator and other supplies; in other cases, the wheelchair must be custom-made if the patient is a paraplegic or quadriplegic)

In addition, many home ventilator patients require the following items, purchased on a one-time basis:

- Suction machines (stationary and portable)
- Communication system or devices (often including special tracheal devices that allow the patient to speak, or sign boards)
- Battery and battery charger
- Nebulizer
- Oxygen analyzer
- Oxygen sensor
- Pressure manometer (for ambu bag)
- Respirometer
- Weight scale, if patient is an infant
- Air compressor
- Disposable resuscitator bags
- Stethoscope
- Bandage scissors
- Tracheostomy cuff pressure-monitoring device
- Power generator, if applicable

Depending on the patient's healthcare coverage and the healthcare payor's requirements, the following items may be rented by the month, if they have not been previously obtained:

- Portable ventilator
- Pulse oximeter
- Liquid oxygen
- Liquid oxygen base unit and portable unit

The final case management plan for the ventilator-assisted patient must also include plans for procurement and purchase of the following soft good items on a monthly basis. Note: if clean technique can be used, homemade supplies can be made, or other substitutes can be used if allowed by the ordering physician; in such cases, some of the costs associated with the following items can be reduced:

- Half-inch twill tape
- Suction catheters
- Ventilator circuits
- Nonsterile gauze dressings (4 × 4)
- Split sponges (4 × 4 and 2 × 2)
- Nonsterile gloves
- Micropore tape
- Cotton-tip applicators
- Saline packets or solutions

- Syringes (10 cc, 60 cc)
- Positive end-expiratory pressure (PEEP) valves
- Oxygen sensor (for oximeter)
- Additional tracheostomy tubes, including inner cannulas

Other miscellaneous supplies that must also be purchased include:

- Nasal oxygen catheters
- Tracheostomy swivel adapters
- Tubing connector or adapters
- In-line temperature probe
- Flexible tracheostomy connector
- Tracheostomy moisture exchanger
- Pressure limiter valve

COMPLICATIONS

Complications are a reality with ventilator-assisted patients. Consequently, complications must be anticipated, and plans for their immediate resolution must be included in the case management plan. To keep complications to a minimum, families must be taught all aspects of care, including all necessary emergency measures. The most common problems encountered include:

- Mucus plugging
- Displacement or accidental removal of tracheostomy tube
- Tracheostomy cuff failure
- Failure of any or all equipment
- Ventilator disconnection
- Failure of ventilator alarm to signal
- Respiratory infection or failure
- Inadequate ventilation
- Power failure
- Caregiver burnout
- Inability to adequately provide care in the home

BARRIERS TO DISCHARGE AND ACCESS TO CARE

Because of the intensity and complexity of the care required by the ventilator-dependent patient, the greatest barrier and challenge is probably the difficulty of locating a caregiver. Other barriers include:

- Facilities unavailable for admission of ventilator-dependent patient, especially pediatric patient.
- Home not available (e.g., persons who rent

may be subject to landlord restrictions regarding oxygen or barrier corrections).
- Home health agency's staff inadequate to manage the level of care required.
- Home conditions inadequate (e.g., water, heat, air conditioning, cleanliness, electric wiring, or other structural barriers).
- Transportation for follow-up care not available or reliable.
- Local physician unavailable or unwilling to assume responsibility for care.
- No telephone access in home.
- Patient or family unable to cope (i.e., they are unaccepting of the condition or cannot cope with the responsibilities of the care required).
- Respite or back-up caregiver not available.

☙ S U M M A R Y

Respiratory disease patients are one of the most common diagnoses found in most medical case management caseloads. Because of their medical condition, these patients are prone to a host of complications. These complications are the prime culprit for inpatient readmissions and increases in the amount, frequency, intensity, or complexity of care.

Many respiratory conditions last for the remainder of the patient's life and are debilitating. These characteristics result in an extremely costly category of patients. Costs are also increased if the patient cannot be cared for at home and requires long-term care in a skilled nursing facility.

CASE MANAGEMENT OF THE CARDIAC PATIENT

Cardiac conditions, whether alone or in combination with other diseases or underlying body system problems caused by the cardiac condition, warrant mention because they are frequently the reason for referral and case management intervention. Like the other conditions described in this manual, they are among the most common diagnoses found in medical and geriatric case management caseloads.

The reasons for case management of a cardiac patient are many and varied. While the ideal case management process starts at the onset of the disease, many case management organizations target these cases only when they reach the end stages of the disease. Early intervention allows the case manager to link the patient to the appropriate resources where he or she can gain an understanding of the disease and the importance of making lifestyle changes. It is at this time that the patient should learn how to make the necessary changes (e.g., dietary changes, proper exercise, smoking cessation, energy conservation techniques).

Typical Diagnoses

Although it is not all-inclusive, the following list indicates the most typical cardiac diseases and conditions followed by case management: myocardial infarction, pulmonary stenosis, ventricular septal defects, any variety of heart or valve defects, valvular heart disease, mitral stenosis, aortic insufficiency, infective endocarditis, coronary heart disease, angina pectoris, any kind of cardiac arrhythmia, cardiac arrest, cardiac failure, cardiomyopathy, and pulmonary hypertension and heart disease. Other diagnoses may include such conditions as neoplasms of the heart, congenital anomalies, extensive invasive surgical procedures, and complications of a heart disorder.

Like patients with respiratory disease, patients with the more severe cardiac problems are likely to have multiple admissions or outpatient procedures. Although some admissions are related to the cardiac condition and corresponding treatments, many are due to noncompliance with the treatment regimen or other complications. The primary (although not the only) focus of treatment for the cardiac patient is designed to prevent further cardiac complications, prevent further myocardial or ischemic loss, reduce pain, alleviate anxiety, maintain PO_2 and oxygen levels, and monitor and control arrhythmias.

To quantify activity limitations in cardiac patients, physicians often refer to the New York Heart Association's classification system in their chart notes. This classification allows documentation of specific activities that produce symptoms. As such, case managers should be familiar with the system because it may be the driving force behind the type of services and resources established at discharge. The New York Heart Association classification is as follows:

Class I: No limitations of physical activity. Ordinary physical activity does not cause undue fatigue, dyspnea, or anginal pain.

Class II: Slight limitation in physical activity. Ordinary activity results in symptoms.

Class III: Marked limitations in physical activity. Comfortable at rest, but less than ordinary activity causes symptoms.

Class IV: Unable to engage in any physical activity without discomfort. Symptoms may be present at rest.

Diagnostic Testing and Procedures

As case managers review charts of cardiac patients, they will see orders for the following tests or studies: exercise electrocardiography (ECG), ambulatory ECG monitoring, echocardiography, blood testing (e.g., chemistry panels, any combination of blood serum testing, electrolytes), chest x-rays, renal function or liver function tests, myocardial perfusion scintigraphy, coronary angiography, cardiac catheterization, myocardial biopsies, magnetic resonance imaging, positron emission tomography (PET) scans, computed tomography (CT) scans, radionuclide flow studies, and angiography.

The cardiac patient's actual treatment course (mode, type, and frequency) is based on the results of these studies. Although the test results may lead to many noninvasive treatments, other treatments are invasive. Among these treatments are: cardioversion, pacemaker insertion, coronary artery bypass graft, percutaneous transluminal coronary angiography (PTCA), intra-aortic balloon counterpulsation, and transplantation. Just as important is the prescription of multiple medications, including such drugs as beta blockers, calcium channel blockers, nitrates, vasodilators, digitalis preparations, diuretics, platelet-inhibiting agents, antiarrhythmic medications, and anticoagulation and thrombolytic therapies.

Nonpharmaceutical orders may include cardiac rehabilitation, dietary restrictions, weight loss, physical therapy for establishment of an exercise program or energy conservation techniques, and counseling (by psychologist, social worker, or support group services) for management of the psychological responses to the diagnosis and disability.

Psychological Factors and Cardiac Rehabilitation

As with any illness that has long-term complications or imposes lifestyle changes, the psychological issues experienced by cardiac patients are often problematic. Typical psychological responses include anger, frustration, depression, and anxiety. As a result, all case management plans must include provisions for linkage of the patient with appropriate counseling resources as soon as needs are identified. Even if psychological factors are not evident, the patient and family should be informed of potential support and psychological resources.

In many cases the most cost-effective resources and the ones that offer patients the greatest benefits are the support services offered by church, ethnic, or disease-specific support groups (e.g., American Heart Association). If support groups are available, their services are free. However, for patients with more serious psychological problems, a referral to a licensed professional may be in order. When this occurs, the patient must use the benefits allowed by his or her mental healthcare benefit coverage. If professional counseling is required, the case manager may have to assist the patient or family in obtaining access to approval for the services.

Although it is rarely seen in the actual orders, an excellent resource to which all cardiac patients and their families should be linked is the American Heart Association. This agency is invaluable for the resources it offers to patients and families. Although the focus of the national organization is on research, the local units offer support groups and educational literature, among other benefits. Other services to which the patient might be linked or made aware of are:

- Chore worker or homemaker services (private pay programs and the county-paid chore worker program)
- Church, ethnic, and community social service agencies (for volunteers and transportation)
- Emergency response systems
- Handicapped transportation services
- Hospital or independent dietitian
- Laboratory or radiologic outpatient centers; if patient is homebound, those that offer portable services to the home should be identified
- Organ procurement coordinators
- Medical alert identification system

Depending on the seriousness of their cardiac condition, many patients are candidates for cardiac rehabilitation. These programs focus on teaching the patient and family how to live within the constraints of the disease. If a cardiac rehabilitation program is identified as a treatment option, case managers must make every effort to ensure that approval is granted. Fortunately, cardiac rehabilitation is a benefit of many healthcare benefit packages. If it is not, the case managers on the case must collaborate to ensure that every attempt is made to obtain approval for it via the extra contractual process.

Barriers to Discharge and Access to Care

Fortunately, many cardiac patients are discharged to home. The actual resources arranged for post-acute care hospitalization depend on the intensity and severity of the illness and the need for skilled care. Many patients need short-term skilled nursing care from a home health agency for monitoring of their condition and teaching about their medications, wound care, and dietary restrictions, while many others need nothing more than custodial or personal care. The first category of care is reimbursable by the healthcare payor, but the latter is not. Unfortunately, because of the other out-of-pocket expenses associated with copayments, deductibles, medications, and so forth, many patients do not have the financial capabilities to pay for the private chore worker or attendant care services they may require. If the patient is not eligible for any alternative funding (e.g., SSI), the case manager must be as creative as possible in establishing a plan that will cover these needs. In most cases, the family must be trained to care for the patient, or volunteers must be recruited and trained.

If the cardiac patient is admitted to a skilled nursing facility or other post-acute care facility (acute rehabilitation or subacute care facility), it is generally because very severe disabilities (e.g., stroke, aneurysms, cardiac arrest, ventilator dependency) have resulted from complications of a procedure. Again, care can range from skilled to custodial care, and reimbursement from the healthcare payor is related to these two factors. Unfortunately, many patients admitted to a skilled nursing facility will need custodial care for the long term. When this occurs, the family must be fully informed about the financial expectations.

Equipment Needs

Durable medical equipment needs are related directly to the patient's physical condition and functional abilities. Occasionally, a hospital bed and bedrails are required, but the most common equipment ordered for cardiac patients includes such items as:

- Oxygen systems (stationary and portable and back-up E tanks) and all supplies
- Pulse oximetry
- Suctioning equipment (stationary and portable) and related supplies
- Feeding pumps (stationary and portable) and related supplies
- Infusion therapy pumps (stationary and portable), all solutions, and medications and all related supplies
- Wheelchair, walker, or other mobility device
- Bedside commode or toilet rails or elevated toilet seat
- Other assistive devices that contribute to energy conservation

Alternate Funding

Assessments and referrals to alternate funding program are critical. It is absolutely necessary to include these in the case management plan because many patients with cardiac conditions are so debilitated that they cannot work. Therefore, they may have no income, nor can they afford to pay for continued healthcare coverage even under the provisions allowed by the Consolidated Omnibus Reconciliation Act (COBRA). As a result, they may be eligible for such income programs as unemployment, state disability insurance (if it is available), Medicaid, or Supplemental Security Income (SSI).

Many cardiac patients can qualify for Social Security Disability Insurance (SSDI) and eventually for Medicare for the disabled under age 65. Similarly, children with cardiac disease must be referred as soon as possible to the local Title V Children's Medical Services program. Depending on their needs and disabilities, they may also be eligible for services from the state agency responsible for handling developmental disabilities. If their cardiac condition imposes restrictions on their ability to learn, they may be eligible for services from the Department of Education and any of its Special Education programs.

Depending on their cardiac condition, some patients may require a heart transplant. In this case, referrals are in order to the appropriate transplant center for, at minimum, a cardiac transplant evaluation. Heart transplantation in most cases is considered a standard of care,

and there is no need to seek research funding. However, if the patient for some reason (e.g., experimental drugs) is enrolled in a clinical trial, the feasibility of inclusion in a research program may be necessary. In such cases, the healthcare payor most often does not assume the costs. If it does, authorization is only granted after sufficient medical information has been submitted to justify the reasons.

In patients with any transplant, all case managers must constantly be communicating with each other and collaborating on the final plans. This is necessary to ensure that all charges will be paid and that all resources are in readiness for discharge. More important, it ensures that provider selection is appropriate. If these details are not watched, the patient may find that he or she is responsible for payment of charges from non-network providers until the care can be transferred to one of the healthcare payor's network providers. Possibly more errors are made on discharge in establishing patients with home healthcare agencies, durable medical equipment companies, infusion therapy services, laboratory testing facilities, and pharmaceutical suppliers.

Anticipated Teaching

All case management plans for cardiac patients must contain provisions for teaching and the teaching-monitoring processes that are necessary. At minimum, cardiac patients and their families must be taught:

- An understanding of the disease process.
- The importance of recognizing signs and symptoms and when to call for help.
- All aspects of skilled care.
- All aspects of care related to the operation, care, and maintenance of any equipment used, such as that needed for suctioning, infusion, or ventilation.
- Proper positioning and skin care.
- Dietary requirements and restrictions.
- The importance of compliance with treatment regimens.
- The importance of prudent exercise and energy conservation techniques.
- Smoking cessation.

Barriers to Discharge or Access to Care

Although barriers to discharge vary with the individual, the following barriers are commonly encountered in attempting to gain access to care for patients with severe cardiac conditions:

- No home or the home is inadequate (e.g., stairs).
- Caregiver is not available or is unwilling to manage the home care program.
- Local community resources (e.g., home health agency) cannot manage the level of care required or are unwilling to assume responsibility for care.
- Transportation is not available.
- Family is unwilling to accept placement.
- Family is unwilling to accept responsibility for home care or caregiver responsibilities.
- Respite services are not available.
- Patient is financially unable to qualify for Medicaid but does not have the financial reserves to pay privately for care or to assume out-of-pocket expenses.
- Physician is unavailable or unwilling to assume responsibility for care.

🎇 SUMMARY

Cardiac diseases and the complications resulting from these diseases are commonly encountered by case managers. Because of their medical condition, these patients can find themselves involved in a host of other medical conditions and complications, leading to costly outcomes in terms of both healthcare expenditures and the quality of life the patient and family must endure. Many cardiac conditions are debilitating, and the patient will need care and services lifelong.

In many instances, early referral to support agencies or select professional disciplines (therapists, dietitians) is critical. These support programs are necessary if the cardiac patient is to be taught how to make lifestyle changes whenever possible.

CASE MANAGEMENT OF PATIENTS REQUIRING TECHNOLOGICALLY COMPLEX ANTIBIOTIC THERAPY

For most patients requiring intravenous (IV) antibiotic therapy, home is the primary alternate setting for their ongoing care, although naturally the final site chosen depends on all case variables. In most cases, infusion therapy companies recommend establishment of a central intravenous line prior to discharge. However, the duration of the therapy is frequently the determining factor in the selection of the venous access route. Most intravenous antibiotics currently in use can be administered safely at home. Thus, prolonged hospitalization for this purpose is reduced or eliminated.

The feasibility of home administration for the patient requiring intravenous or technologically complex antibiotic care depends on several factors, among them the following: the drug selected, the standards of care associated with that drug, and the disabilities or limitations of the patient or caregiver. The following information is designed to assist the case manager in developing a case management plan for these patients at home.

Readiness for Discharge

Readiness criteria for discharge of the patient requiring technologically complex antibiotic treatment vary from patient to patient depending on the disease course and other medical conditions as well as on such case variables as:

- The financial feasibility and cost effectiveness of the final plan.
- The clinical stability of the patient.
- Recognition of the infection and the selected antibiotic therapy as medically appropriate (per county health and Centers for Disease Control and Prevention [CDC] guidelines for care outside the acute hospital).
- Appropriateness of the antibiotic for home use (it is a nonexperimental drug and can be administered and monitored with intermittent skilled visits from a home health agency or infusion provider once the patient or caregiver has been trained and is proficient in the administration).
- Tolerance by the patient of the initial course of antimicrobial agent without problems.
- Acceptance by the patient and family of home care.
- Adequate learning capacity of patient, family member, or caregiver.
- Adequacy of venous access.
- Adequacy and cleanliness of home environment, and presence of refrigeration.
- Availability of community medical resources.

Alternate Funding

Alternate funding sources are rarely required for this category of patients if their financial need is strictly related to the intravenous antibiotic course. However, individual factors, such as the underlying medical condition and its related care and the patient's actual healthcare benefit coverage for drug therapy may determine whether the patient should apply for alternate funding (e.g., the drug is experimental, the patient has exhausted his or her day or dollar limits offered by the healthcare policy). If the patient is referred to alternate funding sources, the referral will depend on the actual diagnosis and specific details of the case.

Services Required for Discharge

Most patients discharged on intravenous antibiotic therapy require the following professional services:

- Home health agency for skilled nursing care (24-hour availability) for:
  - Monitoring, assessment, and reporting of responses to treatments to the physician
  - Teaching of all aspects of care, and emergency precautions or situations
  - Drawing of blood for laboratory tests
  - Actual provision of skilled care until the patient or family demonstrates proficiency in all aspects of care
  - Peripheral vein restarts or troubleshooting of problems related to the intravenous line
- Registered pharmacist or infusion agency (24-hour availability) for:
  - Delivery of supplies, equipment, and solutions
  - Troubleshooting equipment maintenance and operation
  - Review of the formula with the physician after comparison of cultures and other laboratory results (e.g., kidney function)
- Physician for:
  - Follow-up, monitoring, and readjustment or termination of the treatment plan
- Durable medical equipment company for:
  - Delivery and teaching of use of durable medical equipment and supplies, if applicable
- Laboratory services for:
  - Appropriate laboratory studies and panels

Anticipated Teaching

As with any patient requiring ongoing post-acute care, education of the patient, family, or caregiver in the techniques necessary for complex antibiotic infusion is of critical importance. As the patient is readied for discharge instruction in the following topics is commonly offered:

- Understanding of the disease.
- Knowledge of the drug, signs and symptoms of side effects, and complications.
- Care of intravenous catheter and venous access site as well as any other physical care needs.
- Safe handling and proper storage of solutions and medications, disposal of waste, including disposal of sharps container.
- All aspects of administration of the solutions and medications.
- Clean versus sterile technique.
- Troubleshooting of equipment operation and maintenance.
- Emergency precautions and techniques, including when to call the physician or other healthcare professionals.
- Procurement of all solutions and supplies.

Equipment Needs

The actual equipment ordered varies with the needs of the individual patient. However, all patients in this category require at least the following equipment:

- Infusion equipment (e.g., pole, pump), solutions, medications, and all necessary supplies.
- Medications, together with heparin, syringes, and related supplies.
- Dressings for site care.

Complications

Most complications in patients requiring antibiotics of this type are preventable with meticulous attention to technique, close observation, monitoring, and implementation of corrective actions when problems are identified. Problems commonly encountered include:

- Infiltration or accidental dislodgment
- Infection at the venous entrance or exit site
- Sepsis
- Kinking or occlusion of the infusion line
- Allergic or anaphylactic reaction
- Difficulty in maintaining venous access, if central line is not used
- Major event separation (central line) of tub-

ing and catheter during tubing changes, causing air embolism

- Pneumothorax or hemothorax (if there are central line problems); however, these are rare
- Noncompliant patient or caregiver

Barriers to Discharge

Barriers to discharge of patients requiring technologically complex or dependent antibiotic infusion therapy are common. Among them are the following:

- No home is available, or home is inadequate (e.g., no stove, no running water).
- A skilled nursing facility is not available or is unable to assume responsibility for care for any number of reasons, the most common being that the staff is not certified in intravenous therapy.
- A caregiver is not available or is not teachable.
- Community medical resources are unavailable.
- Transportation is not available for any return trips to the physician or for outpatient laboratory testing or radiologic studies.
- The patient or family is unaccepting of home care.
- The home environment is unsanitary or unsafe.
- The local physician is unavailable or unwilling to accept responsibility of care for the patient.
- The patient has other medical conditions that prevent discharge.
- The antibiotic selected is not recognized as a standard for care outside the acute care facility.

❧ SUMMARY

Patients requiring technologically complex antibiotic therapy are encountered frequently in case management. Intravenous antibiotic therapy for many patients can be managed at home if this is the primary need. However, if it is not, selection of the correct alternate site of care after discharge must address these other considerations.

CASE MANAGEMENT OF THE BURN PATIENT

Although burn cases constitute a small percentage of the cases followed by medical case management (at least by case managers employed in other than a facility with a burn unit), the costs associated with the care of burns are exorbitant. Many burn patients are hospitalized in regional burn centers. If the nonhospital-based case manager is unfamiliar with the burn centers in his or her area, any regional tertiary care center's discharge planner or staff social worker can help in locating the appropriate center for treatment.

Two resources worth mentioning in this section are the burn units of the Shriners hospitals and the burn unit at Brooke Army Medical Center in San Antonio, Texas. The Shriners hospitals are an excellent resource, not only for children for whom funding is limited but also for any child with a burn. Care for these children in most cases is free. The Brooke Army Medical Center is another excellent resource, regardless of whether or not the patient has healthcare coverage by the Civilian Health and Medical Program of the Uniformed Services (CHAMPUS [now TRICARE]).

Discharge from the burn unit (for most patients) does not occur until the wounds are healed or it is thought that the patient can be managed out of a "protective care" environment. Because patients are often cared for in regional burn centers rather than in facilities in their own immediate vicinity, the facility-based case manager and the healthcare payor's case manager must collaborate frequently to ensure that healthcare coverage issues are clear and that the appropriate providers have been selected for discharge.

Two major factors affecting most burn patients are (1) the psychological impact associated with pain and rejection and the social stigma attached to the resulting disfigurement and scarring, and (2) the countless hours of grueling physical and occupational therapy that the patient must endure, often on a long-term basis, to prevent contractures and maintain joint mobility. Every effort must therefore be made to link the patient or family with a support group or professional psychological counseling to handle the first problem and an outpatient rehabilitation or physical therapy program to support the patient's efforts in the second. With this in mind, the case management plan must include a long-term plan to reflect the resources that will link the patient with the necessary services.

Readiness for Discharge

The criteria used to judge readiness for discharge of the burn patient depend on the details of the specific case and the guidelines used by the specific burn center. However, in addition to a medically stable condition, readiness for discharge is shown by the following signs:

- The patient's wounds are closed or nearly closed.
- The laboratory tests (e.g., complete blood count and chemistry panel) are within the desired limits.
- The family has been trained to care for the wound, or arrangements have been completed for a home health agency or the burn clinic nurses to perform the wound care.
- The patient is not on any intravenous medications or total parenteral nutrition (TPN) (occasionally a patient may require either of these, but this is rare and depends on the extent of the patient's wounds and the burn center's standard of care). If other than normal food is required, the patient may be fed internally, the formula being administered by tube.
- Swelling is within the desired limits, and a time has been established for measuring and fitting the pressure garment. (Note: most patients are fitted after discharge due to body weight changes.)

Alternate Funding

Alternate funding sources should have been explored long before the burn patient is ready for discharge. If the healthcare payor's resources appear to be limited or nonexistent and the patient will require costly dressings, therapies, or psychological services, common alternate funding programs for which the patient may be eligible include Medicaid, Supplemental Security Income (SSI) and Social Security Disability Insurance (SSDI).

Depending on the state and its criteria for eligibility, most children with burns should be referred at minimum to the local Title V Children's Health Services program and Special Education. Depending on his or her status, any child with a developmental delay resulting from the burns may also be a candidate for the state agency responsible for handling services for those with developmental disabilities.

All adult burn patients who were previously employed and anticipate returning to work should be encouraged to apply to any temporary income program to which they may be entitled (e.g., unemployment, state disability services [but note that this program is not available in all states]). All burn patients who wish to return to work but do not expect to be able to return to their previous employment must be referred to the state Department of Vocational Rehabilitation for assistance in job retraining.

Services Required for Discharge

As with all patients followed by case management, the services required for discharge for burn patients are case specific and related to the patient's overall medical condition as well as specific individual details. However, all case management plans for burn patients must identify specific resources or arrangements that will provide the following services:

- Follow-up at the burn clinic at least once a week for monitoring by the attending physician. The frequency of these visits varies with the burn center and the patient (e.g., while some patients are seen weekly, others are seen twice weekly and others daily, so there is no set rule). If the patient lives out of the area, coordination for follow-up by his or her local physician is required at the foregoing frequency, and arrangements must be made for a return to the burn clinic once every month.
- Dressing changes once or twice daily. If the family is unable to change the dressing, home health agency services must be provided, or arrangements must be made for the patient to return to the burn unit or burn clinic for the nursing staff to do them.
- Measurement and fitting of pressure garments. It takes a minimum of 2 weeks to procure most pressure garments, and patients are only fitted after the wounds have healed, swelling has decreased, and their weight has stabilized.
- Physical and occupational therapy for exercises. A home exercise plan should be established that ensures that the patient performs the exercises 7 days a week at the required daily frequency. Note that this may not be

the optimal choice, since pain is a significant factor, and the family may not be aggressive enough in pushing the patient to do the exercises for fear that they will "hurt" the patient, but teaching the patient or family how to do the necessary exercises is a must.

- Arrangements for psychological support needed by the patient or family.

Depending on the situation, other patients may require:

- Referral for diabetic follow-up and monitoring, if patient is a diabetic.
- Preparation of teachers and students for the child's return to school, if the patient is a child. Also, depending on the extent of the burn trauma and its effect on the patient's ability to learn, it may be necessary to apply for Special Education services.
- If nutrition is a problem, the patient may be sent home earlier, but he or she will require a higher level of involvement with the home health agency about nutritional teaching or an appointment with a registered dietitian.

Equipment Needs

The equipment required at discharge varies; while many burn patients may not require anything, others may require such items as:

- A mobility device—walker, wheelchair, crutches, or cane.
- Bathroom devices—grab bars, elevated toilet seat, toilet rails, or shower chair.
- A hospital bed or durable medical equipment if there is a preexisting condition.

Although the burn patient rarely requires durable medical equipment at discharge, all burn patients do require the following supplies:

- Lubricant for softening the skin after bathing and before applying the pressure garment or dressing. (The most common lubricants ordered are Nivea cream, Lanolor, vegetable oil, and solid vegetable shortening; the last has been found to be the best because it is the purest.)
- Soft pressure gloves (e.g., Isotoner) if there are burns on the hands.
- Two to three pressure garments. These must be worn for 24 hours per day for 1 to 2 years following the burn, and the patient must have one or two for back-up because they can only be hand washed and line dried. Despite their

high cost, the patient will need at least two garments at all times.
- Splints for the hands, arms, or feet to prevent deformities.
- Nonirritating shampoo and soap (e.g., Ivory soap and baby shampoo).
- Stretch gauze (e.g., Flexnet), sold by the yard and used to hold the sterile gauze pads in place until the wounds are healed or until the pressure garment arrives.
- If dressing changes are required, gauze may be required for washing the wounds and redressing the burn sites. However, this order varies with the burn center, because in most cases the patient can wash the wounds with a clean wash cloth.
- Creams such as Benadryl for itching.
- Pain relievers for children such as Tylenol with codeine, or other pain medication depending on allergies.
- Pain relievers for adults such as Vicodin or Percocet, or other pain medication depending on allergies.

Laboratory Tests or Radiologic Studies

Laboratory tests or radiologic studies are rarely required on discharge in burn patients. If they are required, the reasons may be related more to other preexisting medical conditions than to the burn wound. If a burn patient is discharged on total parenteral nutrition, laboratory tests will be required to monitor blood sugar levels and the patient's response to treatment.

Barriers to Discharge

As with any case management patient, barriers to discharge are encountered in burn patients. The most common barriers are as follows:

- A home is not available or is inadequate (e.g., no stove, no running water).
- The family or caregiver is not available or cannot be trained.
- There is no transportation for return visits, dressing changes, or supplies.
- No community resources are available.
- No physician is available for follow-up care and monitoring.

Complications

Most complications in burn patients are preventable by paying meticulous attention to the wounds, caring for the skin, wearing the garments, observing and monitoring the situation closely, and implementing corrective actions when problems are identified. Problems commonly encountered include:

- Infections (if the patient is sent home with open wounds)
- Itching
- Major psychological problems and need for peer and family support
- Failure to do exercises, resulting in contractures
- Dependency on others
- Skin changes and breakdown (skin frequently is dry, scaly, discolored, and stiff)
- Tight clothing, causing blisters
- Gastric ulcers (related to stress)
- Intolerance to heat and cold
- Pain associated with exercise and joint movement
- Depression

Anticipated Teaching

Teaching of burn patients, family members, or caregivers varies with the details of the individual case. However, in most cases, instruction should be given in such areas as:

- Clean versus sterile technique
- Importance of and compliance with the exercise program
- Importance of daily bathing, clean clothing, and application of skin lubricant prior to application of pressure garment
- Importance of wearing pressure garment 24 hours per day
- Patient acceptance of new body image and increased self-esteem
- Importance of return to normal living as soon as possible
- Wound care and dressing changes
- Importance of a balanced diet
- Proper care of pressure garment
- Importance of avoiding sun and wearing protective clothing
- Importance of keeping nails clipped short and clean
- Splint care
- Positioning to allow stretching of burn sites

SUMMARY

Teaching and follow-up arrangements for therapy and counseling are imperative in burn patients because successful outcomes often hinge on these elements. Burn patients often have had extensive hospitalizations and numerous surgical procedures, and contractures are the number one complication if the patient does not do the exercises after discharge or does not do them correctly. Also, because of scarring, leading eventually to self-image problems, counseling and linkage to support groups are very important.

Because not every hospital has the facilities available to treat burns, case managers who are not employed by a regional trauma center must be very familiar with the regional burn centers in their area where such care can be obtained. This knowledge is necessary to ensure that burn patients are moved as soon as possible and that the necessary medical information is transferred as well.

CASE MANAGEMENT OF THE PATIENT RECEIVING TOTAL PARENTERAL NUTRITION

Infusion therapy providers require the establishment of a central infusion line before discharge in all patients needing total parenteral nutrition (TPN) (and any solution of more than 10% dextrose), especially if they are discharged to home. This requirement is made to ease self-administration and ensure fewer infiltration problems or complications, since TPN is often required for several weeks, months, or longer. To avoid delays in discharge, teaching of the patient or family must be started as soon as the patient is identified as a candidate for this mode of nutritional therapy.

Readiness for Discharge

The criteria for discharge of the patient who requires prolonged and short-term parenteral nutritional support vary according to the details of the case. However, most patients are ready for discharge when the following signs or situations exist:

- The patient is clinically and mentally stable and is coping with the treatment regimen.

- A central line has been established.
- The patient or family is accepting of home care.
- The home has a physically adequate layout, is clean, and has refrigeration, and the patient has access to a telephone in the event of an emergency.
- The patient, family, or caregiver can be taught the details of the therapy.
- The cost of the treatment program is financially feasible and is more cost effective than inpatient acute care.
- Community resources are available.

Services Required for Discharge

Although the actual amount of services required by the patient needing TPN vary, most patients require:

- Skilled nursing care (from a home health agency or infusion provider that offers 24-hour availability) for:
  - Monitoring, assessment, and reporting of responses to the physician.
  - Teaching of all aspects of skilled care and emergency precautions and situations to the patient, family, or caregiver.
  - Drawing of blood for laboratory tests.
  - Actual provision of skilled care until the patient or family is proficient in administration.
  - Peripheral vein restarts and troubleshooting of infusion-related issues if a central line is not present.
- Registered pharmacist or intravenous or infusion agency (24-hour availability) for:
  - Delivery of supplies, equipment, and solutions.
  - Troubleshooting of equipment maintenance and operation.
  - Evaluation and review (with physician) of laboratory values, weight gain or losses, formula changes, or recommendations.
- Physician for:
  - Follow-up, monitoring, and revisions to treatment plan.
- Durable medical equipment (DME) company for:
  - Delivery of other durable medical equipment and supplies, when applicable.
- Laboratory services for:
  - Appropriate laboratory tests and panels.

Alternate Funding

By the time discharge arrives, most parenteral nutritional patients should already have been evaluated for any alternate funding resources to which they may be entitled. However, if this has not been done, the three most important programs for which such patients may be eligible are:

- Medicaid
- Supplemental Security Income (SSI)
- Title V Children's Medical Services program

Anticipated Teaching

Teaching of the patient requiring TPN varies with the case. At minimum, instruction for these patients should include:

- Central line care and all aspects of administration.
- Understanding of the disease process and the rationale for receiving nutrition through this route.
- Techniques for coping with illness and long-term TPN use, and psychosocial changes or limitations.
- Importance of monitoring weight, and maintaining a weight record and an accurate intake and output record.
- Importance of keeping scheduled laboratory visits, and of performing glucose monitoring and urine testing and recording.
- Signs and symptoms of infections and other potential problems.
- Equipment operation, maintenance, and troubleshooting.
- Emergency measures and when to call for help.
- Procurement of supplies and solutions.

Equipment Needs

At a minimum, TPN patients require the following equipment at discharge:

Infusion equipment (stationary or portable), tubing, supplies, and solutions
Dressings and supplies for venous site care
Heparin and supplies

Complications

Most complications associated with the administration of TPN are preventable with meticulous attention to details and close observation and monitoring. Potential complications include:

- Pneumothorax or hemothorax (rare)
- Major event separation of tubing and catheter during tubing changes, causing air embolism
- Infection at catheter site
- Sepsis
- Metabolic imbalance, severe dehydration, fluid overload, electrolyte imbalance, or post-infusion hypoglycemia and hyperglycemia

Barriers to Discharge and Access to Care

Barriers to discharge are rare if the patient's only need is for TPN. When barriers are present, they may be related to other medical conditions or to such factors as:

- Unavailability of caregiver, or unwillingness or inability of patient, family, or caregiver to learn
- Difficult or unavailable access to nearest emergency care facility
- Unsanitary home environment or lack of refrigeration
- Dangerous home environment for either patient or professional

SUMMARY

Although not every patient requires total parenteral nutrition, the information provided gives important details about the resources that may be considered in the case management plan when this treatment modality is ordered.

CASE MANAGEMENT OF PATIENTS NEEDING COMPLEX WOUND CARE

Patients with extensive wounds requiring complex post-acute care are frequently seen in medical or geriatric case management caseloads. Not only do these patients require varying degrees of nursing care and supplies, many also need antibiotic infusion therapy, pain medications, and a variety of outpatient services. Consequently, the treatments ordered depend on the severity of the wound and its location, depth, and size as well as on other case variables. The case management plan must address all resources needed to manage the level of care required by the patient.

Possibly one of the best allies of a nonfacility-based case manager for consultation about wound care is the clinical nurse specialist or other healthcare professional who is trained in high-technology wound care techniques. Usually these professionals are nurses, but wound expertise is not limited to nurses. Professionals who deal with wound care generally have had specific training in the most up-to-date techniques and resources. They are invaluable resources for physicians and other members of the healthcare team when questions about wound care arise. If in doubt about how to obtain access to one of these professionals, contact the nearest large tertiary medical center or university hospital, which usually employs them; their names and phone numbers should then be added to the case manager's list of networking contacts.

Although the following diseases or conditions are the most common reasons for high-technology wound care, they are not the only ones. Complex wound care is frequently associated with such conditions as:

- Multiple traumatic wounds and infections
- Amputation and any complicating after-care conditions
- Surgical wounds complicated by infections, dehiscence, or fistulas
- Stoma care after a tracheostomy, ileostomy, colostomy, or urostomy
- Cancerous lesions, with complications
- Necrotizing fasciitis
- Arterial, diabetic, or venous ulcers
- Pressure sores

Readiness for Discharge

Case variables dictate when the patient with complex wounds is actually ready for discharge. In most situations, patients with complex wounds are ready for discharge when:

- The patient is medically stable.
- The infection and treatment are medically appropriate for care outside the acute care facility.

- The patient has tolerated the initial course of antimicrobial agent without problems.
- The home environment is adequate and clean.
- The cost of the plan is financially feasible and cost effective.
- The family member, patient, and caregiver are capable of learning the techniques required.
- The patient and family are accepting of home care.
- Community resources are available and accessible.

Services Required for Discharge

The following services are commonly required for persons with ongoing wound care needs on discharge:

- Skilled nursing care from a home health agency (24-hour availability) for:
  - Monitoring, assessment, and reporting response to treatments
  - Teaching of all aspects of care, including emergency precautions when pertinent
  - Drawing of blood for laboratory testing
  - Actual provision of skilled care until patient, family member, or caregiver can demonstrate proficiency in all aspects of the actual care
  - Peripheral vein restarts for intravenous administration of medications
- Registered pharmacist or, when applicable, infusion agency for:
  - Delivery of supplies, equipment, and solutions
  - Troubleshooting for problems or maintenance of equipment
  - Review of medications (with physician) for response to cultures and other laboratory results
- Physician for:
  - Monitoring of treatment plan and changing orders in response to changing patient's medical needs
- Durable medical equipment company for:
  - Delivery and teaching of use of all equipment and supplies, when applicable
- Medical supplier for:
  - Delivery or supply of all dressings, solutions, and consumable wound care products
- Laboratory services for:
  - Appropriate laboratory studies, chemistry panels, and other tests
- Outpatient facilities for:

- Whirlpool treatments
- Physical therapy or other therapies
- Hyperbaric oxygen treatments
- Outpatient surgical center or other treatment facility capable of performing wound debridement

Anticipated Teaching

Teaching complex wound care depends on many factors. If teaching of all wound care techniques is required, all factors such as the teacher, the caregiver's abilities and limitations, the resources used, the time frame available for teaching, and so forth must be included in the case management plan. In most cases, teaching of wound care covers, at minimum, the following components:

- Importance of sterile technique (although some care and supplies can be "clean," the majority must be sterile).
- Care of catheters, tracheostomy tubes, and supplies.
- How to cope with the illness, psychosocial changes, limitations, and physical changes.
- Importance of a well-balanced diet, high in protein.
- Importance of cleanliness and dryness and adherence to instructions specific for the wound.
- Importance of proper positioning and repositioning changes every 2 hours.
- Physical therapy techniques, especially range-of-motion exercises, endurance, and how to minimize pain with movement.
- Pain control and a bowel elimination regimen.
- Signs and symptoms of complications or problems and when to call the physician.
- Safe handling of solutions and supplies.
- Safe handling of waste and its disposal.
- Procedures necessary for procurement of supplies.
- Venous site care and infusion pump care.
- Emergency precautions and when to call the physician or seek emergency care.

Equipment Needs

Equipment needs depend on the patient, the wound, and any patient limitations. However, the following equipment and related supplies are commonly needed by patients with complicated wounds:

- Water- or air-filled bed or alternating pressure mattress
- Sponge rubber "egg crate" mattress
- Silicone-, air-, water-, or gel-filled pads
- Sheepskin or synthetic equivalent
- Suction equipment (stationary and portable) and supplies—tracheal or gastric, when applicable
- Infusion pump (stationary and portable) and supplies, when applicable
- Pillows and repositioning devices
- Specialized heel or other extremity protection devices
- Alternating compression stockings
- Bedboard
- Trapeze
- Wheelchair or other mobility device

DRESSINGS AND SUPPLIES

As with equipment, the actual supplies required depend on the wound and the treatment regimen. In most cases, voluminous amounts of supplies are required. In addition, many items must be sterile as opposed to merely "clean." When sterile supplies are needed, storage space must be considered as well as their source and cost and the process that will be used to identify their expiration date. At minimum, the following wound care supplies may be necessary:

- Irrigating syringes and supplies
- Scissors and forceps or suture removal sets
- Gloves (sterile, if sterile technique is required)
- Specific gels, powders, or other typical agents (hydrocolloids, transparent dressings)
- Sterile dressings, gauze pads
- Tape
- Support dressings, conforming gauze bandage to hold wound dressings in place
- Irrigating solutions
- Wound and irrigating stoma bags and supplies
- Tracheal care supplies

Alternate Funding

In most cases, alternate funding sources are not necessary if the referral is related specifically to wound care. If a referral is needed, it is frequently related to other underlying medical conditions. The primary reason for a referral to an alternate funding source is because the patient's healthcare coverage limits or excludes the required care (e.g., if the care is needed long-term, this may be excluded from coverage, or the patient may have exhausted his or her day or dollar limit on home care).

A referral may be required if the patient's or family's out-of-pocket expenses for wound care supplies or skilled nursing visits are beyond their financial means yet are medically necessary. For instance, many healthcare payors have a set copayment for each visit, and if the patient requires daily visits for a month or more, this can amount to a substantial outlay of unexpected costs that may be beyond the family's financial means. In such cases, a referral to Medicaid or, in the case of a child, to the local Title V Children's Medical Services program may be necessary. However, these referrals vary with the details of the case. Also, such referrals depend on the alternate funding program's eligibility criteria and the specific criteria covering the benefits available for such services.

Services Required for Discharge

The actual services required for ongoing wound care vary with the case, but the following tests and treatments are likely to be ordered in any combination or any frequency:

- Ultrasound examinations and Doppler ultrasound examinations
- Wound debridement
- Skilled nursing care (most often ordered daily but may be twice daily or even more often)
- Whirlpool therapy
- Wound cultures
- Complete blood counts, cultures, and other laboratory tests to monitor the response to treatment
- Hyperbaric oxygen treatments

The physician's actual written treatment orders are the primary driving force behind the final case management plan specifying the resources and the frequency and intensity of services required.

Complications

Most wound care complications are preventable if adequate training has occurred and meticulous attention to detail has been paid to the care required. If complications do occur, they are often the result of:

- Infiltrates, if the patient is on infusion therapy
- Further deterioration of the wound site
- Allergic or systemic reactions
- Malnutrition
- Progression of the disease
- Noncompliance with care

Barriers to Discharge and Access to Care

Barriers to discharge occur frequently in patients with complex wounds. In most cases they are related to the actual infection, type of drainage, and type and frequency of treatments required and whether facility placement is necessary. The following barriers to discharge or access to care are encountered most frequently in patients requiring complex wound care:

- The wound is repulsive, and the caregiver is unable to manage the care required.
- The home environment is unsanitary.
- There is no home or the home is inadequate (e.g., no stove or running water).
- A caregiver is not available or is untrainable.
- The infection or wound care is not manageable in a subacute care facility or skilled nursing facility because of the frequency and scope of treatments required or because the facility cannot accept an infectious patient. This may be the most common reason for refusal to accept care, because many skilled nursing facilities were built before infection control standards were developed, and thus their ventilatory systems are not equipped to manage such patients.
- Transportation for return visits to the outpatient setting is not available.
- Community resources (e.g., home health agencies) are not available or are inadequate to handle the care required.
- A physician is not available for follow-up care.
- The patient's healthcare benefits are exhausted or limited.

SUMMARY

Complex wounds can have potentially serious consequences, including death, if they are not treated immediately and effectively. The need for complicated wound care is a reality in many case-managed patients. As a result, case managers must be familiar with the professional resources that can offer assistance with recommendations for the latest treatment modalities that have proved effective in caring for wounds.

REFERENCES

1. Berkow R, Fletcher AJ (1992). The Merck Manual of Diagnoses and Treatment, 16th ed. Rahway, NJ, Merck Research Laboratories, pp. 364-594.
2. Tierney LM Jr, et al (eds) (1996). Current Diagnoses and Treatment, 35th ed. Appleton-Lange, pp. 295-402.
3. Berkow R, Fletcher AJ (eds) (1992). Op. cit., pp. 1293-1378.
4. Tierney LM Jr, et al (eds) (1996). Op. cit., pp. 719-767.
5. Berkow R, Fletcher AJ (eds) (1992). Op. cit., pp. 737-930.
6. Tierney LM Jr, et al (eds) (1996). Op. cit., pp. 489-613.
7. Berkow R, Fletcher AJ (eds) (1992). Op. cit., pp. 1753-1912.
8. Tierney LM Jr, et al (eds) (1996). Op. cit., pp. 671-693.
9. TOKOS Medical Corporation (1993). High Risk Clinical Considerations in Pregnancy. Santa Ana, CA, TOKOS Medical Corporation.
10. Berkow R, Fletcher AJ (eds) (1992). Op. cit., pp. 931-1134.
11. Tierney LM Jr, et al (eds) (1996). Op. cit., pp. 972-1111.
12. Berkow R, Fletcher AJ (eds) (1992). Op. cit., pp. 1913-2316.
13. Berkow R, Fletcher AJ (eds) (1992). Op. cit., pp. 1379-1530.
14. Tierney LM Jr, et al (eds) (1996). Op. cit., pp. 858-914.
15. Berkow R, Fletcher AJ (eds) (1992). Op. cit., pp. 1645-1752.
16. Tierney LM Jr, et al (eds) (1996). Op. cit., pp. 795-857.
17. Berkow R, Fletcher AJ (eds) (1992). Op. cit., pp. 595-736.
18. Tierney LM Jr, et al (eds) (1996). Op. cit., pp. 214-294.
19. Berkow R, Fletcher AJ (eds) (1992). Op. cit., pp. 1-364, 1135-1292, 2317-2716.
20. Tierney LM Jr, et al (eds) (1996). Op. cit., pp. 1-213, 403-488, 1112-1438.
21. United Network for Organ Sharing (1996). Facts and Statistics 9/96. Richmond, VA, UNOS.
22. Nolan MT, Augustine SM (1995). Transplantation Nursing: Acute and Long-Term Management. Appleton-Lange, pp. 109-140.
23. Smith S (1990). Tissue and Organ Transplant: Implications for Professional Nursing Practice. St. Louis, Mosby-Year Book, pp. 210-243.
24. Nolan MT, Augustine SM (1995). Op. cit., pp. 141-163.
25. Smith S (1990). Op. cit., pp. 245-259.
26. Nolan MT, Augustine SM (1995). Op. cit., pp. 141-163.
27. Smith S (1990). Op. cit., pp. 260-272.
28. Nolan MT, Augustine SM (1995). Op. cit., pp. 165-199.
29. Smith S (1990). Op. cit., pp. 273-299.
30. Smith S (1990). Op. cit., pp. 301-311.
31. Nolan MT, Augustine SM (1995). Op. cit., pp. 201-237.
32. Smith S (1990). Op. cit., pp. 176-209.
33. Nolan MT, Augustine SM (1995). Op. cit., pp. 239-288.
34. Smith S (1990). Op. cit., pp. 312-337.
35. Nolan MT, Augustine SM (1995). Op. cit., pp. 319-351.

BIBLIOGRAPHY

Achaver BM (1987). Management of the Burned Patient. Stamford, CT, Appleton & Lange.

Ackley BJ, et al (eds) (1995). Nursing Diagnosis Handbook: A Guide to Planning Care, 2nd ed. St. Louis, Mosby–Year Book.

AIDS day health care centers: Next step in outpatient options (1992). Case Manag Advisor 3(3):38.

Allen K (1996). Nursing Care of the Addicted Client. Philadelphia, J.B. Lippincott.

American Spinal Injury Association (1996). Standards for neurological and functional classifications of spinal cord injury. *In* Dobkin BH (1996). Neurologic Rehabilitation. Philadelphia, F.A. Davis, p. 221.

Andrews MM, Boyle JS (1995). Transcultural Concepts in Nursing Care, 2nd ed. Philadelphia, J.B. Lippincott.

Anthony WA (1993). Recovery from mental illness: The guiding vision of the mental health service system in the 1990's. J Psychosoc Rehabil 16(4):11–24.

Areman E, et al (1992). Bone Marrow and Stem Cell Processing: A Manual of Current Techniques. Philadelphia, F.A. Davis.

Arras JD (1995). Bringing the Hospital Home: Ethical and Social Implications of High Tech Home Care. Baltimore, Johns Hopkins University Press, pp. 35-145.

Ashley BW, Cross-Skinner S (1992). Oncology nursing care delivery issues in the ambulatory setting. Curr Issues Cancer Nurs Updates 1(1):1–10.

Ashwanden P, et al (1990). Oncology Nursing Advances, Treatments and Trends into the 21st Century. Gaithersburg, MD, Aspen.

AWHONN (Association of Women's Health Obstetric and Neonatal Nurses) (1993). Core Curriculum for Maternal and Newborn Nursing. Mattson S, Smith JE (eds). Philadelphia, W.B. Saunders.

AWHONN (Association of Women's Health Obstetric and Neonatal Nurses) (1993). Core Curriculum for Neonatal Intensive Care Unit Nursing. Beachy P, Deacon J (eds). Philadelphia, W.B. Saunders.

Barry PD (1996). Psychosocial Nursing Care of Physically Ill Patients and Their Families, 3rd ed. Philadelphia, J.B. Lippincott.

Bartlett RH, Gazzeniga AB, Huxtable RE, et al (1982). Extracorporeal circulation (ECMO) in neonatal respiratory failure. Surgery 92:425-433.

Becker KL (1995). Principles and Practices of Endocrinology and Metabolism, 2nd ed. Philadelphia, J.B. Lippincott.

Bergstrom N, et al (1994). Pressure Ulcer Treatment: Clinical Practice Guidelines (AHCPA Publication No. 95-0653). Rockville, MD, U.S. Department of Health and Human Services.

Berkow R, Fletcher AJ (eds) (1992). The Merck Manual of Diagnosis and Therapy, 16th ed. Rahway, NJ, Merck & Co.

Bernard GR, et al (1994). The American-European consensus conference on ARDS: Definitions, mechanisms, relevant outcomes and clinical trial coordination. Am J Respir Crit Care Med 149:818-824.

Bille D (1981). Practical Approaches to Patient Teaching. Boston, Little, Brown.

Bleile KM (1993). The Care of Children with Long-Term Tracheostomies. San Diego, Singular Publishing Group.

Blumenfield M, Schoeps M (1993). Psychological Care of the Burn and Trauma Patient. Baltimore, Williams & Wilkins.

BMTs for breast cancer case management: Caught in the middle of controversy (1993). Case Manag Advisor 4(1):1–5.

Bontke CF, Boake C (1996). Principles of brain injury rehabilitation. *In* Braddom RL (1996). Physical Medicine and Rehabilitation. Philadelphia, W.B. Saunders.

Braddom RL (1996). Physical Medicine and Rehabilitation. Philadelphia, W.B. Saunders.

Bryant RA (1992). Acute and Chronic Wounds: Nursing Management. St. Louis, Mosby–Year Book.

Buckley K, Kulb NW (1990). High Risk Maternity Nursing Manual. Baltimore, Williams & Wilkins.

Burns SM, et al (1995). Weaning from long term mechanical ventilation. Am J Crit Care 4:4–22.

Burrow G, Ferris TF (1995). Medical Complications During Pregnancy, 4th ed. Philadelphia, W.B. Saunders.

Buchsel PC, Whedon MD (1995). Bone Marrow Transplantation Administration and Clinical Strategies. Boston, Jones and Bartlett.

Cahill MS (1996). Managing IV Therapy. Springhouse, PA, Springhouse Publishing.

Camp-Sorrell D (1990). Advanced central venous access, solution, catheters, devices and nursing management. J IV Nurs 13(6):361-370.

Carnevali DL, Patrick M (1993). Nursing Management of the Elderly, 3rd ed. Philadelphia, J.B. Lippincott.

Carson VB, Arnold EN (1996). Mental Health Nursing—The Nurse Patient Journey. Philadelphia, W.B. Saunders.

Case managing HIV-infected pregnant women requires extra level of sensitivity (1991). Case Manag Advisor 2(11):161-165.

Cassel CK, et al (1990). Geriatric Medicine, 2nd ed. New York, Springer-Verlag.

CDCP's new definitions for AIDS could increase case management caseloads (1993). Case Manag Advisor 4(1):5-7.

Cerille GJ, et al (1988). Organ Transplantation and Replacement. Philadelphia, J.B. Lippincott.

Chacho BP, Kotula C (1995). Perinatal case management: Foregoing short-term limitations for long-term savings. Continuing Care 14(7):28-37.

Chemotherapy and You: A Guide to Self-Help During Treatment (1995). NIH Publication No. 95-1136. Bethesda, MD, National Cancer Institute.

Children's needs determine types of case manager assigned to families (1991). Case Manag Advisor 2(10):152-153.

Chin-Chu L, et al (1993). The High Risk Fetus: Pathophysiology, Diagnosis, Management. New York, Springer-Verlag.

Churg J, et al (1995). Renal Disease Classifications and Atlas of Glomerular Disease, 2nd ed. New York, Igaker-Shoin.

Ciraulo DA, Shaders RI (1991). Clinical Manual of Chemical Dependency. Washington, DC, American Psychiatric Press.

Clemen-Stone S, et al (1995). Comprehensive Community Health Nursing: Family Aggregate and Community Practice, 4th ed. St. Louis, Mosby–Year Book.

Conners RB, Winters RW (1995). Home Infusion Therapy: Current Status and Future Trends. Chicago, American Hospital Publishing.

Curtan S, et al (1996). Case management in home TPN: A cost identified analysis. J Parenter Enter Nutr 20(2):113.

Daugirdas JT, Ing TS (1994). Handbook of Dialysis, 2nd ed. Boston, Little, Brown.

Davidson L, Strauss JS (1992). Sense of self in recovery for severe mental illness. Br J Med Psychol 65(Pt 2):131-145.

Davidson MB (1991). Diabetes Mellitus: Diagnosis and Treatment, 3rd ed. New York, Churchill Livingstone.

Davis H (1991). Counseling families of children with disabilities. *In* Davis H, Fallowfield L (eds) (1991). Counseling and Communication in Health Care. New York, John Wiley and Sons.

Davis T, et al (1990). The gap between reading comprehension and the readability of patient educational material. Fam Pract 31(5):533-538.

Dellasega C, et al (1994). Use of home health services by elderly persons with cognitive impairment. J Nurs Admin 24(6):20-25.

DeLisa JA, et al (1993). Rehabilitation Medicine: Principles and Practice, 2nd ed. Philadelphia, J.B. Lippincott.

Develop protocols to ensure quality placements for mental health clients (1992). Case Manag Advisor 3(6):73-79.

Dobkin BH (1996). Neurologic Rehabilitation. Philadelphia, F.A. Davis.

Divon MY (1991). Abnormal Fetal Growth. New York, Elsevier.

Early aggressive case management gives patient the key to survival with HIV (1996). Case Manag Advisor 7(1):1-4.

Errico TJ, et al (1991). Spinal Trauma. Philadelphia, J.B. Lippincott.

Evans R (1996). Neurology and Trauma. Philadelphia, W.B. Saunders.

Falvo DR (1994). Effective Patient Education: A Guide to Increased Compliance. Gaithersburg, MD, Aspen.

Finances often are elderly women's greatest long term care problem (1991). Case Manag Advisor 2(10):149-151.

Flaskerud JH, Ungvarski PJ (1995). HIV/AIDS: A Guide to Nursing Care, 3rd ed. Philadelphia, W.B. Saunders.

Flye MW (1995). Atlas of Organ Transplantation. Philadelphia, W.B. Saunders.

Fisher M (ed) (1994). Cerebrovascular Disorders. St. Louis, Mosby-Year Book.

Foley GV, et al (1993). Nursing Care of the Child with Cancer, 2nd ed. Philadelphia, W.B. Saunders.

Foreman MD, Fletcher K (1996). Assessing cognitive function. Geriatr Nurs 17(5):228-232.

Foreman MD, Zane D (1996). Nursing strategies for acute confusion in elders. Am J Nurs 96(4):44-52.

Fraley AM (1992). Nursing and the Disabled Across the Life Span. Boston, Jones and Bartlett.

Fuchs AR, et al (1993). Premature Birth: Causes, Prevention and Management, 2nd ed. New York, McGraw-Hill.

Gaedeke MK (1996). Pediatric and Neonatal Critical Care. St. Louis, Mosby-Year Book.

Gaedeke-Norris MK, House MA (1991). Organ and Tissue Transplantation: Nursing Care from Procurement Through Rehabilitation. Philadelphia, F.A. Davis.

Gale D, Charette J (1995). Oncology Nursing Care Plans. El Paso, TX, Skidmore-Roth.

Geniusz G (1995). Future trends affecting the home infusion therapy industry. Caring 14(5):58.

Gerson V (1996). Pediatric case management. Case Review 2(1):20-62.

Glass C, et al (1996). Collaborative support for caregivers of individuals beginning mechanical ventilation at home. Clin Care Nurse 16(4):67-72.

Gogia PP (1995). Clinical Wound Management. Thorofare, NJ, Slack.

Gokal R, Nolph KD (1994). The Textbook of Peritoneal Dialysis. Norwell, MA, Kluwer Academic Publishers.

Graham DR (1993). Nosocomial infections: Complications of home intravenous therapy. Infect Dis Clin Pract 2(2):158-163.

Gralnick A (1985). Build a better state hospital: Deinstitutionalization has failed. Hosp Commun Psychiatr 36:738-741.

Graves D (1995). Home infusion therapy: Meeting a need. Nurs Manag 26(8):32.

Groth CG (1988). Pancreatic Transplantation. Philadelphia, W.B. Saunders.

Guralnik J, Simonsick E (1993). Physical disability in older Americans. J Gerontol 48:3-10.

Haggard A (1989). Handbook of Patient Education. Gaithersburg, MD, Aspen.

Hall KM, et al (1993). Characteristics and comparisons of functional assessment indices: Disability rating scale, functional independence measure, and functional assessment measure. J Head Injury Rehabil 8(2):60-74.

Hall P (1996). Providing psychological support. Am J Nurs 96(10):16N-16P.

Hanneman SK, et al (1994). Weaning from short term mechanical ventilation: A review. Am J Crit Care 3:421-443.

Harris JA (1996). Recording brain injury rehabilitation. Continuing Care 15(7):41-44.

Haynes VL (1996). Caring for the laryngectomy patient. Am J Nurs 9(5):16B-16K.

Heidrich S (1993). The relationship between physical health and psychological well-being in elderly women: A developmental perspective. Res Nurs Health 16:123-130.

Henrick W (1994). Principles and Practices of Dialysis. Baltimore, Williams & Wilkins.

Hickey JV (1992). The Clinical Practice of Neurological and Neurosurgical Nursing, 3rd ed. Philadelphia, J.B. Lippincott.

Hirsch IB, et al (1990). Intensive insulin therapy for treatment of type I diabetes mellitus. Diabetes Care 13(12):1265.

Hochschuler SH, et al (1993). Rehabilitation of the Spine: Science and Practice. St. Louis, Mosby-Year Book.

Holland JC, Rowland JH (1989). Handbook of Psychooncology: Psychological Care of the Patient with Cancer. New York, Oxford University Press.

Holloway NM (1993). Nursing the Critically Ill Adult, 4th ed. Reading, MA, Addison-Wesley.

Home and community-based options expand for psychiatric cases (1993). Case Manag Advisor 4(6):75-78.

Home infusion therapy: Know what you're getting for the money (1993). Case Manag Advisor 4(8):108-112.

Hoobs N, et al (1985). Chronically Ill Children and Their Families. San Francisco, Jossey-Bass.

Hurt SW, et al (1991). Psychological Assessment, Psychiatric Diagnoses and Treatment Planning. New York, Brunner/Mazel Publishers.

Identifying at-risk seniors prevents costly admissions (1996). Case Manag Advisor 7(1):4-8.

Ignatavicius DD, Hausman KA (1995). Clinical Pathways for Collaboration. Philadelphia, W.B. Saunders.

Iyers PW, Camp NH (1995). Nursing Documentation. St. Louis, Mosby-Year Book.

Jackson DB, Saunders RB (1993). Child Health Nursing: A Comprehensive Approach to Care of Children and Their Families. Philadelphia, J.B. Lippincott.

Jackson KL (1988). Smith's Recognizable Patterns of Human Malformations. Philadelphia, W.B. Saunders.

Jackson PL, Vessey JA (1996). Primary Care of the Child With a Chronic Condition, 2nd ed. St. Louis, Mosby-Year Book.

Johnson BS (1993). Adaptation and Growth: Psychiatric Mental Health Nursing. Philadelphia, J.B. Lippincott.

Johnson T (1991). Mental health, social relations, and social selection: A longitudinal analysis. J Health Soc Behav 32:408-423.

Kanter JS (1987). Mental health case management: A professional domain? Social Work 32:461-462.

Katzung BG (1995). Basic and Clinical Pharmacology, 6th ed. Stamford, CT, Appleton & Lange.

Kenner C, et al (1993). Comprehensive Neonatal Nursing: A Physiologic Perspective. Philadelphia, W.B. Saunders.

Kersten LD (1989). Comprehensive Respiratory Nursing. Philadelphia, W.B. Saunders.

Klaus MH, Avroy AR (1993). Care of the High Risk Neonate, 4th ed. Philadelphia, W.B. Saunders.

Knebel AR (1996). Ventilator weaning protocol and techniques: Getting the job done. AACN Clinical Issue 7(4):550-559.

Krach P (1992). Discovering the secret: Nursing assessment of elderly alcoholism in the home. J Gerontol Nurs 16(11):32-38.

Krach P (1993). Assessment of depressed older persons living in a home setting. Home Healthcare Nurse 13(3):61-64.

Krasner D (1990). Chronic Wound Care: A Clinical Source Book for Healthcare Professionals. King of Prussia, PA, Health Management Publications.

Kropfelder L, Winkelstein M (1996). A case management approach to pediatric asthma. Pediatr Nurs 22(4):291-295.

Lanterman F (1986). Developmental Disabilities Act and Developmental Disabilities Assistance. Bill of Rights. California Welfare and Institutions Code, Sections 4-5. Sacramento, CA, Office of State Publishing.

Lawrence JC (1994). Dressings and wound infection. Am J Surg 167(1A):215-245.

Lebowitz H, et al (1994). Therapy for Diabetes Mellitus and Related Disorders, 2nd ed. Alexandria, VA, American Diabetic Association.

Lee M (1996). Drugs and the elderly: Do you know the risks? Am J Nurs 96(7):25-31.

Leninger M (1995). Transcultural Nursing Concepts: Theories, Research and Practice. New York, McGraw-Hill.

Leon RL (1988). Psychiatric Interviewing: A Primer, 2nd ed. New York, Elsevier.

Levin HS, et al (1987). Neurobehavioral Recovery from Head Injury. New York, Oxford University Press.

Lewis CB (1990). Aging: The Health Care Challenge, 2nd ed. Philadelphia, F.A. Davis.

Lilley LL, Guanci R (1996). Educate the patient. Am J Nurs 96(4):14-16.

Lindeman CA (1988). Individual characteristics such as age, social status and education level influence teaching effectiveness and long-term behavior. Ann Rev Nurs Res 6:29-60.

Locas AB (1992). A critical review of venous devices: The nursing perspective. Curr Issues Nurs Pract Updates 1(7):1-10.

Loeb S, et al (eds) (1992). Teaching Patients with Chronic Conditions. Springhouse, PA, Springhouse.

Loeb S, et al (eds) (1994). Handbook of Medical-Surgical Nursing. Springhouse, PA, Springhouse, pp. 252-258.

Long CJ, Ross LK (eds) (1992). Handbook of Head Trauma: Acute Care to Recovery. New York, Plenum Press.

Martyn JA (1990). Acute Management of the Burned Patient. Philadelphia, W.B. Saunders.

Masoocli S (1996). Home IV therapy comes of age. RN 10:23-26.

McConville BJ, et al (1990). Pediatric bone marrow transplants: Psychological aspects. Can J Psychiatr 35:769-775.

McCubbin HI, Patterson JM (1982). Family adaptation to crisis. *In* McCubbin HI, et al (eds) (1982). Family Stress, Coping and Social Support. Springfield, IL, CC Thomas, pp. 24-47.

Miaskowski C (1997). Oncology Nursing: An Essential Guide to Patient Care. Philadelphia, W.B. Saunders.

Milkovick G (1993). Outpatient parenteral antibiotic therapy: Costs and benefits. Hosp Pract 28(1):39.

Miller CA (1995). Nursing Care of Older Adults: Theory and Practice. Philadelphia, J.B. Lippincott.

Miller JF (1992). Coping with Chronic Illness: Overcoming Powerlessness, 2nd ed. Philadelphia, F.A. Davis.

Miller MP, Duffey J (1993). Planning and program development for psychiatric home care. J Nurs Admin 23(11):35-41.

Moore EE (ed) (1990). Early Care of the Injured Patient. Philadelphia, B.C. Decker.

Murray RB, Zenter JP (1993). Nursing Assessment and Health Promotion Strategies Through the Life Span, 5th ed. Stamford, CT, Appleton & Lange.

National Cancer Institute (1988). What are clinical trials all about? Office of Cancer Communications (NIH Publication No. 88-2706). Bethesda, MD, National Cancer Institute.

National Cancer Institute (1993). Radiation Therapy and You: A Guide to Self-Help During Treatment. (NIH Publication No. 95-2227). Bethesda, MD, National Cancer Institute.

National Cancer Institute (1996). Taking Time to Support People with Cancer and the People Who Care about Them. (NIH Publication No. 96-2059). Bethesda, MD, National Cancer Institute.

National Coalition for Cancer Survivorship (NCCS) Patient/ Doctor Communication Committee (1991). Teamwork: The Cancer Patient's Guide to Talking with Your Doctor. National Coalition for Cancer Survivorship and Lederle Laboratories. Wayne, NJ.

New options emerge in cost-conscious mental health arena (1991). Case Manag Advisor 2(5):68-70.

Oeth K (1996). Care for Children at Home. Continuing Care 15(7):35-48.

Ostrow DG (ed) (1990). Behavioral Aspects of AIDS. New York, Plenum Publishers.

Otto SE (1994). Oncology Nursing, 2nd ed. St. Louis, Mosby-Year Book.

Pachter LM (1994). Culture and clinical care: Folk illness, beliefs and behaviors and their implications for health-care delivery. JAMA 271(9):690-694.

Paniagua FA (1994). Assessing and Treating Culturally Diverse Clients. Thousand Oaks, CA, Sage Publications.

Peter JW, et al (1990). Diabetes and Its Management, 4th ed. Cambridge, MA, Blackwell Scientific Publishers.

Pheneuf C (1996). Screening elders for nutritional deficits. Am J Nurs 96(3):58-60.

Pollack ML, Schmidt DH (1986). Heart and Disease and Rehabilitation. New York, John Wiley and Sons.

Pollack S, et al (1990). Responses to chronic illness: Analysis of psychological and physiological adaptation. Nurs Res 37:300-304.

Porter RR, et al (1991). Stress during the waiting period: A review of pre-transplantation fears. Crit Care Nurs Q 13:25-31.

Portez DM, et al (1982). Intravenous antibiotic therapy in an outpatient setting. JAMA 248:336-339.

Portez DM (1993). Models for delivery: Infusion center, office and home. Hosp Pract (Suppl) 2:40-43.

Proper assessment of medications can stave off a host of problems in frail, elderly clients (1991). Case Manag Advisor 2(5):65-68.

Radde IC, MacLeod SM (1993). Pediatric Pharmacology and Therapeutics. St. Louis, Mosby-Year Book.

Rector WG (1992). Complications of Chronic Liver Disease. St. Louis, Mosby-Year Book.

Reilly BM (1991). Practical Strategies in Outpatient Medicine, 2nd ed. Philadelphia, W.B. Saunders.

Reynolds JM, et al (1991). Changes in psychosocial adjustment after renal transplantation. Arch Dis Child 66:508-513.

Rice R (1995). Manual of Home Health Nursing Procedures. St. Louis, Mosby-Year Book.

Rizzo M, Tranel D (1996). Head Injury and Postconcussive Syndrome. New York, Churchill Livingstone.

Robin NI (1996). The Clinical Handbook of Endocrinology and Metabolic Disease. Pearl River, NY, Parthenon.

Robertson C, Cerrato PL (1993). Managing diabetes mellitus: A major study injects good news. RN 10:26-29.

Rorden JW, Taft E (1990). Discharge Planning Guide for Nurses. Philadelphia, W.B. Saunders.

Roth EJ, Harvery RL (1996). Rehabilitation of stroke syndromes. *In* Braddom RL (1996). Physical Medicine and Rehabilitation. Philadelphia, W.B. Saunders.

Sanderson RG, Kurth CL (1983). The Cardiac Patient: A Comprehensive Approach, 2nd ed. Philadelphia, W.B. Saunders.

Schielke C (1996). Finding the key to recovery. Continuing Care 15(8):24-42.

Schover LR, Randers-Pehron M (eds) (1988). Sexuality and Cancer. New York, American Cancer Society.

Schultz JM, Videback SD (1994). Manual of Psychiatric Nursing Care Plans, 4th ed. Philadelphia, J.B. Lippincott.

Segatore M (1994). Understanding chronic pain after spinal cord injury. J Neurosci Nurs 26:230-235.

Shapiro J (1983). Family reactions and coping strategies in response to the physically ill or handicapped child: A review. Soc Sci Med 17(14):913-931.

Shurman SA (1987). A model of case management of mental health services. Q Rev Bull 13:314-317.

Siegler EL, Whitney FW (1994). Nurse-Physician Collaboration. New York, Springer Publishing.

Sigardson-Poor KM, Haggerty LM (1990). Nursing Care of Transplant Patients. Philadelphia, W.B. Saunders.

Sinaki M (ed) (1993). Basic Clinical Rehabilitation Medicine, 2nd ed. St. Louis, Mosby-Year Book.

Sivak ED, et al (1995). The High Risk Patient: Management of the Critically Ill. Baltimore, Williams & Wilkins.

Skewer SM (1996). Skin Care Rituals that Do More Harm than Good. Am J Nurs 96(10):33-35.

Smith CM, Maurer FA (1995). Community Health Nursing: Theory and Practice. Philadelphia, W.B. Saunders.

Smith R (1996). RCP's in case management. Case Review 2(1):65-71.

Smith SL (1990). Tissue and Organ Transplantation: Implications for Professional Nursing Practices. St. Louis, Mosby-Year Book.

Snyder B (1996). An easy way to document patient education. RN 59(3):43-45.

Snyder M (1991). A Guide to Neurological and Neurosurgical Nursing. Charlotte, NC, Delmar Publications.

Stanhope M, Knollmueller RN (1992). Handbook of Community and Home Health Nursing. St. Louis, Mosby-Year Book.

Steele J (1996). Practical IV Therapy, 2nd ed. Springhouse, PA, Springhouse.

Stone CS, et al (1995). Community Health Nursing: Family Aggregate and Community Practice, 4th ed. St. Louis, Mosby-Year Book.

Stoves SL, et al (1995). Spinal Cord Injury: Clinical Outcomes from the Model Systems. Gaithersburg, MD, Aspen.

Swenson JP (1981). Training patients to administer intravenous antibiotics at home. Am J Hosp Pharm 38:1480-1483.

Taylor RB (1991). Difficult Medical Management. Philadelphia, W.B. Saunders.

Terry J, et al (1995). Intravenous Therapy: Clinical Principles and Practices. Philadelphia, W.B. Saunders.

Thal LJ, et al (eds) (1992). Cognitive Disorders: Pathophysiology and Treatment. New York, Marcel Dekker.

Thompson RC (1995). Protecting "human guinea pigs." *In* FDA Consumer From Test Tube Patient: New Drug Developments in the United States, 2nd ed. (DHHS Publication No. 95-3168). Washington, DC, Department of Health and Human Services, pp. 14-18.

Tierney LM Jr, et al (1996). Current Medical Diagnosis and Treatment, 35th ed. Stamford, CT, Appleton & Lange.

Thoene JG (1995). Physician's Guide to Rare Diseases, 2nd ed. Montvale, NJ, Dowden.

Thomas DO (1996). Assessing children: It's different. RN 4:38-44.

Tobin MJ (1994). Principles and Practice of Mechanical Ventilation. New York, McGraw-Hill.

TOKOS Medical Corporation (1993). High Risk Clinical Considerations in Pregnancy. Santa Ana, CA, TOKOS Medical Corporation.

Tollison CD, et al (eds) (1994). Handbook of Pain Management. Baltimore, Williams & Wilkins.

Transplant case management increasing in complexity (1995). Case Manag Advisor 4(7):95-98.

Trella RS (1993). A multidisciplinary approach to case management of frail, hospitalized older adults. J Nurs Admin 23(2):20-26.

Trofino RB (1991). Nursing Care of the Burn Injured Patient. Philadelphia, F.A. Davis.

Ulrich SP (1995). Nursing Care Plans and Documentation, 2nd ed. Philadelphia, J.B. Lippincott.

Ulrich BT (1989). Nephrology Nursing: Concepts and Strategies. Stamford, CT, Appleton & Lange.

Ungvarski PJ (1995). Adults and HIV/AIDS: Clinical considerations for care management. J Care Manag 1(3):40-63.

Waechter EH, et al (1985). Nursing Care of Children. Philadelphia, J.B. Lippincott.

Walker D (1996). Choosing the correct wound dressing. Am J Nurs 96(9):35-39.

Watch for signs of neglect when helping elderly clients (1992). Case Manag Advisor 3(3):39-40.

Watkins PJ, et al (1990). Diabetes and Its Management, 4th ed. Cambridge, MA, Blackwell Scientific Publications.

West P, Sieloff-Evans CL (1992). Psychiatric and Mental Health Nursing with Children and Adolescents. Gaithersburg, MD, Aspen.

White AH, Schafferman JA (1995). Spine Care: Diagnoses and Conservative Treatment. St. Louis, Mosby-Year Book.

Whyte J (1986). The care and rehabilitation of the patient in a persistent vegetative state. J Head Trauma Rehabil 3:39-53.

Wickwire PA (1990). Nutrition and HIV: Your Choices Made a Difference. New York, National Hemophilic Foundation.

Williams JW (1990). Hepatic Transplantation. Philadelphia, W.B. Saunders.

Williams SR (1994). Essentials of Nutrition and Diet Therapy, 6th ed. St. Louis, Mosby-Year Book.

Winkelstein MA (1995). Case management approach to pediatric asthma. Pediatr Nurs 22(4):291-295.

Wong DL (1995). Waley and Wong's Nursing Care of Infants and Children, 5th ed. St. Louis, Mosby-Year Book.

Workman ML, et al (1993). Nursing Care of the Immunocompromised Patient. Philadelphia, W.B. Saunders.

Yarkony GM (1994). Spinal Cord Injury, Medical Management and Rehabilitation. Gaithersburg, MD, Aspen.

Yen P (1994). Boosting intake when appetite is poor. Geriatr Nurs 15(5):294.

Zaloga GP (1994). Nutrition in Critical Care. St. Louis, Mosby-Year Book.

Zejdlik CP (1992). Management of Spinal Cord Injury, 2nd ed. Boston, Jones and Bartlett.

Zook R (1996). Take action before anger builds. RN 4:46-49.

Chapter 11

Post-Acute Care

PRINCIPLES FOR DETERMINING SKILLED VERSUS CUSTODIAL SERVICE

The purpose of this section is to highlight the basic issues that help a case manager to determine whether a service is skilled or custodial (Fig. 11-1). In many cases the answer is not clear cut—this may be one of the most problematic areas case managers encounter—and all factors of the case must be taken into consideration before a final determination is made. When in doubt, it is wise always to review the case with the medical director or a physician advisor from a related specialty (i.e., a neurologist for neurology cases). Also, denials can never be issued by a nurse or case manager, only by a physician.

In making the determination that a patient requires skilled or custodial care, one must examine the current level and complexity of care and whether the patient needs medical supervision or direct care. This done, one must then ask, if these services were discontinued would there be a significant probability (as opposed to possibility) that the patient would be at risk for complications or further need for acute

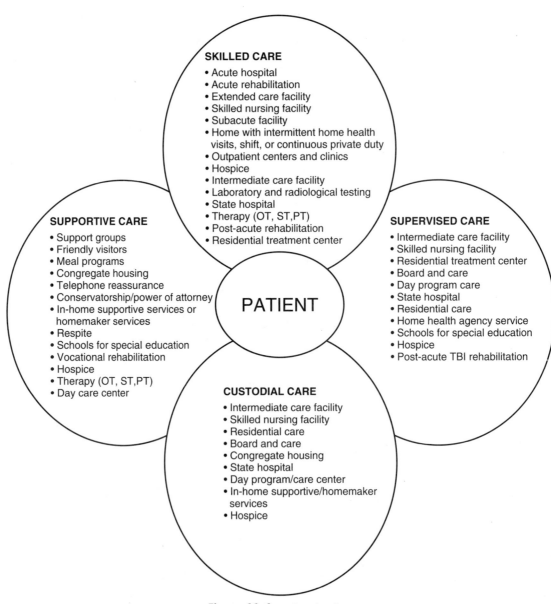

Figure 11-1 • Levels of care.

care? Just because a patient has a caregiver who is trained to provide the care does not necessarily mean that the care is not skilled. Similarly, just because a patient has a spouse or other relative or significant other does not mean that person can provide the required care. In both cases, skilled professionals may be required indefinitely for either supervision or actual provision of direct care.

Decisions for coverage of skilled care must not be based on diagnosis, number of diagnoses, type of condition, degree of functional limitations, rehabilitation potential or prognosis, or the fact that someone is living with the patient. Decisions must be based on medical necessity, the complexity of prescribed service, and the fact that it can be performed safely or effectively under the general supervision or by direct involvement of licensed nursing or rehabilitation professionals.

Definitions

To be considered skilled, a service must be so inherently complex that it can be performed safely and effectively only by or under the supervision of a licensed healthcare professional—a registered nurse, licensed vocational or practical nurse, physical therapist, occupational therapist, or speech therapist—to ensure that care is rendered safely and the desired results achieved.[1]

In contrast, custodial care can be defined as care rendered to a person who is mentally or physically incapable of providing the care to himself. It is also appropriate for any person who requires a protected, monitored, or controlled environment, whether at home or in an institution.[2] In most cases, custodial care is the care that is required to support or sustain a person and allow the person to have activities of daily living (ADL) provided. Activities of daily living are activities associated with safety, food preparation, feeding, toileting, grooming, mobility, and positioning. Just because a caregiver has mastered the techniques to render the skilled care does not mean the services are no longer skilled or the patient is custodial.

Examples of Skilled Nursing Services

The following are examples of skilled care:

- Observation and assessment when a patient's condition requires the expertise of licensed personnel to identify and evaluate for possible modifications of the treatment plan. Observation may be required for initiation of medical procedures or for stabilization of the patient. It is also necessary for reporting findings to the physician for possible adjustments to orders and to the treatment plan (e.g. for a patient taking anticoagulant therapy, the medication continues to be adjusted in response to laboratory data).
- Treatments for open wounds or ulcers that require both objective and subjective evaluation and documentation of size, depth, amount and frequency of drainage, signs of granulation, and evidence of further infection. This also includes (1) application of dressings involving prescription medication or requiring aseptic technique and other wound care, and (2) initial care of ostomies and associated care (as a rule, skilled care is necessary only during the early postoperative [learning] period or until the patient demonstrates proficiency).
- Positioning and transfer of a patient with a newly repaired hip fracture or as outlined by the physical therapist in the therapy treatment plan.
- Intravenous, intramuscular, and subcutaneous injections (as a rule administration of insulin is considered a skilled-care activity only when diabetes is newly diagnosed or frequent dosage adjustments are necessary).
- Nasogastric feedings are considered custodial, whereas gastrostomy or jejunostomy findings may be considered custodial, as there is no risk for aspiration or complications as with a nasaogastric tube.
- Insertion, sterile irrigation, and replacement of urinary catheters (excluding general maintenance of such catheters).
- Heat treatments that require direct application of heat and supervision and evaluation of progress or results.
- Rehabilitative nursing or therapy for self-care skills, ambulation or mobility, communication, or other needs or as outlined by the physical therapist, occupational therapist, or speech therapist for the treatment plan.
- Initial phases of medical gases, inhalation, or bronchodilator therapy.
- Initial phases of intravenous chemotherapy or other intravenous medications.
- Nasopharyngeal or tracheal suctioning.
- Teaching and training of patient, family, or other caregiver in any of the foregoing activities.

Examples of Skilled Rehabilitation Therapy

The following are examples of skilled rehabilitation modalities:

- Services directly and specifically related to the patient's condition.
- Services so technical or complex and sophisticated that they require the judgment and expertise of a licensed professional therapist.
- Services that cannot be carried out by therapy aides or other unlicensed personnel.

The deciding factor in skilled therapy coverage should not be the patient's potential for recovery alone. For example, patients with a diagnosis of terminal cancer can still be taught to be as independent as their pain allows.

Other factors that must be considered when determining if rehabilitation services are skilled include:

- The patient is medically stable and able to participate consistently in a therapy program.
- The patient has an appropriate diagnosis or recently experienced an acute change in functional status or onset of a condition or trauma that requires rehabilitation.
- There is an expectation that the patient's condition will improve significantly within a reasonable (and generally predictable) time.

Responsibilities of the Three Therapy Disciplines

Basically, the three therapy disciplines perform the following:

Physical therapy serves patients with neuromuscular and functional disorders from a cardiovascular accident, transient ischemic attack, spinal cord injury, head injury, Guillain-Barré syndrome, total hip or other joint replacement, closed or open reductions of fractures, diabetic neuropathy, amputation, a congenital anomaly, or another neurologic condition.

Speech therapy aims to restore speech or teach an alternative communication technique or to treat swallowing disorders (only when there is a coexisting communication disorder) or cognitive deficits.

Occupational therapy is intended to retrain for ADL and instruct in the use of adaptive devices, safety, neuromuscular reeducation and fine motor coordination, toilet and tub or shower transfer, positioning and splinting, oral or bulbar exercises, retraining and diet progression, and sensory or perceptual retraining.

TREATMENT MODALITIES

Some of the most common skilled modalities rendered by physical, occupational, or speech therapists are:

- Assessment and initial evaluation for rehabilitation needs and potential (tests are conducted to measure range of motion [ROM], pain, strength, balance, coordination, endurance, safety, self-care dependence, mobility dependence, perceptual or motor loss, need for ambulatory, mobility, or self-help devices, muscle spasticity, and functional ability).
- Development of a therapeutic exercise and gait training or rehabilitation program (if ambulation is impaired by a neurologic, muscular, or skeletal disorder and significant improvement in the patient's mobility is expected) and ongoing performance of therapeutic exercise or mobility treatments.
- Development of an ROM or maintenance program to prevent or minimize atrophy. (Once this assessment is accomplished, if ROM is the only treatment modality identified by the therapist and is not related to the restoration of a specific loss of function and if the patient has no other skilled nursing needs, the care level is most often classified as custodial.)
- Ultrasound, short-wave, or microwave diathermy treatments.
- Hot packs, infrared treatments, paraffin baths, whirlpool treatments, and débridement.

FUNCTIONAL LIMITATIONS

Functional capabilities may be limited by physical, mental or cognitive, social, or economic factors.[3] Such criteria are usually utilized by the rehabilitation team to evaluate whether a patient is ready for the next level of care or discharge. Thus, it is common to hear the healthcare team discuss functional abilities, independence, limitations, and disabilities as they measure the patient's physical functioning and ability to perform ADL.

Examples of Custodial or Unskilled Care and Supportive Services

The services related to ADL are considered custodial, unskilled, or supportive and include:

- Administration of routine oral medications, eye drops, and ointments.
- General maintenance of ostomies.
- Routine care of indwelling bladder catheters and self-catheterization.
- General maintenance and methods for treating incontinence, including use of diapers.
- Wound care for uninfected postoperative or chronic conditions.
- Prophylactic and palliative skin care, including bathing, application of creams or lotions, and repositioning.
- Use of heat for palliative purposes.
- General administration of oxygen and other inhalation treatments after the initial phase of teaching and treatment adjustments are completed.
- General supervision of exercises including ROM.
- Assistance with eating, dressing, and toileting.
- Long-term feeding by gastrostomy tube.

Unfortunately and often erroneously, healthcare payors often view any skilled care that has been mastered by caregivers to be custodial, and then usually terminate benefits. The designation of custodial care in no way implies that the care being rendered is less than skilled; it means only that such care is not reimbursable. When termination of benefits occurs, the case management plan must include some form of monitoring, to ensure that family members or other caregivers stay abreast of the skilled care techniques that may have to be implemented as the patient's condition changes.

Documentation—The Key to Support Decisions

When conducting chart reviews for discharge planning needs, key data that support *skilled care* are as follows:

- Physician orders, progress notes, nursing or therapy notes that reveal the following facts:
  - Medical necessity for skilled care.
  - Date of initial treatment.
  - Number or frequency of treatments.
  - Response or tolerance to treatment.
  - Evidence of deterioration, instability, or change of condition that necessitates close skilled monitoring or calls to a physician.
  - Necessity for teaching.
  - Evidence of current functional limitations and capabilities.

- Requirement for skilled services.
- Short- and long-term goals.
- Adjustments or changes to the care plan, when a change of condition is evident and orders support such adjustments.
- Amount, specific characteristics, odor, depth, size, involved area, and type of drainage or secretions, and frequency of suctioning or dressing changes.
- Problems with treatments or teaching.
- Frequent medication adjustments.
- Caregiver's skills.
- Patient or family noncompliance or indifference to treatment.

In contrast, *custodial care coverage* can often be determined by facts such as these:

- Patient is clinically stable.
- A routine of self-care or taking medications has been mastered.
- A plateau or maintenance level of care has been achieved.
- The procedure can safely be done by someone at a less skilled level of care, or the care has been mastered by the patient or a caregiver.
- Assistance is required only for ADL.
- Medication changes, if any, are infrequent and laboratory values are stable and indicate a response to treatment.

When documentation is poor and continued benefit coverage or coverage for the next level of care is in question, it may be helpful to interview staff and conduct on-site evaluation of the patient to observe firsthand what the patient can and cannot do.

Documentation is the key to coverage when services might be considered skilled. In such cases, the medical complication and special services required must be performed, supervised, or observed by a professional and documented not only by the physician's orders but also in the nursing and therapy notes; otherwise there is nothing to support and justify skilled care. *(If it's not documented, it didn't happen!)*

Skilled care benefits may be terminated once the patient reaches a plateau and further significant functional gains are minimal or cease, the condition stabilizes, a pattern of care is established, or the patient or other caregiver has learned to provide the care. Documentation plays a key role in termination of benefits when the patient reaches a custodial level. For instance, the healthcare payor may deem a patient on a ventilator custodial if a patient's blood gases and all vital signs remain stable and the frequency of suctioning and the level of care do not vary. In cases like this, care is deemed custodial because the patient's condition is probably "as good as it will get."

HOME PLACEMENT VERSUS OUT-OF-HOME PLACEMENT

Returning a patient to home and to normal functioning is the ultimate goal of any case management plan, although, unfortunately, it is not always possible.

Overview of Home Care

Much has been written about the benefits of a home environment to a patient's recovery and quality of life, but in some cases one must ask, at whose—and at what—cost? Home care for a "technology dependent" patient is not only complex; there are times when the quality of care can be compromised, and it is not safe to send a patient home. To further complicate the issue, at times home care costs far more than placement. How can this be? When various services must be provided by multiple providers, each bills at a different rate, so it is difficult to obtain services at a capitated or per diem rate. In essence, services are "unbundled."

Here are two examples of unbundling. In the first one, a patient is discharged to a rehabilitation or skilled nursing facility, which may be reimbursed at a capitated rate, a contracted rate, or one that is individually negotiated. This rate includes all services that will be provided while the patient is hospitalized. If the same patient were to go home, contracted rates might be in place, but separately with each provider and not as a single rate that would make the home care package more affordable (i.e., "a package deal"). In the end, each service must be paid for individually, and, thus, costs are "unbundled."

Why is one rate important? First, with high-tech home care it is common for patients to require a minimum of three different providers: (1) a home health agency, (2) an infusion agency, and (3) a durable medical equipment company. Three different companies and three different rates. It is impossible to negotiate an all-inclusive rate, as one might if the patient were a candidate for placement. Fortunately, a trend is emerging toward national vendors (i.e., home health, respiratory therapy, durable medi-

cal equipment, and infusion company) that offer billing under one service. This has tremendous cost containment advantages.

Although costs are often the bottom line for most organizations, it must not be for case-managed patients. Quality must always be paramount, lest the patient's condition deteriorate. So, case managers evaluating a provider must examine not only its ability to render care but also its credentials, accreditation, and internal quality management programs. Most important, there must be a mechanism to verify or validate what process the provider utilizes to effect change when quality of care is jeopardized or other such problems are identified.

For home care or post-acute services, many "technologically dependent" or complex care patients will have their care established "in lieu of hospitalization." In-lieu-of care must be offered or established if that can, quantitatively and qualitatively, replicate the patient's current level of care. More important, it must meet community standards of care for the diagnosis or condition. For instance, in the case of home care, all skilled nursing duties must conform to standards of care established by a state's administrative codes utilized to enforce licensure of home healthcare providers or resources.

Although some families feel compelled by guilt to attempt home care, this is not always a wise option for technology-dependent patients. Should such a situation arise, the case manager must have ready an alternate plan, in the event home care fails. If the patient or family demands home care and the care is complicated and potentially unsafe, the case manager should seek guidance from his or her employer's legal counsel. Should the patient or family continue to insist upon discharge to home most physicians discharge only "against medical advice," as the liability risks are not worth the tradeoff.

In such cases case managers must take a strongly proactive stance and attempt to dissuade the family and impress on them the associated risks. A home health assessment by a reputable agency can often support the case manager's position. Documentation is also vital for the case manager's professional protection.

A case of limited high-technology resources was that of ventilator-dependent twins who lived on the Mexican border. Although the family wanted both children at home, the cost for bringing in ventilator-trained staff exceeded the cost of a critical care unit. After extensive counseling of the family by the social work staff, the children were placed in a specialty post-acute care setting. Even had costs been reasonable, the remoteness of the home and the unavailability of resources to support the children and their medical needs would have made this case impossible for home care.

Barriers

Home healthcare is proliferating and is now an acceptable alternative to placement or acute care. Theoretically, if funds are available, even a "mini-intensive care unit" can be set up in the home. In reality, since funds and benefits are limited, there can be many barriers to successful high-technology home care:

- Living quarters are not environmentally safe (e.g., lacking heat, water, refrigeration, or structural or electrical sounders).
- Durable medical equipment company or the other home healthcare agencies are not geographically accessible. Many home providers will not accept responsibility if they are more than 45 to 60 minutes away from the patient. (Travel time during inclement weather is taken into consideration).
- The home health agency in the immediate area or the staff is unfamiliar or inexperienced with the needed care and must be trained or experienced staff hired.
- Primary caregiver is unavailable or absent or has limited physical or mental capacity.
- Parents of child patients may be themselves too immature to accept responsibility for the care demands.
- The home environment is known to be abusive.
- A local physician is unwilling to accept the patient and responsibility for his or her care.

One key to identifying barriers is to conduct the initial family interview in the home. Case managers must stay attuned to facts by listening, asking questions, and following through when potential barriers are identified. The most common result of ignoring barriers is costly delays caused by prolonged hospitalization.

Home health, infusion, and durable medical equipment agencies focus on the insured population who require short-term episodic care and services (i.e., dressing changes, teaching, observation, chemotherapy, respiratory therapy, short-term equipment support). Consequently, finding a qualified agency to accept the high technology–dependent patient may be a barrier to care. Also, many cases in a case manager's caseload are costly and long term. If the case

manager is not careful in the selection process, the provider may see the case as an opportunity to make money. In cases such as these, the agency's interest is opportunistic rather than for quality as they do not have the capability to manage so complex a case.

Here are two examples of opportunistic interest by a provider. In the first case, a ventilator patient required long-term facility care. After a long search, a provider was found who was willing to render the care if the insurer would increase its per diem reimbursement rate, but that provider refused to hire registered nurses on the afternoon and night shifts. As a result the search for a qualified provider began again. The second case was one of head injury to whom the provider promised multiple services for a post-acute rehabilitation plan, which, however, were never rendered once the patient had been admitted. The patient was transferred to another facility within a relatively short time; benefits were not wasted; and the rehabilitation continued as originally planned.

Types of Care Provided and Authorization Criteria

Regardless of the provider's name and reputation, if the case manager's organization does not allow on-site case management services for close monitoring, policies and procedures must be in place that set limits on the number of visits per authorization or that a mechanism is in place to ensure close monitoring of the provider's activities. This ensures that payment is made only for skilled care.

The same is true when hospital providers are capitated by a healthcare payor and in turn the hospital has its own capitated arrangements with other providers. However, when the hospital is capitated, administrators who want to control their costs have their utilization management departments—rather than the healthcare payor—authorize service. If more care is required, the home care provider must submit an evaluation and treatment plan for additional visits for approval by the discharge-planning unit of the capitated hospital, not the healthcare payor.

If the case manager is in a position to establish how many visits are allowed, a good rule to follow is to grant authorizations in increments, requiring the agency to submit seven to ten consecutive days of notes that reflect the actual skilled care provided. This not only allows close supervision to ensure that only skilled care is provided, it also allows appropriate management of the patient's home health care and many post-acute care benefits, which often have day or dollar limits. Incremental authorizations are also an excellent way to decrease any "right of expectancy" that care will continue indefinitely.

Although home health care agencies are generally referred to as the visiting nurse, many are Medicare certified and offer a full range of skilled professional services provided by registered nurses, licensed vocational or practical nurses, physical, occupational, or speech therapists, nutritionists, respiratory therapists, and social workers. Many also employ home health aides who administer custodial care such as bathing and toileting. Care for most patients is provided on an intermittent or daily basis to persons who are homebound; however, many home health agencies also offer private duty nursing, hospice care, and a variety of specialized nursing and skilled services.

Cases in a case manager's caseload will have various requirements for nursing hours. Some require only daily or twice daily skilled visits from the home health agency; others require 24-hour care. The criteria for the amount, frequency, and level of skilled care must be the intensity and severity of the illness or injury and the intensity and complexity of needed services.

Because of limits placed on home care by healthcare payors (workers' compensation is an exception) and individual policies, when a patient requires hourly skilled nursing care, the extracontractual process is frequently the way approval for such care is gained. Regardless of whether hourly skilled care is a benefit or is negotiated separately, every attempt must be made to approve only what is necessary and what allows the skilled care to be rendered or affords the caregiver time to be trained and to master the techniques.

Placement

If the patient's care is too complex or is affected by any case variables that preclude home care, facility placement is the appropriate option to consider (Fig. 11–2). Note, this is facility placement, not strictly skilled nursing facility placement. Any healthcare professional involved with discharging patients must be keenly aware of the multitude of types of post-acute care facilities. More important, these same professionals must be aware that the patient must be placed in the least restrictive environment that meets his or her needs. With this in mind, the following is a list of types of post-acute care providers (they can be employed in whatever sequence responds to the patient's needs) when out-of-home placement is required:

- Acute rehabilitation facility.
- Subacute, extended care, or acute facility step-down unit.
- Skilled nursing facility.
- Intermediate care facility.
- Post-acute care rehabilitation facility.
- Day treatment facility or care center.
- Board and care home.

Acute Rehabilitation

Naturally, not every patient is appropriate for acute rehabilitation. Most who fall in this category have suffered trauma or a severe neurologic insult (e.g., stroke, subarachnoid bleed, hemorrhage).

To qualify for an acute rehabilitation unit, patients must usually be able to tolerate a minimum of 3 hours' therapy daily and must be coherent enough to participate. Those who cannot tolerate or participate in an intensive rehabilitation regimen or do not require rehabilitation but need skilled care may be considered for the next level, on a subacute care facility, extended care facility, or step-down unit.

Subacute Care Facility

Subacute care facilities, extended care facilities, and step-down units generally are affiliated with an acute care hospital. All facilities in these categories offer more intensive skilled care than does a general skilled nursing facility. This level of care is an alternative for patients who are medically stable but do not require continuous availability of the diagnostic and therapeutic services of an acute facility. However, such patients do continue to require more technical skilled services that can be provided by a skilled nursing facility.

Skilled Nursing Facility

Once the patient is ready for discharge, the next question is, can the patient be discharged

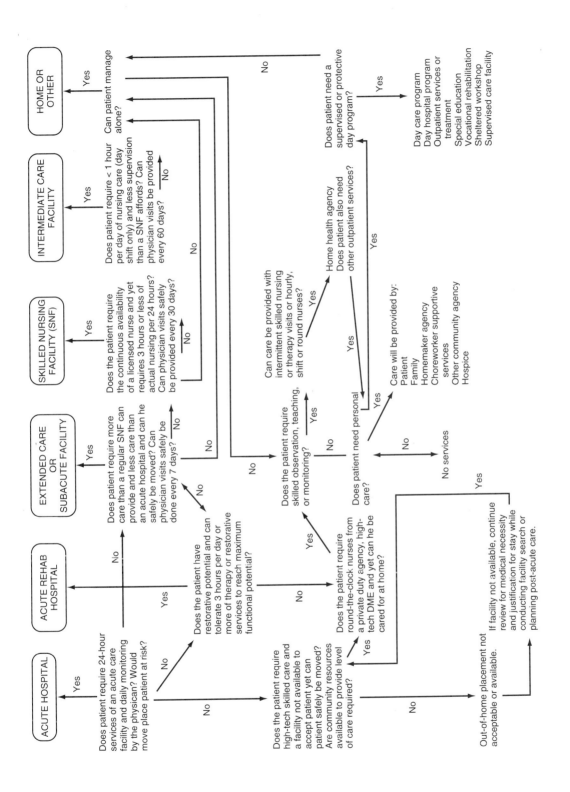

Figure 11–2 • Decision tree.

to home or be placed in a skilled nursing facility? Unfortunately, placement in a skilled nursing facility frequently carries a stigma. Many patients and families regard these "nursing homes" as the last resort, a place to go to die, a warehouse for the elderly. This often delays placement, as the case manager must take the time to educate everyone in pros and cons of placement.

To help families get past their fears, case managers have several resorts. One is to be very familiar with local facilities and their special features. Families must be encouraged to visit several facilities, make notes, visit favored ones at various times of the day, and attend to their senses of smell, sight, and hearing to make their placement decisions. Another technique is to collaborate with a social worker trained in counseling, to educate the family in the benefits of placement.

Historically, skilled nursing facilities have not been reimbursed directly by healthcare payors, Medicare and Medicaid being exceptions. This has changed over the past several years; however, many healthcare payors have only a small number of skilled nursing facilities in their panel or network. It is also common to find that these skilled nursing facilities can meet the care needs of the majority of patients but not those of case-managed patients. Consequently, the case manager must explore the capability of "nonnetwork" skilled nursing facilities in the area and negotiate an acceptable rate before the patient is admitted.

Naturally, the ideal out-of-home placement should be located as close as possible to the family, to prevent social isolation. Unfortunately, some communities have no local skilled nursing facilities available or ones equipped to handle certain levels of care. Then, the patient must be relocated to another community. Such placements are hardest when a child is involved. Again, the case manager must take a proactive role, explaining the positive aspects of the remote facility.

Although initial skilled nursing facility placement must be viewed as a short-term undertaking, long-term plans must also be made. Consequently, patient and family must be prepared for the expenses of long-term placement in the event such care becomes necessary, especially since few people have long-term care benefits.

Alternative Funding

Few patients need skilled services over the long term. Also, depending on any number of factors, a patient may move quickly from skilled to custodial care. When this happens, the healthcare payor often terminates coverage. Consequently, the family must be prepared to pay privately or to enroll in Medicaid, to ensure continued payment of long-term care costs.

The wisest plan always is to prepare the family with an open and honest approach discussion of actual costs of care and what the family's financial responsibilities are likely to be. Those hardest hit are in the income bracket of "too little and too much." The patient or family must exhaust its assets before qualifying for Medicaid. Families who have too many assets to qualify but not enough to pay privately are the ones who really struggle. It thus behooves case managers to encourage families to apply as early as possible for Medicaid, especially since in some states the eligibility process takes weeks to months.

Most healthcare payors cover only short-term skilled care and no custodial care. A patient can be "total care" but also "custodial" if the patient merely needs someone to assist in ADL. Hardest to visualize is the fact that even long-term infusion and ventilator patients can be classified by the healthcare payor as custodial, especially if the primary caregiver has been trained to render the care.

Custodial care is a classification healthcare payors use to denote the point at which coverage is terminated. At this point, coverage from the payor ceases because a caregiver has been trained, but continues for all supplies and solutions. If termination occurs for other reasons (e.g. exhaustion of benefits, patient reaches maximum day limit), other funds must be sought to continue payments for required services.

In most cases, alternative funding comes from Medicaid. It is very difficult for families to accept the end of the insurance benefits, especially for a helpless, total care patient. They must nevertheless be prepared for the financial burdens that follow cessation of healthcare benefits.

Post-Acute Care Facilities and Services

In addition to acute rehabilitation and subacute care facilities, other post-acute rehabilitation and outpatient facilities can be considered as the case manager's plan is researched and formulated. Post-acute rehabilitation and outpatient facilities focus on therapy and retraining for reentry into the community. Post-acute rehabilitation units provide a full range of professional medical care and training in reentry skills. This level of care is most often appropriate for traumatic brain injury (TBI) patients who continue to require rehabilitation. The focus of post-acute rehabilitation is to provide therapy in a noninstitutional environment. As such, many of these facilities are licensed under a state's board and care or small community home licensure law rather than those used for skilled nursing facility license since they can maintain a home-like rather than a hospital environment. For this reason, many healthcare payors do not reimburse this level of care.

Post-acute rehabilitation units have many advantages. If a patient can benefit from this level of care, but it is excluded from coverage, the case manager should pursue the extracontractual route, if that is allowed.

ADULT DAY CARE

One often overlooked and underutilized level of care is adult day care. Unfortunately, these facilities are not designed, staffed, or licensed to accept high technology–dependent patients, but they are ideal for those who require minimal care. They are useful for families who elect to care for their loved one at home but who also must continue working: in adult day care someone watches and cares for the loved one during working hours.

Unfortunately, very few communities have day care units for children with special needs. If they are provided, such units can range from high-technology care to supervised care.

Costs for both adult day care and pediatric units are rarely paid, in whole or in part, by healthcare payors. Most costs are paid privately or by the state Medicaid program. Depending on the person's disabilities, this level of care may be reimbursed by the state agency that is responsible for developmental disability services.

OTHER TYPES OF CARE

If home- or facility-based care is inappropriate, other areas case managers might wish to explore are these:

- Group homes (often called board and care homes).
- Residential care homes for the elderly or disabled, often with assistive living arrangements.
- Intermediate care facilities.
- State hospitals.

To be accepted into a group or board and care home a patient must be able to ambulate, dress, and feed herself and must be continent of bowel and bladder. Many states require group homes of six or more clients to be licensed and to observe fire codes.

The principal services provided by a group home are room and meals. A few offer recreational activities. Others are designed for clients with specific disorders (e.g., alcohol or drug addiction, head injury). Some offer medical assistance such as medications and personal care; others do not. For the most part, to enter this level of care patients must be fairly self-sufficient. These facilities are rarely covered by healthcare payors, as care is custodial.

In addition to board and care homes where care may be limited to small numbers of patients, some communities have residential care units offering services to large numbers of residents. These units vary in type of care and services. Most offer meals and a room, and services are very similar to those provided by their smaller counterpart. Most are set up to provide services and housing for elderly or mentally impaired persons. Some offer limited medical care; others do not. For the most part, persons entering these units must also be fairly independent, with many residential care units strictly limited to active seniors. Being custodial, this level of care is not covered by healthcare payors.

Many states allow licensure of what are called intermediate care facilities. These are similar to skilled nursing facilities, but they offer fewer care hours than those provided by a skilled nursing facility. In many cases, skilled care is minimal—often an hour or less per day (or week). Most patients are ambulatory and fairly independent. The principal criteria for persons entering this level of care are bowel and bladder control and sufficient mobility. This level of care is rarely covered by healthcare payors, as skilled care is rare.

In most instances state hospital placement is reserved for the mentally ill or very severely handicapped persons (i.e., those with severe cerebral palsy or profound mental retardation). Although this level of care may be covered on an interim basis by a healthcare payor if care is skilled, it is rare. Most patients in state hospitals need long-term care and, thus, must resort to Medicaid as they are custodial and require a protective setting that meets their needs. State hospital care costs some $40,000 to $50,000 per year per patient.

SUMMARY

Return to home is the goal of every case management plan; however, not all patients can go home. Case managers must stay abreast of local facilities and providers and with levels of care they provide. Knowledge of licensure laws and state administrative codes for healthcare providers is equally important. This knowledge is critical if quality of care is to be maintained. Most placements (except state hospital care and certain skilled nursing facilities) should always be regarded as temporary, moving the patient from one level of care to another, depending on how his or her condition progresses or regresses.

Many levels of care are excluded from the patient's benefit package and from payor coverage; however, if the patient absolutely needs care of an excluded level the case manager may need to seek approval for it through the extracontractual process.

Because the care level can plateau or change to custodial, families must be prepared for the fact that they may be expected to assume responsibility for payment. If they are unable to pay, Medicaid or another resource for funding must be sought.

REHABILITATION

Rehabilitation aims to restore functional capacity—mental or physical—to the highest level consistent with a patient's illness or injury. It consists of treating and training a patient to maximize his potential for normal living— physically, psychologically, socially, and vocationally.[4]

Until recently, the importance of rehabilitation was not recognized.[5] Consequently, many seriously compromised patients were moved to a skilled nursing facility or a state hospital without benefit of a proper evaluation for the formal, structured environment and intensive training an acute rehabilitation program offers. These patients never were afforded the benefit of any attempts at rehabilitation.

Disabled persons constitute a significant proportion of the population in the United States and of case managers' caseloads. Because not all disabling conditions are handicapping or permanent, every patient's potential for recovery of some degree of independence must be considered. Consequently, all case managers who will be involved with the patient, regardless of their employer affiliations, must be involved as early as possible, so they can plan accordingly with the patient, family, and healthcare team to select a rehabilitation facility or alternate level of care that is appropriate.

Case managers must be very familiar with all phases of rehabilitation and with local rehabilitation facilities. To this end, they must maintain a current listing of rehabilitation units and their capabilities and limitations. Not all hospitals have a separate licensed rehabilitation unit appropriate for acute rehabilitation. Many freestanding rehabilitation units are very specialized and accept only persons with certain levels of neurologic involvement or spinal cord injury.

Equally important, case managers must be very familiar with both physical medicine and rehabilitation procedures and TBI or acquired brain injury (ABI) rehabilitation, as not all patients are candidates for acute rehabilitation. Thus, a TBI patient may require a temporary move to a skilled nursing facility or home before formal rehabilitation can be undertaken. There, the patient's therapy can continue as the patient is readied for admission to the rehabilitation unit. In such cases, the patient must be reevaluated at regular intervals for acceptance into a formal inpatient rehabilitation program.

Not all healthcare payors offer acute rehabilitation as a benefit, and others have strict day and dollar limits. Thus, case managers, from both the facility and the healthcare payor, must collaborate to ensure that rehabilitation is available. The earlier rehabilitation is started, the greater is the likelihood that the patient can regain some function and avoid institutionalization or dependency.[6] The overall course of rehabilitation varies—with the patient, the premorbid personality, intelligence, education level, and community resources for follow-up care.

Physical Medicine and Rehabilitation

The spinal cord injuries, other neuromuscular injuries, and insults such as stroke, amputation, and Guillain-Barré syndrome require an acute inpatient medical model for the majority of the treatment program. Many physical medicine and rehabilitation (PMR) units specialize in and offer services for particular types of injury or levels of involvement. Thus, length of stay varies with and depends on such factors as level of injury, severity of the illness or injury, complexity of care, and factors peculiar to the patient or family.

Depending on a patient's needs and the capabilities of the facility, it may be necessary to place some patients on several facility waiting lists or to move them to a facility outside the immediate area. This is especially true for ventilator-dependent and high cervical spinal cord–injured patients, even more so for pediatric trauma patients. Facilities for all these categories of patients are limited. To evaluate the patient's needs and determine which rehabilitation unit is appropriate, a comprehensive functional assessment is essential. The assessment goes beyond disease categories and functional impairments to address the resultant disability that rehabilitation efforts target. Functional assessment is a common screening tool for rehabilitation, to set therapeutic goals and monitor the clinical course of the disease while providing objective criteria for treatment planning and progress monitoring.

Various PMR units specialize in certain levels and types of injury and in the services they provide. For instance, whereas many of these units are equipped and staffed to manage strokes, certain other neurologic disorders, and paraplegia, others are not. Also, many quadriplegics, especially those who are ventilator dependent, may be admitted to only a few facilities nationwide.

GOALS

Unrealistic goals established too early produce frustration, despair, anxiety, and withdrawal and can have a negative effect on the entire process and the outcome. When goals are realistic and therapy is paced appropriately for the patient, they are motivators. Without properly set goals therapy is ineffective. Goals should be reevaluated at each case conference.[6]

The short-term goals of a PMR program are these:

- Prevent or correct deformities or complications.
- Retrain patients to walk, speak, or otherwise function at the maximum level consistent with their impairments.
- Train the affected body system to its maximum level of usefulness.
- Teach patients to perform ADL as independently as possible.[7]

The long-term goals aim to return the patient to one of these four levels:

- Return to full-time employment (either resume previous job or retrain for a new one).
- Return to part-time work (as a previous job, a sheltered environment, another occupation, or working from home).
- For those unable to work, to assume self-care.
- For those who require full care, placement in an appropriate facility or caregiver training for home care.[7]

Variables critical to the success of a rehabilitation program include these:

- Location and extent of the injury.
- If a head injury, duration of coma.
- Age at time of injury.
- Preinjury level of intelligence, personality development, and maturity.
- Home environment.
- Availability of rehabilitation services and insurance benefit structure for rehabilitation.
- Motivation to recover.
- Quality and quantity of family support.
- Early assessment and management of complications.

MODELS

Inpatient PMR is often provided in traditional inpatient facilities such as (1) acute rehabilitation, (2) subacute care facility, (3) extended-care facility, and (4) skilled nursing facility.

PHASES OF REHABILITATION

PMR has four phases: (1) initial identification, (2) evaluation, (3) treatment, and (4) follow-up or outpatient treatment. Timing and realistic goals are critical to the success of the patient during each phase of rehabilitation.

Identification

Rehabilitation starts with identification of patients who can benefit from it. This process starts either at the time of admission to the acute care facility or shortly after the patient's condition stabilizes. At this time, rehabilitation may consist simply of splinting, ROM exercises, or other preventive measures. If this is overlooked permanent, irreversible contractures can result and that can make return to functional status impossible or more difficult to achieve.

For persons with a traumatic or acquired brain injury, simple commands are introduced soon after they awaken from a coma. These commands must be appropriate for the patient's level of awareness and ability to respond. It is generally accepted that, the longer a person is in a coma, the longer the rehabilitation process will be and the less likely is full recovery.

Evaluation

Once the patient exhibits readiness to move to another level of care, the physiatrist or an interdisciplinary rehabilitation team conducts an intensive evaluation. It is best for the patient to be evaluated initially by the physiatrist in the acute hospital setting before transfer to the rehabilitation unit. When circumstances do not allow this, the patient's medical records must be forwarded to the rehabilitation facility for review by the physiatrist and other team members. Depending on the physiatrist's findings, the patient may be transferred to the rehabilitation unit for completion of the evaluation, where a team examination is conducted.

If the patient is found to be a potential candidate, the patient is moved to the rehabilitation unit, as the evaluations and formulation of the final recommendations take several days. Each member of the team conducts a comprehensive evaluation of the "whole patient," and the family and the findings are integrated into the final plan. If the patient is ultimately found not to be a candidate for rehabilitation, placement in a skilled nursing facility, a state hospital, or at home may be recommended. Such placement can be permanent or temporary (until recovery reaches a stage at which reevaluation for acute rehabilitation is feasible).

ASSESSMENTS

The cornerstone of rehabilitation medicine is a thorough evaluation—an assessment that goes beyond the traditional medical workup.[8, 9] In addition to medical assessment, tools such as the Functional Assessment Measure (FAM) may be used. Whatever the tool, the patient is assessed for the following variables:

- Motivation.
- Premorbid functional level and pertinent medical history.
- Perception of illness, injury, and expectation for recovery.
- Current physical and cognitive functional limits and capabilities, medical condition and stability, dependence on support for feeding, breathing and swallowing, seizure activity, pain, and mobility.

- Psychosocial and socioeconomic factors, personality, values, coping skills, and attitudes that figure importantly in affecting the desired outcomes.
- Ability to tolerate at least 3 hours of therapy per day.
- Prognosis for recovery.
- Plans for corrective surgery or reconstruction.

During this time the family is also assessed for pre- and postmorbid dynamics, expectations, legal and financial concerns, willingness to be trained as caregivers (should one be needed), coping skills, and attitudes toward the rehabilitation process. Although the primary focus is the patient, the family must not be forgotten. For the reasons listed below and others, they must participate in the process and be included in all decision making. It is common to observe a large variety of reactions in affected families[10]: anger, guilt, depression, helplessness and hopelessness, anxiety, denial, and withdrawal or unreasonable demands.

Families need support to help them deal with their initial and ongoing reactions. They need to know that resource information is available, as well as advice on placement, discharge options, alternative funding for long-term care, and community resources. As the reality of the situation sets in, or as the patient approaches discharge and the prospect of long-term care looms, many other fears and anxieties surface that must be addressed.

Treatment Plan

During the rehabilitation process the treatment plan and goals are continually reevaluated and revised.[11] This is necessary to ensure that treatments are constantly tailored to the patient's needs and level of functioning and that progress toward goals is being achieved within the established time frame. The rehabilitation treatment plan is updated at regularly scheduled team conferences where each team member reports on the patient's progress or on problems. Adjustments may be made and new short-term goals established. Most rehabilitation units offer regularly scheduled family conferences as part of the treatment planning, at which goals are determined and the family is encouraged to actively participate in decision making. Documentation at all phases of rehabilitation is key to coverage determinations.

The total rehabilitation course is often prolonged, and predictions for prognosis, date for program completion, and some form of recovery are often uncertain. It is usual for stroke patients and amputees to be hospitalized 1 to 2 weeks, whereas a person with quadriplegia or a head or brain injury may require rehabilitation for a longer period of time. Diseases of the brain or neuromuscular system such as stroke, tumors, or spinal cord injuries tend to affect certain areas and thus have more predictable outcomes. With TBI or acquired brain injury outcomes are less predictable.

Case managers must collaborate and work closely with patient, family, and healthcare team during all phases of rehabilitation so that post-acute rehabilitation alternatives will be in place when the patient is ready for discharge. Also, because a patient can "plateau" at any time, the family must be prepared for discharge and a postdischarge plan must be ready for immediate implementation. Patients of this category are frequently discharged to home or to a skilled nursing facility. It is during this phase of the rehabilitation process that a home assessment is done by a rehabilitation team member to identify barriers that can be eliminated or modified before discharge.

As the day of discharge nears, it is common for the patient to get a weekend pass or a trial period at home. A pass can last 2 days (48 hours). After each pass, the patient and family or caregiver report problem areas that require further therapy or adjustments before the actual discharge. Despite the fact that such passes are important to the rehabilitation process, many healthcare payors do not cover them. The cost must then be assumed by the patient or family, via the extracontractual process, or in some instances, by the hospital. Should these options not be available, the patient may be discharged directly to home without the benefit of a trial period.

Most patients are discharged, when the short-term hospital-related care goals have been met. On occasion, if the patient does not progress as anticipated, placement may be indicated—at skilled nursing facility, a long-term care psychiatric facility, or a state hospital. Other patients may be discharged to a community care facility such as board and care, a group home, or another safe and structured environment, should a private home be unavailable or inappropriate. Fortunately, most persons with quadriplegia, hemiplegia, or paraplegia can be discharged home with ongoing outpatient therapy. If the home is equipped, the family is trained, and there is coverage from the healthcare payor, even respirator-dependent persons can be discharged home.

Discharge does not mean patients have reached their maximum potential nor that all goals have been reached. It means only that they have reached a stage at which rehabilitation can continue at a less intensive level.

Outpatient Care and Follow-Up

Once the acute inpatient portion of the rehabilitation is completed, ongoing therapy from an outpatient setting is almost always necessary. Outpatient or post-acute rehabilitation for spinal cord injuries and other neurologic insults can take many forms. Usually, the patient goes home and returns to the rehabilitation or outpatient therapy unit several times per week. If the patient is considered homebound, therapy may be established using a home health agency. Such service continues until the patient can be transferred and treated in an outpatient setting.

THE TEAM

Intensive PMR and TBI rehabilitation programs use an interdisciplinary approach, patient and family being the most important—and most intensely engaged—members of the team, which is directed by a physiatrist. The PMR team, at a minimum, is comprised of professionals from nursing; physical, occupational, and speech therapy; and durable medical equipment, orthotics, or prosthetic device companies. The brain injury rehabilitation team consist of these plus specialists for case management, cognitive retraining and behavior modification, community reentry, basic living skills, and educational or vocational retraining.[5]

Each team also offers a variety of other specialists who enhance program objectives[12]—neurologist, neuropsychiatrist, psychologist, respiratory therapist, dietitian, social worker, case manager, discharge planner, vocational rehabilitation specialist, recreational or activity therapist. Because of the long-term nature of rehabilitation, out-of-facility case managers must be included in the team as soon as the patient is identified as a candidate for rehabilitation.

🕮 S U M M A R Y

PMR is an important aspect of recovery from neurologic insults. When a patient is identified as a candidate for rehabilitation, every effort must be made to provide this opportunity. To ensure that this happens, all case managers, regardless of their employer, must become integrated into the rehabilitation team as soon as possible.

This process not only affords opportunities for communication among the whole team but also ensures that the patient reaches the goals established. More important, it ensures that healthcare coverage and benefits will be available when the patient needs them. Because benefits for rehabilitation are frequently limited or not covered at all, case managers must collaborate to submit requests for approval (including by extracontractual process) for all levels of rehabilitation when the patient demonstrates readiness to move on, so she may reach maximum functional potential.

Traumatic Brain Injury or Acquired Brain Injury Rehabilitation

Many healthcare professionals can remember how, before the development of TBI rehabilitation, many patients with cognitive or behavioral impairments were subjected to overmedication, wrongly institutionalized in skilled nursing facilities or state hospitals, or remanded to a family ill-equipped for the future. This was so, because it was believed that brain injury was irreversible and that significant gains were rare. With the advent of new treatment modalities for brain-injured persons it has been proven that specific stimulation, simple repetition, and retraining are essential for cognitive improvement. For these reasons, new treatment methods are now being used successfully.

Because recovery from brain injury is often slower than other forms of recovery, case managers whether facility or nonfacility based must be involved as early as possible. In many cases, the out-of-facility case managers may have to remain involved with the patient or family for months after the injury if the continuum of care resources is to be negotiated appropriately. It is also necessary to ensure that health benefit coverage is available and approvals are issued as plans are ready for implementation at the next phase. This also ensures that the patient is moved to an appropriate provider recognized by the healthcare payor or that the provider that accepts the patient is prepared and can manage the required level of care.

GOALS

The principal goal of a brain injury rehabilitation program is cognitive retraining that teaches the patient to live and function safely and independently and to be a useful and productive member of society. For this reason, many brain injury rehabilitation programs are based in the community rather than in hospitals (i.e., a non-medical milieu). Additionally, many have strong vocational and educational components.[13]

TREATMENT PROGRAMS AND PHASES OF TRAUMATIC BRAIN INJURY REHABILITATION

Rehabilitation of brain-injury patients involves relearning old skills and learning new ways to compensate for deficits. Expressive, receptive, and cognitive deficits must be thoroughly evaluated to determine what functional communication and survival skills retraining must be incorporated into the treatment plan.

Treatment programs for brain-injured patients are frequently conducted in multiple settings and in four phases (different from the phases of PMR programs discussed earlier). At every phase safety awareness and premorbid personality or disposition play key roles.[14]

Phase I. A very structured environment that offers one-on-one supervision. This is very important for development of the overall plan of care.

Phase II. A less structured setting that allows the patient to function with less direct supervision.

Phase III. An even less structured environment that offers little direct supervision.

Phase IV. Outpatient rehabilitations, during which the patient lives at home and may work or attend school. Therapy continues in the outpatient rehabilitation department.

Although determining prognosis may be difficult, the patient's clinical status must be monitored continuously throughout the recovery course to ensure that treatment planning is appropriate.[14] Thus, as the patient progresses, she must be transitioned to the different phases of the program, where further learning can take place. At each phase, treatment and supervision must conform to these criteria:

• Provided that are appropriate to the patient's level of mental involvement.
• Consistent, repetitive, and structured.
• Provided in such a way that task difficulty is

upgraded at appropriate times and supervision or structure is provided according to the patient's level of mental functioning.

- Provided so that there is consistent feedback and reinforcement and the patient is constantly encouraged.
- Provided so that more than one sensory stimulus can be given at any one time, to enhance learning.
- Provided so that the goals established change as the patient progresses.

How long a patient is comatose has significant implications for overall recovery time.[15] In general, recovery is most rapid during the first weeks and months after the brain injury or after the person awakes from the coma. Unfortunately, the overall recovery process is slow and often has plateaus.

The duration of both coma and posttraumatic amnesia has implications for outcome.[16, 17] For instance, patients long in a coma make gains much more slowly than those whose coma was shorter lived. Out-of-facility case managers must realize that gains are made in weeks or months, not days. Overall, recovery to maximum potential can take years.

TBI literature specifies that persistent vegetative state (PVS) should not be identified as such until it has persisted at least 12 months. Before any final long-term placement is chosen, PVS patients should be given the benefit of a sensory or coma stimulation program.[18] This type of program could last months or until the patient shows no evidence of progress despite consistent and repeated efforts at stimulation. This level of care is best accomplished in a skilled nursing facility that specifically offers this level of care.

Treatment programs for brain injury are best offered in a calm and structured milieu. More often than not, these units are designed to resemble a home rather than a hospital atmosphere. This is necessary as behavioral problems and agitation escalate in brain-injured persons, especially when they are exposed to noise, altercations, threats, confrontation, restrictions, and changes in environment. To minimize agitation and behavior problems, many brain injury rehabilitation units emphasize: (1) a calm approach, (2) removal of known sources of agitation, (3) concrete and tangible rewards, (4) redirection of attention (distraction), (5) formation of trusting relationships, (6) shorter treatment sessions, and (7) familiar surroundings and minimal restrictions.

TRADITIONAL LOCATIONS FOR BRAIN INJURY REHABILITATION

Historically, TBI facilities have specialized in various levels of cognitive deficits as they relate to the Glasgow Coma Scale and the Disability Rating Scale. In these instances, the Coma Scale was the principal tool for measuring extent of injury and cognitive function. Another tool utilized was the Rancho Los Amigos Cognitive Levels, which both describes the patient's status and recommends appropriate treatment (e.g., Level II–III is appropriate for sensory or coma stimulation, Level IV for sensory moderation, and Level V–VIII for cognitive retraining). It is useful for identifying which brain injury unit is appropriate for a given patient's cognitive level of functioning.

Until recently, these coma and rating scales were the ones most often used. Over the past 5 years, however, the number of assessment tools designed for severely brain-injured patients has increased significantly. Now, such scales as the Coma or Near Coma Scale, the Coma Recovery Scale, Sensory Stimulation Assessment Measure, and the Western Neurosensory Stimulation Profile, and other standardized assessment instruments are being used.[18] As a result, case managers who work with brain-injured patients must be familiar with these tools and which providers can render the care appropriate to the level of head injury so identified.

As treatment modalities for brain-injured patient have changed, so have the types of resources now utilized. For successful integration of a patient into the community, coordination with multiple community resources may be necessary. It is common for persons with brain injury to require many different services as they recover.[19] Entry into the following models, with the exception of a home plan, depends on the facility's level of specialization and the Coma Scale or cognitive level of functioning it accepts. The traditional sites for rehabilitation of the brain injured patients are these:

- Acute rehabilitation facility.
- Subacute care facility.
- Extended care facility.
- Skilled nursing facility (traditional long-term or specialized for brain injury).
- Transitional living centers (with supervised and independent living).
- Outpatient or day treatment programs.
- Behavioral rehabilitation.
- Group homes and other safe environments.

- Psychiatric facilities.
- State hospitals.

Depending on the program and the facility's licensure, case managers frequently have to request or utilize the extracontractual process to obtain coverage and allow the patient to participate in the treatment program that is best for his or her condition. Psychiatric facilities and state hospitals should be the last resort and utilized only after all attempts at brain injury rehabilitation have failed.

Because many brain injury units do not conform to the medical model and licensure is similar to that granted community board and care homes, many programs are not accepted for healthcare reimbursement. In contrast, a similar brain injury program offered in a skilled nursing facility may be covered. This is true when the patient meets skilled care criteria and the patient's healthcare benefit plan pays for skilled nursing facility care.

An emerging trend for brain-injured patients is specialty subacute skilled nursing facilities as an alternative, cost-effective approach to an acute rehabilitation-based program. These facilities employ highly trained specialists and provide intensive therapy designed to treat specific degrees of cognitive function; however, caution must be exercised to ensure that a particular skilled nursing facility actually has a program for TBI rehabilitation. This caveat is necessary to ensure that the facility is not a regular skilled nursing facility whose administrator sees an opportunity for financial gains.

PHYSICAL AND MENTAL CHANGES

Except in coma patients and the PVS, it is common to see certain physical and mental changes after a brain injury.[20] When these are identified specialty physician referrals may be necessary:

- Motor deficits leading to poor coordination, decreased strength, immobility, decreased ROM, tremor, and self-care problems.
- Emotional problems such as denial, frustration, depression, flat affect, euphoria, irritability, and redundant mood swings.
- Regulatory disturbances in toileting, digestion, and sleep patterns.
- Traumatic epilepsy or seizures.
- Visual field limits, perceptual deficits, diplopia, and optic atrophy.
- Vertigo.
- Speech and language disorders.

- Localized headaches.
- Tremors.
- Behavior problems or drastic personality changes.
- Overdependence.
- Cognitive deficits.
  - Decreased or increased sensation.
  - Safety awareness.
  - Memory and concentration.
  - Loss or gross distortion of perception.
  - Cognitive functions (slowed or decreased sequencing, recall, abstracting or thinking, learning or grasping of details, problem solving, planning, or organization).
  - Verbal, visual, and nonverbal abilities.
  - Social skills.

Any of these manifestations has the potential to affect discharge planning and selection of appropriate post-acute rehabilitation program or services.

ADDITIONAL RESOURCES

After a brain injury families are often in crisis, and, owing to the emotionally charged atmosphere, it is very important that families be informed of community support groups where they can learn mechanisms for coping and for navigating the system.[21] Role reversal and related effects on household financial stability are common aftermaths of brain injury. As a result, emotions can range through anger, anxiety, frustration, and depression for the significant other suddenly placed in charge of the family. When this occurs, if support groups cannot offer the support the family needs, professional counseling must be recommended.

Because brain injury recovery is a lengthy process, families must be apprised of community resources to which they or the patient might be entitled, for example, the Easter Seal Society, national or local head injury foundation, independent living centers, sheltered workshops and training programs, legal centers for the disabled, and vocational rehabilitation.

ALTERNATIVE FUNDING AND RESOURCES

Because brain injury recovery is often prolonged and payment for many programs (e.g., coma stimulation, cognitive therapy) is excluded or limited by healthcare payors, case managers must encourage patients and families to apply for any alternative funding to which the patient is entitled, which may be:

- Medicaid.
- Supplemental Security Income.
- Social Security Disability Income.
- Workers' Compensation, if applicable.
- Title V Children's Medical Services Program.
- Agencies responsible for providing services to the developmentally disabled (if the injury occurs before the 22nd birthday).
- Third-party liability insurance.
- Victims of violent crimes.
- State or local rehabilitation authorities.

In addition, all insurance policies must be explored for coordination of benefits. This is necessary to supplement or extend coverage for treatment programs and to enable the patient to regain some level of functional independence.

SUMMARY

Brain injury rehabilitation differs from traditional PMR programs in that once patients complete the acute rehabilitation program, they often require continued rehabilitation in a post-acute program. There, the emphasis is on re-training in cognitive skills to allow them to function as independently as possible. Unfortunately, many of these programs do not fit the traditional medical model and, so, are often excluded from payor coverage. Also, because patients progress more slowly, they can exhaust their rehabilitation benefits. In some cases, reimbursement for post-acute rehabilitation may be disallowed because the patient is classified as chronic or the care as long term.

For all of these reasons, case managers must be very knowledgeable about brain injury rehabilitation programs, at a minimum in the area where they practice. Because of limitations or exclusions in the patient's healthcare benefits, payments for traumatic brain rehabilitation are frequently disallowed or allowed only if the extracontractual process is pursued. Thus, case managers must know this process, what is required, and when and how to request it.

Pulmonary Rehabilitation

Outpatient pulmonary rehabilitation programs have evolved over the past decade. They focus on evaluation, treatment, and management of breathing difficulties associated with the following diagnoses:

- Chronic obstructive pulmonary disease.
- Asthma.
- Emphysema.
- Chronic bronchitis.
- Bronchiectasis.
- Any respiratory disease that decreases quality of life.
- Restrictive lung disease (e.g., pulmonary fibrosis).
- Lung transplantation.
- Respiratory arrest.
- Cor pulmonale.

One of the case manager's best guidelines for selecting such programs is to look for ones that are Medicare certified, accredited by the Joint Commission on Accreditation of Healthcare Organizations (JCAHO), or paneled by the state's Title V Children's Medical Services Program (since many of these also accept children with respiratory disorders).

GOALS

The goals of pulmonary rehabilitation are to achieve an optimal functional level, prevent hospitalizations, and shorten lengths of stay. Unfortunately, with the exception of Medicare and a few other healthcare payors, these programs are often excluded from coverage.

PROGRAM COMPONENTS

Pulmonary rehabilitation is the process of restoring a pulmonary disease patient to optimal physical and psychological status. The program has three basic components:

- Exercise and energy conservation in ADL.
- Education in the disease process so they can understand the rationale behind techniques taught and the need to comply with them.
- Lifestyle modifications techniques.

ADMISSION CRITERIA

Although respiratory or pulmonary rehabilitation can be offered on an inpatient basis, it is most often provided to outpatients.[23] Programs vary in length, but most last several weeks, and sometimes a total of 18 sessions, depending on the patient's needs. Admission criteria are based on the following considerations:

- The patient must have a diagnosis of chronic pulmonary disease or restrictive lung disease that causes symptoms and impairs function.
- The patient must be medically stable and not have acute-stage disease.

- The patient must be mentally and emotionally able to comprehend the treatments and to set and achieve personal goals.
- The patient must not have a history of chemical abuse.
- The patient must desire and be motivated to achieve symptomatic and functional improvement, such as greater walking distance, less shortness of breath, a more independent lifestyle, and better control of symptoms.
- The patient must be strongly motivated to stop smoking. Although most programs recommend the program be restricted to nonsmokers, this is not a prerequisite.[29]

TEAM MEMBERS

Pulmonary rehabilitation is offered in a multidisciplinary team approach design. It aims to minimize or reverse the symptoms of lung disease. The team is comprised, at a minimum, of the following healthcare professionals:

- A medical director, generally a pulmonologist.
- Respiratory therapist.
- Occupational therapist.
- Physical therapist.
- Dietitian.
- Social worker.
- Pharmacist.
- Nurses.

Each healthcare professional has responsibility for specific components of the program:

- The respiratory therapist is responsible for teaching the patient about home equipment such as nebulizers and oxygen systems. He also develops a home care and preventive maintenance program.
- The physical therapist teaches breathing exercises and designs a special exercise program for use at home that allows the patient to conserve energy while performing ADL.
- The occupational therapist teaches proper body mechanics and energy conservation techniques related to ADL and designs a home program to help the patient conserve energy while performing tasks.
- The dietitian advises patient and caregivers on proper diet and food preparation.
- The pharmacist teaches the patient about the medication regimen.
- The nurses monitor the patient's response to treatments and provide any necessary teaching.
- The social worker provides psychological support for patient and family. In addition, she educates and helps the patient gain access to community resources (e.g., alternate funding and support groups).

Many of these programs include educational lectures, meals, and educational audiovisual materials. Unfortunately, as a rule, this type of education is not reimbursed by healthcare payors. Therefore as rates are agreed upon, it is important to seek coverage for these programs, either through an all-inclusive rate negotiation or via the extracontractual process. Otherwise costs for these services must be assumed by the patient.

✂ SUMMARY

Pulmonary rehabilitation has emerged over the past several years as a modality for improving the quality of life for patients with chronic lung disease. Programs are administered by a multidisciplinary team, the overall program lasting about 18 sessions and its goal being to enable the patient to function at maximum potential.

Cardiac Rehabilitation

Many cardiac patients can benefit from an intensive rehabilitation program that teaches them how to live within the limitations imposed by their disease. Typically, cardiac rehabilitation has four phases. Phase one is the inpatient portion, following the acute insult. Phase two, the outpatient portion, generally takes some weeks. Phase three starts approximately 9 months after phase two. Phase four is the maintenance program, which extends indefinitely.

Case managers must be familiar with cardiac rehabilitation programs, their admission criteria, and most important, whether they are reimbursed by the healthcare payor. One of the best mechanisms for selecting a cardiac rehabilitation program is to look for ones that are Medicare certified or accredited by the JCAHO.

GOALS

The goals of cardiac rehabilitation are to reduce symptoms and improve function.[25-27] Thus, they have these objectives:

- To return the patient to optimal physiologic and psychological functioning.

- To prepare the patient and family for a lifestyle that reduces the risk of cardiovascular events (much emphasis is placed on changing dietary habits, exercise practices, work and play habits, and self-destructive habits).
- To reduce the emotional factors (depression, anxiety, anger) associated with severe cardiac events.
- To reduce the cost of care by decreasing hospitalizations and dependence on cardiac medications.
- To return the patient to work or increase the likelihood she can remain at work or have a more active lifestyle.

PROGRAM COMPONENTS

Cardiac rehabilitation is the process by which a person is restored to optimal physical and psychological status after suffering a life-threatening cardiac event.[28] They include such services as these:

- An exercise component and teaching in energy conservation.
- Patient education in the disease process and the importance of compliance with instructions and restrictions.
- Lifestyle and behavior modification techniques.

Without cardiac rehabilitation, it is common for feelings of depression and helplessness to overwhelm the patient, and, as in many illnesses, a full range of psychological problems can occur, which, left untreated, can result in costly outcomes. Patients lose their motivation and self-esteem and become more dependent on others. Certainly, motivation for follow-through, personal ambition, age, and the extent of cardiac damage affect decisions and outcomes, but it is important to consider any cardiac patient's rehabilitation potential.

Cardiac rehabilitation programs vary in components, intensity, and duration. Although they are divided into three phases—inpatient, outpatient, and maintenance—for the most part, programs are conducted in an outpatient setting and are conducted several hours per day or several times per week for a total of 2 to 12 weeks. Most programs are hospital based, and admission is by physician's order.

ADMISSION CRITERIA

As a rule, cardiac rehabilitation programs are for persons who have experienced one of the following insults during the preceding 12 months:

- Myocardial infarction.
- Coronary artery bypass graft.
- Coronary angioplasty.
- Percutaneous transluminal coronary angioplasty.
- Chronic stable angina (chest pain that has not changed in character, frequency, intensity, or duration for at least 60 days).
- Heart valve surgery.
- Heart transplantation.
- Heart-lung transplantation.[29]

Although some conditions are more specific to the respiratory system, patients with a diagnosis of lung transplantation, respiratory arrest, or cor pulmonale may also be candidates for cardiac rehabilitation (especially if their healthcare coverage allows cardiac rehabilitation but not pulmonary rehabilitation).

TEAM MEMBERS

Cardiac rehabilitation programs take a full multidisciplinary approach. The team consists of the following professionals:

- Nurses.
- Physical and occupational therapists.
- Medical social workers.
- Psychologists.
- Dietitians.
- Recreational therapists.
- Physicians.
- Respiratory therapists.
- Pharmacists.[29]

PROGRAM COSTS

Because many such programs are offered only for fee for service, case managers must be prepared to request an all-inclusive per diem rate if the rehabilitation program is not in the healthcare payor's network. Otherwise, costs can be exorbitant, and in some cases, certain professionals who are important to the overall success of the program may not be covered by the healthcare payor if the services they provide are billed separately (i.e., unbundled).

If rate negotiation is necessary, the case managers must work together to ensure that the rate is finalized and is acceptable to the healthcare payor before the time of admission. If a rate must be agreed upon, it is important to ensure that it includes the following services:

psychological testing and therapy, medication adjustments and related medication teaching, dietary teaching, and other self-care education programs (e.g., smoking cessation, exercise).

SUMMARY

Any cardiac patient who has experienced a life-threatening cardiac event within the past 12 months should be considered for cardiac rehabilitation. Although these programs can be offered to inpatients, most are outpatient services from a full multidisciplinary team.

Pain Management

Possibly the most difficult patients a case manager deals with are in pain. Pain can be acute or chronic. Acute pain can be alleviated, in most cases, by modern technology or drugs. Chronic pain, however, presents significant challenges, but this is not to say that acute pain is not a challenge and can be ignored.

Unfortunately, not all physicians and healthcare professionals are well-versed in pain and appropriate treatments. It is necessary in situations of inadequate treatment of acute pain, that the case manager advocate for the patient in seeking solutions for relief of the pain. If acute pain is not treated properly, it can develop into chronic pain.

If the case manager sees that pain is not being managed adequately, consultation with the healthcare organization's medical or pharmacy director may be in order. If a patient is taking intravenous or intrathecal analgesics one of the most valuable resources is a pharmacist. Professionals such as these not only afford an opportunity to discuss treatment options but are an avenue to the patient's attending physician.

Although many conditions can cause acute pain, two frequently seen in the post-acute care setting are multitrauma and terminal cancer. The key in both cases is to ensure that the patient is kept as comfortable as possible. Every attempt must be made to spare cancer patients a horrifically painful death. Similarly, pain associated with multitrauma or another medical condition or injury must not be allowed to progress to chronic pain.

ACUTE VERSUS CHRONIC PAIN

Acute pain is usually of brief duration, subsides as healing takes place, and ranges from mild to severe.[30] In contrast, chronic pain usually lasts longer than 3 to 6 months.[30]

FACTORS RELATED TO PAIN

Although treatment of chronic pain is a multibillion-dollar annual healthcare expense, in relation to human suffering its cost cannot be measured. Chronic pain sufferers and those with persistent pain are often chemically dependent and plagued with psychological and physical problems like the following ones[31, 32]:

- Physical, emotional, and affective personality disorders.
- Physical deterioration secondary to sleep and appetite disturbances.
- Decreased physical activity.
- Fatigue.
- Debility.
- Anxiety.
- Depression.
- Hypochondriasis.
- Somatic preoccupation.
- Denial.
- Manipulation and lying.
- Weight gain.

In the case of chemical abuse, the case manager may find it necessary to enlist the assistance of the primary care physician and the patient's family to conduct an intervention. When noncompliance is the issue, the physician may require the patient to sign a contract with a commitment to obtain care only from the physician and to comply with any program presented. Often, this process is necessary when the healthcare payor has agreed to pay for the program and the patient only half-heartedly agrees to enter into treatment.

COMMON CHARACTERISTICS

In their attempt to gain relief it is common for chronic pain patients to take multiple medications in large doses. In addition to drug intoxication, such large doses can cause major behavior changes—and in many patients "drug-seeking behavior." Many withdraw from all social activity, reduce their activity, and spend much of their time in bed or lying down. Chronic pain patients are often very manipulative of their families, peers, and physicians, and many go from doctor to doctor or from one emergency room to the next in their quest for drugs. The end result can be a desperate substance abuser who frequently has no job or family. Unfortunately, many consent to operation after operation but get no relief, or they seek relief from quacks or, worse yet, commit suicide. In contrast, healthcare professionals must not pigeonhole patients: research to date indicates that chronic pain patients are very different from one another and that there is no such thing as typical pain.[33]

Despite the fact that chronic pain is a major problem, many healthcare payors (including Medicaid) do not cover this level of care. When it is covered, it is often allowed as a mental health substance abuse benefit and may be piecemealed with various components of the process covered individually or not versus coverage of the program as a whole. Pain management programs are not substance abuse programs but a vital component of the rehabilitation continuum, as the underlying cause for the problem is physical, not mental.

PROGRAM COMPONENTS AND COSTS

Pain management is an evolving specialty. Many providers offer a vast variety of what are called pain management programs. These can be anything from an individual provider that offers one or more treatments to clinics and facilities that offer inpatient and outpatient and multidisciplinary approaches to treatments. As a result, it is common to find the following services in a pain management program:

- Patient education.
- Acupuncture.
- Physical therapy.
- Speech therapy.
- Pool therapy or aquatics.
- Individual counseling or psychotherapy.
- Group counseling.
- Family counseling.
- Instruction in biofeedback and relaxation.
- Medication management.
- Case management services.
- Social worker services.
- Steroid injections.
- Nerve blocks.
- Vocational counseling.
- Nutritional counseling.
- Transcutaneous electrical nerve stimulation.[34]

The efficacy of a program depends largely on the thoroughness of the initial evaluation, the patient's complaints, and the final treatment plan. Average costs vary from pain management program to program and from region to region but can range from several hundred dollars a day to a thousand or more.

A case manager who has a chronic pain patient who needs help must make every effort to place the patient in an appropriate treatment program. If the patient's healthcare coverage has no mental health benefit (for substance abuse) and does not recognize pain management under its medical benefit, the case manager must seek approval for a formal pain management program via the extracontractual process. If the extracontractual process fails, review of the patient's coverage may reveal areas of potential coverage, and a cafeteria plan may be established.

"Cafeteria plans" are often necessary because pain management has not been clearly defined nor actual "programs" allowed as benefits by most healthcare payors. For instance, in such situations the patient is afforded as many services as his healthcare policy permits (e.g., physical therapy, steroid injections, nerve blocks, psychotherapy). Each professional discipline bills separately or for fee for service. Rather than being billed at a flat rate, services are unbundled. As a result, the program may be more expensive, disorganized, and of less benefit in the long run.

MEDICAL VERSUS MENTAL HEALTH BENEFITS

Because pain management is primarily a medical measure, the most effective approach is to make every attempt to allow coverage under the traditional medical benefit structure rather than a mental health benefit. This practice, however, is healthcare payor specific. What are the advantages? At a minimum, they include avoidance of claims issues consequent on claims processing by two entities (medical payor and mental health payor) and one case manager, rather than two, on the case.

Before being approved for a pain management program, the patient is often evaluated by the pain management team. This initial evaluation includes a thorough history and a comprehensive review of systems and psychosocial history. This evaluation is not only critical for determining the appropriateness of the referral, it also allows the business office staff to determine who will accept financial responsibility for the treatment program. For example, if the pain is the result of a motor vehicle accident, a third-party liability payor is often responsible for reimbursement and must approve the coverage. When the cause of the pain is a work-related injury, costs of care must be approved by the appropriate workers' compensation carrier. Unfortunately, what often happens with both of these scenarios is that the patient has already accepted a settlement and the case has been closed by workers' compensation or an auto insurer. Reimbursement for the pain program then shifts to the patient's private healthcare payor, although such care may not be included in that benefit package. The facility's social worker or case manager may have to help the patient seek another source of reimbursement.

Once the initial evaluation is completed and the patient is determined to be a candidate, a coverage determination review must be made by the healthcare payor who will assume financial responsibility. This review affords an opportunity to determine whether the plan is appropriate to the patient's history and whether the proposed provider is qualified to deliver the treatment. If the claims are to be paid by the patient's private coverage, this review helps to determine which benefit structure—mental health or medical—will assume responsibility. Because pain management programs frequently are not a benefit, the case manager or social worker working with the patient and family must be prepared to request that it be covered through the extracontractual process.

INPATIENT VERSUS OUTPATIENT TREATMENT

The first program for pain management was established at Emory University in 1983, as an inpatient program.[35] Over the past 10 to 12 years, significant advances have been made. Treatment programs are now available as inpatient and outpatient offerings or as a combination of the two. Today, there are several hundred programs throughout the United States.

To ensure reimbursement, many healthcare payors require that the pain management program be an accredited inpatient program developed according to criteria of the Commission on Accreditation of Rehabilitation Facilities. This commission sets minimum standards for these programs, and the commission clearly recognizes that pain management requires a multidisciplinary team approach. The commission,

at a minimum, requires that the core team be composed of such specialists as the program medical director, the patient's treating physician, a psychologist or psychiatrist, physical therapists, occupational therapists, and sometimes other professionals (i.e., nursing staff, vocational counselors).

There are advantages and disadvantages to both inpatient and outpatient programs, one being cost.[36] Despite the fact that inpatient programs may cost more, there are times when they are the program of choice. A formal, structured environment allows for intensive treatment. Such programs are also designed for clients who have deteriorated physically owing to their pain and inactivity or for persons who are noncompliant with their treatments. Most of these cases are more complex and often require an inpatient program of approximately 4 weeks' duration followed by several more weeks of outpatient therapy. Similarly, outpatient programs can last 4 weeks or more, although the treatment may be less intensive (in frequency and duration).

Inpatient programs not only help to restore patients to an appropriate functioning level, they are also useful for detoxification. Regardless of whether detoxification is required, both inpatient and outpatient programs are designed to (1) rid the person of assistive devices, which are thought to perpetuate the idea of disability, and (2) educate the patient in alternatives for pain relief and how to prevent further injury.

GOALS AND OBJECTIVES

Treatment whether inpatient or outpatient must be flexible, individualized, and goal oriented.[34] Both programs are useful for treating the psychological problems and behavior manifestations that are commonly associated with pain and dysfunction. Program goals are as follows:

- To interrupt the chronic pain cycle.
- To optimally rehabilitate the patient physically, behaviorally, avocationally, vocationally, and socially.
- To teach responsibility, control, awareness of possible reinjury, and total independence from drugs, appliances, and the system.
- To return the patient to home and work with minimal limitations.[37]

Generally, admission to either program is based on the patient's ability to understand and follow instructions and motivation to comply with the program and the treatment regimen. Patients who are disruptive or aggressive or who have a severe psychiatric disorder frequently are not considered candidates, as they are too disruptive to the treatment setting. This variable is program specific. The principal objectives of either program are these:

- Detoxification.
- To relieve or decrease pain.
- To restore the person to an appropriate functional level.
- To eliminate use of assistive devices by restoring physical abilities and conditioning and to correct gait and posture.
- To return patient to work and leisure activities.
- To educate patient in preventing reinjury, weight control, ergonomics, body mechanics, energy-saving techniques, wellness, and alternatives for pain relief.
- Modification through biofeedback, family and group therapy, relaxation techniques, assertiveness training, and stress management.
- To provide vocational retraining when applicable.

CASE REVIEW

Although frequent review of each patient's case should always be the rule, it is best to do it at regular intervals for patients with chronic pain. The case review may include working with the healthcare payor's case manager, to review claims actually paid to date. At a minimum this addresses drugs paid for by the healthcare payor, all visits to other physicians, and all emergency and urgent care visits. (It would not reveal that drugs had been obtained from others or purchased privately or illegally.) Nevertheless, case review can enhance development of strategies for further case planning.

CASE MANAGEMENT INVOLVEMENT

The involvement of case managers in the actual pain management program depends on case variables and what sort of employer (i.e., facility-based case manager, healthcare payor) the case manager represents. Certainly, when the case manager is based outside a facility her involvement does not cease while the patient is in the program. The outside and facility-based case managers will work closely to keep the team apprised of healthcare benefits and limitations or exclusions and to ensure that the family

has made plans for when the patient is ready for discharge.

SUMMARY

Pain is a very debilitating problem, yet many healthcare payors do not cover formal pain management programs. Case managers must monitor their clients to ensure that acute pain is treated effectively, lest it progress to chronic pain. Case managers must make every attempt to help patients with chronic pain who seek treatment to obtain it whether through the extracontractual process, medical benefit coverage, or substance abuse benefits available as mental health coverage.

SKILLED NURSING FACILITY

When a patient no longer needs acute care, the first question is whether the patient needs skilled or custodial care. The case manager must also examine whether the patient requires services daily or intermittently and whether between nursing visits the patient can manage safely at home.

Medicare Criteria

Many payors utilize the best-recognized and utilized criteria for determining skilled or custodial care, those developed by Medicare, to certify providers. Often they will reimburse only services from Medicare-certified facilities.

To ensure compliance with Title XVIII of the Social Security Act and Medicare's Federal Conditions of Participation, each state has developed Administrative Codes that set minimum criteria and standards. The state's regulating bodies use these for licensure and standardization of service. As a rule, the regulating body designated to enforce these conditions is a state Department of Licensing and Certification or a similar agency under the state's Department of Health and Human Services. Under this department's guidance, standards are monitored through regularly scheduled facility surveys, and anyone can request copies of the findings, of citations for violations, and details of what corrective action was taken. These findings are a matter of public record and, as a rule, are posted at the facility or are available for review at regional licensing and certification offices. Case managers must know how to access this information.

What Is It?

A skilled nursing facility provides care for patients who do not need the full range of services available in an acute care hospital but who may need 24-hour services or daily treatments provided or supervised by professional licensed nursing or rehabilitation staff.

Skilled Care

Medicare defines skilled care thus: "The service must be so inherently complex that it can be safely and effectively performed only by or under the supervision of, professional or technical personnel."[38] At a minimum, these licensed professionals include the registered nurse, licensed vocational or practical nurse, and physical, occupational, or speech therapist. To qualify for reimbursement, the patient must be cared for in a skilled facility daily or at least 5 days per week. Because most skilled facilities offer services only 5 days per week this frequency constitutes "daily skilled care" under Medicare criteria.[39] Healthcare payors use similar criteria to develop policy guidelines for review and coverage.

Skilled nursing care or skilled rehabilitation therapy involves observation, assessment, judgment, supervision, documentation, teaching, or direct specific tasks and procedures necessary to establish and execute the treatment plan. For coverage to continue, the patient must make steady and significant functional improvement. In addition, Medicare and healthcare payors impose the following constraints on services or treatments:

- Performed in accordance with a physician's written order.
- Reasonable and necessary for the illness or injury.
- Consistent with the nature and severity of the client's illness or injury.
- Provided according to acceptable standards of medical practice.
- Reasonable in terms of duration and quantity.

In addition, case managers must be aware of the following facts:

- A physician is required to see the patient no more than every 30 days. Thus, the physician's progress notes are not as helpful as nursing and therapy notes in determining the need for skilled (versus custodial) care.
- Each state has its own administrative codes for enforcement of Title XVIII and XIX of the Social Security Act that establish minimum standards for care and other regulations for skilled nursing facilities.

Therefore, case managers must be familiar with minimum staffing patterns and frequency of physician visits as set forth in their state. These two variables most often decide whether a facility can or cannot accept a patient. For example, Title XXII is California's Administration Code for enactment of Title XVIII and XIX of the 1965 Social Security Act. Basically, these codes stipulate that skilled nursing facilities need provide only one licensed registered nurse for every 99 patients in any 24-hour period. Also, a skilled facility must provide the appropriate ratio of professional nurses for the number of patients they are licensed to admit. As a rule, nursing aides are the largest complement for all three shifts.

Other factors case managers must know are:

- Many skilled nursing facilities have a designated Medicare or skilled nursing unit to which skilled care patients are admitted. If that unit is full, the "new potential skilled patient" is placed on a waiting list.
- A skilled nursing facility is not obligated to admit any patient it feels it cannot care for.
- Many do not accept private insurance (bill only Medicaid or Medicare), and the family must pay up front and then seek reimbursement from their insurer.
- Financial eligibility for alternative funding (such as Medicaid) must be explored well in advance of any move to a skilled nursing facility if delays are to be avoided, and it is known beforehand that the family cannot afford skilled nursing facility costs. Costs for a skilled nursing facility average $3000 to more than $4000 per month, depending on where they are located.
- Most therapy is provided once a day. Only a few skilled nursing facilities offer it twice a day.
- In many facilities physical, speech, and occupational therapists are independent contractors and are not employed by the facility. The therapist develops a therapy plan, but much of the actual treatment is performed by therapy aides.

- If a skilled nursing facility is to maintain its profit margin, it needs a high ratio of private payors. Unless the family can demonstrate ability to pay private rates after payor benefits terminate, the facility may place the patient on a waiting list.
- Because many patients are confined to skilled nursing facilities total care beds are in short supply. Thus, case-managed patients who need total care must be placed on one or several waiting lists. This wait can be the single greatest cause of costly delays and of transfer to an alternate level of care.

General Selection Criteria

The following suggestions may help case managers facilitate discharge of the patient to skilled nursing care:

- Proximity of the facility to the family is a consideration, to prevent social isolation. As a rule, 30 to 40 miles is the accepted distance, but this must not interfere with placement if the only facility that can provide the needed level of care is farther away.
- The capabilities of the staff to provide the needed level of care must be explored, to ensure they can manage care on all shifts.
- Adequacy of staffing to manage the level of care (and willingness of the administration to add additional or specific licensed staff when warranted) must be evaluated before admission.
- Willingness of the administration to train staff when special training is necessary.
- Care rendered in accordance with state and federal regulations and conditions of participation.

Custodial Care

Custodial, or personal, care is defined as "the services or personal care that is necessary to assist the patient in meeting ADL." Assistance with ADL does not require trained medical or paramedical personnel.

ACTIVITIES OF DAILY LIVING

Activities of daily living are:

- Getting into and out of bed or a chair.
- Turning over in bed.

- Exercises to enhance overall fitness.
- Toileting.
- Bathing, dressing, and other personal hygiene activities.
- Feeding (including gastrostomy feedings) or preparation of special diets.
- Supervision or giving of medications that normally could be self-administered.

The custodial care level can also be appropriate when a patient has ceased to make functional improvements, for whatever reason or when there are no longer any changes in the frequency or type of care for a technology-dependent patient. In other words, the needed care is maintenance. In many cases, custodial care patients require a protected, monitored, and controlled environment.

As a rule, a custodial care determination is not precluded by the fact that the patient is under the care of a physician; that services are ordered to support the patient's condition; or that care or services must be supervised by a licensed professional nurse.[40]

Family Involvement

Finding a skilled nursing facility to manage all types of patients in a case manager's caseload is frequently a labor-intensive undertaking. For optimal results, the family must be involved in the process: they must be encouraged to visit, evaluate, and report back to the case manager or discharge planner. Because most skilled nursing facilities require admission paperwork to be completed before admission, the family must take the time to do this.

With any patient, but especially one who will be admitted to a facility outside the immediate area, communication must be open and as frequent as necessary to educate the patient and family of the positive aspects of the placement.

Barriers to Placement

Although barriers to placement are case specific, any discharge planner can confirm that the ones that are commonly encountered—and that most often cause delays—are these:

- Diagnosis related to human immunodeficiency virus or acquired immunodeficiency syndrome.
- Stage three or more severe decubitus ulcer.
- Infected wounds.

- Weight over 200 pounds.
- Contagious disease.
- Child patient.
- Age less than 50 years.
- Tracheostomy that needs frequent (usually at least three times per shift) suctioning or care.
- Ventilator dependency.
- Lack of family or other party responsible for financial follow-through once insurance coverage terminates.
- Need for total care (depending on the intensity and frequency of care).
- Psychiatric problems in addition to physical ones.
- Alcohol or drug abuse.
- Combative or abusive (physical or verbally) behavior.
- Need for equipment or supplies over and above what the facility provides.
- Need for dialysis or special diets. (These patients require the locations of a dialysis center and a skilled nursing facility and arrangements for transportation from one to the other.)
- Need for infusions and related services.
- Need for extensive dressing changes.
- Need for more than one complex treatment.
- Need for more hours of nursing care per day than the facility is licensed or staffed to provide.

In any of these circumstances it is common for the discharge planner or case manager to call many facilities before an appropriate one is located. It is also not uncommon to have to place patients outside their immediate area. Case managers must be familiar with the levels of care available, not only in a given community but throughout the state, and sometimes throughout the nation.

Subacute Care Facilities

Subacute care facilities have slowly emerged over the past decade, and such facilities provide both comprehensive medical nursing and rehabilitation services. The principal difference from a skilled nursing facility is that the subacute care facility offers (1) a higher nurse-patient ratio; (2) a larger number of nursing hours per day for skilled care (set by the state licensing codes); and (3) more frequent physician visits. For instance in California Title XXII sets the minimum criteria and standard for skilled care at less than 4 hours per day. In contrast, the nursing ratio for skilled care for a subacute care facility is almost 5 hours per day for nonventilator-dependent patients and much more for ventilator-dependent ones. Title XXII further stipulates that physicians must see their patients every 30 days in a skilled nursing facility, whereas patients in a subacute care facility must be seen at least every 7 days.

Certainly, some subacute care facilities are located outside the acute hospital setting; however, facility-based subacute care facilities, extended care facilities, and step-down units have several advantages over free-standing skilled nursing facilities—and even over other free-standing subacute care facilities. In addition to physicians' being more receptive to utilizing facility-based subacute care (the patient can be moved quickly back to the acute care setting if the patient's condition suddenly changes), other advantages are these:

- Staffing ratios and expertise are greater and in case of staffing shortages, staff may be available from the acute hospital inpatient pool.
- Visits from the patient's personal physician or attending physician team are more frequent, as the patient is more accessible.
- Radiologic and laboratory services are readily available 24 hours a day, 7 days a week.
- Surgery services, postanesthesia care, follow-up, or more intensive treatment are readily available 24 hours a day, 7 days a week.
- Review by the utilization review nurse is more frequent, as the patient is readily accessible.
- Physicians are often more receptive to using facility-based subacute units early, because the patient can be quickly returned to an acute care setting in the event of a sudden change in condition.

At this writing, subacute facility care is still in its infancy. Unfortunately, not all communities have access to this type of care. Another drawback is that payor networks do not always routinely include this level of care, so arrangements must be negotiated.

Although the cost for subacute care may at first glance seem greater, often, when all the pros and cons are considered, it is not. This level of care frequently is the more cost effective when one must choose between home care and facility-based care. The average cost of skilled nursing facility care averages $3000 to $4000 per month, whereas a subacute care facility, after rate negotiations, may cost $500 to $700 per day. Costs for home care, if private duty nursing is required, can be $100 or more per hour, or $2400 per day. Adding to the other costs associated with care, home care charges can exceed $20,000 per month for some high-technology patients.

What is the difference between a skilled nursing facility and a subacute care facility? A skilled nursing facility can be used for long-term placement and care. In contrast, a subacute care facility is designed for short-term care, until the patient stabilizes further and can safely be discharged to a lower level of care.

When transfer to a community-based subacute care facility is considered, the patient's personal physician or attending physician must have privileges at that facility. Otherwise, arrangements must be made for another physician to cover the patient. This alone can be a barrier to discharge for a complex-care patient. Many physicians who are unfamiliar with a patient's history and needs are reluctant to accept responsibility for the care. Often the case manager supplies the attending physician with a list of physicians who have patients at the subacute care facility and the physician must persuade a colleague to accept the case.

Admission Criteria

As a rule, most subacute facilities have admission criteria that require the patient to need three or more types of skilled care. Patients who need subacute care often have the following characteristics:

- They continue to need frequent laboratory testing or radiographic examinations.
- They continue to require frequent changes in orders and treatment planning, necessitating frequent physician visits.
- Treatments are too complex to be administered at a skilled nursing facility. (For instance, if the patient needs frequent suctioning or infusions a skilled nursing facility may not have sufficient numbers of staff or trained staff on all shifts to manage this.)
- Patients are ventilator dependent and were admitted for a weaning program.
- Patients have multiple skilled needs plus rehabilitation needs and cannot tolerate the intensity and demands of therapy in an acute rehabilitation unit.

Because care is short term, discharge planning and coordination for the next level of care must always be foremost in the case manager's mind. Lengths of stay vary and are case specific,

and there is no set rule about how long certain categories of patients remain at a specific level of care. Thus, medical necessity and the intensity and complexity of the treatment rendered are among the criteria used to justify continued stay and healthcare reimbursement. Once the care level stabilizes, consideration must be given to transfer to one of the following facilities:

- Acute rehabilitation unit.
- Skilled nursing facility.
- Home.

SUMMARY

Case managers must be keenly aware of available skilled nursing facilities, their capabilities, and any problems or licensing issues. For questions about licensing and care the best source of information is the state agency responsible for licensing and certification of healthcare facilities.

Not every patient requires the services of skilled nursing facility, but for those who do, careful coordination must take place to ensure that the patient is placed appropriately and rehospitalization is avoided. For optimal results, the family must be involved in all aspects, especially facility selection. Planning must start as soon as the patient is identified as a candidate for placement.

Finding an appropriate facility is often a labor intensive process, and the patient may be placed on several waiting lists until a vacancy is found. Also because of multiple conditions or illnesses or the intensity or complexity of their needs, not all patients are candidates for a skilled nursing facility. In situations such as these, the patient may require short-term placement in a subacute care facility; while in other cases, care may be possible at home.

All families must be counseled and prepared for the financial impact (and often guilt) associated with long-term skilled nursing facility placement. They also must be assured that such placement is frequently the only alternative to home care and that there is nothing wrong with admitting that they are not capable of managing the patient at home.

HOME HEALTH AGENCY CARE

Once a patient no longer requires acute care, the case manager must decide, based on the chart findings and physician's orders, whether or not the patient can go home. During the review the following questions may arise: Can the patient be managed safely at home with intermittent skilled visits? Is the patient "custodial"? If placement is necessary, which facility provides the least restrictions but can provide the required level of care? Can care in the home safely be arranged?

When Required and Provided by Whom?

Most healthcare payors require, at a minimum, that the home health agency be Medicare certified; others require the agency to be accredited by the JCAHO. Home health agency care is required when the skill and proficiency of a technical or professional health service provider is required to achieve the medically desired results for a homebound patient. Home health agencies provide these skilled technical and professional services:

- Licensed practical nurses and licensed vocational nurses.
- Occupational therapists.
- Physical therapists.
- Registered dietitian.
- Registered nurses.
- Social worker.
- Specialty care professionals (i.e., mental health professionals, chemotherapy nurse, pediatric nurse, respiratory therapist).
- Speech or language pathologists or audiologists.
- Other.

Definitions

Medicare defines a homebound person as one "who is essentially confined to the place of residence due to illness or injury and who can be ambulatory or otherwise mobile but is unable to safely be absent from the residence except for periods of relatively short duration." Intermittent or part-time skilled care is defined as, "the services of licensed professionals that is required daily (i.e., a daily visit or several times per week)."[1] Skilled home care can also be provided by more than one licensed professional, and some cases may require two visits from different licensed professionals in one day. Still, these constitute intermittent, or part-time, care.

Primary Functions

The principal functions of the home health agency are to provide skilled nursing or other therapeutic services to homebound patients on a part-time, intermittent, or visiting basis. Home health agency care can be preventive, diagnostic, therapeutic, rehabilitative, or long term. Each case must be assessed for the complexity of needed care, to prevent deterioration of the patient's condition and unnecessary hospitalization, and the type and extent of teaching or direct care required. Once the assessment is completed, a treatment plan is developed and submitted for the attending physician's approval.

Home healthcare that requires skilled nursing or rehabilitation services is frequently provided in lieu of continued hospitalization, confinement in a skilled nursing facility, or an outpatient center. Services include these:

- Evaluation and management of the care plan.
- Teaching and training activities.
- Direct skilled services.

Types of Services

There is no set rule as to what type of services a patient may require. For example, some patients may require varying arrangements for intermittent care at home (i.e., they may require skilled nursing on a very intermittent basis but rehabilitation therapy more frequently, or vice versa). The same patient may also need to hire unlicensed staff to assume personal care or homemaker duties (i.e., cleaning, laundry, cooking, shopping). Yet another patient may need hourly, shift, or live-in professionals. Home health can also be used to provide the terminally ill patient and family with hospice service.

Referral

Before referral to a home health agency the following variables must be considered:

- Attitudes of patient, family, or caregiver toward home care.
- Adequacy and suitability of the agency personnel to manage the complexity of care.
- Comparative benefits of home care and an extended care facility, subacute care, skilled

nursing, or intermediate care facility (cost and skilled care capabilities).

- Reasonable expectation that the patient's medical, nursing, and social needs can adequately be provided for at home.
- The availability, ability, and willingness of patient, family, or caregiver to participate in the care.
- The availability of a home setting.
- Adequate physical facilities in the home to provide proper care.
- Adequate structural and electrical capabilities to handle all equipment.

Medicare and many healthcare payors require that home health agency care meet these criteria:

- Be provided in accordance with written physician orders and the written treatment plan.
- Be provided by or supervised by a licensed professional (nurse or therapist).
- Relates directly and specifically to a treatment regimen.
- Is reasonable and medically necessary.
- Meets standards of practice and is safe and effective for treatment of the particular condition.

In addition to offering intermittent skilled services, many home health agencies also provide "registry" or private-duty nursing for patients who require hourly, shift, or live-in registered nurses, licensed vocational or practical nurses, certified home health aides, homemaker aides, or companions.

Case managers must know the various agencies, their capabilities, and the healthcare payor's policy on home benefits. At times they may have to seek an extracontractual waiver when a combination of cost-effective staffing is found to be adequate to manage the patient's level of care but is excluded from or limited by the patient's policy. For example, many policies cover only the registered nurse and not a home health aide, even though the aide might be more cost effective.

Professionals Involved and Their Services

The professional nursing services offered by a home health agency include these:

- Evaluating and reevaluating patient needs.
- Developing and implementing the plan of care.

- Providing direct nursing services, treatments, and preventive procedures.
- Observing for signs and symptoms, problems, and progression or regression and reporting all to the attending physician.
- Educating, supervising, and counseling patient, family, or caregiver about nursing care and related problems.
- Supervising and training other nursing personnel (aides).

Home health agency skilled physical therapists' duties include these:

- Evaluating and reevaluating patients and their therapy needs. (Tests are conducted to establish baseline data for functional impairment, abilities, and development of the care plan.)
- Providing direct treatments to relieve pain, develop or restore function, and maintain maximum performance.
- Use of equipment such as ultraviolet lights, diathermy, ultrasound, whirlpool and contrast baths, moist packs, and other durable medical equipment (e.g., walkers, braces, wheelchairs).
- Educating patient, family, or caregiver in care and use of durable medical equipment and therapy modalities.
- Instructing other health team personnel, including nurses, aides, patient, family, and caregiver in the therapy program.

Home health agency skilled speech therapists' duties include the following:

- Evaluating and reevaluating the patient for speech, hearing, and language disorders.
- Determining, recommending, or providing appropriate speech and hearing services.
- Instructing other health team personnel, including aides and caregiver, in the therapy program.
- Helping families to develop communication techniques (i.e., communication boards, signaling).

Home health agency occupational therapists' duties include these:

- Evaluating and reevaluating the patient's level of functional impairment and ability to perform self-care, including ADL.
- Instructing other health team personnel, including nurses, aides, and caregivers in the therapy program.

Home health agency social workers' duties include the following:

- Helping the healthcare team to understand

the social and emotional factors related to the patient's health and care.

- Assessing the social and emotional factors to estimate the caregiver's capacity and potential, including but not limited to coping with the problems of daily living, acceptance of the illness or injury or its impact, role reversal, sexual problems, stress, anger or frustration, and make the necessary referrals to ensure that the patient receives the appropriate treatments.
- Helping the caregiver to secure or utilize other community agencies as needs are identified.
- Helping the patient or caregivers to submit paperwork for alternative funding.

Home health agency home health aides' duties include these:

- Helping the patient with all aspects of personal or custodial care.
- Performing incidental household services essential to the patient's healthcare (e.g., the bed making, laundry, cooking, shopping, transportation to and from the physician's office).
- Helping with medications that ordinarily are self-administered.
- Helping with exercises as outlined by therapists.
- Reporting changes in condition to the supervising professional nurse.

Duration of Treatment

The actual frequency, type, and duration of the skilled services provided depend on multiple case variables. In most cases, skilled services are no longer considered medically necessary or appropriate for reimbursement purposes when the following conditions occur:

- Documentation indicates that patient or caregiver can safely and effectively administer or perform the skilled service that has been taught without direct supervision.
- Documentation reveals no significant change in the patient's status and it appears that none is expected; there has been no significant change in the therapeutic regimen; or, there is no indication of deterioration of the patient's condition for at least the last several weeks.
- Services are solely for observation and assessment of the patient.

- Services are ordered by a physician without any indication for skilled care.
- The patient has reached a plateau where no continued improvement and restorative potential can be reasonably predicted.

Documentation

To support coverage by the healthcare payor, home health agency documentation of services must, at a minimum, include these:

- Diagnosis and all existing conditions that are relevant to the care plan.
- Level of need, frequency of visits, and by which discipline (i.e., special care, need for special dressings or supplies, laboratory testing, observations, teaching, long- and short-term goals).
- Any changes in condition and related physician's orders and changes in the care plan.
- Responses to treatments and recommendations for changes in care plan.
- Referrals and coordination with other community agencies and reasoning.
- Medications, type, frequency, and any side effects.
- Type of diet, hydration, and response.
- Rehabilitation plan, ADL.
- Social or other problems.
- All teaching.

Barriers

The biggest barriers to establishing home care are the lack of a caregiver, financial limitations, and limited community resources to support the level of care. Others barriers are:

- There is no home (landlord restrictions are common for renters) or the home is structurally or electrically unfit to accommodate needed equipment.
- Patient or family does not accept a home care plan.
- The home environment is inadequate (e.g., lack of water, heat, air conditioning, electricity, refrigeration, phone, cleanliness, lack of space for special equipment).
- The home care plan is inadequate in terms of staffing, specialty, or the ability or willingness of the agency to hire and train necessary staff.
- Patient, family, or caregiver is unable or unwilling to learn care techniques.
- Caregiver has physical or mental limitations.

- Home situation is abusive.
- A physician is unavailable or unwilling to assume responsibility for the care.
- Transportation to the nearest resources is unavailable.
- No local agencies or resources are available to provide the required level of care.
- An agency is available, but staffing is limited and available nurses do not have necessary specialty training.
- A conservatorship is required prior to move or the conservatorship proceedings have been started but the patient cannot be moved until the final or temporary conservator is appointed.
- The physician refuses to approve a transfer.
- Cultural, ethnic, perceptual, or language factors preclude or delay a move.
- Other problems encountered are with teaching and relate to patient or caregiver issues: (1) patient or family readiness is inhibited by emotions, perceptions, stress, or role reversal; (2) inability to read and comprehend instructions; (3) visual impairment; (4) altered coping ability.

Private Duty Nursing

It is common for mechanically dependent patients to require private duty nursing. This is especially true on initial discharge and during periods of crisis or to give the caregiver respite. Examples of patients who need private duty nursing follow:

- Ventilator-dependent persons.
- New tracheostomy patients who require frequent suctioning and teaching.
- Terminally ill patients with multiple skilled nursing needs.
- Patients with multiple skilled care needs that require professional nursing interventions for several extended periods per day or a medical condition that requires continuous skilled care.

The need for private duty care must be assessed individually. The actual number of hours of skilled nursing is based on frequency and duration of care (i.e., several times in each eight hour shifts, sporadically, or instantly required at any time during a 24 hour period). If private duty nursing is allowed, the number of hours requested or approved should be contingent on the family's or caregiver's competence at providing the care and on other case variables

such as the intensity and complexity of the care. In some cases it is established to provide the skilled care the patient needs and to allow the caregiver time to sleep or attend to personal matters or business.

It is common on discharge of a technology-dependent or complex-care patient to provide 24-hour private duty nursing for the first week, at least while the caregiver learns skilled care techniques. As the caregiver develops proficiency, the nurse's hours can be reduced; however, this factor is case specific.

PRIVATE DUTY MEDICAID (IN-HOME WAIVERS)

When benefits are exhausted or the extracontractual process fails, the case manager may wish to consider applying for acceptance into a Medicaid In-Home Waiver program, Medicaid's version of private duty nursing. Unfortunately, application for a waiver program is an arduous process, and unless application is made months earlier it may not be a viable option. Case managers must be familiar with the Medicaid programs and waiver programs, including eligibility requirements and the appropriate procedures in their state. This is especially true if it appears the patient will require 24-hour care and this level of care is excluded by the healthcare payor. Application must be made as soon as possible.

If the patient is eligible and appropriate for a Medicaid in-Home Waiver, the healthcare payor retains responsibility for all other services or benefits not related to the services provided by the waiver (i.e., for benefits to which the patient is entitled by virtue of the health plan benefits). For instance, if the Medicaid waiver covers skilled care for a ventilator-dependent patient who requires gallbladder surgery, the surgery would be covered by the patient's healthcare payor, not by Medicaid. Medicaid is the payor of last resort, and if the patient is eligible for the Medicaid waiver, the waiver covers only services the payor disallows.

OTHER ALTERNATIVE FUNDING PROGRAMS

For technology-dependent children with special needs the case manager must work closely with the state's Title V Children's Medical Services Program and the agency responsible for administering services to persons with developmental disabilities to gain broader benefits, especially when hourly private duty nursing is required but is excluded from the child's health coverage. This level of service varies from state to state.

A key to a cohesive, nonredundant, and thorough care plan is joint development of the child's case management plan with the healthcare payor and each alternative source of funding for which the child might be eligible. Alternative funding or entitlement programs are payors of last resort, so any benefits available from the healthcare payor must be utilized or exhausted before other funding "kicks in."

Another key to working with alternate funding programs to deliver coherent care is to utilize their vendored private duty registries or home health agencies. Although often the vendored or paneled providers are not the ones in the healthcare payor's network, the case manager may need to request approval for their usage either through the normal review processes or extracontractually.

COSTS

Costs for private duty and skilled nursing vary from region to region, but case managers should expect a quote of approximately $100 per hour. Many agencies are willing to negotiate a daily or shift rate discount, but others are not. Despite the cost, private duty nursing is appropriate for the following situations:

• Technology-dependent patients whose physician agrees to home care and whose family, once trained, can assume a portion of the responsibilities for care.
• Patients unacceptable for post-acute care facility placement owing to the complexity of skilled care needs.
• Patients at risk for frequent acute-care readmissions or emergency room use and whose intermittent or daily home health agency care is insufficient.

Private duty nursing is also useful for technology-dependent patients who refuse any option except home. If such a patient is competent, out-of-home placement cannot be forced, as it violates the patient's rights.

APPROVAL

Because of limitations many healthcare payors place on home care benefits, skilled nursing facility level of care is often the most cost-effective alternative. If this level of care is not possible, approval may have to be obtained for private duty nursing or some combination of home health services.

It is common for many technology-dependent patients to require 16 to 24 hours of private duty nursing for several weeks or until the family or caregiver is proficient in all skilled techniques or the patient's medical condition has stabilized. All ventilator-dependent patients, once they are stabilized and comfortable in their home, can eventually have private duty nursing decreased to 8 hours per day. Such an arrangement affords the primary caregiver respite to sleep before resuming his or her normal 16-hour shift.

When the extracontractual process is utilized, the case manager may have to seek approval for ongoing private duty nursing in weekly increments. This allows better case control and monitoring of the situation. It also avoids the expectation that care will continue indefinitely. Getting approvals in this way takes more of the case manager's time but in the long run it is the best way because the case manager stays apprised of problems and progress. More important, it allows gradual decrements in the level of care.

One technique for seeking continued home health or hourly skilled care is to request 5 to 7 consecutive days of nursing or therapy notes. This gives the reviewer a better idea of the skilled level of care required and of the patient's response to treatment and expedites approval.

SUMMARY

Home health agencies are the most frequently utilized post-acute providers. They provide services for patients who are homebound and require continued skilled care. In addition, many technology-dependent patients need hourly private duty nursing.

If hourly private duty nursing is required, hours of care are case specific, but many patients require a minimum of 8 hours per day to allow the primary caregiver time to sleep. It is wise to seek or approve hourly care in increments, lest blanket approval set up the right of expectancy that this level of care will be a long-term service. Because many healthcare payors limit home care benefits, the extracontractual process may be a last resort, especially if private duty nursing is required.

REFERENCES

1. St. Anthony's Medicare Coverage Manual (1996). Reston, VA, St. Anthony's Publishing, pp. 181-214.
2. CHAMPUS Regulations. (1991). Aurora Co, Department of Defense Publications, pp. 2-8 to 2-9.
3. Granger CV, et al (1996). Quality and outcome measures for medical rehabilitation. *In* Braddom RL (ed). Physical Medicine and Rehabilitation. Philadelphia, WB Saunders.
4. Sinaki M (ed) (1993). Basic Clinical Rehabilitation Medicine. St. Louis, Mosby-Year Book, p. 3.
5. Sinaki M, Ibid., p. 4.
6. Granger CV et al (1996). Quality and outcome measures for medical rehabilitation. *In* Braddom RL (ed). Physical Medicine and Rehabilitation. Philadelphia, WB Saunders, p. 245.
7. Roth EJ, Harvery RL (1996). Rehabilitation of stroke syndromes. *In* Braddom RL (ed). Physical Medicine and Rehabilitation. Philadelphia, WB Saunders, pp. 1053-1081.
8. McPeak LA (1996). Physiatric history and examination. *In* Braddom L (ed). Physical Medicine and Rehabilitation. Philadelphia, WB Saunders, pp. 3-65.
9. Sinaki M, Ibid., pp. 9-16.
10. Sinaki M, Ibid., pp. 415-423.
11. Sinaki M, Ibid., p. 15.
12. Roth EJ, Harvery RL, Ibid., p. 1071.
13. Horn LJ, Zasler ND (1996). Medical Rehabilitation of Traumatic Brain Injury. St. Louis, Mosby-Year Book, p. 71.
14. Bontke CF, Boake C (1996). Principles of brain injury rehabilitation. *In* Braddom RL (ed). Physical Medicine and Rehabilitation. Philadelphia, WB Saunders, pp. 1027-1052.
15. Glacino JT, Zasler ND (1995). Outcome after severe traumatic brain injury: Coma, the vegetative state, and the minimally responsive state. J Head Trauma Rehabil 10 (1):40-56.
16. Whyte J, Gleason MB (1986). The Care and Rehabilitation of the Patient in a Persistent Vegetative State. Gaithersburg, MD, Aspen.
17. Cope ND (1990). The rehabilitation of traumatic brain injury. *In* Kottke FJ, Lehman JF (eds). Krusen's Handbook of Physical Medicine and Rehabilitation, 4th ed. Philadelphia, WB Saunders, pp. 1217-1251.
18. Cope ND, Ibid., p. 1217.
19. Bontke CF, Ibid., p. 1039.
20. Glacino JT, Ibid., p. 44.
21. Hosack KR, Roccbio CA (1995). Serving families of persons with severe brain injury in an era of managed care. J Head Trauma Rehabil 10(2):57-65.
22. Kersten LD (1989). Comprehensive Respiratory Nursing: A Decision Making Approach. Philadelphia, WB Saunders, p. 501.
23. Kersten LD, Ibid., p. 503.
24. Sinaki M (ed) (1993). Basic Clinical Rehabilitation Medicine. St. Louis, Mosby-Year Book, pp. 294-297.
25. Sanderson RG, Kurth CL (1983). The Cardiac Patient. A Comprehensive Approach, 2nd ed. Philadelphia, WB Saunders, p. 507.
26. Sinaki M, Ibid., p. 291.
27. Wenger NK. Cardiac rehabilitation components of a rehabilitation program for coronary patients. *In* Goodgold J (1988). Rehabilitation Medicine. St. Louis, Mosby-Year Book, pp. 217-225.
28. Sanderson RG, Ibid., p. 509.
29. Sanderson RG, Ibid., pp. 507-508.
30. McCaffery M (1996). The Scientific Method. Continuing Care 15(3):18-20.
31. Waldman SD, Winnie AP (1996). Interventional Pain Management. Philadelphia, WB Saunders, pp. 119-127.
32. Hinnat DW (1988). Psychological evaluation and testing. *In* Tollison CD (ed). Handbook of Pain Management, 2nd ed. Baltimore, Williams & Wilkins, pp. 18-35.
33. Chapman S (1988). Outpatient pain management. *In* Tollison CD (ed). Handbook of Pain Management, 2nd ed. Baltimore, Williams & Wilkins, p. 679.
34. Chapman S, Ibid., p. 684.
35. Chapman S, Ibid., p. 676.
36. Chapman S, Ibid., p. 678.
37. Rosomoff RS, Rosmoff HL (1989). Hospital based inpatient treatment programs. *In* Tollison CD (ed). Handbook of Pain Management, 2nd ed. Baltimore, Williams & Wilkins, p. 688.
38. St Anthony's Medicare Coverage Manual, Ibid., p. 184.
39. St. Anthony's Medicare Coverage Manual, Ibid., p. 186.
40. CHAMPUS Regulations. Ibid., pp. 2-8 to 2-9.

BIBLIOGRAPHY

Appleton M (1996). Hospice and skilled nursing facilities. Am J Hosp and Palliative Care May/June:11-12.
Aronoff G (1992). Evaluation and Treatment of Chronic Pain, 2nd ed. Baltimore, Williams & Wilkins.
Arras JD, et al (1995). Bringing the Hospital Home: Ethical and Social Implications of High-Tech Home Care. Baltimore, Johns Hopkins University Press.
Bernstein LH, et al (1987). Primary Care in the Home. Philadelphia, JB Lippincott.
Braddom RL (1996). Physical Medicine and Rehabilitation. Philadelphia, WB Saunders.
Bontke CF, Boake C (1996). Principles of brain injury rehabilitation. *In* Braddom RL (1990). Physical Medicine and Rehabilitation. Philadelphia, WB Saunders, pp. 1027-1051.
DeLisa JA, et al (1993). Rehabilitation Medicine: Principles and Practices, 2nd ed. Philadelphia, JB Lippincott.
Dobkin BH (1996). Neurologic Rehabilitation. Philadelphia, FA Davis.
Dorland's Illustrated Medical Dictionary, 28th ed. (1994). Philadelphia, WB Saunders.
During CG (1996). Learning to say no. AJN 96(4):62-64.
Farr A (1991). Medical halfway houses. Continuing Care 10(8):14-17.
Feldman C, et al (1993). Decision making in case management of home healthcare clients. J Nurs Admin 23(1):33-38.
Gill HS (1995). Home care's place within an integrated delivery system. J Care Manag 1(3):17-22.
Hall KM, et al (1993). Characteristics and comparisons of functional assessment indices: Disability rating scale. Functional independence measure, and functional assessment measure. J Head Inj Rehab 8(2):60-74.
Harris JA (1996). Recording brain injury rehabilitation. Contin Care 15(7):41-44.
HCFA clarifies home care regulations. (1991). Case Manag Advisor 2(12):181-182.
Hoeman SP (1996). Rehabilitation Nursing Process and Application, 2nd ed. St. Louis, Mosby-Year Book.
Hyer K, Rudick L (1994). The effectiveness of personal emergency response systems in meeting the safety monitoring needs of home care clients. J Nurs Admin 24(6):39-44.

Kataja G, Leonard N (1996). Coordinating long term care. Contin Care 15(3):26–28.

Kersten LD (1989). Comprehensive Respiratory Nursing: A Decision Making Approach. Philadelphia, WB Saunders.

Kottke FJ, Likmann JF (1990). Krusen's Handbook of Physical Medicine and Rehabilitation, 4th ed. Philadelphia, WB Saunders.

Lesko M, et al (1993). What to Do When You Can't Afford Healthcare: An A–Z Sourcebook for the Entire Family. Kensington, MD, Information USA.

Levin HS, et al (1987). Neurobehavioral Recovery for Head Injury. New York, Oxford University Press.

Lindaman C (1995). Talking to physicians about pain control. Am J Nurs 95(1):36–37.

Long CJ, Ross LK (eds) (1992). Handbook of Head Trauma: Acute Care to Recovery. New York, Plenum Press.

Lutz S (1993). Hospitals continue to move into home care. Modern Healthcare. Jan 25:28–32.

MacDonell C (1996). Defining home rehabilitation. Case Review. 2(1):87–88.

Matthews J (1990). Eldercare: Choosing and Financing Long-Term Care. Berkley, CA, Nolo Press.

Matthews J (1993). Beating the Nursing Home Trap: A Consumer's Guide to Choosing and Financing Long-Term Care, 2nd ed., Berkley, CA, Nolo Press

Medicare: Conditions of Participation of a Home Health Agency (1988). Washington, DC, U.S. Department of Health and Human Services. Health Care Financing Administration.

Medicare Conditions of Participation of a Skilled Nursing Facility (1988). Washington, DC, U.S. Department of Health and Human Services. Health Care Financing Administration.

Medicare Conditions of Participation for Extended Care Facilities and Skilled Nursing Facilities (1988). Washington, DC, Health Care Financing Administration.

Medicare Part A Intermediary Manual: Part 3 Skilled Nursing Facility Care Manual (1985). Bulletin 85-46. Washington, DC, Health Care Financing Administration.

Medicare Skilled Nursing Facility Manual (1988). U.S. Department of Health and Human Services. Washington, DC, Health Care Financing Administration.

Milhorn TH (1990). Clinical Dependence, Diagnosis, and Treatment Prevention. New York, Springer-Verlag.

Miller MS (ed) (1995). Health Care Choices for Today's Consumer. Washington, DC, Living Planet Press.

Mitchell PH, et al (1988). AANN's Neuroscience Nursing.

Phenomena and practice: human responses to neurologic health problems. Norwalk, CT, Appleton and Lange.

Moore EE (ed) (1990). Early Care of the Injured Patient. 4th ed. Philadelphia, BC Decker.

Pasero C, McCaffery M (1996). Managing postoperative pain in the elderly. Am J Nurs 96(10):39–45.

Pollack ML, Schmidt DH. Heart Disease and Rehabilitation. Boston, John Wiley & Sons.

Poretz DM (1991). High Tech Comes Home. Am J Med 91(5):453–454.

Raj PP (1992). Practical Management of Pain, 2nd ed. St. Louis, Mosby-Year Book.

Retzlaff K (1996). Assisted living. Contin Care 15(8):30–36.

Rice R (1995). Manual of Home Health Nursing Procedures. St. Louis, Mosby-Year Book.

Rizzo M, Tranel D (1996). Head Injury and Postconcussive Syndrome. New York, Churchill Livingston.

Rosenthal MG, et al (1983). Rehabilitation of the Head Injured. Philadelphia, FA Davis.

Roth EJ, Harvery RL (1996). Rehabilitation of stroke syndromes. In Braddom RL (ed). Physical Medicine and Rehabilitation. Philadelphia, WB Saunders, pp. 1053–1081.

Sanderson RG, Kurth CL (1983). The Cardiac Patient: A Comprehensive Approach, 2nd ed. Philadelphia, WB Saunders.

Sinclair BJ (1992). Alternative Health Care Resources: A Directory and Guide. West Nyack, NY, Parker.

Stahl DA (1996). Clinical assessment algorithm: Subacute care admission decisions. Nurs Manag 27(1):16–17.

Stanhope M, Knollmueller RN (1992). Handbook of Community and Home Health Nursing. St. Louis, Mosby-Year Book.

St. Anthony's Medicare Coverage Manual (1996). Reston, VA, St. Anthony Publishing, p. 187.

Thal LJ, et al (eds) (1992). Cognitive Disorders: Pathophysiology and Treatment. New York, Marcel Dekker.

U.S. Agency of Healthcare Policy and Research. Management of Cancer Pain Guideline Panel (1986). Management of Cancer Pain: Clinical Practice Guidelines. (AHCPR Pub No 94-0592). Washington, DC, U.S. Department of Health and Human Services.

Waxman JM (1994). A new wave of regulations for subacute care. Subacute Care 1(3):23–25.

Whyte J, Rosenthal M (1986). Rehabilitation of the patient with head injury. In DeLisa JA, Rehabilitation Medicine: Principles and Practice, 2nd ed. Philadelphia, JB Lippincott, p. 585.

Appendix
Community Resources

SYNOPSIS OF COMMUNITY AGENCIES

The community resources listed in the following pages are included primarily for case managers who might not have access to a community directory. As with all communities, the names, eligibility criteria, and type and level of services provided vary from state to state and often from county to county within a state.

The value of many of these resources cannot be underestimated. In most cases, they are a wonderful addition to the case management plan and an invaluable resource to the patient and family. Any of these agencies are excellent sources of:

- Information
- Assistance with referral
- Education through literature, educational classes, or public speaking forums
- Support groups in which patients and families can share tips on how to use and navigate the system, how to perform tasks better, and how and where to obtain supplies
- Opportunities for social outings
- Opportunities for peer support from others who have been there and experienced similar events or feelings
- Specialized services (e.g., transportation, advocacy, crisis intervention)

While many of the resources listed on the following pages are community-specific, others are affiliates of national groups; and while many agencies are listed in the local phone directories, national organizations may not be. In most cases, the national agencies concentrate their efforts on developing educational programs and literature and participating in research studies for the development of better techniques. They also provide information and referral services. Most of the national organizations can be reached by a toll-free telephone number. Many community-specific agencies offer case management services and other direct patient-related services or loan closets.

Most of these resources operate from Monday through Friday, and many offer traditional business hours of 8 AM to 5 PM. In most cases, there are no charges for the services provided. Some agencies charge a nominal fee; in these organizations, repayment charges are based on a sliding scale and the patient's ability to pay.

Community agencies and the services and information they provide to clients are a wonderful addition to any case management plan.

Not only can they supply callers with information and referral tips, many can also offer the emotional support and socialization opportunities that patients, families, and caregivers require.

The following has been provided to allow case managers to write in phone numbers for various agencies in their communities when a community-specific directory is not available.

SERVICES AVAILABLE FROM COMMUNITY AGENCIES

Adult Protection Services

Round-the-clock casework services from the county social services department.

- Advocacy
- Crisis intervention
- Investigation of complaints of abuse or neglect
- Placement

Local Telephone # _____

AIDS Foundation

May or may not provide home health and support services.

- Assistance in locating housing or caregiver
- Counseling
- Education
- Information and referral
- Case management
- Support Groups

Local Telephone # _____

National 800 Telephone # _____

Alcohol and Drug Abuse Programs

- Alternate programs
- Counseling
- Crisis intake or intervention
- Detoxification
- Maintenance or medication programs

- Residential and inpatient treatment program information

Local Telephone # ⎯⎯⎯⎯⎯⎯⎯

National 800 Telephone #

Alcoholics Anonymous

- Programs for family members
- Self-help recovery programs

Local Telephone # ⎯⎯⎯⎯⎯⎯⎯

National 800 Telephone #

Alzheimer's Aid Society

- Caregiver information
- Day care information
- Educational literature
- Respite information
- Support groups
- Skilled nursing facilities or nursing home information

Local Telephone # ⎯⎯⎯⎯⎯⎯⎯

National 800 Telephone #

American Cancer Society

- Counseling
- Sources of dressings and supplies
- Durable medical equipment (loan closets and local DME companies)
- Educational literature and programs
- Hospice information, bereavement outreach, or volunteers
- Support groups
- Transportation
- Visitor programs (for patients with laryngectomy, mastectomy, stoma, etc.)
- Wigs or hair bank

Local Telephone # ⎯⎯⎯⎯⎯⎯⎯

National 800 Telephone #

American Diabetes Association

- Camps (for diabetic youths)
- Educational literature or classes
- Foot screening
- Information and referral
- Newsletter
- Nutritional counseling
- Support groups

Local Telephone # ⎯⎯⎯⎯⎯⎯⎯

National 800 Telephone #

American Heart Association

- Dietary information
- Educational literature
- Information and referral
- Professional and lay training in cardiopulmonary resuscitation
- Stroke and cardiac support groups or clubs

Local Telephone # ⎯⎯⎯⎯⎯⎯⎯

National 800 Telephone #

American Lung Association

- Counseling
- Durable medical equipment (limited) may be available for loan
- Educational literature
- Free lung testing at local health fairs
- Information and referral
- Self-help classes
- Smoking cessation programs
- Support groups (better breathers, family asthma)

Local Telephone # ⎯⎯⎯⎯⎯⎯⎯

National 800 Telephone #

American Lupus Society

- Educational literature
- Information and referral

- Support groups

Local Telephone # _____

National 800 Telephone #

_____

American Red Cross

Offers many services.

- Casework services to the military, veterans, and their families
- Nursing and health programs
- Volunteers

Local Telephone # _____

National 800 Telephone #

_____

Arthritis Foundation (Local Chapter)

- Education
- Research
- Self-help classes

Local Telephone # _____

National 800 Telephone #

_____

Assistive Device Center

- Assessment and measurement for assistive devices
- Educational literature, slides, and videos

Local Telephone # _____

Blind Society

- Glaucoma screening (free)
- Preschool vision screening (free; groups only)
- Referral to local groups
- Information about special schools for the blind

LOCAL CENTERS FOR THE BLIND

- Braille training
- Educational literature
- Family counseling
- Glaucoma testing
- Information and referral
- Orientation and mobility training (limited)
- Sale of special visual daily living aids (adaptive games, Braille supplies, canes, electronic aids, special adaptive aids, preschool sensory development aids)
- Canine companion information
- Talking books and readers for the blind
- Weekly outings
- Volunteers

Local Telephone # _____

Library of Congress National 800 Telephone #

_____

EYE AND CORNEAL DONATIONS

- Registry and referral for organ donations

National 800 Telephone #

_____

EYE AND CORNEAL TRANSPLANTATION SERVICES

- Coordination of organ donations
- Education
- Literature

National 800 Telephone #

_____

Brain-Impaired Regional Center

California only. Serves patients with Alzheimer's disease, Parkinson's disease, multiple sclerosis, stroke, traumatic brain injuries, brain tumors, and other degenerative disorders of the brain.

- Conservatorship or power of attorney
- Counseling
- Diagnostic assessment
- Educational literature
- Financial advice

- Information and referral
- Legal advice
- Respite
- Support groups

Local Telephone # _____

Bereavement Outreach

Call the local information and referral system or the American Cancer Society.

- Educational literature
- Information and referral
- Support groups

Local Telephone # _____

Camps for Handicapped

Call specific disease agency for availability of camps (e.g., American Diabetes Association, American Cancer Society)

- Educational literature
- Recreational opportunities
- Therapeutic

Local Telephone # _____

Center for Deafness

- Advocacy
- Children's recreational programs
- Education
- Hearing aid clinic or loan of aid
- Hearing dog information
- Information and referral
- Independent living skills
- Interpreters
- Job development or counseling
- Lip reading instruction
- Mobile van for testing
- Sale of assistive devices
- Sign language instruction
- TTY information

Local Telephone # _____

National 800 Telephone # _____

Center for Independent Living

- Assistance in recruiting attendants or caregivers
- Screening and referral
- Training in basic self-care, functional skills, or independent living skills
- Crisis intervention
- Peer counseling
- Retrofitting of an apartment for accessibility
- Sex education
- Support groups
- TTY message relay services
- Use of attendants or in-home supportive services
- Use of community resources
- Use of transportation system

Local Telephone # _____

Children's Liver and National Liver Foundation

- Educational literature
- Organ procurement
- Support groups

Local Telephone # _____

National 800 Telephone # _____

Child Protection Services

- Advocacy
- Crisis intervention
- Investigation of complaints of neglect and abuse
- Placement

Local Telephone # _____

National 800 Telephone # _____

Conservator's Office

- Investigation of all referrals for public conservatorship for persons who cannot afford to pay a private attorney to perform the process

- Performs the duties of public guardianship and conservatorship for persons who are unable to manage their financial resources or personal affairs, when legally appointed by the court to do so, there being no family member willing or able to assume these duties

Local Telephone # _____

Consumer Credit Counseling Services

- Budget preparation and money management
- Counseling
- Creditor payment (check distribution) and negotiations
- Education
- Family income management

Local Telephone # _____

National 800 Telephone #

_____

Corporate Angel Network

- Provides air transportation for cancer patients on corporate airplanes when space is available (based in White Plains, NY)

National 800 Telephone #

_____

County Department of Health

ALCOHOL AND DRUG DIVISION

- Advocacy
- Counseling and rehabilitation information
- Detoxification
- Education
- Inpatient, outpatient, and residential treatment facility information
- Referral

Local Telephone # _____

MENTAL HEALTH DIVISION

- Mental health centers
- Mobile outreach
- Referral to regional inpatient and outpatient mental health centers
- Special programs for children, adults, and minorities
- Suicide prevention programs

Local Telephone # _____

PUBLIC HEALTH DIVISION

- Epidemiologic information about communicable or infectious diseases and rabies

Maternal and Child Health Program (Title V)

- Child health and disability program
- Prevention programs
- Women, Infants, and Children (WIC) nutrition programs

Local Telephone # _____

Primary Care Clinics

- Medical care
- Immunizations
- Venereal disease (diagnosis and treatment)
- AIDS (diagnosis and treatment)
- Tuberculosis (diagnosis and treatment)
- Family planning
- Well-child care

Local County Health Department

Local Telephone # _____

Public Health Chest Clinic

Local Telephone # _____

AIDS Clinic

Local Telephone # _____

Public Health Nursing

- Counseling
- Referrals
- Teaching or classes

Local Telephone # _____

Well-Baby or Well-Child Clinics

- Counseling about normal growth and development, nutrition, and health
- Physical examinations
- Immunizations
- Referrals as needed to Women, Infants, and Children (WIC) nutrition programs

Local Telephone # _____

County Department of Social Services (Welfare Department)

WELFARE DIVISION

- Financial assistance (general assistance)
- Food stamps
- Medical assistance (Medicaid)
- Supplemental Security Income (SSI)

Local Telephone # _____

CHILD DIVISION

- Adoptions
- Licensing of child day care centers
  - Child protective services (CPS—24-hour hotline)
  - Dependent services (court-ordered care)
  - Licensing of foster homes
  - Out-of-home placement services

Local Telephone # _____

ADULT AND AGING DIVISION

- Adult protective services (APS—24-hour hotline)
- In-home supportive services (homemakers, personal care, etc.)
  - Licensing of adult board and care homes
  - Out-of-home placement and alternative information

Local Telephone # _____

Crisis Center

- Counseling
- Crisis intervention
- Information and referral
- Inpatient care

- Mobile outreach (home assessment of patient)

Local Telephone # _____

DOMESTIC VIOLENCE HOTLINE

Call the local sheriff or police department if the name of the local unit is unknown.

- Advocacy
- Assistance
- Counseling
- Crisis intervention
- Education
- Emergency transportation
- Food and clothing
- Housing
- Legal information and referral
- Resettlement
- Social services
- Support groups
- Transportation

Local Telephone # _____

Cystic Fibrosis Foundation

- Educational literature
- Support groups
- Information and referral to tertiary or regional medical center programs

Local Telephone # _____

National 800 Telephone # _____

Department of Developmental Disabilities (state or county)

- Advocacy
- Behavior modifications
- Casework or case management
- Counseling
- Court-ordered evaluations
- Day care placement
- Guardianship, conservatorship, or payee services
- Medical and dental care
- Placement in state or residential treatment facilities

- Recreational planning
- Respite services
- Skilled nursing care
- Therapy (occupational, physical, or speech therapy)
- Training and vocational planning
- Transportation

Local Telephone # _____

State Telephone # _____

Department of Rehabilitation

Also called vocational rehabilitation.

- Advocacy
- Job training, skill training, or job placement
- Sheltered workshops
- Situational assessments
- Social and vocational counseling
- Speech therapy
- Work experience

Local Telephone # _____

State Telephone #

_____

Easter Seal Society

- Creative adult living programs or functional integrated living skills
- Loans of equipment (limited)
- Information and referral
- Medical social services
- Peer visiting programs
- Pool exercises
- Resident camps
- Skill training and employment preparation
- Support groups
- Therapy (occupational therapy, physical therapy, speech therapy)

Local Telephone # _____

National 800 Telephone #

_____

Emergency Response System (ERS) or Lifeline Systems

Call the nearest local ERS or the local Area on Aging.

- Electronic telephone system that alerts the local emergency room when the device worn by the patient is activated, setting off a pre-arranged emergency plan.

Local Telephone # _____

Fraternal Organizations

Shriners, Lions Club, Elks-Moose clubs, etc.

- Animals for patient use (e.g., seeing eye dogs, hearing ear dogs, monkeys)
- Assistive devices
- Equipment
- Fund raisers for special patient needs
- Organ and tissue banks
- Special projects
- Special Olympics
- Special hospitals and programs for handicapped children

Local Telephone # _____

Handicapped Transportation Services

Call the local or regional public bus services or the local area on aging.

- Coordination of transportation services with other agencies
- Door-to-door transportation services
- Mobility training for use of public buses
- Taxi coupon service

Local Telephone # _____

Hemophilia Foundation

- Annual camp
- Information and referral
- Scholarships for hemophiliacs
- Psychological and emotional support

Local Telephone # _____

National 800 Telephone #

_____

Hospice Groups

- Information
- Bereavement outreach and support
- Emotional support
- Pain and symptom management
- Respite care
- Skilled nursing care
- Trained volunteers

Local Telephone # _____

American Cancer Society

National 800 Telephone #

_____

Information and Assistance Services

Call United Way or the local or state department of aging or the local Directory Assistance service of the phone company.

- Telephone service that maintains lists by name and phone number of services and agencies available in the local area

Local Telephone # _____

Interpreter Services

- Ethnic groups or local church groups whose parishioners are of a specific ethnic origin
- Staff at nearest major regional or tertiary medical center who are available to act as interpreters
- AT & T (can be accessed by calling AT & T operator)

Local Telephone # _____

Legal Service Centers

Clients must meet income and disability criteria. These agencies offer free legal services but do not handle criminal cases.

- Advice and assistance with small claims issues, bankruptcy, and administrative laws
- Discrimination

- Domestic relations
- Health
- Social Security
- Unemployment

Local Telephone # _____

Leukemia Society of America

- Information and referral
- Educational literature
- Possible financial aid for:
  - Blood transfusions
  - Some medications
  - Transportation
  - X-ray treatments
  - Information and referral

Local Telephone # _____
National 800 Telephone #

_____

Library Services

- Bookmobile
- Books by mail
- Books in Braille
- Dial-a-book (or story [children])
- Large print books or magazines
- Readers for the blind
- Talking books

Local Telephone # _____

Library of Congress National 800 Telephone #

_____

Make-A-Wish Foundation

- Fulfills wishes of children aged 2 to 18 battling a life-threatening illness.

Local Telephone # _____

National 800 Telephone #

_____

Maternal-Child Health Programs

Eligibility and program components vary from state to state.

- Federal alternate funding program that can provide healthcare benefit coverage to certain persons under the age of 21 who have a catastrophic illness or injury that will result (or has resulted) in a chronic crippling disorder.

Local Telephone # _____

National 800 Telephone #

_____

Meal Programs

Call the nearest community information and referral service or the local state department of aging.

- Congregate meal sites
- Home-delivered meals

Local Telephone # _____

Mental Health Groups

- Advocacy
- Assessment and treatment
- Case management
- Counseling
- Crisis intervention
- Emergency evaluation and treatment
- Employment and training
- Independent living skills
- Inpatient or outpatient treatment
- Medication management
- Outreach and prevention services
- Patients' rights advocacy
- Protective services (adults and children)
- Residential treatment facilities
- Special education programs

Local Mental Health Association

Local Telephone # _____

Adult Protective Services

Local Telephone # _____

Alcohol and Drug Abuse

Local Telephone # _____

Child Protective Service

Local Telephone # _____

Crisis Clinic

Local Telephone # _____

County Conservator's Office

Local Telephone # _____

Developmental Living Center

Local Telephone # _____

Mobile Outreach

Local Telephone # _____

Toughlove

Local Telephone # _____

Muscular Dystrophy Association

- Camps
- Diagnostic and evaluation clinics
- Educational literature
- Loans of wheelchairs and other hospital equipment

Local Telephone # _____

National 800 Telephone #

_____

National Foundation for Ileitis and Colitis

- Educational literature
- Support groups

Local Telephone # _____

National 800 Telephone #

_____

National Handicapped Sport and Recreation Association

- Ski instruction for handicapped
- Other sports instruction and events

National 800 Telephone # _____

National Marrow Donor Program (St. Paul, MN)

- Created to improve efficiency and effectiveness of donor searches for unrelated bone marrow transplants

National 800 Telephone # _____

National Multiple Sclerosis Society

- Educational literature
- Home healthcare classes
- Loans of wheelchairs and other standard equipment
- Newsletter
- Peer counseling
- Referrals to social service agencies
- Social activities
- Support groups

Local Telephone # _____

National 800 Telephone # _____

Opportunities for the Handicapped

- Speech therapy
- Survival skill training (self-care, mobility, socialization, and leisure development)
- Training and work experience
- Vocational education

Library of Congress National 800 Telephone # _____

Organ Procurement or Transplant Services

- Coordinates donations through national computer from organ bank and hospitals
- Education

Local Telephone # _____

Parkinsonian Foundation

- Educational literature
- Support groups

Local Telephone # _____

National 800 Telephone # _____

Planned Parenthood

- Abortions
- Birth control
- Counseling
- Family planning
- Information and referral
- Pregnancy testing

Local Telephone # _____

Pregnancy Hotlines

- Counseling
- Education
- Free pregnancy testing
- Information and referral
- Support groups (child care available)

Local Telephone # _____

Protection and Advocacy (Ombudsman)

- Investigates and resolves complaints for persons confined to licensed facilities
  - Abusive situations
  - Dietary complaints
  - Finances
  - Medical and nursing care complaints

- Patients' rights
- Quality of care

Local Telephone # _____

Rape Crisis Centers

- Advocacy
- Counseling
- Crisis intervention
- Emergency referral

Local Telephone # _____

Regional Centers

For developmentally disabled persons; available only in California.

- Advocacy
- Assistance with alternate funding
- Assistance with obtaining a public official's statement (POS) needed for the CHAMPUS Program For The Handicapped (PFTH)
- Counseling
- Education
- Genetic counseling
- Guardianship
- Information and referral
- Placement
- Preventive services for high-risk couples and infants

Local Telephone # _____

Religious or Ethnic Social Service Agencies

- Advocacy
- Clothes closets
- Counseling
- Crisis intervention
- Forms (assistance with)
- Group activities
- Information and referral
- Loan closets
- Nutrition sites, food closets, or home-delivered meals
- Outreach
- Parenting classes
- Telephone reassurance services
- Visitation programs

- Vouchers for food, housing, and employment
- Transportation

Asian

Local Telephone # _____

Hispanic

Local Telephone # _____

Other ethnic groups

Local Telephone # _____

Catholic social services

Local Telephone # _____

Lutheran social services

Local Telephone # _____

Other religious social services

Local Telephone # _____

Respite Services

Call the nearest community information and referral service for lists of agencies or facilities.

- Caregiver relief
- Care for patient
- Day care (24 hour)
- Support network

Local Telephone # _____

Retarded Association

- Advocacy
- Conservatorship or payee services (money management)
- Education
- Employment (evaluation and training)
- Information and referral
- Sheltered workshops

Local Telephone # _____

Senior Centers

- Advocacy
- Blood pressure screening

- Information and referral
- Legal services
- Nutrition
- Outreach to the homebound
- Recreation
- Socialization
- Tax preparation

Local Telephone # _____

Sickle Cell Anemia Foundation

- Clinics
- Education
- Genetic counseling

Local Telephone # _____

Spina Bifida Association of America

- Information and referral

Local Telephone # _____

National 800 Telephone # _____

Sudden Infant Death

- Information and referral

Local Telephone # _____

Suicide Prevention

- Counseling
- Crisis intervention (24-hour hotline)
- Emergency aid dissemination
- Training program for volunteers

Local suicide prevention unit

Local Telephone # _____

Crisis Clinic

Local Telephone # _____

Mobile Health Outreach

Local Telephone # _____

Mental Health Association

Local Telephone # _____

United Cerebral Palsy Association

- Advocacy
- Education
- Information and referral
- Support groups
- Transportation

Local Telephone # _____

National 800 Telephone # _____

Utility Companies

- Braille knobs and markings
- Discounts for seniors or the handicapped
- Extended billing and discounts for the disabled
- Special phones, communication devices, and interpreter services
- TTY services
- TDD services

Gas company

Local Telephone # _____

Electric company

Local Telephone # _____

Phone company

Local Telephone # _____

Water company

Local Telephone # _____

Veterans Affairs or Services

- Alcohol and drug abuse treatment
- Assistance with claims and location of services for veterans and their dependents

- Educational benefits for eligible veterans
- Information and referral services
  - Agent Orange
  - Benefits
  - Delayed stress and other war-related maladies
  - Educational benefits
  - Home and farm low-interest loans
  - Veterans' homes, hospitals, and outpatient clinics

Local Telephone # _____

State Telephone # _____

National 800 Telephone #

_____

Victim and Witness Assistance Program (for victims of violent crimes)

- Claim filing assistance
- Crisis and short-term counseling
- Liaison between victim and court system
- Referral to private or public service agencies as needed

Local Telephone # _____

National 800 Telephone #

_____

Visual Aid Center

- Individual living skills
- Prism glasses
- Visual assistive devices

Local Telephone # _____

Vocational Rehabilitation

- Advocacy
- Assessment
- Counseling
- Information and referral
- Job placement or work experience
- Job retraining or training
- Sheltered workshops

POSSIBLE SITES FOR VOCATIONAL REHABILITATION OR JOB RETRAINING

- Desert Industries
- Goodwill Industries
- PRIDE Industries
- Purple Heart
- Salvation Army
- Other

Local Telephone # _____

State Telephone # _____

Glossary

In attempting to coordinate benefits with those of other insurance policies, the case manager may encounter unfamiliar terms used by healthcare payor employees. Another area that often confuses utilization reviewers or new case managers is the field of neurologic impairment and rehabilitation; the progress notes for these patients often contain very specialized terms. Therefore, the following list of basic insurance, rehabilitation, and continuum of care terminology should prove helpful.

Abstract Concept. Refers to concepts that may be very difficult to understand (theoretical or detached).

Abstract Reasonings. Process of generalizing from concrete examples and experiences to larger, broader principles.

Acalculia. Dysfunction or inability to perform mathematical operations, recognize numbers, or count.

Accreditation. Accreditation is the most reliable indication that an agency meets basic standards and levels of performance. To be accredited, an agency voluntarily undergoes an investigation of its services and management practices by a professional organization whose purpose is to accredit or monitor agencies or healthcare organizations. Depending on the organization being accredited, this might be the Joint Commission for Accreditation of Healthcare Organizations (JCAHO) or, for rehabilitation facilities, the Commission for Accreditation of Rehabilitation Facilities (CARF), among many others.

Activities of Daily Living (ADL). The activities associated with daily life, including such activities as personal hygiene, elimination, ambulation, getting in or out of a bed or chair, and eating.

Actuary. A statistician who computes insurance rates and premiums.

Acuity. Sharpness or acuteness of sensation.

Adaptive Equipment. Ordinary utensils that have been specially adapted for a person with a disability.

Adjudication. Settlement of a claim for payment.

ADL. See *Activities of Daily Living (ADL).*

Administrative Services Only (ASO). Contract between a self-insured plan and an insurance company whereby the insurance company performs the administrative services such as claims processing, actuarial analysis, utilization review, and sometimes case management.

Adult Day Healthcare (ADHC). Centers that provide health, recreation, and social services to the disabled or frail elderly during the day from Monday to Friday. Most patients served by such day centers would be at risk of placement in a skilled nursing facility or intermediate care facility if the day center were unavailable. Health services may be provided at these agencies but are not as intense as those provided in a day hospital, intermediate care facility or skilled nursing facility. There are two day care models: the "social" model, in which the emphasis is on socialization (supervision and services are primarily for mental health patients), and the "medical" model, in which care is provided for persons with physical or functional impairments.

AFO. Ankle or foot orthotic. See also under *Orthotic.*

Agnosia. Loss of ability to recognize familiar people, places, and objects and inability to recognize a sensory stimulus.

Agraphia. Loss of ability to express thoughts in writing.

Aid to Families with Dependent Children (AFDC). A federal-state program administered by the county that provides financial assistance and medical care. Food stamps are granted as specified in the Social Security Act to children and their parents or caretakers who meet eligibility criteria. The amount of money received is computed according to the number of persons who reside in the home. The program is also available to children in foster homes and to those who are wards of the juvenile court or have been referred to the social welfare department for placement.

Aide. A nonlicensed person who performs custodial nursing care for a patient such as bathing, grooming, dressing, ambulating, and toileting.

Alexia. Inability to read or recognize words.

Allowable Charge. The amount derived from averaging a region's charges or prevailing rates for specific diagnoses and procedures over a period of time.

ALOS. Average length of stay.

Amnesia. Lack of memory for periods of time. Several varieties exist:

Anterograde amnesia: Inability to remember events beginning with the onset of the injury; severely decreased ability to learn.

Retrograde amnesia: Loss of memory for events preceding the injury.

Post-traumatic amnesia (PTA): The period of anterograde amnesia following a head injury. Patient is unable to store new information.

Ankle Foot Orthotic (AFO). See under *Orthotic.*

Anomia. Dysfunction or inability to name objects or recall individual names. Inability to find the correct word.

Anosognosia. Inability to recognize disease or disability in oneself.

Anoxia. Lack of oxygen to the brain, resulting in brain damage.

Aphasia. Loss of ability to express coherent ideas in speech or understand spoken language. The impairment of some aspects of language is not due to defects in speech or hearing but to brain dysfunction. Aphasia may be described specifically as:

Receptive: Inability to understand what has been said. Also called Wernicke's aphasia (temporal lobe).

Expressive: Inability to express oneself. Also called Broca's aphasia (frontal lobe).

Global: Both expressive and receptive aphasia.

Appeal. Disagreement in writing about an issue that involves payable benefits.

Apraxia. Loss of ability to carry out habitual movements or acts that were previously automatic. This inability to plan and execute a learned voluntary movement smoothly is not due to muscle weakness or failure to understand directions. Verbal apraxia is impaired control of the proper sequencing of the muscles used in speech. Constructional apraxia is an inability to assemble, build, draw, or copy accurately that is not due to apraxia.

APS. Adult Protective Services. See also under *Protective Services.*

Areflexia. Loss of reflex action.

ASO. Administrative services only.

Assignment or **Assignment of Benefits.** Agreement by the healthcare provider to accept the amount paid by the insurer as full payment for the services rendered, requiring the insured person to pay only his or her cost shares or deductible. Generally, assignment requires a contract between the provider and the healthcare payor; the provider is paid directly by the health plan.

Astereognosis. Inability to recognize objects or shapes by touch.

Asymmetry. Discrepancy in function or appearance between sides or organs.

Ataxia. Dysfunction in motor coordination and balance.

Attention. Ability to sustain focus on task for a period of time to allow coding and storing of information in memory. There are three components:

Alertness: The degree of generalized readiness of the central nervous system to receive information.

Selection: The ability to choose the information that deserves the effort of further analysis while simultaneously suppressing irrelevant stimuli. Selection reflects the qualitative aspect of attention.

Effort: The amount of attention needed for a task. Concentration, persistence, and the ability to maintain focus over long periods of time are examples of effort. Effort reflects the quantitative aspect of attention.

Authorization or **Preauthorization.** Approval required prior to claims payment or the rendering of services or admissions.

Autonomic Dysreflexia. "Crisis" condition usually caused by a distended bladder or bowel and resulting in headache, sweating, flushing, or high blood pressure. This can result in stroke and can be fatal.

Average Wholesale Price (AWP). Price of a drug from the manufacturer before dispensing fees and other charges are added.

Balance Billing. Practice (by providers) of charging the patient for any amounts between what was billed and what was actually paid by the the healthcare payor. Balance billing is generally prohibited by managed care plans except for normal copayments, coinsurances, and deductibles or when coverage is denied by the healthcare payor and the patient elects to have the procedure performed regardless.

Balanced Forearm Orthotic (BFO). See *BFO.*

B & B Training. Bowel and bladder retraining for normal use, or to establish a "habit" or a specific time for elimination.

Bed Mobility. Rolling or getting into or out of bed.

BFO. Balanced forearm orthotic, which assists the patient in feeding and grooming activities as it supports the arms.

Bill Audit. Process conducted after discharge on large bills in which the actual billed amounts are verified and compared against the written orders and the documentation in the patient's chart that supports the fact that tests or procedures were actually performed.

Binder. Abdominal support that aids circulation (by preventing blood pooling) and breathing.

Board and Care Facillities. See *Residential or Board and Care Facilities.*

Bolsters. Specially sized mattress sections arranged to promote good skin care through proper positioning.

Bonding. A financial arrangement, something like an insurance policy, that pays any penalties levied against an agency or individual that result from a lawsuit. Some states require bonding before they will issue an agency's license. Bonding is actually a method of protecting the agency against consumer claims, not an assurance of the agency's or individual's quality.

Brain Stem-Evoked Response. Auditory brain stem responses provoked by stimulating the brain with painless sound waves using headphones.

Capitated Rates. Rates based on the number of persons enrolled. These rates generally remain the same regardless of the level of services delivered and represent payment of a set amount of money.

Caregiver. Generally a family member, friend, volunteer, or medical professional who provides care to the patient in the home.

Carrier. An insurance company.

Catastrophic Cap. The upper limit that the insured or patient must pay out-of-pocket in any fiscal year for covered medical care. Often this amount is $1000 to $10,000. Once this cap is reached, the healthcare payor pays 100% of the charges rather than the lower percentage it had paid before the cap was reached. As a rule, there is no catastrophic cap if a patient is enrolled in a health maintenance organization (HMO) or in some other managed care plan.

C-Clip. Assistive device worn on the hand that has a pocket for utensils.

Centers for Disease Control and Protection (CDC). Federal agency in charge of protecting the public's health by administering national programs intended for the prevention and control of communicable and vector-borne diseases. This agency has nine subagencies: (1) Epidemiology, (2) International Health, (3) Public Health Practice, (4) National Center for Prevention Services, (5) National Center for Environmental Health and Injury Control, (6) National Institute for Occupational Safety and Health, (7) National Center for Chronic Disease Prevention and Health Promotion, (8) National Center for Infectious Diseases, and (9) National Center for Health Statistics.

Centers for Independent Living. Units that offer services to physically disabled or challenged individuals. Many offer services such as peer counseling, advocacy, attendant recruitment, screening and referral, retro-fitting of the residence, information and referral, TTY message relay, crisis intervention, mobility training for use of public transportation, training in activities of daily living, and use of community resources.

Certification. Process that ensures that an agency meets certain basic standards for patient care. The state Department of Health or a similar state agency assumes responsibility for the certification process. Certification allows the agency to qualify for Medicare and some Medicaid reimbursement. Individual professionals such as social workers and therapists may also be certified by their professional organizations. Although certification indicates that certain standards have been met, it is not an assurance of quality, nor does it guarantee that the agency provides good care.

Cervical Thoracic Orthotic (CTO). See *CTO Brace.*

CBI. Continuous bladder irrigation.

Claim. The bill for medical care or services rendered to a particular patient that is submitted by the provider to the healthcare payor or claims processor for payment.

Claim Cycle Time. The period of time, recorded in calendar days, that elapses from receipt of the claim to the printing of the check and explanation of benefits (EOB).

Clinical Nurse Specialist. A licensed professional nurse who has successfully completed a training program (Master's level) in a specific or specialized area of nursing. Often the clinical nurse specialist fulfills multiple roles such as clinical practice, consultation, education, research, and administrative support.

Clonic. Rapid muscular spasms in which contractions alternate with relaxation.

Clonus. Involuntary rhythmic series of spasms.

Closed Panel. A managed health plan that contracts with a group of physicians on an exclusive basis; patients are not allowed to see physicians outside this panel for routine care. See also under *Health Maintenance Organization (HMO).*

CMG (Cystometrogram): A test that evaluates bladder capacity and expulsive response.

Cognition. The process of knowing or being aware of thoughts and perceptions, including thinking, reasoning, problem solving, and understanding.

Cognitive Flexibility. The ability to shift one's cognitive or perceptual reference points or mind-set.

Cognitive Retraining. A fairly new specialty developed to meet the special needs of the traumatic brain-injured patient or persons with acquired brain injury. Although all members of the rehabilitation team are responsible for cognitive retraining, some rehabilitation programs actually use the professional expertise of a cognitive retrainer. Cognitive retraining addresses problems in orientation, concentration, memory, judgment, problem solving, and other cognitive skills necessary to function in our society.

Coinsurance or **Cost Share.** The provision that limits the amount of coverage by a healthcare plan to a certain percentage, often 80%, of the charge; any remaining amount is paid out-of-pocket by the patient.

Coma. A state of unconsciousness from which the patient cannot be aroused, even with deep stimulation.

Coma Stimulation Program. Program that offers a specialized therapeutic milieu to the traumatic brain-injured patient who is in a coma. In these programs, consistent, repetitive stimulation techniques are used over a period of time to arouse the patient. Coma programs are considered a skilled nursing facility level of service rather than rehabilitation. The patient should not be considered for custodial care until he or she has shown no progress in arousal from coma within a specified period of time.

Commission on Accreditation of Rehabilitation Facilities (CARF). The body responsible for reviewing and accrediting rehabilitation facilities and related treatment centers to ensure that they meet basic established standards and levels of performance.

Commission on Aging. Focal point for senior concerns in a particular community. Primary advisory board and communication conduit between the county board of supervisors and senior advocates. This commission studies, evaluates, and makes recommendations about senior services within a county.

Complete Lesion. Spinal cord injury leading to total loss of motor ability and sensory function. Also called a Frankel class A lesion of the cord. See also *Incomplete Lesion; Lesion*.

Comprehension. The ability to understand or draw meaning from what is seen, heard, or touched.

Comprehensive Alcohol Abuse Prevention, Treatment and Rehabilitation Act of 1970. Regulates the use and disclosure of information pertaining to drug and alcohol abuse; supersedes the Privacy Act. Protected are records about the identity, diagnosis, prognosis, and treatment of any person in a drug or alcohol abuse program. Information can be disclosed only if such disclosure is authorized by the person or his or her legal guardian.

Concentration. Ability to remain attentive to a task at hand over a period of time and to resist distraction or diversion.

Concrete Thinking. Thought patterns centered primarily on objects, events, or attributes that can be easily imagined.

Concurrent Review. The review that occurs during the course of treatment by the healthcare payor or department responsible for utilization review; usually refers to any review that occurs while the patient is hospitalized or receiving treatment.

Confabulation. Verbalization about people, places, and events that have no basis in reality. May be detailed and delivered with apparent confidence by the patient.

Congregate Housing. A residence that resembles a boarding home. The residents may or may not share a room and bath; meals are served in a central dining room, and activities may or may not be planned. Many congregate housing units are designed for the elderly or mentally disabled. Medical care is not provided, and readmission to such units after a hospital stay depends on the patient's ambulatory ability and independence. Some facilities allow patients who need intermittent nursing care to be followed by a home health agency, but others, owing to licensing restrictions, may not allow the patient to be readmitted until the person can function independently.

Congregate Meals. Group meals that may be offered by a church group, social service agency, or low-income housing complex. These programs are designed to facilitate socialization and to ensure that the participants receive a healthy meal. Most programs serve one meal per day from Monday to Friday, primarily to ambulatory or independent wheelchair-bound persons. Costs for this program are nominal.

Conservatorship. Legal process whereby a conservator is appointed by the local county probate court for persons (principal) who are declared mentally incompetent. Conservatorship can be obtained for either financial needs (estate) or health needs (person), or both. The "conservator of the person" is responsible for making decisions about the patient's care as well as the place where he or she is to live or receive treatment. The "conservator of the estate" is the financial guarantor and manages the person's financial affairs. Conservatorship, once issued, remains valid indefinitely. Once conservatorship proceedings have been started, the patient frequently cannot be moved to another location until a "temporary conservator" has been appointed.

Consolidated Omnibus Reconciliation Act (COBRA) of 1985. This act contained many Medicaid and Medicare Amendments. The most important portion of this act requires employers to offer employees who have been terminated the option to purchase and continue their medical coverage for a minimum of 18 months after termination.

Constructional Apraxia. Inability to assemble, build, draw, or copy accurately; it is not part of apraxia or inability to make single habitual movements.

Contact Guard. Term used in rehabilitation medicine to indicate that the patient requires physical contact by the caregiver or therapist throughout the activity.

Contracted or **Network Provider.** Provider that signs a contract to provide services to the healthcare payor's members for a specified rate. See also *Provider*.

Contrecoup. Bruising of brain tissue opposite the side where the blow was struck.

Coordination of Benefits (COB). Method used by healthcare payors when a patient has more than one policy and it is necessary to coordinate benefits to prevent overpayment or duplication of payment. When patients have more than one insurance policy, one policy is considered the primary payer and has the first responsibility to pay or deny the claim.

Copayment. The out-of-pocket expenses (usually a fixed amount) that must be assumed by the patient at the time each service is rendered. In health maintenance organizations (HMOs) the charge is often a nominal amount ($5 to $10) for an office visit or prescription.

Coping Skills. The ability to deal with problems or difficulties whereby the person attempts to resolve, accept, or overcome them.

Cost Containment. Formal active attempts to control healthcare costs through such efforts as improved efficiency, utilization review, claims review, prospective review, rate negotiations, and rate reviews.

Cost Share. See *Coinsurance or Cost Share*.

Court-Ordered Care. Medical care or services ordered by a court of law, which may direct a person to obtain or a professional entity to provide. The services ordered may or may not be reimbursed by the healthcare payor. In most instances, the costs are paid by the state or county agency that ordered or requested the services. (For example, recently the state of Texas passed a law requiring a healthcare payor to continue coverage for a dependent child if such coverage is court ordered regardless of where the child resides, even if he or she lives out of the payor's service area. [This action can occur during a divorce proceeding.])

CPS. Child Protective Services. See also under *Protective Services*.

Credé's Maneuver. Method of emptying the bladder by applying pressure on the suprapubic area.

Credentialing. The most common process used to review the information provided by professional healthcare providers. Credentialing involves reviewing and validating such documents as licenses, certificates, documents relating to accreditation, insurance, evidence of malpractice insurance and malpractice history, and so forth. This process is necessary to ensure that the information supplied by the provider is complete and accurate and maintains quality within the provider network.

CTO Brace. Cervical thoracic orthotic or brace used to immobilize the upper spine.

Current Procedural Terminology (CPT). Manual of five-digit codes used by healthcare providers to classify procedures or medical services to simplify billing. The numerical figure listed after the title indicates which edition has been used (e.g., 4 indicates the fourth edition).

Custodial Care. The services or personal care necessary to assist the patient in performing the activities of daily living (ADLs). The provision of custodial care does not require the skills and expertise of professional or trained medical or paramedical personnel. Patients need custodial care when they can no longer make functional improvements and when the family or caregiver has been adequately trained to provide the care or services required.

Cystometrogram: See *CMG (Cystometrogram)*.

Day Hospital or **Partial Program.** A program that offers medical or psychiatric nursing or rehabilitation services to persons who generally spend only the day hours at the facility, returning home at night. Patients in need of this type of care do not require 24-hour care but could require an inpatient stay if a day program were unavailable.

Days Per Thousand. Unit of measure used in utilization review to measure the number of hospital days used in any year for every thousand insured persons.

Deductible. A form of cost share; the amount paid each year by the patient out-of-pocket toward his or her medical care, or the amount allowable before the healthcare payor assumes responsibility for coverage. Patients are commonly responsible for specific amounts such $75 to $200.

Defensive Medicine. The practice of medicine by physicians who order a variety of tests and treatments that are not really required or indicated to protect themselves against possible malpractice suits.

Denial. Inability to admit or recognize the existence or severity of problems.

Denial or **Noncertification.** Withholding of approval of services rendered or actual payment for such services because either procedural requirements or coverage criteria were not met.

Dependent. Term used in rehabilitation to indicate that the patient requires approximately 75% or more assistance to complete an activity.

Developmental Centers. Centers that provide care to persons with the more severe developmental disabilities (e.g., disabilities attributable to mental retardation, cerebral palsy, epilepsy, autism, or other neurologic disorder that originated before the individual attained the age of 22 and are expected to last indefinitely). These institutions are often referred to as state hospitals or state schools; the actual name for this type of provider varies from state to state. Entrance to such centers is gained through the state agency responsible for providing services to the developmentally disabled; often this agency is the state department of mental health or mental retardation, whereas in California the local Regional Center assumes this responsibility.

Diagnostic and Statistical Manual of Mental Disorders (DSM). A manual of five-digit codes used by providers to classify mental diagnoses in order to simplify billing. The numerical figure after the title specifies which edition has been used (e.g., IV indicates the fourth edition).

Diagnostic Related Group (DRG) Rates. Rates paid to a facility to reimburse them for the care of patients with certain diagnoses. As a rule, these rates have been determined to be the maximum amounts necessary to provide care for patients with that diagnosis regardless of complications, and they are specific for the region in which the facility is located.

Dietitian. A professionally trained individual who specializes in nutrition. Duties include evaluating the person's nutritional needs, taking into consideration the patient's premorbid weight and eating habits as well as his or her status following the illness or injury. The dietitian is also responsible for teaching patients and families how to calculate dietary needs according to activity level, recommending certain foods and supplements, and noting any dietary restrictions.

Diffuse Brain Damage. Injury to the brain in many different sites rather than in one specific location.

Diffuse Cerebral Lesion. Insult involving multiple areas of the brain in both hemispheres; it may not be possible to identify all areas affected.

Diplopia. Double vision.

Discharge Coordinator. Hospital resource person responsible for coordination and implementation of the resources necessary to manage the patient once he or she has been discharged. To be effective, discharge coordination must start at the time of admission.

Disinhibition. Inability to suppress impulsive behavior or emotions.

Disorientation. Confusion about one's identity and about time and place.

Distractibility. Inability to separate stimuli, to concentrate, or to make judgments.

Domestic Violence Units. Offer temporary shelter and support to battered women and their children in crisis situations who need a safe place to stay. These shelters offer counseling, social service advocacy and referrals, emergency transportation, food and clothing, identification and intervention in child abuse situations, legal information and referral, and, when requested, assistance with relocation.

Double Coverage. Benefit coverage by more than one insurance policy for the same services or supplies. In double coverage situations a primary payor is distinguished, and benefits are coordinated to avoid double payments.

Drug Utilization Review. Process used to monitor the frequency and use of prescriptions.

Durable Power of Attorney. A signed document that allows the patient to control his or her life even after he or she is incapacitated because it is based on the principal's (patient's) expressed wishes if decisions must be made about such things as whether to remove life-sustaining equipment or to maintain life through extraordinary means. Differs from the traditional power of attorney in that it does not terminate when the principal becomes incapacitated because it contains specific language that remains valid indefinitely. When properly executed and used, the durable power of attorney may make the more expensive conservatorship process unnecessary.

Dysarthria. Disruption or dysfunction in the articulation of speech. Difficulty with pronunciation due to weakness or poor coordination of the muscles of the lips, tongue, and jaw.

Dysesthesia. Abnormal sensations, such as the feeling of numbness, tingling, prickling, burning, or cutting pain.

Dysphagia. Difficulty in swallowing

Dysphasia. Impairment of the ability to speak.

Easter Seals Society. Chapters of this society vary in capabilities, but many offer comprehensive outpatient rehabilitation therapy, brain trauma reintegration programs, creative adult living programs, functional integrated living skills (skills that are taught and incorporated into the patient's therapy program), integrated employment services, and a rehabilitation work center. Additionally, many offer a variety of support groups (e.g., Stroke Club, Brain Trauma Programs, and programs designed for a specific neurological disorder such as multiple sclerosis). Programs are aimed at patients with severe neurologic disorders of whatever cause—cerebrovascular accidents, trauma, or birth defects. Referrals are accepted from any source, and services are reimbursed through private healthcare insurance coverage, Medicare, Medicaid, or, in some cases, by sliding scale. The program components and services provided vary with each chapter.

Educational or Vocational Specialist. Person responsible for evaluating the patient's educational or vocational abilities and coordinating or structuring a training program containing whatever activities are necessary to retrain the person. This specialist works closely with schools and the Special Education department, sheltered workshops, or other vocational training sites and may be a member of the rehabilitation team.

ELOS. Estimated length of stay.

Emergency Response System (ERS). A communication system for disabled patients and the frail elderly. In this two-part system, one part (a portable emergency response unit) is attached to the patient's telephone, and the other unit is stationed in the nearest emergency room. The patient wears an electronic device that, when activated, secures the phone line, routing the emergency signal to the local emergency room, where a predetermined emergency action plan is executed.

EMG (Electromyogram). An electrical test of the muscles and nerves.

Employee Retirement Income Security Act (ERISA). Multiprovisional act that, among other things, requires the healthcare payor to issue an explanation of benefits (EOB) statement to members stating when and how much of a claim was paid or, alternatively, why it was denied, and informing them of their appeal rights.

Enterostomal Therapist. Person, frequently a professional nurse or other healthcare professional, who is specially trained in ostomy care and all types and aspects of wound care and treatment. These professionals not only administer the actual care of wounds and ostomies, they are frequently consulted by physicians about recommendations for wound care. In most cases, they are responsible for teaching patients and monitoring their care until the patient or family has mastered all techniques required to manage and monitor the wound or ostomy care.

Environmental Control Unit. Breath-activated unit that performs a variety of functional tasks, such as controlling the temperature by use of an electronic device that is activated by breath.

Exclusive Provider Organization (EPO). Like a health maintenance organization in that primary care physicians are used as gatekeepers and prior authorization is required for services. However, the exclusive provider organization frequently capitates rates, and their provider panel is very limited.

Experience Rated. A procedure of the healthcare payor whereby premiums for a particular group of enrollees are based on the utilization record of the enrollees.

Experimental or Investigational. Procedures, treatments, drugs, devices, or equipment that have not yet proved their medical effectiveness. The treatment regimen or drug does not meet generally accepted standards by the medical community because it is still undergoing clinical trials or studies and therefore has not yet been approved by the appropriate authorizing body. As a rule, the experimental or investigational process can take years from concept to final approval.

Explanation of Benefits (EOB). A document or statement issued by the fiscal intermediary or claims processor (FI) that informs the patient who provided the care, what kind of covered service or supply was received, the charge allowed, the amount billed, and the amount paid to date toward the deductible or cost share. If the claim is denied, the explanation of benefits statement also includes the reason for the denial and a statement informing the patient of his or her right to appeal.

Explanation of Check (EOC). A document or statement issued by the fiscal intermediary (FI) or claims processor that informs the provider which patient and services are covered by payment of the check.

Extended Care Facility (ECF). Generally, a hospital-based skilled nursing facility that is licensed by the state Department of Health or a similar agency. Extended care facilities provide "subacute" nursing or restorative care. The services are designed to provide a significantly higher level of care than that offered by a skilled nursing facility. Patients admitted to the extended care facility or subacute care facility are expected to be discharged home or to another level of care once their condition is stable or their progress has reached a plateau. Physician visits are required at least every 7 days, and nursing hours and ratios per patient are significantly higher than those provided by a skilled nursing facility.

Extended Role Nurse. Nurse who has been specially trained to provide or perform certain services or procedures in the absence of a physician. These nurses are often found in large medical or trauma centers.

Extra Contractual Process (also called **Waiver of Benefits**). Process by which some healthcare payors pay for services or supplies that are normally excluded from the written policy. This process is often used when services are necessary to avoid hospitalization and limited or excluded by the healthcare payor, and all alternate funding resources have been explored and found to be unavailable. In this situation, studies have shown that if the extra contractual process

can be used, cost-effective care can be established elsewhere "in lieu of hospitalization." Not all healthcare payors are prepared to offer this service, nor are all employers (policy holders) willing to consider it or the cost-effective alternatives.

Facilitation. External stimuli applied to a muscle or group of muscles to elicit a response.

Family. The most important members of the healthcare team.

Fasciculations. Involuntary twitching of muscle groups.

Federal Insurance Contribution Act (FICA). Taxes deducted from a worker's paycheck and paid to the Social Security Administration trust fund. This fund is then used to pay monthly checks to persons over age 65 and to the disabled under age 65 who qualify for Social Security benefits.

Fee-for-Service Rate. Fee billed by a healthcare provider and paid in full by a healthcare payor for services rendered.

Figure-Ground Discrimination. The ability to recognize and respond to given stimuli, focusing on the essential and ignoring the irrelevant.

Fiscal Intermediary (FI). The organization that is responsible for processing and denying or paying claims.

Fiscal Year. A 12-month accounting period. Differs from the calendar year that starts in January.

Flaccid. Totally limp and lacking in muscle tone.

Flexed Funded. Special fund or claim reserve, established by the policy holder, from which claims up to a predefined amount, are paid. Claims in excess of this amount are paid from the healthcare payor's funds.

Focal Cerebral Lesion. Insult involving a specific identifiable area or areas of the brain.

Focused Review. A review of predetermined diagnoses, procedures, or providers to determine utilization issues, quality of care, and community standards. This review is conducted by the healthcare payor or utilization review department retrospectively or after services are rendered.

Food and Drug Administration (FDA). Federal agency responsible for protecting the nation from impure or unsafe drugs, foods, and cosmetics. There are eleven divisions of this agency: (1) Office of Operations, (2) Center for Drug Evaluation and Research, (3) Center for Biologic Evaluation and Research, (4) Center for Food Safety and Applied Nutrition, (5) Center for Veterinary Medicine, (6)

National Center for Devices and Radiological Health, (7) National Center for Toxicological Research, (8) Regional Operations, (9) Office of Policy, (10) Office of External Affairs, and (11) Office of Management and Systems.

Freestanding or **Community Based.** Not institution based or institution affiliated.

Frog Breathing. See *Glossopharyngeal Breathing or Frog Breathing.*

Frustration Tolerance. The ability to deal with frustrations.

Fully Insured. Status of a policy holder that pays a premium (computed yearly) in monthly installments to the healthcare payor, which then assumes responsibility for payment of all claims.

Function. Ability to perform work or any activity.

Functional Activity. An activity that accomplishes a useful or purposeful task.

Functional Limitations or **Abilities.** A term commonly used by the rehabilitation team to describe the abilities or limitations of a patient. Functional limitations or abilities result from physical or cognitive deficits. The deficits may be motor, perceptual, speech and language, cognitive, or psychological. These limitations or abilities are often further influenced by circumstances affecting the patient's life such as economic, social, or ethnic status, motivation, denial, self-esteem, coping ability, and family support. Several measurement scales are used to measure a person's limitations and capacity for rehabilitation; possibly the most frequently used are the Functional Assessment Measurement (FAM) scale, the Functional Independence Assessment (FIM) scale, and the Disability Rating scale. These scales are also used in treatment planning.

Gait Training. Instruction in walking, with or without equipment such as a cane, walker, crutches, or braces. Often the rehabilitation notes use the following terms to rate the patient's independence:

Contact guard: Term used in rehabilitation medicine to indicate that the patient requires physical contact by the caregiver or therapist throughout the activity.

Independent: Patient is able to walk safely consistently without supervision or assistance.

Minimum assistance: Patient needs only slight assistance in transferring or moving.

Moderate assistance: Patient needs moderate assistance in standing, transferring, maintaining balance, or walking.

Maximum assistance: Patient needs total help, which may mean the assistance of one or more persons.

Standby assistance: Another person must stand by as the patient walks or transfers to ensure his or her safety.

Gatekeeper. The primary care manager or physician who must authorize all specialty referrals.

Gel Pad. A special pad used in wheelchairs or on beds to provide additional skin protection.

Generic Substitute. Nonproprietary drugs (e.g., not protected by a trademark). Often managed care organizations and Medicaid mandate the use of a generic substitute rather than the brand name substance.

Glasgow Coma Scale. A scale describing various levels of cognitive function developed by the Rancho Los Amigos Rehabilitation Hospital in Downey, California. This scale is possibly the most widely recognized and used tool for rating cognitive abilities in brain-injured patients. The seven levels in the scale depict the patient's responses and are as follows:

Level I: No response to stimulation.
Level II: Generalized irregular response to stimulation.
Level III: Localized response; appears alert for short periods and responds consistently to stimulation.
Level IV: Confused-agitated: alert, very active; often aggressive and unable to cooperate, but can pay attention for a very short period.
Level V: Confused-nonagitated; appears alert and responds to commands but is distractible; cannot concentrate, is easily agitated in response to external stimuli, and uses verbally inappropriate language.
Level VI: Confused-appropriate: gives confused but appropriate responses; follows simple directions and is able to perform routine activities; memory for recent events is poor but shows greater awareness of time and place.
Level VII: Automatic-appropriate: Memory for past events is good, although current memory is fuzzy; slow learning is possible, but judgment in emergencies or unusual situations is still poor.

Most transitional rehabilitation units that treat brain-injured patients accept patients at level

VII, and some accept patients with lower levels of function. If the patient is placed in such a rehabilitation facility, care must be taken to ensure that he or she is placed in a facility that matches the patient's level of cognitive function. Once the person has been placed, close monitoring is essential to ensure that continued progress at the desired rate is being made; if not, placement in another facility may be necessary. This monitoring process is especially necessary for patients for whom rehabilitation benefits are limited.

Glossopharyngeal Breathing or **Frog Breathing.** Gulping extra air into the lungs to expand the chest and achieve a functional cough.

Grace Period. A stated period of time, usually 31 days, after the due date for payment of a renewal premium, during which time the policy remains in force.

Gravely Disabled. A person who, regardless of age, is a serious danger to himself or others due to a mental or alcoholic disorder (this definition does not include those who are mentally retarded). Frequently patients classified as gravely disabled cannot provide food or shelter for themselves, nor can they take part in basic activities of daily living.

Grievance. Disagreement or complaint in writing about an issue that does not involve money. See *Appeal*.

Group Health Association of America (GHAA). A health maintenance organization (HMO) trade association that voices the concerns of HMOs. Recently changed their name to American Association of Health Plans (AAHP). This group works with government representatives and officials to make and shape legislation and regulations that affect HMOs.

Group Model. A version of a closed panel healthcare payor in which a health maintenance organization (HMO) contracts with a medical group to provide healthcare services. See also under *Health Maintenance Organization (HMO)*.

Halo. A metal ring that screws into the patient's skull; it is used for patients with spinal cord injuries. The unit encircles the patient's head and aligns the neck and spinal column properly.

Hand Splint. A metal, plaster, or plastic support for the hand, wrist, or fingers. It allows greater function or prevents deformity.

Healthcare Financing Administration (HCFA). Federal agency responsible for administering and enforcing the Social Security Act and other laws as they pertain to health and human services for the United States.

Healthcare Financing Administration 1500 (HCFA-1500). Commonly used claims forms used by professional providers to bill for services.

Healthcare Financing Administration Common PROCEDURAL Coding System (HCPCS). A coding system used to code durable medical equipment, ambulance services, and other services and procedures.

Healthcare Payor. The insurance entity that pays the healthcare claim.

Health Maintenance Organization (HMO). An organization that provides healthcare services for persons in a specific geographic area, charging them a predetermined amount in advance. Typically, HMOs are organized in the form of various models: closed panel or group model; staff model; independent practice association (IPA); network model, and mixed model.

Hemianopsia (Homonymous). Lesion of the right or left optic tract resulting in a visual field cut.

Hemiparesis. Weakness on one side of the body.

Heterotrophic Ossification. Abnormal bone deposit in the muscles around a joint.

Home Health Agency (HHA). Home health agencies provide skilled nursing or restorative services to elderly, disabled, or recuperating persons who live at home or in residential care or board and care units on a daily or intermittent basis. Home health agency services must be prescribed by a physician and are provided by registered nurses, therapists, home health aides, and medical social workers. These services range from prescribed medical treatments and therapies to personal care. Fees are paid by Medicare, Medicaid, other entitlements, private insurance, or private funds. Some agencies offer services on a sliding scale based on the patient's assets, income, and ability to pay.

Homemaker or **Companion.** A nonlicensed person who offers companionship or performs light housekeeping duties such as cooking, shopping, or cleaning.

Homemaker Services. Personal in-home chore and housekeeping services for chronically ill or incapacitated individuals. Services are available from (1) private homemaker agencies, which offer services to clients on a fee-for-service basis, or (2) local social service programs, which provide services to low-income persons who are eligible for welfare benefits. Availability of the latter programs varies from community to community.

Home Visitors. Volunteers who act as friendly visitors, providing companionship to home-bound elderly people according to an established agreement for home visits. These visitors are generally found through local departments of aging because services are designed for elderly individuals who live alone.

Hospice Care. Services that range from interest and support groups to agencies that provide complete nursing, palliative, and supportive care and bereavement services. Although hospice is primarily a concept of care rather than a specific place for care, it is usually provided in the home environment but can be provided to inpatients in a hospital facility or skilled nursing unit. Hospice services are provided only to patients who are known to be terminally ill and in the last 6 months of life.

Hospital Day. A confinement or inpatient stay that lasts beyond midnight. The term is also applied to a stay by patients who are admitted and assigned a bed with the intent of remaining hospitalized overnight.

Hypalgesia. Diminished sensitivity to pain.

Hyperesthesia. Increased sensitivity to pain and touch stimuli.

Hypertonicity. Increased muscle tension.

Hypertrophic Scars. Increase in bulk of tissue or structure as a burn heals and scar tissue forms. To prevent hypertrophic scars the burn patient wears pressure garments for approximately 2 years after the burn.

Hypotonicity. Reduced muscle tension.

ICD: See *International Classification of Diseases (ICD)*.

Impulsivity. Inability to control impulses.

Incomplete Lesions. Partial or variable loss of motor ability and sensory function.

Indemnity. Traditional type of healthcare insurance in which claims are paid without regard to the actual cost of the services or length of the confinement.

Independent. In rehabilitation usage, the patient can function by himself with no assistance from others, although he may require the use of assistive devices. See also under *Gait Training*.

Independent Practice Association (IPA). An organization that has a contract with a managed care system to deliver services for a capitated rate. The IPA, in return, contracts with individual providers to provide the services on either a capitated basis or a fee-for-service basis to the enrollees.

Indian Health Services. This agency provides comprehensive healthcare to American Indians and Alaskan Natives. It focuses on health programs, vocational training, and health planning activities.

Individual Educational Plan (IEP). A technique used by school districts to establish a written educational plan for pupils who require Special Education.

Individual Program Plan (IPP). A technique used by the state agency responsible for administering the state's services for persons with developmental disabilities. A plan is developed based on a patient's assessed level of functional development. The plan includes recommendations for achieving immediate and long-term goals. The IPP may include recommendations for a variety of services, such as coordination of infant development programs, behavior management, and training, skilled nursing care, respite care, and educational and vocational planning. The IPP is modified as the patient's needs change.

Individuals with Exceptional Needs. Terminology used most often by the Department of Education to identify persons who need Special Education. These persons are disabled and require intensive instruction or training. Such persons include those with blindness, autism, deafness, severe orthopedic impairments, emotional disturbances, and mental retardation.

Infant Stimulation Program. Program designed to provide consistent and repeated stimulation to infants or small children under the age of 3 with exceptional needs. The program also trains parents or caregivers in providing such stimulation. The goal of the program is to allow these children to reach the developmental milestones established for their age group and disability. Stimulation may be offered in the areas of touch, sight, hearing, smell, taste, and motor control (movement, coordination, and sucking).

Inflexibility. Inability to adjust to changes.

Information and Referral or **Assistance (I & R).** Special program designed to provide information about and referral to services available in a community. These services are available by telephone. The formal Information and Referral or Assistance programs are primarily sponsored by the Older Americans Act and United Way; many disease-specific agencies, community or ethnic centers, or other health-related service agencies also offer information and referral services to their clients.

In-Home Supportive Services (IHSS). A program provided by some county social service departments for persons eligible for Supplemental Security Income (SSI). This is a state-funded, county-administered program intended to enable aged, blind, or disabled individuals to live in the residence of their choice. Services vary from state to state, but if they are available, the patient is assessed for the number of service hours per month required to permit him or her to function at home and for which the program will pay. Typical services include meal preparation, shopping, cleaning, transportation, and personal care. The hours granted for care are limited to a few hours a day, week, or month.

Insight. The ability to understand comprehensively the true nature of a situation.

Intermediate Care Facility (ICF). Facilities designed to provide supervision and assistance to ambulatory patients who need less supervision and care than patients in a skilled nursing facility. They offer limited hours of nursing supervision per day; many stipulate that individual patients require skilled nursing care for 1 hour or less per day. In addition, many require that their patients be ambulatory and continent of bowel and bladder. As with the number of nursing hours required, the frequency of physician visits is also regulated (e.g., the physician may be required to see the patient no less than every 60 days). These facilities are licensed by the state Department of Health Services or a similar state agency, and the level of care they offer is rarely covered by healthcare payors.

International Classification of Diseases (ICD). A three- to five-digit coding system used to classify medical diseases by diagnosis numbers in order to simplify billing. The numerical figure after the title indicates which edition is being used (e.g., 9 indicates the 9th edition). DHHS Publication No (PHS) 91–1260 U.S. Department of Health and Human Services, Public Health Service, Health Care Financing Administration.

Intracranial Pressure Monitor. A monitoring device used to determine the pressure in the brain.

Involuntary Hold (5150) or **Order of Protective Custody.** A 72-hour involuntary psychiatric hold for persons deemed to be gravely disabled due to a psychiatric or alcoholic disorder when the person refuses intervention, treatment, or evaluation. The process can be initiated by the police or physician and requires that the person be hospitalized until a psychiatric evaluation can be made.

Island Graft. A flap that is surgically attached and contains both nerves and blood vessels.

Jewett Brace. A brace used to immobilize the lower spine.

Joint Commission for the Accreditation of Healthcare Organizations (JCAHO). A nonprofit organization responsible for reviewing healthcare facilities and related services and determining whether they have met established basic standards and practice patterns for the type of service they provide. This commission accredits such healthcare organizations as acute care facilities, outpatient facilities, home health agencies, and other healthcare providers.

Judgment. The process of forming an opinion based on evaluation and comparison with personal values, preferences, and insights.

Lability. Loss of emotional control, resulting in inappropriate or exaggerated emotional expressions or outbursts, such as laughing or crying.

LE. Lower extremity; leg.

Learning Disabled. Disorder primarily associated with school-aged children in which one or more of the basic mental processes involved in understanding or using language is affected. This disorder often becomes manifest as an imperfect ability to listen, think, speak, read, write, spell, or perform mathematical calculations and includes such conditions as perceptual handicap, brain-injury, minimal brain dysfunction, dyslexia, and developmental aphasia. This term does not include learning problems that result primarily from visual, aural, or motor defects, mental retardation, emotional disturbance, or environmental, cultural, or economic disadvantages.

Legal Service Centers. Centers that serve the disabled, low-income, and frail elderly, providing legal aid, information and referral, advocacy, and advice on civil matters (e.g., housing, Social Security, welfare, Medicaid, and consumer issues and problems). These centers do not handle criminal or fee-generating cases.

Length of Stay (LOS). Number of days a person is hospitalized.

ELOS: Estimated length of stay.
ALOS: Average length of stay.

Lesion. Change in or damage to tissue. For lesions of the spinal cord, see also *Complete Lesion; Incomplete Lesion*; for lesions of the brain, see also *Diffuse Cerebral Lesion*; *Focal Cerebral Lesion*.

Liability Limits. The stated sum beyond which a healthcare payor is not liable or will not pay.

Licensure. Official or legal permission by the state to operate a healthcare facility. Most states use the state Department of Health or a similar state agency to implement the certification process; in addition, this department is responsible for performing yearly inspections to ensure that the facility continues to comply with licensing standards. In addition to licensing acute-care facilities and outpatient units, most states require home health agencies and skilled nursing facilities to meet basic standards for licensure as well. Although licensure does not necessarily mean that an agency or skilled nursing facility provides a high quality of care, it is inadvisable to use any home health agency or skilled nursing facility that is not licensed. A reputable agency or skilled nursing facility must also ensure that its staff members are properly licensed or certified.

Licensed Vocational or **Practical Nurse (LVN, LPN).** A person who has successfully completed a required number of hours in a designated program and is licensed in the state to practice as a vocational or practical nurse. In most healthcare organizations, these nurses work under the general supervision of a registered nurse.

Life Care Communities. Complexes designed to offer a full range of services for retired persons or persons over a specified age. Complexes may consist of apartments, townhouses, mobile homes, or private residences. Some life care commodities also offer the services of an infirmary, a clinic, or a nursing home. As a rule, any recreational or medical costs are included in the general charges levied to join the community.

Loan Closets. Used durable medical equipment that has been donated to a church group, ethnic center, or disease specific agency that is free as a "loaner" to persons in need.

Long-Term Care Insurance. Insurance issued to a group or individual that covers the cost of skilled nursing facility care or private duty nursing in the home.

Long-Term Psychiatric Facilities. Skilled nursing facilities (which may also include state hospitals or state schools) that are designed to treat persons with severe mental illness over an indefinite period of time or lifelong. These facilities are licensed by the state Department of Health. To enter a long-term psychiatric facility a person must either enter voluntarily or enter involuntarily under conservatorship.

LOS. Length of stay, or the number of days a person is hospitalized. There are two types: ELOS, estimated length of stay, and ALOS, average length of stay.

Loss Ratio. The ratio of claims to premiums.

Lower Motor Neuron Lesion. Lesion that occurs at the level of the spinal cord injury. Reflex patterns are absent, and flaccid paralysis occurs at this level.

Major Medical Max. The maximum amount paid by the healthcare payor during the course of an illness, injury, the person's lifetime, or the period of insurability with the healthcare payor.

Managed Care. Association or organization of healthcare payors such as health maintenance organizations (HMOs), independent practice associations (IPAs), or preferred provider organizations (PPOs) in which preadmission or prior authorization requirements and concurrent review or other forms of reviewing services or supplies are intended to control inappropriate healthcare use. These groups also make use of contracted or network providers that provide services at lower prearranged rates.

Mandated Benefits. Services that a healthcare payor is required by law to provide.

Maximum Allowable Charge (MAC). The highest amount a provider can charge for its services. This rate is set by the healthcare payor and is the maximum amount it will reimburse.

Maximum Assistance. Amount of assistance from another person required by the patient to perform all necessary care needs or to achieve mobility. In most cases, this term implies a need for assistance from another person in more than 50% of his or her activities. See also under *Gait Training*.

Meals on Wheels. These programs (or other similar programs offering home-delivered meals) are offered by social service or ethnic-specific agencies or church groups. The programs are designed to meet the nutritional needs of the homebound and offer, at minimum, one hot meal and possibly one cold meal per day, Monday to Friday. Income, age, and the actual location of the residence are frequently the most common barriers to access to these services. Many of these meal programs are funded through the Older

Americans Act and are restricted to the low-income elderly.

Medicaid (Title XIX of the Social Security Act). Federal-state program in which the state pays for medical care for public assistance recipients and other low-income persons. Minimum benefits are established at the federal level. However, benefits as well as eligibility and categories of patients served vary from state to state. Persons eligible are those deemed medically needy who are receiving Supplemental Security Income (SSI) or Aid to Families with Dependent Children (AFDC) and meet income eligibility requirements.

Medicaid Waiver. In essence, this is Medicaid's extra contractual process. The Consolidated Omnibus Budget Reconciliation Act allows states to make exceptions for Medicaid's traditional scope of benefit coverage. Under the waiver program, benefit coverage is epanded for certain categories of persons with special needs, who under normal conditions would be excluded from Medicaid coverage. Criteria for coverage are often based on the fact that long-term institutionalization will be prevented if the coverage is allowed through the waiver.

Medicare (Title XVIII of the Social Security Act). Federal health insurance program for persons over age 65, those under age 65 who are permanently disabled (disabled longer than 2 years), those with end-stage renal disease, or legal aliens who have resided in the United States for 5 years or more. Eligibility for the program is based on contributions to the Social Security or Railroad Retirement fund having been made during the appropriate number of employment quarters. Medicare is divided into two parts. Part A covers hospital, skilled nursing facility, and home health agency charges and occurs automatically once the beneficiary applies and is deemed eligible. Part B covers physician, durable medical equipment, and outpatient charges and has a monthly premium that is adjusted yearly. Beneficiaries may be covered by either one or both parts. If they are not eligible for Part A, they can purchase it, but the premiums amount to an average of several hundred dollars per month.

Medicare-Certified Provider. Provider who meets Medicare's standards for provision of care. Most healthcare payors recognize Medicare's providers and require that all providers used be Medicare-certified at minimum.

Medically Necessary. Medical care or services that have been accepted by qualified medical professionals as reasonable, needed, or adequate for the treatment of the illness or injury.

Medigap Policies. Insurance polices that supplement the coverage provided by Medicare. These polices cover deductibles and copayments primarily. Some cover pharmaceuticals.

Memory. Stored recollections of experiences, events, feelings, and dates from the recent and distant past. There are three types:

Immediate recall: Ability to recall information from moment of reception up to 1 minute after its reception.

Short-term memory: Ability to recall information from 1 minute to 1 hour after its reception.

Long-term memory: Ability to store and retrieve information for more than 1 hour to days and weeks.

Mentally Incompetent. Cognitive or physical impairment that does not allow the person to comprehend, understand, or make correct decisions; provide properly for personal needs for food, clothing, or shelter; manage finances appropriately; protect against fraud, undue influence, or loss of property; or permit assistance from friends, relatives, or service agencies.

Minerva Jacket. A molded plastic jacket that provides support for the neck and extends from the back of the head to the hips with a detachable front section.

Minimum Assistance. Amount of assistance from another person required by the patient for his or her care or mobility. This term implies that assistance from another person is needed in less than 25% of the patient's activities. See also under *Gait Training*.

Mixed Model. A health maintenance organization (HMO) that combines two or more types of delivery systems (e.g., closed panel and open panel).

Mobility. Ability to move.

Motor Control. Regulation of the timing and amount of contraction of the muscles to produce smooth and coordinated movement.

Muscle Tone. Resistance of a muscle to stretching.

Nanny Nurse. Healthcare professional, frequently a clinical nurse specialist, who has a background in growth and development. Duties include direct services in helping families make the transition from the neonatal intensive care unit to home. The nanny nurse may act as a consultant or resource person to community agencies, physicians, or other health professionals in making appropriate referrals.

National Committee on Quality Assurance (NCQA). A nonprofit organization that accredits and reviews organizations for quality assurance.

National Institutes of Health (NIH). Biomedical research agency for the federal government. The agencies under the NIH include: (1) National Cancer Institute, (2) National Heart, Lung and Blood Institute, (3) National Institute of Diabetes and Digestive and Kidney Disease, (4) National Institute of Allergy and Infectious Diseases, (5) National Institute of Child Health and Human Development, (6) National Institute on Deafness and other Communicative Disorders, (7) National Institute of Dental Research, (8) National Institute of Environmental Health Science, (9) National Institute of Neurological Disorders and Stroke, (10) National Eye Institute, (11) National Institute on Aging, (12) National Institute of Arthritis and Musculoskeletal and Skin Disease, and (13) National Institute of Nursing Research. The National Institutes of Health also include the National Library of Medicine, the National Center for Research Resources, the National Center for Human Genome Research, the Clinical Center, the Division of Computer Research and Technology, and the Fogarty International Center.

NCQA. See *National Commission on Quality Assurance*.

Nerve Grafts. Grafts that bridge a gap to allow regeneration of a nerve.

Neurodevelopment Treatment (NDT). A therapeutic approach based on normal development of movement with emphasis on restoring normal movement and function. Treatments are common with patients with neurological disorders, such as cerebral palsy.

Network Model. A healthcare plan that contracts with many physician groups, especially large or mixed specialty groups, to deliver healthcare to its members. Differs from group model plans, in which contracts are made with a single medical group.

Network Provider. See *Participating Network Provider*.

Neuralgia. Intermittent but intense pain due to disease of the nerve.

Neuropsychiatrist. Medical doctor who specializes in the relationship between the neurologic system and psychiatric or psychological disturbances. This physician may direct individual and family therapy sessions and may order the appropriate drugs to control behavior, agitation, depression, or moodiness.

Neuropsychologist. Psychologist who has a doctorate in philosophy (Ph.D) and has specialized training and expertise in the interrelationships between the brain and behavior. In addition to other responsibilities, the neuropsychologist performs a number of tests to determine the patient's intellectual, cognitive, and personality function; these test results are then used by other members of the rehabilitation team as they develop and implement the treatment plan.

NIH. See *National Institutes of Health (NIH)*.

Nurse's Aide or **Certified Nurse's Aide.** Person who has successfully completed a program of study and received a certificate indicating that he or she can perform such activities as custodial care, observation and monitoring for changes in condition, taking vital signs, or assistance to the patient for self-administered medications.

Nurse Practitioner. Nurse who has completed special schooling (at the Master's level) and receives further training under the direction of a preceptor physician. After the training has been completed and the nurse is licensed as a nurse practitioner, the nurse practitioner practices in an expanded nursing role under the direct supervision of a licensed physician.

Occupational Therapist (OT). Therapist who has special training in the physical retraining of the upper extremities and in cognitive, perceptual, and swallowing deficits that influence the patient's ability to eat or perform functional tasks. This healthcare professional not only evaluates the patient and develops a treatment plan specific to the level of deficit, he or she also performs any actual therapy and teaches the family or caregiver whatever they need to know to ensure that the goals established for the patient are reached. Areas often assessed and treated are the patient's ability to perform fine motor tasks, use the hands and fingers, swallow, coordinate eye and hand movements, and perform self-care tasks such as bathing and dressing. This therapist makes recommendations for splinting or the use of self-care devices that allow independence and evaluates the person's functional ability to cook or work with tools.

OHI. Other health insurance.

Ombudsman or **Patient Rights Advocate.**

Agency that responds to and investigates complaints about patient rights, the existence of abuse in facilities, the quality of care, or abuse of the person's financial resources.

Omnibus Reconciliation Act (OBRA). Multiprovisional act of 1981 & 1986 that allowed states to expand their coverage of Medicaid for certain categories of patients. This act was a major cost-containment law that greatly impacted services provided by health and welfare programs in the United States.

Open Enrollment. A period when employees can change their choice of healthcare payor—generally once a year during a specific month.

Open Panel. A managed healthcare plan in which healthcare payors contract with private physicians to deliver care in their own offices.

Order of Protective Custody. See *Involuntary Hold (5150) or Order of Protective Custody.*

Organizing Ability. Ability to establish a consistent relationship between objects, events, or features.

Orthotic. External supportive device or brace. There are ankle-foot orthotics (AFOs) and cervical thoracic orthotics (CTOs), among others.

Orthostatic Hypotension. Low blood pressure caused by changes in position.

Other Health Insurance (OHI). Term used when a patient has more than one health insurance policy.

PAR. See under *Preadmission Review.*

Parallel Bars. A set of bars or rails placed an equal distance apart that allows the patient to practice walking while gripping the rails.

Participating Network Provider. A provider who makes a contract with a healthcare payor in which it agrees to furnish medical services or supplies to patients in return for predetermined amounts for these services; these amounts are accepted as total payment for the services. The healthcare payor usually reimburses the provider directly, whereas nonparticipating providers charge the patient for payment in full or for any amounts that remain after the healthcare payor has paid its share.

Parts to Whole Relationships. Ability to integrate or analyze whole or component parts in speaking, reading, or writing.

PAS (Professional Activity Study) Norms. Regional length of stay statistics published by the Commission on Professional and Hospital Activities.

Pass. Permission for the patient to leave the hospital for a few hours to a day or so. The pass allows a trial period at home so that the rehabilitation team can assess the components of the discharge plan. It is often allowed as the patient nears the time of discharge and is an integral part of the rehabilitation process.

Patients' Rights. Patient rights are protected under the Civil Rights Act of 1964, and each state has administrative codes that mandate protection of such rights. The Civil Rights Act is designed to forbid discrimination and ensure fair and equal treatment for all.

Patients' Rights Advocate. See *Ombudsman or Patients' Rights Advocate.*

Patterned Movement. Movement that is not completely under the person's control.

Payee (Money Management) Services. Money management services are provided by county social service workers or other agencies to persons who are at risk of being exploited or who, because of failing health or organic mental health disorders, are unable to manage their financial resources by themselves.

Per Diem Rate. Fee paid to a healthcare provider based on a set amount per day or per service as opposed to a fee-for-service rate.

Peer Review. A group of professionals, usually physicians, who review the care provided to determine whether it complies with the standards of care and acceptable practice.

Perception: Ability to recognize and distinguish objects. There are three main types of perception:

Perception of form: Ability to distinguish stimuli based on touch, shape, or structural details.

Perception of sequence: Ability to understand the order, concepts, or numerical progression of visual or other material in meaningful sequence.

Perception of space or relationships: Ability to visualize, move, or organize points in space without bumping into objects or spilling liquids and to find starting and stopping points.

Per Member Per Month (PMPM). Refers to the revenue or costs associated with each enrolled member each month.

Per Member Per Year (PMPY). Refers to the revenue or costs associated with each enrolled member each year.

Perseveration. Inability to control persistent repetition of verbal responses or motor activity, or to switch back and forth from one activity to another or to move to another idea, word, or task (e.g., eating continuously owing to inability to interrupt feeding motion).

Philadelphia Collar. A molded plastic collar used to provide firm support and to maintain the neck in proper alignment.

Phrenic Nerve Stimulation. Electrical stimulation of the nerve to the diaphragm.

Physiatrist or **Doctor of Physical Medicine and Rehabilitation.** Licensed physician who has specialized in the field of physical medicine and rehabilitation, with emphasis on orthopedics and neurology. A physician with this background often directs the therapy services offered in the rehabilitation unit.

Physical Therapist (PT). Person who has specialized training in teaching or treating the patient to return to his or her maximum level of physical motor functioning. The physical therapist evaluates the patient extensively for muscle tone, ability to ambulate or move, and muscle strength and coordination. Once the evaluation is completed, the therapist devises a program of exercises and movements to develop or retrain the patient's motor abilities and recommends the necessary durable medical equipment, splints, braces, or prosthetic devices that will allow the patient to function or prevent deterioration.

Physician Advisor. Physician who provides advice or review. Generally, utilization review and claims administration staffs maintain panels of practicing physicians who are willing to participate in the review process. These physicians are most often consulted to review cases involving their specialty or a similar specialty.

Physician Hospital Organization (PHO). A version of a healthcare payor model in which hospitals and their attending medical staff contract as with each other and then as an organization contract with healthcare payors to provide healthcare.

Plateau. Absence of significant functional improvement.

Point of Service (POS). Customized managed care plans that allow members to choose providers in exchange for higher out-of-pocket costs.

Policy Holder or **Plan Sponsor.** The employer or company, union, or sometimes an individual who determines what services are allowed in the insurance benefit package. The policy holder assumes responsibility for the major portion or all of the premium.

Pooling. Employers or other groups of insured people who combine their resources into one insured group. Fluctuations in costs can therefore be smoothed, stabilized, or eliminated and premium costs reduced.

Posey Roll. A protective device that surrounds the ankle and elevates the heel off the bed.

Positioning. Changes of position or alignment of the body, whether in bed or in a wheelchair, to prevent the development of contractures or pressure sores and to promote function.

Positive Resistive Exercise. Progressive resistive exercise using weighted resistance to increase muscle strength.

Postresidual Voiding. Catheterization after voiding to determine the amount left in the bladder.

Power of Attorney (POA). Process that allows a competent person, known as the "principal," to appoint an "attorney in fact" to conduct his or her financial affairs. Although this term is frequently confused with conservatorship, power of attorney is a simple process, and the necessary papers are available at most stationery stores and banks. To be legal, the appointment of the person to act as the attorney in fact must be notarized, and the notary must attest to the fact the the principal was competent at the time the forms were signed.

Preadmission Review, PAR, Precertification, Prior Authorization, or **Prospective Review (PR).** A function used by most managed care plans whereby cases are reviewed before the services are performed and an authorization for such services is granted, often in the form of an authorization number. This process does not guarantee payment; it merely certifies that the patient meets the medical criteria for the service at the time of the request.

Preauthorization. See *Authorization or Preauthorization*.

Premorbid. Characteristics of the person before the the injury or illness.

Primary Care Physician (PCP) or **Primary Care Manager (PCM).** Physician who acts as the gatekeeper for most health maintenance organizations. These physicians are usually family practitioners or general practitioners, internists, pediatricians, obstetricians, or gynecologists.

Primary Payor. Healthcare payor that has been determined to be responsible for first payment or denial of benefits. For example, a wife's policy would be primary if the wife was insured by her employer and also by her husband's insurance.

Prior Authorization. See under *Preadmission Review.*

Privacy Act (1974). Federal law intended to preserve the personal privacy of individuals and to permit them to know what records pertaining to them are collected, maintained, used, and disseminated. The information disseminated must be lawful and necessary, must not be misused, and must not be unauthorized. The law also ensures that information collected is accurate, relevant, timely, and as complete as reasonably necessary. Personal information cannot be shared without prior consent, must be accessible to the individual concerned, and must be maintained in a manner that ensures confidentiality. The following information is protected under the act: home address, phone number, race, Social Security number, medical records, and photographs. While this law protects privacy, the Comprehensive Alcohol Abuse Prevention, Treatment and Rehabilitation Act of 1970 and the Drug Abuse and Treatment Act of 1972 are much more restrictive in the information that can be disclosed.

PRO. See under *Professional Standards Review Organization.*

Problem-Solving. Ability to select the most advantageous solution to a problem or to consider probable factors that will influence the outcome.

Processing Time. Speed with which information is assimilated.

Professional Activity Study (PAS) Norms. See *PAS (Professional Activity Study) Norms.*

Professional Review. Retrospective review of claims for medical appropriateness and benefit determinations before claims are payed.

Professional Standards Review Organization (PSRO). Organization that is usually contracted by a government agency to review criteria or procedural performance of healthcare providers.

Prone. Lying flat on the stomach.

Proprioception. Awareness of body position in space without a visual point.

Prospective Payment. A contractual agreement for payment before services are rendered.

Prospective Review (PR). See under *Preadmission Review.*

Protective Services (APS, CPS). Services for adults (APS, age 18 or older) and children (CPS, under age 18) are available through the county department of social services. These services are designed to assist children, adults, and frail elderly people who are living in abusive or neglectful situations or are in danger of being exploited. Intensive counseling and alternative placement as well as an array of other social services are offered.

Provider or **Vendor.** A hospital, physician, durable medical equipment company, home health agency, or other supplier of medical care or healthcare services. Many healthcare payors, alternate funding programs, and case managers refer to providers as vendors.

Proximal Instability. Weakness of the trunk, shoulder girdle, or hip girdle muscles that causes poor posture, abnormal movement of the arms or legs, or inability to hold the head up.

Public Health Clinics. Although public health clinics and services are often associated with the poor, these clinics may also be used for patients who have limited benefits or who have exhausted their benefits. Public health nursing services and clinics are provided by the county primarily to serve needs in maternal and child health, communicable diseases, and adult health. To foster maternal and child health, classes are offered in parenting and preparation for childbirth, and well-baby clinics offer physical examinations and immunizations to children aged 6 and under; counseling is provided to parents about normal growth and development, nutrition, and other health-related matters. Outpatient primary care clinics are also available and may offer services in general medical care, immunizations, venereal disease diagnosis and treatment, diagnosis, treatment, and confidential testing for AIDS and tuberculosis, family planning and counseling for health-related problems, treatment and information as well as epidemiologic study of communicable diseases, dental services, alcohol and drug abuse prevention and treatment, and health services for the homeless. Some clinics charge a nominal fee for immunizations, whereas tuberculosis and AIDS services are provided at no cost. Other clinic charges are based on a sliding scale and the client's ability to pay. Although contact with the public health department will probably be infrequent, case managers must be familiar with the services provided by this department and the location of clinics if patients or families wish to obtain access to care. Similarly, if the case manager needs information, especially about communicable diseases, these clinics and their staffs can be invaluable aids.

PVD. Percussion, vibration, and drainage, a process used to clear secretions from the lungs.

Reasoning. Ability to draw logical conclusions from supporting facts and use of analytical abilities.

Recreational Therapist. Person responsible for evaluating the patient's leisure interests and skills as well as his or her ability to interact with other individuals in a group or in the community or to date. This therapist also evaluates the patient's ability to take the initiative and make decisions, and teaches him or her how to make use of community services and transportation.

Reflex. Involuntary or uncontrolled movement or muscle response.

Regional Center. Regional Centers are found only in California. They are nonprofit organizations that contract with the state department of developmental services and with private agencies to evaluate developmentally disabled patients and determine their eligibility or direct their entrance into a state Developmental Center (state hospital). Regional centers are designed to determine the person's eligibility for services, make diagnoses, and secure funding; they have the primary responsibility for coordinating and facilitating the services clients require. Persons must be residents of the state to use the services of the centers.

Registered Nurse (RN). Licensed professional nurse who has successfully completed the required number of hours of study, has graduated from an accredited school of nursing, and is licensed in the state to practice as a registered nurse

Rehabilitation Facility (often referred to as a PM & R [Physical Medicine and Rehabilitation Unit]). An institution or distinct part of a hospital licensed by the state Department of Health and often accredited by the Commission for Accreditation of Rehabilitation Facilities to provide acute rehabilitative services to patients who require an intensive program of restorative therapy after an illness or injury. With the help of this interdisciplinary program, patients are expected to be able to return home within a given period of time. The primary goal of a rehabilitation program is to restore patients to their maximum functional level.

Reinsurance. See *Stop Loss.*

Reinsurer. Insurance company that insures healthcare payors against large claims.

Reserve. Sum set aside by a healthcare payor to cover known or anticipated claims payments and expenses.

Residential or **Board and Care Facilities.** Facilities that provide room and board and also sometimes assistance with activities of daily living, supervision of prescribed medications, and recreational activities. This type of facility is not reimbursed by healthcare payors and is designed to serve patients who cannot live alone owing to safety factors or for other reasons. Depending on the facility, patients who need intermittent nursing care may be followed by nurses from a home health agency. Patients see their physician as often as necessary in the physician's office.

Residential Treatment Center (RTC). Facility or distinct part of a facility that provides a 24-hour therapeutically planned group living and learning environment to children or adolescents with mental disorders who have sufficient intellectual potential to respond to active treatment. These facilities also provide individualized psychotherapy and other psychiatric services.

Respiratory Therapist. Healthcare professional specifically trained in respiratory care. The respiratory therapist is often involved in the early stages of recovery of patients who have experienced difficulty with breathing. The therapist is responsible for administering respiratory treatments, including oxygen or ventilation, monitoring the patient, assisting the patient in managing secretions, and teaching the patient or family any phase of respiratory or ventilator care necessary to permit discharge or aftercare.

Respite Care. Short-term care for severely disabled or frail elderly persons that permits the primary caregiver to take a break from their everyday care responsibilities. Because respite care is rarely funded by healthcare payors, it is paid for primarily by the caregiver or family from their own funds. If the patient is terminally ill and is receiving hospice care, respite care may be included in the patient's hospice benefit package.

Reston. Adhesive-backed foam used to protect the skin.

Retroactive Review. Review that occurs after the service is rendered to determine whether the services received were medically appropriate.

Rider. Document that modifies the original policy.

Rigidity. Lack of flexibility or inability to conform or change attitudes or actions.

Risk. Contractual agreement to share the financial burden or uncertainty associated with delivery of medical care services.

Roho Cushion. Special type of wheelchair cushion.

ROM. Range of motion or amount of movement available to the joint.

Active ROM: Accomplished by the patient
Passive ROM: Accomplished by the therapist.

SCI. Spinal cord injury.

Scissors Walk. A walk in which one foot is passed in front of the other, using a cross-legged progression.

Second Opinion. Requirement of many healthcare payors that another physician in the same specialty give his or her opinion about the patient's diagnosis or treatment before any service is performed to ensure the medical necessity of the service.

Self-Funded or **Self-Insured.** A method of providing insurance to employees in which benefits are financed entirely by the company.

Senior Retirement Home or **Housing Complex.** A housing arrangement designed for a specific age group of persons (often 55 years or older). In this type of setting, the residents generally rent, lease, or own their own unit. Restrictions on independence, dependency, and the level of services and activities provided vary. In most cases, these units are designed for active independent people, and care of various kinds may or may not be provided.

Sheltered Workshops. Special training sites or programs used by vocational rehabilitation facilities that offer training to the disabled. This training allows disabled persons to return to regular or sheltered employment. Services provided by these programs consist of work and job skill evaluation, job training, work tryout, job placement, and psychological and social services. Many of these programs are offered by such agencies as the Salvation Army and the Volunteers of America.

Short Leg Brace. Metal, plastic, or leather leg support that fits below the knee and extends to the ankle or foot. Also called an ankle-foot orthotic (AFO).

Slide Board. A smooth lightweight board used to ease the transfer of nonambulatory patients between bed or chair and wheelchair and to and from the toilet or the car.

Skilled Care. Services that require the direct skills or supervision of a qualified licensed healthcare professional to ensure the safety of the patient and achieve the medically desired results. Skilled care is often a process that combines necessary observation, assessment, judgment, supervision, documentation, teaching, or direct performance of specific tasks and procedures.

Skilled Nursing Facility (SNF). Facilities licensed by the state Department of Health services or a similar state agency to provide medical, nursing, and restorative services to patients who are not in the acute phase of their illness or injury but require the continuous availability of a licensed nurse or professional healthcare team. These facilities historically have been called nursing homes or convalescent hospitals. Patients can stay indefinitely if their care needs cannot be met by another level of care within the community. Once the patient no longer requires skilled care, however, payment for care in the SNF must come from either private funds, Medicaid, or another alternate funding source, since healthcare payors will not pay for such care. Physicians are required to visit at least every 30 days.

Social Security Administration. Federal agency that administers Title XVI (Supplemental Security Income [SSI]) and Title XVIII (Medicare) of the Social Security Act. This office establishes eligibility for Medicare benefits, assists in the completion of applications for Social Security benefits, and determines disability payments (for those receiving Social Security Disability Insurance [SSDI]) and monthly payments for those receiving SSI.

Social Security Disability Insurance (SSDI). Federal program paid for from the Social Security trust fund (which is funded by FICA payroll deductions) and available to those who are totally disabled. Persons who are eligible are the blind, disabled workers under age 65, and their dependents. To be eligible, the worker must have contributed the appropriate number of credits to the Social Security trust fund. Application is made at the nearest Social Security office. Criteria are consistent nationally, and there is no income criterion as there is with Medicaid. If the person qualifies and remains on SSDI for 24 months, he or she is eligible for Medicare.

Social Worker. Healthcare professional who can be a medical social worker (MSW) or a licensed clinical social worker (LCSW). These professionals at minimum serve as a liaison between the patient and the healthcare team; they conduct assessments to obtain background data from the patient, family, and friends or support systems, and perform counseling or referral tasks to provide emotional, social, and financial support often needed by the disabled.

Somatosensory Evoked Potentials. Electrical activity in the brain recorded at various levels in the central nervous system in response to stimuli.

Space Boots. Lambs' wool padded support devices used to align the muscles or tendons to prevent contractures or drop foot.

Spasticity. Involuntary, rapid tightening of the muscles that results in increased muscle tone and resistance to movement.

Special Education Programs. Specially designed instruction that meets the unique needs of a child who has exceptional educational needs (physical or mental) that cannot be met by the regular school program even if it is modified. This instruction is provided at no cost to the parents and is mandated by federal law (public law 94-142 and, more recently, the Individuals with Disabilities Education Act of 1991). Special Education programs provide a full range of options to meet the educational and service needs of individuals in the least restrictive environment. Individuals with exceptional needs are grouped for instructional purposes according to their instructional needs.

Speech Therapist or **Pathologist (ST).** Healthcare professional with specialized training in evaluating the patient's motor-speech skills and his or her abilities in swallowing, use of expressive and receptive language, memory, concentration, attention span, hearing, writing, and reading. The information gathered by the speech therapist is valuable and useful for the entire team because it influences the methods they use to communicate with the patient and to teach the concepts necessary for retraining. The speech therapist provides instruction, makes recommendations for evaluation by an audiologist or an ear, nose, and throat specialist; and carries out the actual training or teaching of the skills necessary to communicate. Both patient and family may have to learn or improve their skills in this area.

Spinal Shock. A period of complete areflexia occurring at or below the level of injury.

Spontaneous Recovery. Recovery that takes place as the brain heals (early recovery process).

Standards of Care. Treatment modalities recognized by authorizing bodies or the medical community as safe and efficacious for the illness or injury. These standards are used as guidelines to define appropriate types and levels of patient care that should be implemented.

Standby Assistance. Assistance given a patient in which the caregiver or therapist remains within arm's length of the patient to ensure his or her safety. See also under *Gait Training*.

Standing Frame. Frame that allows a person with a spinal cord injury to stand with the hands free. If the lesion is at the T7 level or below, a manual frame is preferred to a hydraulic frame.

State Department of Aging. Department that administers the funds provided to states under the federal Older Americans Act that are intended to develop a variety of social services and home and community-based long-term care programs. This department develops and coordinates programs and services for older persons through the various local Area on Aging agencies.

State Department of Alcohol and Drug Prevention. Develops the statewide plan and budget for the prevention, identification, and treatment of alcohol and drug abuse, administers state and federal funds allocated to the county programs, and adopts rules and regulations relating to standards of service. This agency also evaluates the effectiveness of programs, offers technical assistance, administrative oversight, and cost control for local programs, as well as education, literature, and information and referral services. The drug services division in addition approves, licenses, and regulates methadone maintenance programs.

State Department of Health Services. Administers health programs at the state level to ensure a safe environment and provision of adequate healthcare and treatment to all state residents. This agency is responsible for licensing, certifying, and maintaining surveillance of health facilities to ensure their compliance with all federal and state laws and regulations. It also investigates complaints against health facilities and administers family health services (Title V Children's Medical Services programs, genetic disease prevention and treatment, and infant health and family planning programs) and rural and community health programs (e.g., Indian healthcare; medically underserved rural areas; financial support; technical assistance and liaison with local health agencies, county hospitals and facilities, and indigent care programs; toxic substances; and environmental and public health programs).

State Department of Mental Health. Ensures a statewide compensation system for preventive treatment, rehabilitative programs, and uniform accessibility to mental health services. Offers educational literature and information and referral to inpatient and outpatient mental health services. Outside of California, the Department of Mental Health or Department of Mental Retardation is the point of entry for the developmentally disabled to the continuum of care.

State Department of Rehabilitation. State agency (also known as DR, Voc rehab, or, in some states, the Bureau or Office of Vocational Rehabilitation) that offers services to persons (or their spouses) with medically diagnosed, stable physical or mental conditions that have resulted in moderate to severe functional limitations. These services include vocational testing, assessment, guidance, and counseling for potential employment or assistance in establishing living arrangements for the disabled person to facilitate employment of the spouse. If a person becomes an active client and has the potential to return to work, vocational rehabilitation may at times assist with the purchase of selected medical equipment, modifications to the home, drivers' evaluation, purchase or modifications to a van, and other job-related expenses.

State-County Department of Social Services (Welfare Department). Supervises and regulates financial aid and food stamps to needy families in conformity with both state and federal regulations. This department is also responsible for supervising Medicaid services as mandated by the Social Security Act, licensing community care facilities, evaluating disability claims, and supervising adoption services.

State Hospitals. Hospitals designed to provide care and treatment for patients suffering from a severe psychiatric illness or a severe developmental disability who cannot be cared for in a less restrictive long-term care facility or at home.

State Schools. Facilities designed to provide care and treatment to school-aged children who suffer from a severe psychiatric illness or exhibit severe behavioral outbursts that prevent them from participating in family or peer relationships.

Stop Loss. The ceiling or limit set on claims payments by a healthcare payor before the claim passes to a reinsurer who will accept liability for payments above this limit. Often the ceiling is set at $75,000 to $100,000 per claim. If a claim exceeds this amount and the reinsurer has not been notified of the claim before this point, the healthcare payor must assume responsibility for all payments for the case and risks losing a great deal of money. Stop loss means the catastrophic cap or point at which the patient reaches the limit on out-of-pocket expenses per calendar year; the healthcare plan assumes responsibility for 100% of the costs for that patient for the remainder of the calendar year.

Subacute Care Facilities. Facilities licensed under the regulations established for skilled nursing facilities. However, the regulations for these facilities require more nursing hours per patient per day, lower numbers of patients in relation to nursing personnel, and more frequent physician visits. Most subacute care facilities are hospital based and offer a higher level of care than community-based skilled nursing facilities.

Subarachnoid Screw or Bolt. Measuring devices that rest on the surface of the brain.

Subrogation. A clause that gives a healthcare payor plan the right to recover payments after the patient has received money from third party liability or legal damages.

Supervised Care. The patient requires only verbal cues from the caregiver or therapist to judge his own movements or orient himself.

Supplemental Security Income (SSI; Title XVI of the Social Security Act). Federal-state cash assistance program that provides additional monthly income to persons ages 65 or older or to those under 65 who are blind or disabled. This program is funded by income taxes and not from the general Social Security trust fund. Eligibility is based on income, savings, and proof of age, disability or blindness. If the patient is eligible for the program, he or she is also eligible for Medicaid. This program is administered by the Social Security Administration.

Suprapubic Rhythmic Manual Pressure (SRMP). Stimulation technique used for patients with neurogenic bladders to maintain continence.

Swan-Ganz Catheter. Catheter that is similar to a central venous pressure (CVP) line. It allows measurement of blood pressure and monitoring of the blood in the lungs as well as both sides of the heart.

Swing Beds. Beds, usually found in small or rural hospitals, that may be used to serve patients requiring either long-term skilled nursing care or acute care.

Tactile Defense. Oversensitivity to touch.

TAR. See *Treatment Authorization Request*.

Tax Equity and Fiscal Responsibility Act (TEFRA). Multiprovisional act that contains one key provision that is important to case managers. This provision prohibits healthcare payors from requiring employees between the ages of 65 and 69 to use Medicare rather than the group healthcare plan.

TBI. Traumatic brain injury.

TCU. See *Transitional Care Unit*.

Telephone Reassurance Services. Services available through local senior organizations or volunteer agencies serving seniors. In this service a volunteer calls the subscriber (usually an older person living alone) each day at a predetermined time to chat and make sure the person is all right.

Tendon Grafts. Grafts that replace lost or damaged tendons to restore mobilization.

Tenodesis Splint. Wrist-powered orthosis that enables the patient to produce a pinch grasp (i.e., this splint may improve the grasp of a patient with a spinal cord injury sufficiently to allow self-catheterization).

T Foam. Type of wheelchair cushion that protects the skin and prevents pressure points.

Third-Level Review. Review performed when a determination of benefit coverage is unclear or further physician advice for approval or denial is required. This review is performed by other than the medical director or a physician advisor.

Third-Party Administrator (TPA). A firm or organization that performs claims administration and adjudication and membership enrollment and offers administrative oversight; it is often used for self-funded or managed care plans.

Third-Party Liability (TPL). Those claims for an injury or illness that is liable for payment by another insurance company, generally one providing auto insurance or workers' compensation.

Title V Children's Medical Services. Federally mandated program that provides medical services for children with special needs. Benefits vary from state to state. However, they are intended to meet the medical needs of children or young adults with specific diagnoses who are 21 years old or younger (regardless of marital status) and meet certain eligibility criteria. Eligibility is based on diagnosis, income, and place of residence. The program is frequently administered by the state Department of Health or a similar state agency. These programs are always the payor of last resort.

Tone. Degree of tension in a muscle or group of muscles.

Transitional Care Unit or Program. Community-based housing units offered by many rehabilitation centers serving brain-injured patients. The emphasis is on retraining the individual to allow him or her to care for personal needs and to provide vocational or educational skills that will allow the person to reenter society. These units offer varying levels of supervision and often do not provide the conventional medical model for care. For this reason they are usually excluded from healthcare benefit coverage. The only exceptions occur in cases in which the healthcare payor may allow coverage through the extra contractual process.

Treatment Authorization Request (TAR). The formal written process for seeking approval for Medicaid and mental health services before the service is rendered.

Triple Option Plan. Healthcare payor that provides more than one option to its members or policyholders. These options are often a health maintenance organization (HMO), a preferred provider organization (PPO), a point of service (POS) plan, and an indemnity or traditional plan.

UB 92. Universal or standard billing form used by most hospital providers for submission of claims for inpatient or outpatient care. To simplify claims processing, much of the form is coded using the International Classification of Diseases (ICD), Current Procedural Terminology (CPT), or Diagnostic and Statistical Manual of Mental Diseases (DSM) codes.

Unbundling. The practice of billing the multiple components of a bill separately as several individual services instead of in the typical "bundle" covered by a single fee.

Unilateral Neglect. Unawareness or inattention to one side of the body or the events occurring on one side of the body.

Upcoding. A practice sometimes used by providers of billing for a procedure that pays more than the service that was actually performed.

U.S. Department of Health and Human Services (DHHS). Federal agency responsible for health planning, resource development, research, healthcare delivery, financing, and oversight on a national level. Within this agency are several subdivisions such as (1) Administration for Children and Families, (2) Healthcare Financing Administration, (3) Public Health Services, (4) Social Security Administration, (5) Administration of Aging, (6) Office of Civil Rights, (7) Office of the General Counsel, (8) Office of the Inspector General, (9) Office of Consumer Affairs, and (10) Office of Human Development Services.

U.S. Public Health Service (PHS). Administers many of the familiar federal health functions and is headed by the Surgeon General of the United States. Under the Surgeon General, the Assistant Secretary for Health is responsible for the administration and management of the following federal departments: (1) Agency for Toxic Substances and Disease Registry, (2) Alcohol, Drug Abuse and Mental Health Administration, (3) Center for Disease Control and Prevention, (4) Food and Drug Administration, (5) Health Resources and Services Administration, (6) Indian Health Services, and (7) National Institutes of Health.

Usual and Customary. Method of profiling the prevailing fees of providers (same specialty) in the area and then reimbursing providers standard amounts based on these findings. Often abbreviated as U & C.

Utilization Review. Process used by healthcare payors to evaluate and monitor all care and services rendered by healthcare providers for medical necessity, appropriateness, and efficiency. Review is also performed to ensure that neither overutilization nor underutilization occurs. Review techniques include prospective review, concurrent review, and retrospective review.

Verbal Apraxia. Impaired control of proper sequencing of the muscles used in speech.

Verbosity. Rambling or inability to control verbal comments. The person often talks continuously, and the content is disorganized.

Vestibular Function. The sense of balance.

Veterans Administration or **Veterans Affairs.** Provides information on veterans' benefits such as insurance, home loans, compensation, education, medical services, nursing home or domiciliary care, home care, other outpatient care, dental services, alcohol or drug treatment and rehabilitation, rehabilitation services for the physically impaired, dependents' benefits, pensions, and other related benefits. This agency also assists with filing claims and filling out forms and applications. It also investigates and takes remedial action on claims of nonpayment of benefits and offers information and advice on the effects of Agent Orange, delayed stress, and other war-related maladies.

Victims or **Witness Program.** Offers crisis and short-term counseling and referral to private or public agencies to victims of violent crimes. Some money is available for temporary assistance for victims who have necessary or unexpected expenses. However, the application process is lengthy, and funds are not always available when the need is most critical.

Visual Field Neglect. Inability to perceive information in a specific area of the visual field.

Waiver. In essence, this is Medicaid's extra contractual process. The Omnibus Reconciliation Budget Act allows states to make exceptions for Medicaid's traditional scope of benefit coverage. Under the waiver program, benefit coverage is expanded for certain categories of persons with special needs, who under normal conditions would be excluded from Medicaid coverage. Criteria for coverage are often based on the fact that long-term institutionalization can be prevented if coverage is allowed through use of the waiver.

Wards of the Court. Persons under the age of 18 who come within the jurisdiction of the juvenile court and are judged to be dependent children of the court. Such persons are those who need proper and effective parental care or control but have no parent or guardian willing or able to actually exercise care or control. Children in this category are often destitute and lack the necessities of life, or they may be physically dangerous to the public because of a mental or physical deficiency, disorder, or abnormality. They may come from a home that has been declared unfit by virtue of neglect, cruelty, depravity, or abuse. Wards of the court also include children who have been available for adoption for 12 months or more. Costs for medical care for these children can be paid from private insurance funds, but in most instances they are paid through use of Medicaid funds.

Workers' Compensation. A law that requires employers to pay benefits and furnish needed care to employees injured while on duty. Salary and medical care are available to persons who were injured while working and who meet certain eligibility requirements. There are no payroll deductions because the employer contributes to the state Compensation Insurance Fund, from which benefits are paid. Application for this program should be made through the employer. If a person is eligible for workers' compensation, regular insurance benefits, any state disability income, or unemployment benefits are not applicable.

BIBLIOGRAPHY

Dorland's Illustrated Medical Dictionary, 28th ed. (1994). Philadelphia, W.B. Saunders.

Evashwich CJ, Weiss LJ (1987). Managing the Continuum of Care. Gaithersburg, MD, Aspen.

Gurland BJ, Chacken EE (1989). Meeting the Health Care Needs of the Old—The Columbia University College of Physicians and Surgeons Complete Home Medical Guide, 2nd ed. New York, Crown Publishers.

Zarle NC (1987). Continuing Care: The Process and Practice of Discharge Planning. Gaithersburg, MD, Aspen.

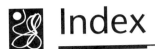 Index

Note: Page numbers in *italics* refer to illustrations;
page numbers followed by t refer to tables.

Abandonment, 138
ABI. See *Acquired brain injury (ABI)*.
Abuse, alcohol and drug, programs
    for. See *Alcohol and drug abuse
    programs*.
  financial, 137
  of children, 226-227
  of healthcare system, 139-140
  of patients, 137-138
    geriatric, 240
  substance. See also *Substance
    abuse programs*.
    chronic pain and, 326-327
Accreditation, defined, 356
Acquired brain injury (ABI), 255-259
  cognitive therapy for, 256
  day training programs for, 259
  day treatment programs for, 258
  home care for, 259
  initial treatment of, 255-256
  post-acute care of, 256-258, 320-
    323
    alternate funding for, 322-323
    benefits termination during, 258
    community resources for, 322
    nonmedical models of, 257-258
    support groups for, 322
  rehabilitation of, 320-323
    admission criteria for, 256
    criteria for, 320-321
    exclusion of benefits for, 255
    goals of, 320
    locations of, 321-322
    phases of, 320
    physical and mental changes in,
      322
  sheltered workshops for, 259
  supported work programs for, 259
Acquired immunodeficiency syndrome
    (AIDS), 198-225
  alternate funding for, 201
  barriers and problems for, 199-200
  case management pros and cons
    for, 198-199
  common diagnoses associated with,
    203
  community resources for, 201-202
  discharge services required for,
    202-203
  durable medical equipment and sup-
    plies for, 200-201
  medications for, 204
  patient/family instructions for, 203
  physical manifestations of, 203-204
  resources for, 198

Acquired immunodeficiency syndrome
    (AIDS) *(Continued)*
  specialists for, 199
  terminal care for, 204-205
Activities of daily living (ADL), 331
  defined, 307, 356
Acute care psychiatric hospitals, 245
Adaptive driving programs, for
    disabled, 149
ADL. See *Activities of daily living
    (ADL)*.
Administrative services only (ASO),
    defined, 14-15, 356
Adult day care, 315
Adult day care centers, 239
Adult day healthcare, defined, 356
Adult protective services (APS), 137,
    342
Advance directives, 136-137
Aeromedical evacuation system,
    CHAMPUS and, 91, 151, 267
Aid to Families with Dependent
    Children (AFDC), 62
  defined, 356
Aide, defined, 356
AIDS. See *Acquired
    immunodeficiency syndrome
    (AIDS)*.
AIDS Foundation, services of, 342
Air ambulances, CHAMPUS and, 91
  for disabled, 151
Airline services, for disabled, 150-151
Alcohol and drug abuse programs, for
    mental health patients, 247
  services of, 342-343
  social security benefits for, 96
  veterans benefits for, 84
Alcoholics Anonymous, services of,
    343
Allogeneic bone marrow
    transplantation, CHAMPUS and,
    270
Alternate funding, 16-17. See also
    under specific agencies.
  eligibility for, delays in, 123
  for AIDS patients, 201
  for brain-injured patients, 322-323
  for cancer patients, 210
  for cardiac patients, 288
  for chronically ill/disabled children,
    220-222
  for common high-risk catastrophic
    cases, 189, 192t, 192-193
  for diabetes, 232
  for durable medical equipment and
    supplies, 156-157

Alternate funding *(Continued)*
  for end-stage renal disease, 217
  for geriatric patients, 239
  for intravenous antibiotic therapy,
    289
  for mental health patients, 245
  for neonates, 228
  for neurologically impaired patients,
    251
  for private duty nurses, 337-338
  for respiratory disease, 280-281
  for total parenteral nutrition, 295
  for transplant patients, 266-267
  for wound care, 298
Alzheimer's Aid Society, services of,
    343
Alzheimer's disease, 254-255
Ambulances, 151-152
  air, CHAMPUS and, 91, 151
  vs. nonemergent transportation,
    151-152
American Cancer Society, services of,
    343
American Diabetes Association,
    services of, 343
American Heart Association, services
    of, 343
American Lung Association, services
    of, 343
American Lupus Society, services of,
    343-344
American Nurses' Association, case
    management definition, 4
American Red Cross, services of, 344
Americans with Disabilities Act,
    defined, 16
Antibiotics, intravenous, 289-291. See
    also *Intravenous antibiotic
    therapy*.
Antirejection drugs, costs of, 274
Antitrust law, 137
Anxiety, in respiratory disease
    patients, 280
Apnea monitoring, home, 158-159
APS (adult protective services), 137,
    357
Arthritis Foundation, services of, 344
ASO (administrative services only),
    defined, 14-15
Assertiveness, of case managers, 6, 41
Assessment, clinical. See *Clinical
    assessment*.
  defined, 32
  for Individuals with Disabilities Edu-
    cation Act, 76-77

Assessment *(Continued)*
 for rehabilitation, 318, 321
 for State Agency for Developmental
  Disabilities, 106
 preliminary, 29-30
  documentation of, 29-30
Assistive Device Center, services of,
 344
Attire, for on-site visits, 36
Attorney(s). See also *Power of
 attorney.*
 role of, in case management, 34-35
Audits, 11-12
Autologous bone marrow
 transplantation, 207

Bathroom(s), self-help devices for use
 in, 165
Bathroom equipment, for spinal cord
 injury, 262
Bedpans, disinfection of, 162
Beds, swing, defined, 378
Beneficence, defined, 41
Benefit modification process. See
 Extra contractual process.
Benefits, termination of, 60
 veterans, 63
 waiver of. See *Extra contractual
  process.*
Bereavement outreach, services of,
 345
Blind, community resources for, 194
 diabetes and, 231-232
 schools for, 78
 veterans benefits for, 84
Blind Society, services of, 344
Board and care homes, 315
Body systems, assessment of, for
 teaching plan development,
 182-183
Bonding, defined, 358
Bone marrow transplantation,
 allogeneic, 270
 autologous, 207
 complications of, 276
 discharge criteria for, 274
 for military personnel, 89-90
 indications for and contraindications to, 272-273
Books, for case managers, 19-20
Braces, care of, 163
Brain-Impaired Regional Center,
 services of, 344-345
Brooke Army Medical Center, burn
 unit of, 291
Burn(s), 291-294
 complications of, 294
 discharge barriers for, 293
 durable medical equipment and supplies for, 293
 laboratory tests for, 293
 patient/family instructions for, 294
 radiologic studies for, 293
Burn unit, Brooke Army Medical
 Center, 291
 Shriners hospitals, 291
Burnout, in caregivers, 18-19
Bus services, for disabled, 150
Button infusor, 231

Camps, for handicapped, services of,
 345
Cancer patient(s), 205-210
 alternate funding for, 210
 barriers to discharge and care access for, 209-210
 case management pros and cons
  for, 205
 centers of excellence/tertiary care
  centers for, 206
 community resources for, 209
 discharge services required for, 208
 durable medical equipment and supplies for, 209
 early intervention in, indications
  for, 205
 experimental/investigational services for, 206-207
 pain management for, 208-209
 treatment of, 205-206, 207-208
Capitation, defined, 13
Cardiac patient(s), 285-289
 activity limitations of, 286
 alternate funding for, 288
 diagnostic testing for, 286
 discharge/care access barriers for,
  287, 288-289
 durable medical equipment and supplies for, 287-288
 patient/family instructions for, 288
 psychological impact on, 286-287
 rehabilitation of, 287, 324-326
 treatment of, 286
Cardiac rehabilitation, 324-326
 admission criteria for, 325
 components of, 325
 costs of, 326
 goals of, 324-325
 team members in, 325
Cardiac transplantation. See *Heart
 transplantation; Heart-lung
 transplantation.*
Care map. See *Case management
 plan.*
Career training, financial resources for,
 76, 80, 102-104
Caregiver(s). See also *Family
 caregiver(s), instructions for.*
 burnout in, 18-19
 care of, 144-145, 189
  peer support vs. professional
   counseling in, 145
  respite, 144-145
 communication with, 32
 defined, 358
 role of, in discharge planning, 113
 supervision of, by healthcare team,
  144
 unavailability of, 122
CARF (Commission on Accreditation
 of Rehabilitation Facilities), 328
 defined, 359
Cars, rental, for disabled, 152
Case(s), catastrophic, 5-6. See also
 Catastrophic cases.
 closure of, 43, 57-58
  criteria in, 57-58
  steps in, 57-58
 reasons for not opening, 30
Case conference(s), as communication
 tool, 37

Case management, auditing of, 11-12
 barriers to, 112-126
  discharge, 115-116, *116*
  overcoming, 116-126
  problem(s) and solution(s) associated with, 118-126
   conflict between organization
    and patient goals as, 124-
    125
   confusion with utilization re-
    view as, 118
   eligibility delays as, 123
   family conflicts as, 122-123
   family coping skills as, 123-124
   inaccessible hospital charts as,
    119
   incapable providers as, 121-
    122
   lack of quality as, 121
   limited resources as, 120-121
   multiple case managers as, 120,
    124
   need for specialist as, 126
   noncompliant patients as, 125-
    126
   unavailable physicians as, 119
   unavailable respite care as, 123
   unavailable/untrainable caregiv-
    ers as, 122
   uncooperative/inaccessible phy-
    sicians as, 118-119
   uninformed providers and fami-
    lies as, 118
 definition of, 4
 demographics affecting, 8
 discharge barriers to, 115-116, *116*
 factors affecting, 7, 8-9, 12
 failure of resulting from caregiver
  burnout, 18
 flow of, 24, *24*
 legal aspect(s) of, 134-141
  abandonment as, 138
  advance directive as, 136-137
  antitrust law as, 137
  confidentiality as, 134-135
  conservatorship as, 135-136
  fraud and abuse as, 139-140
  living will as, 136
  negligent referrals as, 139
  patient abuse as, 137-138
  patient rights as, 135
  power of attorney as, 136-137
  standards of care as, 138
  Wickline case as, 138
 models of, 5
  vs. nursing care delivery models,
   5
 need for, 5
 origins of, 2
 patients served in, 2-3
 principles of, 24-25
 process of, 12, *12*
 referrals in. See *Referral(s).*
 senior management commitment to,
  7-8
 services provided by, 2-3
 tools for, 18-19
 utilization of, 8
 vs. utilization review, 4-5
Case management plan, 37-42

Case management plan *(Continued)*
  basis for, 176
  conflict in, between provider and
      family, 176
  data elements of, 37-38
  development of, 38-39
  establishment of, 176
  final, 39-40
  focus of, 37
  for geriatric patients, 236
  for mental health patients, 243-244
  for neurologically impaired patients,
      248
  implementation of, 40-41, 187
  monitoring of, 187
  reassessment of, 41-42, 187
    frequency in, 41-42, 187
    techniques in, 41-42
  review of, second level, 38
Case manager(s), as guides to
      healthcare system, 2-4, *3*
  certification of, 4
  expertise of, 5-7
  knowledge of, 9
  multiple, 55
    problems with, 120, 124
  new, monitoring of, 8
  patient/family as, teaching of, 185-
      186, 225
  responsibilities of, 6-7
    to healthcare payors, 6-7
    to home health agencies, 6-7
    to hospitals, 6
  sensitivity of, 36
  skills of, 5-6, 30
Case planner(s), 12-13
Caseload(s), activity levels of, 11-12
  acuity rating for, 10
  auditing of, 11
  determination of, 9-12
  diagnoses in, 9
  difficult, 10
  factors affecting, 8
  fluctuation of, 9-10
Catastrophic cases, 5-6, 176-198
  alternate funding for, 189, 192t,
      192-193
  alternate levels of care for, 193
  care of caregiver in, 189
  case management plan for, 176-177
    changes in, 187
  common diagnoses in, 189, 190t-
      191t
  communication in, 179-180
  community resources for, 193-194,
      198
  defined, 8
  discharge and care access barriers
      in, 178-179
  discharge services required in, 195t,
      198
  durable medical equipment and sup-
      plies for, 187-188, 196t-197t
  high risk flags in, 189, 190t-191t
  home care vs. out-of-home care,
      177-178
  multiple diagnoses in, 177
  provider or vendor selection for,
      188-189
  psychological impact of, 180-182

Catastrophic cases *(Continued)*
  teaching in, 182-187
  trial passes in, 185
Catchment areas, defined, 91
CDC (Centers for Disease Control and
      Prevention), defined, 358
Center for Consumer Healthcare
      Information, 19
Center for Deafness, services of, 345
Center for independent living,
      defined, 358
  services of, 345
Center of excellence, for cancer
      patients, 206
Centers for Disease Control and
      Prevention (CDC), defined, 358
Certification, defined, 358
Certification of insurance
      rehabilitation specialist (CIRSC),
      4
Certified case manager, National Case
      Management Task Force criteria
      for, 4
Certified nurse's aide, defined, 370
CHAMPUS (Civilian Health and
      Medical Program of Uniformed
      Services), 86-93, 192-193
  adjunctive dental care and, 90
  aeromedical system and, 91, 151,
      267
  allogeneic bone marrow transplanta-
      tion and, 270
  benefits waivers and, 57
  defined, 15
  eligibility and, 87
  Home Health Care Demonstration
      and, 90
  Home Health Care-Case Manage-
      ment Demonstration and, 90
  mental health and, 90-91
  military treatment facilities and, 88
  nonavailability statement and, 88
  reimbursement and copayments
      and, 88-89
  services of, 88
  terminology of, 91-93
  TRICARE and. See *TRICARE.*
  Wilford Hall Medical Center and,
      89-90
CHAMPUS maximum allowable charge
      (CMAC), 88-89, 91
CHAMPVA (Civilian Health and
      Medical Program of Department
      of Veterans Affairs), 85, 91-92
Chemotherapy, 212-214
  complications of, 213
  discharge and care access in, barri-
      ers to, 214
  discharge requirements for, 212
  discharge services for, 212-213
  durable medical equipment and sup-
      plies for, 213
  patient/family instructions for, 213
Child(ren). See also *Infant(s);
      Neonate(s).*
  abuse of, 226-227
  chronically ill/disabled. See *Chroni-
      cally ill/disabled child(ren).*
Child protective services (CPS), 137,
      345

Children's Liver Foundation, services
      of, 345
Children's Medical Services, 62,
      64-69, 220
  defined, 15, 353
  eligibility requirements of, 66-67
  genetic programs of, 67-68, 222
  names of, by state, 68
  purpose and objectives of, 64-65
  referrals, 66
  services of, 67
  transportation reimbursement of,
      221
Chronic pain, common characteristics
      of, 326-327
  physical and emotional factors of,
      326
  rehabilitation for, 326-329
    case management involvement in,
      329
    case review of, 329
    costs of, 327
    goals of, 328-329
    inpatient vs. outpatient treatment
      of, 328
    medical vs. mental health benefits
      and, 327-328
Chronically ill/disabled child(ren),
      219-230. See also *Infant(s);
      Neonate(s).*
  alternate funding for, 220-222
  caregivers of, care for, 219
  communication about, 224-225
  community resources for, 220-222
  demographics of, 219-220
  developmental delays in, 222-223
  discharge and care access for, barri-
      ers to, 227
  durable medical equipment and sup-
      plies for, 223-224
  emotional support for, 227
  family instruction for, 225-226
  financial resources for, 62, 63, 64-
      69, 73-81, 194
  genetic services for, 222
  home health agency services for,
      224
  psychological impact on, 226-227
  skilled nursing facility care for, 223
CIRSC (certification of insurance
      rehabilitation specialist), 4
Civil Rights Act, defined, 15
Civilian Health and Medical Program
      of Department of Veterans Affairs
      (CHAMPVA), 85, 91-92
Civilian Health and Medical Program
      of Uniformed Services
      (CHAMPUS). See *CHAMPUS
      (Civilian Health and Medical
      Program of Uniformed Services).*
Clinical assessment, 30-35
  attorneys' role in, 34-35
  components of, 33
  cultural sensitivity in, 31
  data elements of, 31
  data sources for, 33-34
  documentation of, 35
  of body systems, for teaching plan
      development, 182-183
  success of, 31-33

Clinical nurse specialist, defined, 358
Clinical pathways, in utilization review, 130
CMAC. See *CHAMPUS maximum allowable charge.*
Cognitive retrainer, defined, 359
Collaboration, 6
Coma scales, 321
Coma stimulation program, defined, 359
Commercial buses for disabled, 150
Commission on Accreditation of Rehabilitation Facilities (CARF), 328
  defined, 359
Commission for Case Management Certification, assessment definition of, 32
  beneficence definition of, 41
  case management principles of, 24-25
  case management values of, 37
  coordination definition of, 40
  definition of, 41
  evaluation definition of, 32-33
  justice definition of, 41
  monitoring definition of, 33
  nonmaleficence definition of, 41
  planning definition of, 38
  veracity definition of, 41
Commission on Aging, defined, 359
Communication, 6
  about chronically ill/disabled children, 224-225
  with mental health care patients, 243
  with patients or family, 13-14, 179-180
    poor, example of, 180
    self-help devices for, 165
    through case conferences, 37
    with caregivers, 32
    with team members, 14, 34, 179-180, 224
Community agencies, services of, 342-354
"Community reentry program," for brain-damaged patients, 257, 322
Community resources, filing system for, 19
  for cancer patients, 209
  for catastrophic cases, 193-194
  for chronically ill/disabled children, 220-222
  for durable medical equipment and supplies, 156
  for end-stage renal disease, 217-218
  for geriatric patients, 238-239
  for hearing impaired patients, 194
  for mental health patients, 245
  for neurologically impaired patients, 254
  for respiratory disease, 281
  for visually impaired patients, 194
  with diabetes, 231-232
  utilization of, 61
Concurrent review, 129, 371
Confidentiality, 134-135
Congregate housing, defined, 359
Congregate meals, defined, 359

Consent form, for experimental transplants, 269
  for investigational/experimental treatment, 207
Conservator, 136
Conservator's office, services of, 345-346
Conservatorship, 135-136
  defined, 359-360
Consumer(s), healthcare. See *Patient(s).*
Consumer Credit Counseling Services, 346
Continuum of care, terminology of, 342-354
Contractual process, extra. See *Extra contractual process.*
Coordination, defined, 40
Corporate Angel Network, services of, 346
Cost(s), of antirejection drugs, 274
  of cardiac rehabilitation, 326
  of chronic pain management, 327
  of healthcare providers, 48
  of healthcare services, evaluation of, 39-40
  of home care, 178, 239, 310-311
  of home health care, 252
  of outpatient therapy, for neurologically impaired patients, 252
  of pharmaceuticals, 170, 368
  of post-acute care, for neurologically impaired patients, 250-251, 252
  of private duty nurses, 338
  of skilled nursing facilities, 239, 330
  of subacute care facilities, 332-333
  of wheelchairs, 252-253
Cost savings, reports for, 53-54
  format of, 53
  frequency of, 53
Counseling, psychological, for families of chronically ill/disabled children, 226
County Department of Health, 346-347
County Department of Social Services, 347
Court-ordered care, defined, 360
CPS (child protective services), 137, 360
Creativity, of case managers, 6, 12
Crisis centers, services of, 347
Cruiselines, for disabled, 152
Culture, sensitivity to, 31
Custodial care, alternate funding for, 314
  defined, 307, 331, 360
  documentation of, 309
  of acquired brain injury, 256
  of geriatric patients, reimbursement for, 234-235, 236
  skilled care vs., *306,* 306-310
Cystic Fibrosis Foundation, services of, 347

Data, collection of, for case management plan, 37-38
  for clinical assessment, 31

Data *(Continued)*
  sources of, for clinical assessment, 33-34
Day hospitals, defined, 360-361
Day training programs, for acquired brain injury, 259
Day treatment programs, for acquired brain injury, 258
Deaf, community resources for, 194
  schools for, 78
Defense Enrollment and Eligibility Reporting System (DEERS), 87, 92
Demographics, affecting case management, 8
  patient, for referrals, 28-29
Dental care, CHAMPUS and, 90
  veterans benefits for, 84
Department of Developmental Disabilities, services of, 347-348
Department of Health and Human Services (DHHS), defined, 379
Department of Rehabilitation, services of, 348
Department of Veterans Affairs, 81
  defined, 379
  services of, 366
Department of Vocational Rehabilitation, for neurologically impaired patients, 251, 259
Dependency, in respiratory disease, 280
Depression, in respiratory disease, 280
Designed Instruction and Services (DIS), 78-79
Developmental centers, defined, 361
Developmental Disabilities Act, defined, 16, 222
Developmental disability, defined, 105, 222-223
Device(s), orthotic, Food Drug and Cosmetic Act definition of, 156
  prosthetic, Food Drug and Cosmetic Act definition of, 156
  veterans benefits for, 84
  self-help. See *Self-help device(s).*
DHHS (Department of Health and Human Services), defined, 379
Diabetes, 230-234
  alternate funding for, 232
  blindness in, community resources for, 231-232
  chronic pain in, management of, 232
  complications of, 230-231
  discharge/care access barriers of, 233-234
  insulin for, 231
  laboratory tests for, 231
  patient/family instructions for, 233
  psychological impact of, 232-233
  services required for, 231-232
  types of, 230
Dialysis, medical management of, 215-216
Diet, discharge planning for, 114
Dietitian, defined, 361
DIS (Designed Instruction and Services), 78-79
Disability, developmental, defined, 105, 222-223

Disabled, adaptive driving programs for, 149
airline services for, 150-151
bus services for, 150
children. See *Chronically ill/disabled child(ren)*.
fast food restaurants for, 152
financial resources for, 63, 75-76, 104-108
gravely, defined, 365
handicapped stickers for, 149
learning, defined, 367
modified vehicles for, 149-150
rental cars for, 152
ships or cruiselines for, 152
trains for, 152
Discharge coordinator, defined, 361
Discharge criteria, bone marrow transplantation and, 274
for neonatal patients, 228
for TPN patients, 294-295
for ventilator-dependent patients, 282-283
heart transplantation and, 274
intravenous antibiotic therapy and, 289
kidney transplantation and, 274
liver transplantation and, 274
wound care and, 296-297
Discharge planning, barriers to, 115-116, *116*, 178-179
conservatorship and, 136
caregivers and, 113
durable medical equipment and, 112-113
for AIDS patients, 202-203
for home placement, 113
for out-of-home placement, 112
for spinal cord injury patients, 263
medications and, 114
nutritional needs and, 114
patient education and, 114
questions for, 112-115
services required for, 195t, 198
to another facility, 114-115
Discharge services, for AIDS patients, 202-203
for cancer patients, 208
for intravenous antibiotic therapy patients, 290
for neonatal patients, 228-229
for TPN patients, 295
for transplant patients, 275
for ventilator-dependent patients, 283
for wound care patients, 297, 298
Discharge/care access barriers, for cancer patients, 209-210
for cardiac patients, 287, 288-289
for chronically ill/disabled children, 227
for geriatric patients, 241
for neonatal patients, 230
for neurologically impaired patients, 254
for TPN patients, 296
for transplant patients, 276-277
in diabetes, 233-234
in respiratory disease, 282
in wound care, 299

Distributive justice, defined, 41
Do not resuscitate (DNR) orders, 240
Doctor of physical medicine and rehabilitation, defined, 372
Documentation, for case management plan, 38
for extra contractual process, 56
of case closures, 43, 58
of clinical assessments, 35, 36
of preliminary assessments, 29-30
Domestic violence units, defined, 361
Domiciliary care, veterans benefits for, 83
Dress, for on-site visits, 36
Dressing, self-help devices for, 164
Drinking, self-help devices for, 164-165
Driving programs, adaptive, for disabled, 149
Drug(s), 168-172
antirejection, costs of, 274
case manager's knowledge of, 169
eligibility for, 168-169
Medicare, 101, 168
experimental, Food and Drug Administration approval of, 169-170
for cancer patients, 206-207
reimbursement of, 170
exclusion in, 168
verification of, 207
for AIDS patients, 204
for geriatric patients, 236-239
for mental health patients, 244-245
intravenous. See *Intravenous antibiotic therapy.*
over-the-counter, provision of, by healthcare payors, 168
utilization review of, 169, 170, 373
wholesale price of, average, 170
Drug abuse programs. See *Alcohol and drug abuse programs.*
Durable medical equipment and supplies, 156-162
alternate funding sources for, 156-157
billing for, by Health Care Financing Administrators Common Procedural Coding System, 161
commonly ordered, 157-158, 196t-197t, 198
costs of, ongoing, 158
customization of, 161
discharge planning for, 112-113
duplicated, 166, 188, 253
eligibility for, exclusion from, 156, 157, 158
requirements of, 157
Food, Drug, and Cosmetic Act definition of, 156
for AIDS patients, 200-201
for burn patients, 293
for cancer patients, 209
for cardiac patients, 287-288
for chemotherapy patients, 213
for common high-risk catastrophic cases, 187-188
for end-stage renal disease, 218
for intravenous antibiotic therapy, 290

Durable medical equipment and supplies *(Continued)*
for neonatal patients, 229
for neurologically impaired patients, 252-253
for respiratory disease, 281
for spinal cord injury, 261-262
for TPN patients, 295
for transplant patients, 276
for ventilator-dependent patients, 284-285
for wound care, 297-298
home evaluation for, 188
home modifications for, 161
home monitors and, 158-159
provision of, by community agencies, 156
purchase vs. rental of, 159-160
service contracts for, 160
veterans benefits for, 84
Durable medical equipment company(ies), selection of, criteria for, 49
Durable power of attorney, 136-137
defined, 362

Early education programs, 79-80
Easter Seal Society, defined, 362
services of, 348
Eating, self-help devices for, 164-165
ECF (extended care facility), defined, 363
Education, early, 79-80
special, defined, 376
financial resources for, 63, 73-81
Education for All Handicapped Children Act, 73
defined, 16
Educational specialist, defined, 362
Egg crate mattresses, care of, 163
Electric wheelchairs, costs of, 262
Eligibility, Children's Medical Services program requirements for, 65-66, 66-67
delays in, for alternate funding programs, 123
for CHAMPUS and, 87
Individuals with Disabilities Education Act criteria for, 74
verification of, 29
Emergency response system (ERS), 165, 194
defined, 362
services of, 348
Emotion(s), of patients and families, 180-182
Emotional abuse, 137
Emotional support, for chronically ill/disabled children, 227
End-stage renal disease, 214-219
alternate funding for, 217
barriers to discharge and care access for, 218-219
community resources for, 217-218
complications of, 216-217
dialysis and, medical management of, 215-216
durable medical equipment and supplies for, 218

End-stage renal disease *(Continued)*
  Medicare and, 101–102
  patient/family instructions for, 218
  psychological impact of, 216
  treatment of, 214–215
  treatment team for, 215
Enteral therapy, 170–172
  administration of, 171–172
    clean vs. sterile technique in, 172
  cost and procurement of, 171
  family/caregiver instruction for, 171
  for infants, 171
  homemade, 172
  medical necessity for, 170
  provision of, by healthcare payor, 168
  reimbursement for, exclusion of, 170
  services required for, 171–172
Enterostomal therapist, defined, 362
EPOs (exclusive provider organizations), defined, 15
Equipment. See *Durable medical equipment and supplies.*
ERS. See *Emergency response system (ERS).*
Ethnic social service agencies, services of, 352
Exclusive provider organizations (EPOs), defined, 15
Extended care facility (ECF), defined, 363
Extended role nurse, defined, 363
Extra contractual process, 55–57
  approval of, 56–57
  defined, 55–56
  documentation for, 56

Families and Medical Leave Act, defined, 16
Family(ies), as employers of home help, 146
  assessment of, 30–35
  communication with, 14, 179–180
  conflicts within, 122
  financial resources for, 62–64
    from fraternal organizations, 62
    from government programs, 62–64
    from research grants, 63
    sliding scale in, 63
  ignorance about case manager's role by, 118
  inability of, to cope, 123–124
  instruction for. See *Family caregiver(s), instructions for; Patient/family instruction(s).*
  involvement of, with geriatric patients, 238
    with skilled nursing facilities, 331
  of chronically ill/disabled children, support groups for, 226
  of geriatric patients, support groups for, 238
  psychological impact on, 180–182
  role of, in case planning, 11–12, 36, 37
Family caregiver(s). See also *Caregiver(s).*

Family caregiver(s) *(Continued)*
  instructions for, 144
    in enteral therapy, 171
    in home monitoring, 159
    with chronically ill/disabled children, 225–226
    with neonates, 229
Fast food restaurants, for disabled, 152
FDA (Food and Drug Administration), defined, 363–364
  experimental drug approval by, 169–170
Federal Insurance Contribution Act (FICA), defined, 363
Feeding bags, 171–172
Feeding pumps, mechanical, 171–172
Feeding tubes, gastrostomy, 171
Feelings, of patients and families, 180–182
FICA (Federal Insurance Contribution Act), defined, 363
Financial abuse, 137
Financial consideration(s), 48–58
  case closure in, 57–58
  cost savings, cost avoidance, or cost benefit analysis reporting as, 53–54
  extra contractual process as, 55–57
  multiple case managers as, 55
  providers' role in, 48–51
  reduced rate negotiations as, 51–52
Financial resource(s), 60–108. See also *Alternate funding.*
  coverage constraints as, 60
  for families, 62–64
  lack of, problems concerning, 122–123
  of healthcare payor, vs. alternate payor, 50
Food and Drug Administration (FDA), defined, 363–364
  experimental drug approval by, 169–170
Food, Drug, and Cosmetic Act, device defined by, 156
  durable medical equipment defined by, 156
  medical supplies defined by, 156
  orthotic device defined by, 156
  prosthetic device defined by, 156
Food preparation, self-help devices for, 165
Fraternal organization(s), as alternate payor sources, 62, 192, 253
  services of, 348
"Friendly visitor" programs, 194
Functional abilities, defined, 364
Functional limitations, 308
  defined, 364

Gastrostomy feeding tubes, 171
Genetic services, for chronically ill/disabled children, 222
  of Children's Medical Services program, 67–68
Genetically Handicapped Persons Program (GHPP), 67
Geriatric patient(s), 234–241
  abuse of, 240

Geriatric patient(s) *(Continued)*
  alternate funding for, 239
  assessment of, 235
  case management plans for, 236
  community resources for, 238–239
  demographics of, 234
  discharge/care access barriers of, 241
  family involvement with, 238
  interviewing, 235–236
  medication needs of, 236–238
  neglect of, 240
  nutritional needs of, 236–237
  on-site visits for, 235–236
  referrals of, 234–235
GHPP (Genetically Handicapped Persons Program), 67
Glasgow Coma Scale, defined, 364–365
Grants, research, 63, 192
Gravely disabled, defined, 365
Grooming, self-help devices for, 165
Group homes, 315

"Habilitation" plan, State Agency for Developmental Disabilities and, 106
Handicapped. See also *Chronically ill/disabled child(ren).*
  camps for, services of, 357
  parking stickers for, 149
Handicapped bus services, for disabled, 150
Handicapped transportation services, 348
HBAs (health benefits advisors), 92
HCFA (Health Care Financing Administration), defined, 365
Health benefits advisors (HBAs), 92
Health Care Financing Administration (HCFA), defined, 365
Health Care Financing Administrators Common Procedural Coding System, for billing of durable medical equipment and supplies, 161
Health Maintenance Organization Act, defined, 16
Health maintenance organizations (HMOs), defined, 14
  for military personnel, 86–87
Healthcare, standards of, 138–139
Healthcare consumer(s). See *Patient(s).*
Healthcare finders (HCFs), 87, 92
Healthcare payor(s), case managers' responsibilities to, 6–7
  coverage constraints of, 60
  defined, 15, 365
  malpractice suits against, 138
  provision of durable medical equipment and supplies, exclusion of, 156, 157, 158
  requirement for, 157
  provision of pharmaceuticals, requirements for, 168–169
  types of, 14–15
  vs. alternate payor, 60
Healthcare provider(s). See also individual provider group, e.g., *Nurse.*

Healthcare provider(s) *(Continued)*
  and ignorance of case manager's role, 118
  and patient's needs, inability to meet, 121-122
  costs of, 48
  for mental health patients, 245-246
  for transplant patients, 266
  fraud and abuse of healthcare system by, 139-140
  information supplied to, 48
  malpractice suits against, 138
  Medicare-certified, defined, 369
  multiple, problems with, 17
  quality standards for, inability to meet, 121
  role of, in case planning, 12
  selection of, 48-51, 188-189
    criteria in, 48-50
    patients' rights in, 12, 38-39
Healthcare resources, access to, problems with obtaining, 17-18, 120-121, 178-179
  evaluation of, 39-40
Healthcare system, complexities of, 2-4, *3*
  fraud and abuse of, by healthcare providers and patients, 139-140
Healthcare team, supervision of, 144
Hearing impaired, community resources for, 194
  schools for, 178
Heart. See also *Cardiac* entries.
Heart transplantation, complications of, 276
  discharge criteria for, 274
  indications for and contraindications to, 270-271
Heart-lung transplantation, indications for and contraindications to, 271
Hemophilia Foundation, services of, 348
HMOs (health maintenance organizations), defined, 14
  for military personnel, 86-87
Home(s), board and care, 315
  group, 315
  modifications to, elimination of architectural barriers as, 167
  for durable medical equipment and services, 161
  residential care, requirements for, 239
  senior retirement, defined, 375
Home apnea monitoring, 158-159
Home care, authorization of, 311-312
  barriers to, 311
  costs of, 178, 239, 252, 310-311
  determining factors for, 177-178
  example of, 178
  for acquired brain injury, 259
  for neurologically impaired patients, 252
    costs of, 252
  hiring help for, 145-148
    employer responsibilities in, 146
    interviews for, 146-147
    problems with, 147
    recruitment methods for, 146

Home care *(Continued)*
  references verification for, 147
  using nursing agencies, 147-148
  vs. out-of-home care, 177-178, 312-316
Home health agency(ies), 333-338
  barriers to, 336-337
  case managers' responsibilities in, 7
  defined, 365
  documentation for, 336
  duration of treatment in, 336
  for chronically ill/disabled children, 224
  for mental health patients, 246
  functions of, 334
  Medicare, 99-100
  nursing services provided by, 335
  occupational therapy services provided by, 335
  physical therapy services provided by, 335
  referrals to, 334-335
  requirements for, 334
  selection of, criteria for, 49
  services of, 334
  social work services provided by, 335-336
  veterans benefits for, 83
Home Health Care (HHC) Demonstration, CHAMPUS and, 90, 92
Home Health Care-Case Management (HHC-CM) Demonstration, CHAMPUS and, 90, 92
Home monitors, 158-159
  family/caregiver instruction for, 159
Home visitors, defined, 366
Home visits. See *On-site visits*.
Homebound, Medicare definition of, 334
Homemade enteral formulas, 172
Homemade solutions, for dissolving urine mineral deposits, 163
Homemade supplies, 162-164
Homemaker, defined, 365
Homemaker services, defined, 365-366
Hospice care, 210-212
  admission criteria for, 211
  defined, 366
  Medicare and, 99-100
  Medicare certification for, 211-212
  services of, 212, 349
  types of, 210-211
Hospital(s), acute care psychiatric, 245
  case managers' responsibilities in, 6-7
  day, defined, 366
  Shriners, burn unit, 291
  state, 315
    defined, 377
    for mental health patients, 246-247
Hospital charts, inaccessibility of, to case manager, 119
Hospital programs, partial, defined, 360-361
  for mental health patients, 245-246

Household tasks, self-help devices for, 165
Housing, congregate, defined, 359
  local, for children/families in tertiary care centers, 221
Hygiene, self-help devices for, 165

I & R. See *Information and referral (I & R)*.
ICF. See *Intermediate care facilities (ICF)*.
IDEA. See *Individuals with Disabilities Education Act (IDEA)*.
IEP (individualized education program), defined, 366
  Individuals with Disabilities Education Act and, 77-78, 220
IHSS (in-home supportive services), defined, 366-367
Incompetent patient(s), 240-241
Incontinent pads, homemade, 163
IND (investigational new drug), for cancer patients, 207
  reimbursement for, 204
Indemnity insurance, defined, 15
  for military personnel, 87
Independent practice association (IPA), defined, 15
Indian Health Services, defined, 366
Individual Program Plan (IPP), defined, 366
Individualized education program (IEP), defined, 366
  Individuals with Disabilities Education Act and, 77-78, 220
Individuals, with exceptional needs, defined, 366
Individuals with Disabilities Education Act (IDEA), 63, 73-81, 220. See also *Education for All Handicapped Children Act*.
  assessments, 76-77
  career and vocational education programs, 80
  defined, 16
  designed instruction and services, 78-79
  early education programs, 79-80
  eligibility criteria, 74
  individualized education plan, 77-78
  purpose of, 73-74
  referrals for, 76
  special program(s) of, 75-76
    extended school year as, 76
    for communicatively handicapped, 75
    for learning handicapped, 75
    for physically handicapped, 75
    for severely handicapped, 75
    in least restrictive environment, 76
    in nonpublic schools, 76
    in state special schools, 76
    infant development program as, 76
    resource specialist program as, 76
    special day classes as, 75-76

Individuals with Disabilities Education Act (IDEA) *(Continued)*
   vocational or transitional programs as, 76
Infant(s). See also *Neonate(s)*.
   enteral formulas for, family/caregiver instruction in, 171
   financial resources for, 76
Infant stimulation program, defined, 366
Information and assistance services, 349
Information and referral (I & R), defined, 366
Infusion company(ies), selection of, criteria for, 49
Infusion pump, insulin, 231
In-home supportive services (IHSS), defined, 366-367
Inpatient care, Medicare, 98-99
Insulin infusion pump, 231
Intensity-Severity-Discharge-Appropriateness (ISD-A) criteria, for utilization review, 130
Intensive care unit nurses, for spinal cord injury, 260-261
Intensive supportive facilities, for neurologically impaired patients, 259
Intermediate care facilities (ICF), 315
   defined, 367
   requirements for, 239
   veterans benefits for, 83
Intermittent skilled care, Medicare definition of, 334
Interpreter(s), location of, 349
   sources of, 31
InterQual criteria, for utilization review, 130
Interview(s), 35-37
   attire during, 36
   case conferences in, 37
   length of time for, 36
   location of, 36
   of hired home help, 146-147
   purpose of, 35
   success of, 36
   with geriatric patients, 235-236
Intestinal transplantation, indications for and contraindications to, 272-273
Intravenous antibiotic therapy, patients receiving, 289-291
   alternate funding for, 289
   complications of, 290-291
   discharge barriers of, 291
   discharge criteria for, 289
   discharge services required for, 290
   durable medical equipment and supplies for, 290
   patient/family instructions for, 290
Investigational new drug (IND), for cancer patients, 207
   reimbursement for, 204
Involuntary hold, defined, 367
IPA (independent practice association), defined, 15

IPP (Individual Program Plan), defined, 366
ISD-A (Intensity-Severity-Discharge-Appropriateness) criteria, for utilization review, 130

Job training, financial resources for, 76, 80, 102-104
Joint Commission for Accreditation of Health Care Organizations (JCAHO), defined, 367
Justice, defined, 41

Kidney disease, end-stage. See *End-stage renal disease*.
Kidney transplantation, complications of, 276
   discharge criteria for, 274
   indications for and contraindications to, 272
Kidney-pancreatic transplantation, indications for and contraindications to, 272

Learning disabled, defined, 367
Least restrictive environment (LRE), 76
Legal defense, guidelines to, 134
Legal service centers, defined, 367
   services of, 349
Legislation, 15-16
Leukemia Society of America, services of, 349
Library services, 349
Licensed practical nurse (LPN), defined, 368
Licensed vocational nurse (LVN), defined, 368
Licensure, defined, 368
Life care communities, defined, 368
Litigation, defense against, guide to, 134
   prevention of, documentation for, 30, 39
Liver transplantation, discharge criteria for, 274
   indications for and contraindications to, 271-272
Living will(s), 136, 240
Loan closets, defined, 368
Local housing, for children/families, in tertiary care centers, 221
Long-term disability (LTD) policies, defined, 15
Long-term insurance, defined, 15
Long-term psychiatric facilities, defined, 368
Loyalty, to organization vs. patient, 124-125, 176
LPN (licensed practical nurse), defined, 368
LRE (least restrictive environment), 76
LTD (long-term disability) policies, defined, 15
Lung(s). See also *Pulmonary; Respiratory* entries.
   transplantation of, complications of, 276

Lung(s) *(Continued)*
   indications for and contraindications to, 271
LVN (licensed vocational nurse), defined, 368

Mail order pharmacies, 169
Maintenance care, of geriatric patients, reimbursement of, 234-235, 236
Make-A-Wish Foundation, services of, 349
Maleficence, defined, 41
Malpractice suits, against healthcare payors and providers, 138
Managed care, Medicaid and, 70
Management services organizations (MSOs), defined, 15
Management techniques, business, required by case managers, 6
Maternal-child health programs, services of, 350
Mattresses, egg crate, care of, 163
Meals, congregate, defined, 359
   programs for, 350
Meals on Wheels, defined, 368-369
Mechanical feeding pumps, 171-172
Medicaid, 62, 69-73
   and skilled nursing facilities, 73
   application process for, 71-72
   defined, 15, 369
   eligibility for, 71
   federally mandated benefits of, 69
   for neurologically impaired patients, 251
   for transplant patients, 268
   key points, 70
   managed care and, 70
   optional state services of, 69
   program administration of, 72
   state variations of, 70-71
Medicaid in-Home Waiver program, private duty nurses and, 337
Medicaid waivers, 57, 72-73
   defined, 369
Medical equipment. See *Durable medical equipment and supplies*.
Medical record(s), 34
Medical supplies. See also *Durable medical equipment and supplies*.
   Food, Drug, and Cosmetic Act definition of, 156
Medicare, 62-63, 96-102
   and certification of hospice care, 211-212
   and criteria for skilled nursing facilities, 329-330
   and criteria for utilization review, 130
   and medications, eligibility for, 101, 168
   defined, 15, 369
   End-Stage Disease Amendment defined by, 16
   end-stage renal disease and, 101-102
   part A, 96-100
      benefit periods, 97-98
      home health agencies, 99-100

Medicare *(Continued)*
  hospice, 100
  inpatient care, 98–99
  skilled nursing facilities, 99
  part B, 100–101
Medicare-certified provider, defined, 369
Medication(s). See *Drug(s)*.
Medigap, defined, 15
Mental abuse, 137
Mental health, CHAMPUS and, 90–91
Mental health groups, services of, 350
Mental Health Parity Act, 244–245
Mental health patient(s), 241–247
  acute care psychiatric hospitals for, 245
  alternate funding for, 245
  case management plan for, 243–244
  communication with, 243
  community resources for, 245
  diagnostic flags for, 242–243
  dual diagnosis of, 243
  healthcare providers for, 245–246
  home health agencies for, 246
  medication needs of, 244–245
  outpatient programs for, 246
  partial hospital programs for, 245–246
  professionals and programs for, 243
  reimbursement for, limitations on, 244–245
  residential treatment centers for, 246
  state hospitals for, 246
  substance abuse programs for, 247
Mental health professionals, 243
Mental health programs, 243
Mental healthcare, changes in, 242
Mentally incompetent, defined, 369
Military treatment facilities (MTFs), TRICARE responsibilities of, 88, 92
Milliman and Robertson's guidelines, for utilization review, 130
Mobility, self-help devices for, 165–166
Money management services, defined, 371
Monitoring, defined, 33
  in reassessments, 41–42
Monitors, home, 158–159
  apnea, 158–159
  family/caregiver instruction for, 159
Mothers, financial resources for, 63
MSOs (management services organizations), defined, 15
MTFs (military treatment facilities), TRICARE responsibilities of, 88, 92
Muscular Dystrophy Association, services of, 350

Nanny nurse, defined, 369–370
NAS (nonavailability statement), 88, 92, 270
National Case Management Task Force, case management definition, 4

National Case Management Task Force *(Continued)*
  Certified Case Manager criteria, 4
National Committee for Quality Assurance (NCQA), defined, 370
National Foundation for Ileitis and Colitis, services of, 350
National Handicapped Sport and Recreation Association, services of, 351
National Institutes of Health (NIH), defined, 370
National Liver Foundation, services of, 345
National Marrow Donor Program, services of, 351
National Multiple Sclerosis Society, services of, 351
National registries, for transplant patients, 265
NCQA (National Committee for Quality Assurance), defined, 370
Neglect, 137
  of geriatric patients, 240
Negligent referrals, 139
Negotiations, for reduced rates, 51–52
  importance of, 51
  requirements for, 52
  steps in, 51–52
Neonate(s), 227–230
  alternate funding for, 228
  complications of, 229
  discharge requirements for, 228
  discharge services for, 228–229
  discharge/care access barriers of, 230
  durable medical equipment and supplies for, 229
  family instruction for, 229
Neurologically impaired patient(s), 248–263. See also specific impairment or disease.
  alternate funding for, 251
  case management plans for, 248
  community resources for, 254
  discharge/care access barriers for, 254
  durable medical equipment and supplies for, 252–253
  extended coverage for, 250
  home care for, 252
  patient/family instructions for, 253
  post-acute care costs of, 250–251
  post-acute care services for, 251–252
  rehabilitation of, 15–18, 249–250
  skilled nursing facilities for, 252
  typical diagnoses for, 248–249
Neuropsychiatrist, defined, 370
Neuropsychologist, defined, 370
New York Heart Association classification system, for activity limitations in cardiac patients, 286
NIH (National Institutes of Health), defined, 370
Nonavailability statement (NAS), 88, 92, 270
Noncompliant patient(s), 125–126, 239

Nurse. See also individual specialty nurse, e.g., *Licensed practical nurse (LPN)*.
  in home health agencies, 335
  primary care, communication with, 14
  role of, in case management, 4
Nurse practitioner, defined, 370
Nurse's aide, certified, defined, 370
Nursing agencies, role in hiring home help, 147
Nursing care, models of, vs. case management models, 5
Nutrition, discharge planning for, 114
  for geriatric patients, 236–237
Nutritional supplements, provision of, by healthcare payors, 168
  reimbursement for, exclusion of, 170

Occupational therapist, defined, 370
  for spinal cord injury, 261
  in home health agency(ies), 335
Occupational therapy, 308
OCHAMPUS, 92
Office of Vocational Rehabilitation. See *State Department of Rehabilitation*.
Older Americans' Act, defined, 15
Ombudsman, defined, 370–371
  offices for, 137–138
  services of, 351–352
Omnibus Reconciliation Act, and Medicaid waivers, 72
  defined, 16
On-site visits, attire for, 36
  for geriatric patients, 235–236
  importance of, 30–31, 32
  safety during, 36
Opportunities for the Handicapped, services of, 351
Order of protective custody, defined, 367
Organ acquisition, costs of, reimbursement for, 269
Organ procurement services, 351
Orthotic device, Food, Drug, and Cosmetic Act definition of, 156
Out-of-home care, barriers to, 179
  discharge planning for, 112
  for geriatric patients, 238–239
  placement in, 311, *312*
  vs. home care, 177–178, 312–316
Outpatient programs, for chronic pain, 328–329
  for mental health patients, 246
  for neurologically impaired patients, costs of, 252
  for rehabilitation patients, 319
  veterans benefits for, 83–84
Over-the-counter (OTC) medications, provision of, by healthcare payors, 168

Pads, incontinent, homemade, 163
Pain, acute, vs. chronic, 326
  chronic. See *Chronic pain*.
Pain management, 326–329. See also *Chronic pain, rehabilitation for*.

Pain management *(Continued)*
  Commission on Accreditation of Rehabilitation Facilities criteria, 328
  for cancer patients, 208–209
  for diabetics, 232
Parkinsonian Foundation, services of, 351
Part-time skilled care, Medicare definition of, 334
Pathway, critical. See *Case management plan.*
Patient(s). See also individual patient group, e.g., *Geriatric patient(s).*
  abandonment of, 138
  abuse of, 137–138, 240
    reports of, agencies investigating, 137–138
  as employers of home help, 146
  assessment of, 30–35
  communication with, 14, 179–180
  empowerment of, 2, 182
  fraud and abuse of healthcare system by, 139–140
  incompetent, 240–241
  noncompliant, 125–126
  psychological aspects of, 180–182
  rights of, 135
  role in case planning, 11–12, 36, 37
  transportation of, 151–152
  with multiple diagnoses, 177
Patient care, standards of, 138–139
Patient demographics, for referrals, 28–29
Patient rights, 135
  defined, 371
Patient rights advocate, defined, 370–371
Patient Self-Determination Act, defined, 16
Patient/family instruction(s), discharge planning for, 114
  for AIDS patients, 203
  for burn patients, 294
  for cardiac patients, 288
  for chemotherapy, 213
  for diabetes, 233
  for end-stage renal disease, 218
  for neurologically impaired patients, 253
  for patients receiving intravenous antibiotics, 290
  for respiratory disease, 282
  for TPN patients, 295
  for transplant patients, 273
  for ventilator-dependent patients, 283–284
Payee services, defined, 371
Payor(s), alternate, 16–17
  vs. healthcare payor, 60
  healthcare, defined, 15
  types of, 14–15
PCMs (primary care managers), 86, 92
  defined, 372
Peer support, vs. professional counseling, for caregivers, 145
Per certification review, 129
Persistent vegetative state (PVS), sensory stimulation program for, 321

Personal hygiene, self-help devices for, 165
Pharmaceuticals. See *Drug(s).*
Pharmacies, mail order, 169
PHOs (physician hospital organizations), defined, 15
Physiatrist, defined, 372
Physical abuse, 137
Physical medicine and rehabilitation. See *Rehabilitation.*
Physical therapist, defined, 372
  for spinal cord injury, 261
  in home health agencies, 335
Physical therapy, 308
Physician, as data source, in clinical assessment, 34
  inaccessibility of, to case manager, 118–119
  role of, in case planning, 12
  unavailability of, 119
Physician hospital organizations (PHOs), defined, 15
Planned Parenthood, services of, 351
Planning, defined, 38
Point of service (POS) plan, defined, 15
  for military personnel, 87
Power of attorney, defined, 372
  durable, defined, 362
  vs. general, 136–137
Preferred provider organizations (PPOs), defined, 15
  for military personnel, 87
Pregnancy, resources for, 194
Pregnancy hotlines, services of, 351
Preliminary assessment, 29–30
  documentation of, 29–30
Preliminary screening, 29–30
Primary care managers (PCMs), 86, 92
  defined, 372
Primary care nurse, communication with, 14
Primary care physician, defined, 372
Prior authorization review, 129
Privacy Act, 134
  defined, 16, 373
Private conservator, 136
Private duty nurse, 337–338
  alternate funding for, 337–338
  approval for, 338
  costs of, 338
  Medicaid in-Home Waiver program, 337
  requirements for, 337
Professional(s), mental health care, 243
Professional counseling, for families of chronically ill/disabled children, 226
  vs. peer support, for caregivers, 145
Program for the Handicapped (PFTH), CHAMPUS and, 89, 92
Prospective review, 129
Prosthetic device(s), Food, Drug, and Cosmetic Act definition of, 156
  veterans benefits for, 84
Protection and advocacy services, 351–352
Protective services, defined, 373
Psychiatric hospitals, acute care, 245

Psychological impact, of cardiac disease, 286–287
  of catastrophic cases, 180–182
  of chronically ill/disabled children, 226–227
  of diabetes, 232–233
  of end-stage renal disease, 216
  of spinal cord injury, 262–263
Public conservator, 136
Public health clinics, defined, 373–374
Public Health Service, U.S., defined, 379
Public Law 94-142. See also *Education for All Handicapped Children Act; Individuals with Disabilities Education Act (IDEA).*
Pulmonary. See also *Lung(s).*
Pulmonary rehabilitation, 323–324
  admission criteria of, 323–324
  components of, 323
  goals of, 323
  team members in, 323–324
PVS (persistent vegetative state), sensory stimulation program for, 321

Quadriplegics, customized wheelchairs for, 166
  durable medical equipment and supplies for, 157

Ramps, 167
Rancho Los Amigos Cognitive Levels, 321
Rape crisis centers, services of, 352
Rate reductions, negotiations for, 51–52
  importance of, 51
  requirements for, 52
  steps in, 51–52
Reassessments, 41–42, 187
  frequency of, 41–42
  techniques of, 42
Recreational activities, 148
Recreational therapists, defined, 374
Recruitment, of hired home help, 146
Reduced rates, importance of, 51
  negotiations for, 51–52
  requirements for, 52
  steps in, 51–52
References, verification, of hired home help, 146–147
Referral(s), 3–4, *25*, 25–29
  appropriateness of, determination of, 27–28
  criteria for, 26–28
  demographics of, 28–29
  early, importance of, 28–29
  for Children's Medical Services program, 66
  for Individuals with Disabilities Education Act (IDEA), 76
  for State Agency for Developmental Disabilities, 105–106
  for State Department of Rehabilitation, 103

Referral(s) *(Continued)*
  for veterans benefits, 81-82
  forms for, 28
  negligent, 139
  of geriatric patients, 234-235
  sources of, *25*, 25-26
  timeliness of, 26
  to home health agencies, 334-335
Referral flags, for cardiac patients, 286
  for common high-risk catastrophic
    cases, 189, 190t-191t
  in utilization review, 131
  for mentally ill patients, 242-243
  for neurologically impaired patients,
    248-249
  for respiratory disease, 277
Regional centers, defined, 374
  services of, 352
Registered nurse (RN), defined, 374
Rehabilitation, 316-329
  goals of, 317
  in skilled nursing facilities, 329-333
  models of, 317
  of cardiac patients, 287, 324-326
  of chronic pain patients, 326-329
  of neurologically impaired patients,
    15-18, 249-250
  of pulmonary patients, 323-324
  phase(s) of, 317-319
    evaluation, 318
    identification, 317-318
    outpatient care and follow-up as,
      319
    treatment plan as, 318-319
Rehabilitation Act, defined, 16
Rehabilitation Commission. See *State
  Department of Rehabilitation.*
Rehabilitation facilities, 312
  defined, 374
Religious agencies, services of, 352
Religious beliefs, impact of, on
  patients, 31
Renal disease, end-stage. See *End-
  stage renal disease.*
Rental cars, for disabled, 152
Reports, 43-44
Research grants, 63, 192
Residential care facilities, defined, 374
Residential care homes, requirements
  for, 239
Residential treatment centers (RTCs),
  defined, 350
  for mental health patients, 246
Respiratory disease, 277-285
  alternate funding for, 280-281
  community resources for, 281
  diagnoses of, 277
  discharge/care access barriers for,
    282
  durable medical equipment and sup-
    plies for, 281
  laboratory tests for, 280
  patient/family instructions for, 282
  psychological impact of, 279-280
  radiologic studies for, 280
  respiratory team for, 277-278
  treatments for, 278-279
  ventilation in. See also *Ventilator-de-
    pendent patient(s).*
  ventilator weaning of, 279

Respiratory team, 277-278
Respiratory therapists, defined, 374
Respite care, 144-145, 352
  defined, 374
  for caregivers of chronically ill/
    disabled children, 219-220
  reimbursement for, 144-145
  unavailability of, 123
Restaurants, fast food, for disabled,
  152
Retarded Association, services of, 352
Retrospective review, 129
"Right of expectation," 41
RN (registered nurse), defined, 374
Ronald McDonald Houses, 221
RTCs. See *Residential treatment
  centers (RTCs).*
Rural areas, healthcare access from,
  problems with, 17-18
Ryan White Comprehensive AIDS
  Resources Emergency Act, 201
  defined, 16

Safety during on-site visits, 36
School bus services, for disabled, 150
Schools, state, defined, 377
SCI. See *Spinal cord injury (SCI).*
Screening, preliminary, 29-30
Second opinions, in utilization review,
  131
Self-care, teaching of, 182
Self-help device(s), 162, 164-166
  emergency response system as, 165
  for communication, 165
  for dressing and undressing, 164
  for eating and drinking, 164-165
  for household or food preparation
    tasks, 165
  for personal hygiene and grooming,
    165
  homemade, 166-167
  in bathroom, 165
  mobility, 165-166
Senior centers, services of, 352-353
Senior retirement home, defined, 375
Sensitivity, of case managers, 36
Sensory stimulation program, for
  persistent vegetative state, 321
Sexual abuse, 137
Sexuality, of spinal cord injured
  patient, 262-263
"Sheet burn," prevention of, 162
Sheltered workshops, defined, 375
  for acquired brain injury, 259
Sherman antitrust law, 137
Ships, for disabled, 152
Shriners hospitals, burn unit, 291
Sickle Cell Anemia Foundation,
  services of, 353
Skilled care, 330-332
  defined, 307, 332, 375
  documentation of, 309
  intermittent, Medicare definition of,
    334
  nursing in, 307
  occupational therapy in, 308
  part-time, Medicare definition of,
    334
  physical therapy in, 308

Skilled care *(Continued)*
  rehabilitation therapy in, 308
  speech therapy in, 308
  treatment modalities in, 308
  vs. custodial care, *306*, 306-310
Skilled nursing facilities (SNF), 312,
  314, 329-333
  barriers to placement in, 331-332
  costs of, 239, 330
  custodial care in, 331
  defined, 375
  family involvement in, 331
  for chronically ill/disabled children,
    223
  for neurologically impaired patients,
    252
  Medicaid and, 73
  Medicare eligibility for, 99, 329-330
  selection of, 331
  veterans benefits for, 83
Sliding scale, 63
Social Security Act, amendments to,
  defined, 15-16
  defined, 15
  Title XIX. See *Medicaid.*
  Title XVI. See *Supplemental Secu-
    rity Income (SSI).*
  Title XVIII. See *Medicare.*
Social Security Administration,
  defined, 375
  programs of, 93-104
Social Security Disability Insurance
  (SSDI), 63, 94-95
  defined, 375
  for neurologically impaired patients,
    251
Social Security Income, 95-96
Social worker(s), defined, 375-376
  in home health agencies, 335-336
Special education programs, defined,
  376
  financial resources for, 63, 73-81
Speech therapists, defined, 376
Speech therapy, 308
Spina Bifida Association of America,
  services of, 353
Spinal cord injury (SCI), 259-263
  complete or incomplete, 260
  discharge preparation for, 263
  durable medical equipment and sup-
    plies for, 261-262
  goals for, 260
  physical manifestations of, 263
  professional disciplines in, 260-261
  psychological impact of, 262-263
  rehabilitation for, 260
SSDI. See *Social Security Disability
  Insurance (SSDI).*
Standards of care, 138-139
  defined, 376
State Agency for Developmental
  Disabilities, 63, 104-108, 220
  appeals to, 108
  assessment by, 106
  "habilitation" plan and, 106
  payment and alternate funding and,
    108
  referrals for, 105-106
  responsible state agencies in, 105
  services of, 107-108

State Department of Aging, defined, 376
State Department of Alcohol and Drug Prevention, defined, 376
State Department of Health Services, defined, 376-377
State Department of Mental Health, defined, 377
State Department of Rehabilitation, 102-104
  assessment and testing by, 103-104
  defined, 377
  eligibility requirements of, 102-103
  goals of, 103
  referrals for, 103
  services, 104
State hospital(s), 315
  defined, 377
  for mental health patients, 246-247
State schools, defined, 377
State-County Department of Social Services, defined, 377
Stomach-intestine transplantation, complications of, 276
Subacute care facilities, 312, 332-333
  admission criteria for, 333
  costs of, 332-333
  defined, 377
  for brain-injured patients, 322
Substance abuse, chronic pain and, 326-327
Substance abuse programs, for mental health patients, 247
  services of, 355
  social security benefits for, 96
  veterans benefits for, 84
Sudden infant death services, 353
Suicide prevention services, 353
Supervised living facilities, for neurologically impaired patients, 259
Supplemental care, CHAMPUS and, 92
Supplemental Food Programs, for Women, Infants, and Children, 63
Supplemental Security Income (SSI), 63
  defined, 377
  for neurologically impaired patients, 251
Supplies. See also Durable medical equipment and supplies.
  homemade, 162-164
  medical, Food, Drug, and Cosmetic Act definition of, 156
Support groups, benefits of, 181
  for families of brain-injured patients, 322
  for families of chronically ill/ disabled children, 226
  for families of geriatric patients, 238
Supported work programs, for acquired brain injury, 259
Supportive care, examples of, 308-309
Swing beds, defined, 378

Teaching182-187. See also Family caregiver(s), instructions for.
  body system assessment for, 182-183

Teaching (Continued)
  checklist for, 183-184
  monitoring of, 226
  of caregivers, 144
  of case management skills, to patients and families, 185-186
  post-discharge need for, 186-187
  responsibility for, 184-185
  timing of, 182
  tools for, 185
  trial passes in, 185
Telephone reassurance services, defined, 378
"Telephone visitor" programs, 194
Terminal care. See also Hospice care.
  for AIDS patients, 204-205
  for children, 221
Terminology, 368-391
  CHAMPUS and, 91-93
  continuum of care, 342-354
Tertiary care centers, for cancer patients, 206
  local housing near, 221
Third-party liability cases, in neurologically impaired patients, 251
"Third-party liability" lien, 17
Title V Children's Medical Services. See Children's Medical Services.
Title XIX, Social Security Act. See Medicaid.
Title XVI, Social Security Act. See Supplemental Security Income (SSI).
Title XVIII, Social Security Act. See Medicare.
Toilets, disinfection of, 162
Total parenteral nutrition (TPN), 294-296
  alternate funding for, 295
  complications of, 296
  discharge criteria for, 294-295
  discharge services required for, 295
  discharge/care access barriers for, 296
  durable medical equipment and supplies for, 295
  patient/family instructions for, 295
TPL cases. See Third-party liability cases.
TPN. See Total parenteral nutrition (TPN).
Tracheostomy care kits, homemade, 163
Trains, for disabled, 152
Transitional care unit, defined, 378
"Transitional living rehabilitation," for brain-damaged patients, 257
Transplant patient(s), 264-277
  after care of, 265-266
  alternate funding for, 266-267
  case management involvement in, 264
  discharge criteria for, 274
  discharge services for, 275
  discharge/care access barriers of, 276-277
  durable medical equipment and supplies for, 276
  financial arrangements for, 269

Transplant patient(s) (Continued)
  healthcare providers for, 266
  laboratory testing for, 275-276
  national registries for, 265
  patient instruction for, 273
  psychological impact of, 267-268
  transplant center evaluation of, 264-265
  transportation for, 267
Transplant services, 351
Transplantation(s), complications of, 276
  denial of, 265
  experimental, 268-269
    consent form for, 269
    reimbursement for, 267
  indications for and contraindications to, 270-273
    bone marrow, 272-273
    heart, 270-271
    heart-lung, 271
    intestinal, 273
    kidney, 272
    kidney-pancreatic, 272
    liver, 271-272
    lung, 271
  types of, 264
Transportation, 149-152
  and adaptive driving programs, 149
  and restaurants, 152
  by airline, 150-151
  by bus, 149
  by modified vehicle, 149
  by rental car, 152
  by ship or cruiseline, 152
  by train, 152
  for chronically ill/disabled children, 221
  for handicapped, 361
  for transplant patients, 267
  medical, 151-152
Traumatic brain injury (TBI). See Acquired brain injury (ABI).
Trial passes, 185, 319
TRICARE, 86-93, 192-193
  authorization for, 87
  defined, 15
  demonstration changes, 89
  eligibility for, 87
  nonavailability statement, 88
  reimbursement and copayments, 88-89
  services of, 88
  through military treatment facilities, 88, 92
TRICARE EXTRA, 87, 93
TRICARE PRIME, 86-87, 93
TRICARE STANDARD, 87, 93

United Cerebral Palsy Association, services of, 353
United Network of Organ Sharing (UNOS), 265
Unskilled care, examples of, 308-309
Urinary catheter, care of, clean technique sterilization in, 163-164
Urine mineral deposits, dissolving with homemade solutions, 162-163

U.S. Department of Health and Human Services, defined, 379
U.S. Public Health Service, defined, 379
Utility companies, services of, 353
Utilization review, 128-131
 collaboration of, with case managers from other companies, 128-129
 concurrent, 129
 criteria of, 129-130
 levels of, 130
 overutilizaiton vs. underutilization, 129
 postpayment, 140
 prepayment, 140
 prospective, 129
 purpose of, 128
 referral flags in, 131
 retrospective, 129
 second opinions in, 131
 types of, 129
 vs. case management, 4-5, 128
Utilization review managers, communication with, 14

VA. See *Veterans Administration.*
Vehicles, modified, for disabled, 149-150
Ventilator(s), rental vs. purchase of, 279
 weaning from, 279
Ventilator-dependent patient(s), 282-285
 complications of, 284
 discharge criteria for, 282-283
 discharge services required for, 283
 discharge/care access barriers for, 285
 durable medical equipment and supplies for, 284-285
 patient/family instructions for, 283-284

Veracity, defined, 41
Verbal abuse, 137
Verification of eligibility, 29
Veterans, disabled, classification of, 82
 financial resources for, 63, 81-86
 organizations of, outside Veterans Administration, 85-86
Veterans Administration, 81
 defined, 379
 services of, 353-354
Veterans benefits, 63, 81-86
 denial of, appeals for, 85
 for alcohol and drug treatment, 84
 for blind, 84
 for dental care, 84
 for domiciliary care, 83
 for durable medical equipment and prosthetics, 84
 for medical care, for dependents or survivors, 85
 for medical center care, in VA facilities, 82
 outside VA facilities, 82-83
 for outpatient medical treatment, 83-84
 for skilled nursing or intermediate care facilities, 83
 overseas, 85
 referrals for, 81-82
Victim or Witness Program, 63-64
 defined, 379
 services of, 354
Visual aid centers, services of, 354
Visually impaired, community resources for, 194
 diabetics, community resources for, 231-232
 schools for, 78
 veterans benefits for, 84
Vocational rehabilitation services, 354
Vocational specialist, defined, 362
Vocational training, financial resources for, 76, 80, 102-104

Volunteer pilot organizations, 267

Waiver of benefits. See *Extra contractual process.*
Walkers, 166
Wards of court, defined, 379
Water, sterilization of, 162
Welfare Department, defined, 377
 services of, 347
Wheelchairs, 166
 costs of, 252-253, 262
 customized, for quadriplegics, 166
 electric, costs of, 262
 for spinal cord injury patients, 261
Wholesale price, of pharmaceuticals, 170, 368
WIC (Women, Infants, and Children), Supplemental Food Programs for, 63
Wickline case, 138
Wilford Hall demonstration, CHAMPUS and, 89-90, 93, 270
Witness program, defined, 379
 services of, 366
Women, Infants, and Children (WIC), Supplemental Food Programs for, 63
Workers' compensation, 64
 defined, 379-380
Wound care, 296-299
 alternate funding for, 298
 complications of, 298-299
 discharge criteria for, 296-297
 discharge services for, 297 required, 298
 discharge/care access barriers for, 299
 durable medical equipment and supplies for, 297-298

Managing the "Drugs" in Your Life

Managing the "Drugs" in Your Life

A PERSONAL AND FAMILY

GUIDE TO

THE RESPONSIBLE USE OF

DRUGS, ALCOHOL, MEDICINE

STEPHEN J. LEVY, Ph.D.

McGRAW-HILL BOOK COMPANY

New York   St. Louis   San Francisco   Auckland   Bogotá   Guatemala
Hamburg   Johannesburg   Lisbon   London   Madrid   Mexico
Montreal   New Delhi   Panama   Paris   San Juan   São Paulo
Singapore   Sydney   Tokyo   Toronto

2 3 4 5 6 7 8 9   DOCDOC   8 7 6 5 4 3

ISBN 0-07-037411-2

LIBRARY OF CONGRESS CATALOGING IN PUBLICATION DATA

Levy, Stephen J.
Managing the drugs in your life.
1. Drugs—Popular works.   2. Medication abuse.
3. Drug abuse.   I. Title.
RM301.15.L48   1983   613.8'3   82–24951
ISBN 0–07–037411–2

Book design by A. Christopher Simon

To my parents
DOROTHY AND MARVIN LEVY
*whose nurturing and love
taught me the fundamentals
of life*

To my loving wife JUDY
my daughter MERYL
and
my son DANNY
*who are teaching the advanced
course*

Contents

Introduction ix

1. Drugs and the Family 1

Early Experiences with Moderation 2
Dealing with Pain 8
Dealing with Pleasure 13
Privacy 20
Talking about Drugs 23
Setting Limits 26
About Alcohol 31
Defining a Drug Problem 37
How to Help Someone in Your Family Who Has a Drug
    Problem 42
Some Common Problems Faced by Families and How
    to Deal with Them 47

2. Drugs and School 58

The Extent of Drug Use 59
Drugs and Studying 74
Peer-Group Pressure 78
Cliques and Popularity 82
School-Based Prevention Programs 87
Some Realities about Dealing Drugs 94
Helping Kids to Help Themselves 99

3. Drugs and the Workplace 106

Rise and Shine 113
America's Nicotine Blues 123
Which Appetites Are We Feeding? 133

Drugs and Sports 140
Health Promotion in the Workplace 144

4. Drugs as Medicine 150

You and Your Doctor 151
Positive Practices Regarding the Use of Medications 158
The Pharmacist 183
The "Dated" Physician 187
Women Beware! 194
Warning: This Drug May Be Habit Forming! 203
Alternatives 211

5. Getting High 216

Don't Put It into Your System Unless You Know What It'll Do to You 217
Cocaine—The High Price of Getting High 224
Ludes 231
Heroin 233
Super Pot 236
Combining Drugs 238
Sex and Drugs 242
Etiquette 252
Drinking, Drugging, and Driving: A Prescription for Death 257
Dealing with Adverse Drug Reactions 261

Appendix A: SUMMARY OF DRUG INFORMATION 271
Appendix B: ADDITIONAL READINGS 290
Appendix C: WHERE TO GET HELP 295
Appendix D: THE MARIJUANA LAWS 298

NOTES 315
INDEX 319

Introduction

Ours is a drug-taking society.

- 1½ billion prescriptions were sold in 1973 in American drugstores.

- Americans spend more than $1 billion per year on tranquilizers (Valium has been the most frequently prescribed drug in this country since 1972).

- The pharmaceutical industry spends $1 billion a year on advertising (the liquor industry spends $100 million).

- $511 million from both public and private sources was used for funding drug-abuse treatment in 1977—some 260,000 drug-dependent people.

- Americans spend over $1 billion a year on over-the-counter (OTC) medications.

- The National Council on Alcoholism estimates that there are 13 million alcoholics and problem drinkers in our society, with an annual cost to business and industry in the neighborhood of $11 billion.

- Drunk drivers kill 25,000 men, women, children, and babies each year on American highways and injure 750,000 more.

- Over 15 million Americans have tried cocaine.

Americans do indeed have a love affair with chemicals.

In our attempts to understand this incredible phenomenon,

we have tried to define the problem in various ways. We speak of many dichotomies—licit versus illicit drugs, soft versus hard drugs, medicinal versus recreational drugs, mind versus body drugs, socially acceptable versus counterculture drugs—and invariably it all seems to fall into the ancient dichotomy "good versus bad." The use and abuse of all drugs is a very complicated affair with physical, mental, spiritual, economic, sociological, and anthropological elements. Polemics and rhetoric on all sides have only served to leave the lay public (and many professionals) in a state of confusion and what I call "rational paranoia" about most drug-related information. For example, concerning the great marijuana debate, Dr. Carlton Turner, President Reagan's White House Special Advisor on Drugs, graphically described this "opinion glut": "In six thousand papers I can support any conceivable idea you may come up with of what marijuana will do or what cannabinoids (61 of a total of roughly 360-odd chemicals in the plant) will do."

The sources of information, each one with its own set of biases, are often at odds with one another. Pressure is exerted on the individual by physicians, pharmacists, other health-care professionals, family members of all generations, friends and lovers (users and non-users), advertising campaigns by drug purveyors of every description, and the portrayal of drug use (with good and bad effects) in the entertainment industry. More and more people are being seduced by emotional appeals to join either the pro-use or the anti-use camp. Slogans range from "Better living through chemistry" to "Drugs are a cop-out." What is one to make of all these conflicting views? Jargonistic scientific reports, pseudoscientific claptrap, rigid and authoritarian pronouncements, all are presently competing not only for our hearts and minds, but for our pocketbooks as well!

This book is based on several premises which are designed to cut through the dense foliage of the drug jungle and clear a rational path to understanding:

1. Drugs have become an integral part of life in modern America.

2. Drugs are neither inherently good nor bad. All drugs have an abuse potential depending on who uses them and how.

3. We must assume full responsibility for what we put in our bodies, and conversely, we must not abdicate this responsibility to others.

4. A core of practical wisdom is already at hand to aid in making informed decisions about the drugs we use.

The main purpose of this book is to share with the reader some pragmatic concepts and caveats to guide you in taking on this personal decision-making process. Neither pro- nor anti-drugs, this book is *pro-health,* with a heavy emphasis on self-awareness, drug awareness, and self-control.

Health is defined here in a holistic context, that is, health as a positive state, not as the absence of illness. To the extent that drugs either enhance or diminish health, they deserve our serious and undivided attention. And in speaking about health, I place equal emphasis on physical, psychological, and spiritual components. Thus, the book is offered in the spirit of seizing control of our own lives and joining in a true partnership with professional experts and providers of health care. The late Dr. John Knowles, former director of Massachusetts General Hospital and Rockefeller University, in his thought-provoking volume *Doing Better and Feeling Worse—Health in the United States,* states:

> When all is said and done, let us not forget that he who hates sin, hates humanity. Life is meant to be enjoyed, and each one of us in the end is still able in our own country to steer his vessel to his own port

of desire. But the costs of individual irresponsibility in health have now become prohibitive. The choice is individual responsibility or social failure. Responsibility and duty must gain some degree of parity with right and freedom.[1]

This book is organized in terms of the various contexts and settings in which drugs of all kinds are used. The central theme, repeated in all chapters, is: *Drugs are not a drug issue—drugs are a people issue!* While specific information is supplied about a wide variety of prescription, OTC, pleasure, and other drugs (alcohol, nicotine, caffeine), the major emphasis is on the human context of drug taking. The book specifically avoids moralistic arguments, political rhetoric, and emotionalism. It is meant to be the eye of the hurricane. It will help you to understand how drugs are used and why; to test your own drug-taking behavior against some rational ideas concerning use and abuse; and will tell you how to handle difficulties without having to resort to outside help. It is not a book for addicts and alcoholics; many of those have already been written. It is a book for the lay person who is at neither extreme of either addiction or drug phobia. It is intended for the millions of Americans who every year cross back and forth over the shifting line between drug use and drug abuse and who need sound and reliable information to keep their lives in order. It is based on the principle that people are responsible for what they put into their bodies and that we are all in grave danger the moment we give up that responsibility.

Chapter 1 is about *drugs and the family* because this is where lifelong health attitudes and practices are first experienced. If parents wait for the fifth-grade science teacher to get to the drug curriculum it will be far too late. Families determine many patterns of behavior regarding drugs, and parents have the opportunity to teach moderation, to teach children how to deal with pleasure and pain, and to create a family setting in which free and open exchanges are possible. This chapter will help you and your children negotiate family rules about privacy, discuss drugs together, and set rational limits for drug-taking behavior. It will help you to define a drug problem, including alcoholism, and tells you how to help someone in your family who has such a problem. It discusses some common issues faced by families and suggests ways of dealing with them.

Chapter 2 deals with *drugs and school*. It will introduce you to the extent of student drug and alcohol use in America (it is quite high). The sometimes hazardous relationship between drugs and studying is examined, with suggestions for avoiding these hazards. It takes a close look at some tough issues like peer pressure, cliques, and popularity, and how drugs play a role in these matters. It contains a frank look at the risks involved in dealing drugs. It goes into some considerable detail about running a good school-based prevention program with suggestions for parental involvement as well as participation by students, teachers, and administrators. And it provides some direct guidelines for kids to help themselves and their friends who are having problems with drugs.

Chapter 3 is about *drugs and the workplace*. Drugs, including alcohol, are costing American business millions of dollars each year. In addition, we describe some of the less obvious but still dangerous kinds of drug use and abuse: nicotine, caffeine, smoking, and obesity. Many people fail to appreciate the profound impact these behaviors have on our health, our work mates, and our careers. Drugs and the world of sports is discussed. How companies can promote health in the workplace and the concept of employee assistance programs are described. You will be able to rate your own use of drugs and how they may be affecting you at work.

Chapter 4 deals with the subject of *drugs as medicine*. It helps you assess and appreciate your own role when it comes to dealing with the two people who should be your active partners, your doctor and your pharmacist. It contains specific advice about drug factors, patient factors, and physician factors—knowing what you are taking, why you are taking it, how to take it, dealing with side effects and adverse reactions, informing your doctor about all the drugs you are taking, drugs and pregnancy and breast feeding, storage and dating, contraindications, food and drink interactions with medications, limited activities, drug-to-drug interactions, stopping medications, drugs and your children, and drugs and older people. You will be warned about a phenomenon called the "dated" physician and shown why they are a problem for us all. There is a section entitled "Women Beware!" which speaks to sexism in drug-prescribing practices. The habit-forming nature of some medications is discussed, and alternatives to standard medical practices are suggested.

Chapter 5 is all about *getting high,* something that millions of Americans are doing every day. The high risks of adulterated and bogus drugs are described, and some advice is given on how to avoid these bummers. Cocaine is examined as the most seductive and expensive—in terms of dollars and risks—drug around. You will learn some of the serious cautions about methaqualone (ludes) and smoking and snorting heroin. Special emphasis is placed on the many hazards of various drug combinations, with particular attention to mixing drugs with alcohol. The seemingly mystical relationship between sex and drugs is examined and a list of drugs that enhance or diminish sexual functioning is included. Your awareness will be heightened regarding sane practices while partying with drugs so that you can have a good time without risking adverse reactions. You will be warned about the dangers of drinking, drugging, and driving, which can equal a prescription for death. And finally there is concrete advice about how to deal with adverse drug reactions when they do occur.

The appendices include an extensive table of commonly used drugs with their indications, contraindications, generic and brand names, street names, possible side effects and adverse reactions, psychological and physical dependence liability, and other information. There is a listing of sources of reliable drug information and literature, with information on finding treatment and self-help agencies across the country. There is also an annotated bibliography of supplemental readings. Lastly there is a listing of the marijuana laws for the fifty states.

By the time you finish this book you will be able to manage the drugs in your life. You will be able to more safely and intelligently integrate drugs into your personal health-care plan. You will develop a more mature and rewarding relationship with your doctor and pharmacist and a more assertive pro-health approach to pleasure drugs.

CHAPTER ONE

Drugs and the Family

The first three years of life form the foundation for all later development. Waiting until the fifth or sixth grade to educate children about the use and abuse of drugs can be disastrous. Parents must begin educating their children at the earliest possible moment.

Attention to the issue of youthful drug use has been overshadowed by a focus on peer-group pressure. Peer pressure *is* central to youthful experimentation with many things—sex, drugs, lawbreaking, outlandish dress styles—but we are neglecting, in a serious manner, attention to the earlier preteen years. Long before children feel the powerful influences of their friends, they are profoundly and indelibly affected by their immediate family. Young people enter their teens already influenced by parents, siblings, and other family members. It is difficult to bring about change later because patterns established in the earliest years of development persist throughout life and are resistant to change.

Family influences have been at work from birth, helping to shape and determine the young person's value orientations, knowledge and attitudes about drugs, feelings of self-worth, sense

1

of moderation, assertive behavior, ability to resist temptation, and body image. Parental emphasis on peer influence is often a cop-out and a smoke screen to hide our guilt and responsibility for our own drug-taking behaviors and the influence of these behaviors on our children.

Attitudes and beliefs about drugs start in the home, and they are effectively communicated to even the youngest member of the household. The family plays a vitally important role in early drug education, one which will help prevent or encourage problems with drugs later on in life.

EARLY EXPERIENCES WITH MODERATION

I took my family out to dinner at a local diner the other night. Seated two tables away from us was a family of four—all obese. My thirteen-year-old daughter was the first to notice them and pointed them out to the rest of us (my wife and ten-year-old son). I asked my kids what they thought of this sight, as the family proceeded to gorge on large desserts after an enormous spaghetti dinner. They were appalled by what they saw. My son said, "I'm glad you and Mom are normal and that we don't eat like that." I realized that by the example of our own physical appearance, the healthful manner in which my wife has fed our children since birth, and our own attitudes about overweight people, we had helped to teach our children about a very important concept—moderation. (Once in a while we will indulge in what the kids call "pigging out," but this is the exception.) As my wife and I discussed this incident in the diner we came to realize how, through a combination of "do as I do" and conscious attention to diet (and exercise), we had shaped our children's attitudes and behavior concerning moderation in food and drink.

The youngest children watch our behavior with fascination and bewilderment. They observe us at times when we are least aware of it. Like a child's version of *Candid Camera*, they will observe us as we grope around the kitchen until we have that first cup of coffee, they watch us light up a cigarette before we

2

eat or brush our teeth, they see us pour a drink before dinner, they see Dad drinking beer in front of the TV set, they watch Mom and her friends sip cocktails at the luncheon, and they watch (depending upon parental guidance and censorship) an endless stream of drug-taking behaviors on television. They experience our lives in a very immediate way, and as they are already deeply emotionally involved with us (parents and siblings), our behavior registers in important ways. Young children learn, in part, by mimicking behavior. They love to imitate us. They put on our clothes, put Daddy's pipe in their mouth, play with an older sister's pompoms, and the like.

Families are powerful social systems where beliefs, opinions, ideals, and attitudes toward inner and outer reality are forged. Families generate their own "myths" much as in Greek or Roman mythology. These myths are a composite of all the belief systems created and reinforced by the family unit. By the time children interact with peers, the myths are firmly established and are accepted without question. Part of the family myth is that what one's own family does is "normal." What other families do that may differ is "deviant." As children interact more and more with the world outside the family, they test the power of the family myths. When their beliefs are challenged, these kids tend to dig in their heels and defend the family honor with a vengeance. But they remember what they have heard and seen and bring it home to us. In an attempt to sort out their own emerging personal sense of "normalcy" and "deviance" they ask us about our eating, drinking, smoking, and drugging behaviors. And this is where primary prevention starts. If we attempt to slough off these questions with vague or evasive answers, then it will be too late by the time the children reach the fifth-grade science teacher's unit on drug-abuse prevention. We as parents can effectively doom the curriculum years before it is taught in school. Kids are very sensitive to hypocrisy and lying in adults, especially their own parents.

Families can support and teach the important concept of moderation. Even in families where alcohol is regularly consumed, problems of abuse need not arise. There are entire cultures that have long histories of relatively safe drinking. They share certain drinking practices:[1]

- Children are exposed to alcohol early in life, within a strong family or religious group.
- Parents present a consistent example of moderate drinking.
- The beverage, normally wine or beer, is viewed mainly as an accompaniment to food.
- Drinking is considered neither a virtue nor a sin and is not viewed as proof of adulthood or virility.
- Abstinence is socially acceptable; excessive drinking or drunkenness is not.
- Alcohol use is not the prime focus of an activity.
- These "ground rules" of drinking are widely agreed upon by all members of the group.

The point is simple: if we model excessive behavior for our children, then we can not reasonably expect them to practice moderation.

Let's examine another area of human behavior where immoderation and compulsive consumption styles can lead to problems in youth and adulthood.

Barbara's Story

At age sixteen my son entered psychotherapy at my urging. He was forty pounds overweight and never participated in sports and had very little to do with girls. He was always eating. I thought it was because he had such a lousy self-image and was lonely. One day he informed me that his therapist wanted to see me. As a concerned mother I went to the session expecting to be asked purely psychological questions. Almost all of the therapist's questions had to do with my son's earliest eating behavior. I learned I had done it all wrong. He was my firstborn and I was never sure what he wanted when he cried. I always thought he was hungry when he cried, so I gave him a bottle which he gladly accepted and drank. I also found

4

out that I had started him on solid foods too early. The food made him thirsty, so then I would give him another bottle. I never dreamed that I was causing a problem which would emerge later on. Chubby babies are so cute. The therapist explained to me that what I had done was to help my son to learn that all or at least many of his discomforts could somehow be alleviated by eating. After all, I didn't just give him food and drink. I held him and kissed him and talked to him while I fed him. So food became associated with love and comfort and gratification. My son is now trying to sort out better ways to meet needs that food can't. I really thought I was doing the right thing at the time.

Barbara learned, in the course of her own psychotherapy, that she had confused her own needs for love and nurturing with eating and then transferred them to her son. This single case can help us to understand that eating behavior, in our society, involves a complex set of social and personal development circumstances. The expression "you are what you eat" tells only part of the story.

Body Weight Standards*[2]

The usual fat content of the body as a percentage of body weight is as follows:

American men	age 25:	14%
	age 55:	26%
American women	age 24:	25%
	age 56:	38%

Male trained endurance athletes usually have less than 12% fat. Female athletes have less than 18%.

Men are considered to be obese if they have more than 25% fat, and women if more than 30% fat.

* These are objective standards. Standing nude in front of your mirror may convince you that you are "fat." If you feel or look fat, then you are fat.

5

Fat children are likely to become fat adults. Both heredity and environment play a role. The "fat cell hypothesis" suggests that there are critical periods in early life when fat cells are formed. If excessive numbers are formed in response to overfeeding, the theory states, they become a lifelong problem. One study has shown that most severely obese people have too many fat cells, while more moderately obese people have too much fat in a relatively normal number of fat cells. Most experts support the theory to the extent that they strongly advise against excessive feeding during early life, particularly the first two years.

While we are not certain of the genetic linkage regarding heredity and obesity, we are aware of the statistical relationships. Dr. Jean Mayer[3] reported in his study in the Boston area that 7 percent of children of thin parents (or at least parents who were not overweight) were too heavy. If one parent was overweight, the proportion jumped to 40 percent. If both parents were overweight, the proportion reached 80 percent. Adopted children do not show this correlation. Overall, about one in eight schoolchildren in America are obese, and 58 percent of them will become obese adults.

Despite the compelling genetic evidence, the influence of the home environment is quite important too, and evidence is mounting which shows that adopted children mimic the behaviors of obese adoptive parents. The fact is that only about 1.6 percent of obese people are that way because of an underlying condition such as problems with metabolism or endocrine function. The rest have learned eating patterns that have led them into obesity.

Our earliest life experiences with eating have a profound effect on later behavior. At birth a baby lives and loves with its mouth. The sucking response in infants is necessary to life (whether the mother employs breast or bottle feeding). How the mother and the father hold the baby during feeding is important. Both parent and baby must be relaxed for feeding to be a pleasurable experience. During the act of feeding a complex series of behaviors occur from which parent and child clearly derive benefits other than the simple transfer of nutrients. Tender words, warm physical contact, a reassuring presence; all of these contribute to emotional well-being and the experiencing of eating as enjoyable. According to Erik Erikson: "The oral stages, then, form in the infant the springs of the basic sense of trust and the basic sense of mistrust which remain the autogenic source of both primal hope and of doom throughout life."[4]

Listed below are some hints for getting your children to eat in a healthful manner.

- Set an example. Eat nutritious foods, avoid junk food, and eat reasonable amounts. Eat with your kids, especially breakfast.

- Know what your kids are eating both in the home and outside and how much they are consuming.

- Avoid sugar-laden products in the home. Check labels of cans and boxes. You'll be surprised how many food-stuffs have added sugar. You can't blame kids for eating such foods if you buy them.

- Substitute healthy snacks. Experiment with different items until you find the ones that your kids like and will eat.

- Educate your kids. Take them with you to the supermarket and let them experience comparison shopping both for pricing and nutrition content.

- Help your kids to acquire good eating health habits. Most food preferences are acquired. My kids didn't even know about sugar in cereals, added or processed, until they were much older. By then they had already developed a taste for unsweetened grain products. The same applies to salt (again read labels and model the appropriate behavior).

- Water, fruit juices and milk are good for you at any age. Soda is not something that is part of a nutritious diet. Especially if you want to avoid sugar and caffeine. Explain the importance of vitamins and minerals.

- Don't be afraid to set up rules and guidelines for family eating behavior. However, avoid rigidity because it invites cheating. You may even want to allow periodic "pig-outs" where everyone "cheats" within reasonable limits.

7

Compulsive immoderate eating has many parallels with compulsive immoderate use of drugs and directly threatens individual and family health.

DEALING WITH PAIN

Life is filled with pain, both physical and psychological, in so many forms: physical illness, mental illness, loss, separation, rejection, criticism, accidents, poverty, racism, sexism. The list is endless. Some pain is acute, that is, sudden and short-lived; some pain is chronic in nature, tending to persist over long periods of time. How we deal with pain is a central issue, as pain, like stress, is unavoidable. Our children look to us to shelter them from pain and to reduce or eliminate it when it occurs. One of the surest ways that life engenders both humility and frustration is in forcing us to realize that we can not ultimately protect our loved ones from pain. A whole new science of pain management is presently being developed, which includes such things as biofeedback, electrical and chemical brain stimulation, autogenic and relaxation training, and meditation. Freud was right in his notion that we are guided by a pleasure principle and seek to avoid pain.

One of the ways that people have sought to pursue pleasure and avoid pain is through the use of drugs, including prescription, over-the-counter (OTC), and so-called illicit or street drugs. A patient of mine who underwent radiation therapy for a cancerous condition described his experience:

> After each treatment I was subject to severe nausea and vomiting. It was so awful. I would vomit until my stomach was empty and then go into dry heaving. My psychologist suggested the use of THC [tetrahydrocannabinol] as an anti-nausea drug. In my case, the THC really helped reduce the nausea and vomiting. The THC had only one side effect—I got stoned!

The radiation treatment was necessary to prevent cancerous tissue growth. The THC (one of the active chemicals found in the marijuana plant and extracted in the laboratory) reduced the side effects associated with the treatments and induced a pleasurable altered state of consciousness. (There are still many states where THC can't be legally prescribed for this purpose. Patients are advised to discuss this treatment with their doctors, as THC doesn't appear to work in all cases.)

Here is another example of drug use to avoid pain:

> My life is one hassle after another. Constant demands from my job. More demands from my kids when I get home. Make dinner, supervise homework, mediate fights. And then my husband wants me to be loving and alluring after the kids go to bed. Thank goodness for my Valium. I don't know how I would get through the day without it.

This woman was suffering from the "superwoman" syndrome and was trying to be all things to all people. Rather than face the basic issues, she retreated into the daily use of a tranquilizer meant for episodes of acute anxiety and stress. While Valium was never intended to be a "maintenance" drug (taken daily), this woman was experiencing pain on a daily basis in the form of anxiety and tension. Therapy consisted of facing the superwoman trip and renegotiating family roles with her husband and kids. Goodbye Valium, hello family support!

And a final example from a very unhappy patient:

> DR. L.: How long have you been experiencing the mood swings you just described?
>
> PATIENT: All through my adolescence and most of my adult life. I'm now thirty-seven.
>
> DR. L.: What kind of treatment have you received before coming to me?
>
> PATIENT: Ten years of group and individual psychotherapy! All to no avail!
>
> DR. L.: How has it been since you started taking lithium [carbonate] prescribed by Dr. Z. [a psychiatrist]?
>
> PATIENT: Well, once you and Dr. Z. helped me to see that I was suffering from manic-depression, I have been

taking my lithium faithfully for three months. I can't tell you how much better I feel. The mood swings are less volatile and my life at home is much happier.

This patient, suffering from a major psychological disorder, manic-depression (or bipolar illness), experienced no relief from his psychic pain by means of talk therapy alone. Without the lithium therapy he was doomed to suffer from an illness which is not under conscious control.

Pain is a symptom which alerts us to the fact that something is not right with ourselves or our world or both. Sometimes the source of the pain is internal and sometimes it is brought about by an external agent. When we take drugs to alleviate pain we often create a psychic state which further prevents us from taking our own inventory to determine the source of the pain. Not knowing or otherwise avoiding the source, the best one can hope for is symptomatic relief—and this can be achieved only by repeating the use of the drug. People facing interpersonal difficulties are the best example of this vicious cycle. Failure to identify and cope with the source of our difficulties can lead to a dilemma: an unresolved problem *and* a drug problem. For example, while many people enjoy using drugs and alcohol for recreational purposes, there are those folks who can't function around other people *without* drugs. The issue is not the drugs so much as the inability to socialize. Here are some "trigger" questions to help you determine how you deal with pain:

- When I hurt, do I feel that I have to tough it out (machismo or machisma) and suffer in silence?
- When I hurt, do I live with the fear of what might be causing the pain or do I check it out with others (family, friends, professionals)?
- Do I consider it unmanly or unwomanly to cry?
- Do I worry about my image and pretend all is well?
- When I hurt, do I bottle it up until I feel like exploding (or actually explode)?

- Do I tend to minimize my pain? maximize (exaggerate) it?
- Do I run to the medicine cabinet?
- Do I use alcohol to alleviate my pain?
- Do I believe that drugs are magic and will make everything okay?
- Do I make an honest appraisal of my situation and try to figure out what is causing my pain?
- Do I believe that I deserve my pain?
- When I know the source of my pain, do I deal with it directly?
- Do I accept pain as a part of life?

One of those aspects of personality which is central to an understanding of how we deal with physical or psychic pain is the disparity between our true self and our image. We all develop an "image" which we use in a conscious manner to impress other people. In our more honest private thoughts we sense a truer self, free of the constraints of our image, a sort of personal bottom line. This is our irreducible essential self. The fears, ambitions, jealousies, strengths, and weaknesses reside here. Sometimes the distinctions between the image and the true self become blurred. The greater the disparity between the true self and the image, the less likely we are to handle pain well and to turn to "artificial" means such as drugs to cope with pain.

Here is a simple exercise you can do to see how aware you are of these distinctions. Take a sheet of paper and draw a line down the middle. Label the left-hand side "my image" and the right-hand side "my true self." Several categories are suggested in the example. These headings are neither good nor bad, just different. List all the traits, attributes, or behaviors that rightfully belong in each column.

Once you have completed the list, you can decide what value to place on the two listings. People who use a lot of drugs have a tendency to live in the world of images more than in the world

Category	My Image	My True Self
friends	I am close to people.	I have trouble trusting.
	I enjoy people.	I'm basically a loner.
sex	I can take it or leave it.	I enjoy sex a lot.
	I'm a real lover.	Women (men) scare me.
feelings	Nothing bothers me.	I'm easily hurt.
	I'm very sensitive.	I use tears to manipulate people.
money	I'm doing real well.	I'm insecure about money.
	Money is unimportant.	Money matters a lot.
power	I'm in charge around here.	Who's really running things?
	I'm not afraid of anyone!	Pushy people scare me.

of the true self. Most relationships are image-to-image. Real friendship and love relationships bring us more into a "core-to-core" orientation. One of the reasons you use drugs may be either a sense of discomfort with your true self or too many image-to-image relationships, which leave one feeling empty. Only you can know for sure. The more you live within your image and the more discrepant the image from the true self, then the more you will fail to handle pain in satisfying ways. Self-honesty is the best route to dealing with pain and discomfort. You are freer to be honest with others when you can break through your image. Sharing pain is one of the best ways to break through.

Within the family context we adults model ways of dealing with pain for our children. If they see us seeking chemical shortcuts instead of squarely facing issues and going through the difficult task of resolving them we have given them a poor example of facing up to reality. From a holistic point of view, when a family member is in pain (of any origin), he or she is suffering on a physical, emotional, and spiritual plane. These planes of experience cannot be separated. There is an emotional component to all physical illness, and physical upsets affect us emotionally. The spiritual area may involve a sense of God or an existential

12

reality or simply our own sense of mortality. We are rapidly learning how loneliness, for example, contributes to the aging process. When you are in pain you need to be healed. Families that can share pain, share feelings, and reach out to their members can heal pain. Families that alter painful reality with drugs alone end up with a dual problem—the original problem plus a drug problem. After a while the two become indistinguishable and pain becomes chronic. Chronic pain requires chronic drug usage! If, as parents, you model the "macho" approach, then don't be surprised when your kids don't share their pain and troubles with you. They are simply feeding back your own behavior. If you pop pills or booze to deal with your problems, don't be surprised when your kids mimic this. You have taught them that this is how your family deals with pain. And when taking prescribed medications to alleviate pain and suffering, take them as prescribed, don't change doses on your own, report side effects to your doctor, and be alert to the effects of combining several drugs. For more on this issue, turn to Chapter 4.

DEALING WITH PLEASURE

> We may put the question whether a main purpose is discernible in the operation of the mental apparatus; and our first approach to an answer is that this purpose is directed to the attainment of pleasure. It seems that our entire psychical activity is bent upon procuring pleasure and avoiding pain, that it is automatically regulated by the pleasure principle.[5]

Very few people would disagree with Sigmund Freud's notion that we seek to avoid pain, but how to pursue pleasure has always been the source of bitter debate. From the hashish-smoking Sufis of ancient Arabia to the pot-smoking hippies of the 1960s; from the drunken revelries of Roman bacchanals to the fraternity and sorority beer blasts of modern times, people have sought out pleasure in the form of drugs of every conceivable description. It is true that there are societies in which certain chemical pleasures are forbidden: alcohol to the Muslims and Mormons, grass and cocaine to the devotees of the "moral majority." How your family defines pleasure and permits or forbids its pursuit will have a profound impact on family attitudes and behaviors regarding drugs. If you were to ask each member of your family to make a list of positive and negative human emotions, you would quickly discover that the negative list is almost twice as long as the positive list. Life is filled with enough pain for us to have developed a vocabulary that reflects this aspect of what we commonly call reality. The pleasure principle is counterbalanced by what Freud called the reality principle. The reality principle also seeks pleasure—but it is a delayed and diminished pleasure, tempered by the harsh facts of life. Chemicals allow us break through delay and pain and can take us to the heights of pleasure, ecstasy, and corporal delights. Disputes about pursuing pleasure via drugs cut deeply into personal belief systems, and often battle lines are drawn along generational lines. Listen to one family attempting a discussion in this volatile area.

SON (AGE 17): When I get high [on grass] I explore parts of my mind and soul that I can't reach any other way. It's like I go more deeply into myself and find both joyous and frightening things. I love being touched when I'm high, and conversations with other people become easy.

FATHER: Someone your age has no business using drugs. When I was your age I was already out working. There was no time for such foolishness. You had better explore your mind by concentrating on serious matters like school.

MOTHER: You should be able to enjoy life without drugs. You don't see me using drugs or alcohol to have a good time. You're just looking for kicks. All you kids today have it too easy.

SON: You don't understand! I take care of my schoolwork and my part-time job. I'm looking to go beyond these simple facts of my daily existence. I'm searching for a higher consciousness—something greater than myself.

MOTHER: You can find that in church!

SON: God is within me as well as without. There are many ways to seek Him and grass does that for me.

FATHER: You spend too damn much time trying to feel good. Who said that life is full of good times? You will have to work hard just like my father and I.

Embedded in this conversation are some bedrock beliefs held by the parents which mitigate against their own pleasure seeking and are projected onto their son. Their statements are heavily value-laden and reflect a rigidity that prevents them from hearing their son. Perhaps the son will have it easier than the parents, working less and playing more. His parents seem threatened by this and, worse, seem embittered in a way that closes off understanding and communication.

Part of the problem is simply that what pleases one person is not necessarily pleasurable to another. One person's pleasure may be another person's idea of pain. But the fact remains that drugs make people feel good or at least ease the way to good feelings. As adults we may seek to deny our children access to certain physical and psychic pleasures, but we can be sure that their friends will tell them about it. Kids are into pleasure and have not yet made bargains with life which call for delay of gratification.

Church and state have sought to govern and regulate the pursuit of pleasure throughout recorded history. Lay and religious laws and precepts have been laid down to control and suppress certain forms of pleasure, most notably alcohol and drugs. In many instances puritanical beliefs have allowed laws to be passed that defy reason and scientific credibility. Harry Anslinger waged a one-man antimarijuana campaign that led to the creation of such laughable products as the film *Reefer Madness,* which depicts the "killer weed" as the source of unbridled sex and violence. No one doubted his sincerity, but his exploitation of the issue may have contributed to pot smoking more than it diminished it.

Among their recommendations, the editors of *Consumer Reports* in their book *Licit and Illicit Drugs* list the cessation of

15

scare tactics and the proper classifying of drugs; moderating two counterproductive aspects of Harry Anslinger's approach. Marijuana to this day is listed by the federal government in the same category (called Schedule I) as heroin and morphine (both narcotics).

In 1970 key federal legislation, Public Law 91–513, the Comprehensive Drug Abuse Prevention and Control Act, was enacted into law. The first major change in the federal law since the Harrison Narcotic Act of 1914, it is more commonly referred to as the Controlled Substances Act of 1970. Various drugs are listed in five categories, called schedules, primarily according to medical usage and abuse potential; the most dangerous in Schedule I, the least in Schedule V.[6]

Schedule I

A. The drug or other substance has a high potential for abuse.

B. The drug or other substance has no currently accepted medical use in treatment in the United States.

C. There is a lack of accepted safety for use of the drug or other substance under medical supervision.

Includes heroin, hallucinogens such as mescaline, LSD, psilocybin, and marijuana. Use is forbidden except for highly restricted research purposes.

Schedule II

A. The drug or other substance has a high potential for abuse.

B. The drug or other substance has a currently accepted medical use in treatment in the United States or a currently accepted medical use with severe restrictions.

C. Abuse of the drug or other substance may lead to severe psychological or physical dependence.

Includes opiates and synthetic opiates such as morphine, methadone, and Demerol, certain barbiturates of the short-acting type, methaqualone, cocaine, and amphetamines. In this schedule, production quotas may be set, import-export quotas are imposed, and telephone and refillable prescriptions are prohibited.

Schedule III

A. The drug or other substance has a potential for abuse less than the drugs or other substances in Schedules I and II.

B. The drug or other substance has a currently accepted medical use in treatment in the United States.

C. Abuse of the drug or other substance may lead to moderate or low physical dependence or high psychological dependence.

Includes Doriden and Noludar 300, barbiturates, and paregoric. No production quotas, looser regulations, and no prescription restrictions except prohibition of refills after six months.

Schedule IV

A. The drug or other substance has a low potential for abuse relative to the drugs or other substances in Schedule III.

B. The drug or other substance has a currently accepted medical use in treatment in the United States.

C. Abuse of the drug or other substance may lead to limited physical dependence or psychological dependence relative to the drugs or other substances in Schedule III.

Schedule V

A. The drug or other substance has a low potential for abuse relative to the drugs or other substances in Schedule IV.

B. The drug or other substance has a currently accepted medical use in treatment in the United States.

C. Abuse of the drug or other substance may lead to limited physical dependence or psychological dependence relative to the drugs or other substances listed in Schedule IV.

Schedules IV and V differ little from Schedule III and from each other. Schedule IV includes long-acting barbiturates such as phenobarbital, Placidyl, and chloral hydrate, and minor tranquilizers meprobamate, Librium, and Valium (manufacturers contested the inclusion of the latter two). Schedule V includes cough medicines with codeine with certain age restrictions.

There are many controversies surrounding what schedule a particular drug or class of drugs is included in. For example, some of the tranquilizers included in Schedule IV have shown themselves far more dangerous in terms of addiction and withdrawal than marijuana, which is listed in Schedule I and has no known physical addiction or established withdrawal syndrome.

While you may agree that laws are needed to control dangerous substances and their distribution, we should all understand that what really is at stake is the legislation of morality. All drug laws exist because powerful members of our society have been able to influence the legislative process to enable government to regulate the pursuit of pleasure. Judging from the fate of Prohibition and the extent of the drug traffic in America today, we are not doing too well in this area. This has prompted some to call for dispensing with all laws prohibiting drug use. The National Organization for the Reform of Marijuana Laws (NORML) is working toward the removal of prohibitions against marijuana. (For a listing of existing marijuana laws on a state-by-state basis, see Appendix D.) The editors of *Consumer Reports* and the former Drug Abuse Council (sponsored by the Ford Foundation) have been among those groups calling for a more rational re-examination of drug laws. At the other end of the spectrum are groups like the Texans War on Drugs, the American Council on Marijuana, and the National Federation of Parents for Drug-Free Youth. These groups seek harsher drug penalities,

18

the establishment of antiparaphernalia laws, and ultimately the cessation of all illicit drug use. Antiparaphernalia laws are probably sitting on constitutional quicksand, because their definitions of drug-using materials tend to be vague. No matter what side you take in these issues, you can be sure that the law of supply and demand will overshadow all else. Ancient and modern history has shown repeatedly that when people want drugs they find ways to get them, and the supply may ebb and flow but it never stops. We have yet to articulate a rational national policy on drugs. The legal one—alcohol—is the leading drug of abuse, even though regulated by the government. The illegal ones are controlled by organized crime. Why we sanction some intoxicants and not others does not seem to be founded on scientific facts. Rather it is the issue of legislating pleasure that is at the heart of this whole controversy. Alcohol influences consciousness as surely as marijuana and cocaine do, and yet we do not think of alcohol as a drug. We have a long way to go in sorting out these issues.

In the meantime, here are some "trigger" questions to help you and your family determine how you conceive of and deal with pleasure.

- Do I consider the pursuit of altered states of consciousness a legitimate pastime in seeking pleasure?
- Do I consider it okay to pursue these altered states with drugs?
- Do I use chemicals to make me feel good? Can I do this without guilt feelings?
- Are words like ecstasy, delight, sweetness, orgasmic, and pleasure-seeking part of my personal vocabulary?
- Is the pursuit of pleasure for its own sake okay with me?
- Am I open to exploring new means of seeking pleasure?
- Do I explore new horizons of pleasure in areas like sex?
- Do I look down on people who seek pleasure in ways that differ from my own?

- Do shame and guilt prevent me from enjoying my life? In what areas?
- Do I have good reasons for allowing or disallowing the people I love to experience pleasure?
- Do I allow myself to feel good?
- Do I feel I always have to be "in control"?
- Do I believe that I deserve to feel pleasure?
- Do I have good reasons for delaying gratification?
- Do I project my own values onto other people, or am I open to what they say and do?

Once you have taken a hard look at how you handle both pain and pleasure, you will be ready to consider other areas such as privacy and limit-setting with less of a risk of hypocrisy or confusion.

PRIVACY

Privacy is one of those terms that everyone thinks they understand until someone's privacy is invaded. Then, in that moment of heat and anger, the parties realize that they may have very different conceptions of just what privacy really is. If you think that all members of your family share a clear agreement about issues of privacy, try this simple test. Tonight, around the dinner table, ask each person to define the term. You go last. Have someone act as recording secretary and write down everyone's definitions and notions. Don't be shocked if there is some real divergence of opinion. By raising the question, you have set the stage for one of the most important issues your family may ever have to face. How does this relate to drug usage? Consider the following aspects of privacy in situations involving drugs.

Controlling access to spaces: "John and I were smoking a joint in my room. My father came in without knocking. I caught hell for smoking dope, but I was furious because he doesn't even respect me enough to knock. I have no rights in my own room."

Controlling access to information: "At dinner last night my parents grilled me for a half-hour about who among my friends is drinking and using drugs. What a drag. I know they are concerned about me, but what my friends do is none of their business."

Being alone: "My wife went off to her usual card party on Thursday night. I finally had a chance to try that piece of hashish that Terry gave me. Well, about three hits into a great head my wife came home early. She did not feel well. She doesn't dig drugs. There went a great high."

Personal property: "I believe that my room and the stuff in it is my personal property and that I have a right to my privacy. Whether it's ludes or condoms, I don't want my mother going through my things. I don't want to have to be paranoid in my own space."

The message about drugs and privacy is that all four of these dimensions have one important and powerful element in common: social control. Whoever controls these various aspects of privacy controls the family unit and its goings and comings. All parents attempt to control their children, and as the children get older, they in turn try to exercise some control over their own lives and the lives of the adults around them. With older children, this attempt to control has a double edge. The parents call the shots; they set down the rules and set limits for the children. The children, on the other hand, can either comply or circumvent the rules.

Privacy can be found in all cultures and societies. There is even major evidence of "privacy" behavior among many species of animals. The need to exercise the freedom of privacy is vitally important to all Americans. As a society we have many concerns about the invasion of privacy by, among other people or groups, the press, the government (federal, state, local), the school system, computers, the clergy, law-enforcement agents, the banks, the credit card companies, and the Internal Revenue Service. We jealously guard our privacy but we rarely define it, negotiate it, and discuss it within the family unit. It usually comes down from parents by direct or indirect fiat. There is one phrase that children abhor hearing their parents speak: "Who ever told you that you could ———!" If you often find yourself saying that, on any variety of topic, it is a strong clue that limits have not been clearly established.

There are parents who, in the name of love and concern, come down very hard on the issue of privacy. They honestly believe that by exercising tight control they can prevent their children from getting into "trouble." Here trouble is defined as doing anything the parents don't like. This works up to a point. If the kids find you inflexible and rigid, they will scheme to get around you. The more you attempt to deny them their privacy, the more their behavior will become secretive; they will "go underground," drugs in tow. The trouble with denying people privacy is that they can turn around and do the very same thing to you. How? you might ask. Let's say you control space and information. You can't keep your kids under constant surveillance no matter how much you "bother them." They can cut off much of their communication to you. Then everyone begins living in separate and narrow corridors within your home. But there are some things you can do, together with all members of your family, to work out this very sensitive issue.

How to Set a Framework for Privacy Within the Family

- Let everyone know that this important topic is going to be discussed. Get a consensus for a time and place free of intrusions. Be prepared to spend more than one session at it before everything is worked out.
- Everyone is going to enter into the discussion with preconceived notions. The first ground rule is that nothing will be decided until everyone has had a chance to be heard and some discussion has taken place.
- A good starting point is to have everyone define "privacy." The next step can be to have each person state his or

22

her concerns about the presence or absence of privacy for them in the household.

- Be sure to cover all four primary areas in the discussion:
  1. controlling access to space
  2. controlling access to information
  3. being alone
  4. personal property
- Once you reach the point where decisions are being made and rules established, write them down, reproduce them, and distribute them to all members. This "contract" on privacy is open to amendments and changes. However, another meeting should be convened before the rules are changed.
- Everyone should be prepared to state his or her rationale for suggested rules. Statements like "because I say so" don't help anyone. Yes, parents may have the ultimate say, but it should not be for arbitrary and capricious reasons.
- While it is not necessary to spell out what will happen each and every time the privacy contract is violated, there should be some notion about redress of grievances. This might start with another family conference. Remember, one member's behavior can have an impact on all other members.

The secret to having this work out well is the willingness of the adults to really involve the kids. Then it's up to everyone to deal with the issue in good faith. No magic here, just something that seems to have disappeared in many families: mutual communication and respect.

TALKING ABOUT DRUGS

In some ways this whole drug thing is like the weather. Everybody talks about it but no one can do anything about it. That's because most of us get lost in sociological generalities, have strong

23

emotional biases, and don't bother to check out the facts. We feel compelled to come down strongly on one side of the issue or the other and to join a camp that has already articulated its position: *Drugs Are a Cop-Out! Better Living Through Chemistry! If You Need a Drink to Be Social, That's Not Social Drinking! Turn On, Tune In, Drop Out! Why Do You Think They Call It Dope? Feed Your Head! Take It Easy! Reefer Madness!* Generalizations and oversimplifications. The whole issue of drug use is complicated and multifaceted, yet users and nonusers alike feel compelled to make extreme statements. People write off each other's views for reasons like "you can't trust anyone over 30," "they don't get high," "he works for a drug treatment program," "he's a cop," and so on. Amidst all the rhetoric and emotionalism, when the National Institute on Drug Abuse announced a few years ago that the U.S. government was cooperating with the Mexican government in spraying Mexican marijuana fields with a deadly herbicide called paraquat, pot smokers began checking their ounces for black burn holes (caused by the paraquat). And with good reason, because paraquat-adulterated marijuana can cause serious pulmonary problems. Between the government's high visibility, public-relations–minded attempts at modifying consumption, and unscrupulous dealers selling the poisoned grass, the consumer is caught.

The most important thing about education (in public schools, private schools, churches and synagogues, camp, the home) is the development of a "learning attitude," an attitude of openness to new information from all sources, a willingness to hear what others are saying, the courage to examine unpopular views, to look at the minority view, and to make up your own mind.

Hints for Parents on Talking About Drugs With Your Children

1. You don't need to be a drug expert to hold a discussion with your kids, only a concerned parent. However, it is a good idea for you to get your drug facts straight (check out resources at the back of the book). Your kids may be able to share informational resources as well.

2. Be honest about your own drug use. Remember, caffeine, nicotine, and alcohol are all powerful drugs. This is an area where many families get into deep trouble. Kids are very sensitive to hypocrisy.

3. All drug experiences teach us something about ourselves. Listen to your kids before reacting.

4. When laying down rules of expected behavior (i.e., no "hard" drug use—no pills, no opiates, no speed), be clear and up front. Don't be wishy-washy and don't make threats you are not prepared to follow through on.

5. Know before you get into this discussion just how much of your own private life you wish to reveal.

6. If you don't want your kids to use certain drugs until they reach a particular age due to differences in physical and emotional maturity, state your case.

7. Don't grill your kids about their friends. You should ask what the local youth drug scene is like, but don't play grand inquisitor when it comes to your children's friends. They will tell you what they think it is important for you to know (usually what they are anxious about).

8. Don't fall into the trap of thinking that all is well if your kids are just drinking. Alcohol in its many forms is just as dangerous as any other drug. Drinking doesn't mean they are not using drugs. Lots of kids do both (so do adults).

9. Try to avoid stereotypes. For example, by conservative estimate, two-thirds of the high-school class of 1981 had tried at least one illicit drug in the year—but that doesn't mean *your* kid did.

10. Recognize that part of being young and growing up is being curious about many things including drugs, pleasure seeking, establishing an identity, copying other kids, rebellion against authority, and the like.

11. The fact is that all you can really do is share your feelings and concerns, state some ground rules and sanc-

tions, and then stand back. You can guide, but you can't really control.

12. Let your kids know that if they have a problem with drugs, any problem, you want them to come to you for help.

13. Remember that drugs are used in a context, and the context can be as important as the drugs themselves.

Since two-way communication is the goal, here are some traps to avoid.

Don't:

    lecture and preach
    forget to listen
    interrupt a lot
    be condescending
    be arbitrary and capricious
    mistake passion for reason
    yell a lot
    exaggerate or lie
    be hypocritical
    insult their intelligence
    refuse to have future discussions on the subject

Good luck!

SETTING LIMITS

Life is full of "shoulds," "oughts," and "have-tos." Children learn them from parents, siblings, friends, teachers, religious leaders, and other authority figures. It starts out with "Thou shalt not" and often ends up with "You'll do it if you know what's good for you!" But here in the United States we value and cherish individual freedom of choice. True, there are some groups, religious fundamentalists foremost among them, who would restrict

26

these freedoms and have us all live our lives according to their narrow interpretation of "right living." The vast majority of Americans, however, will defend to the death their right to individual freedom. Parents reserve the right to raise their children as they see fit, and as long as they don't violate the law, they can exercise this right to govern the lives of their offspring.

Juxtaposed to this parental guidance is a necessary and important fact of life: the only love relationship that must, by definition, lead to separation is the love between parent and child. All other love relationships bring people closer together. Your children, in order to grow into their own maturity, must begin moving further and further away from your parental supervision and influence, until one day they make the physical break with home. We accept this as the natural order of things.

But somehow when it comes to the subject of drug use, our love and concern become tinged with fear and ignorance. We imagine the worst, seeing pushers lurking in schoolyards ready to force drugs upon our children. (The fact is that most kids get their drugs from their friends.) We try to protect our kids by any means possible. We lecture, threaten, cajole, promise, beg, plead, intimidate, and all manner of authoritarian hell tends to break loose. Just about all kids (starting in fifth or sixth grade) will be exposed to the youth drug culture, and most will sample the wares at least once. If primary prevention means never trying a drug, then we as a nation have failed miserably in this regard. I think we must place our emphasis on secondary prevention. That is, accepting that most kids will try drugs, we must help them to not risk toxic or lethal drug effects. This process starts with an honest appraisal of the whole issue of setting limits. Let us begin by stating a maxim: *Parental authority is never absolute!*

You may choose to go to the ends of the earth to see that your children obey you, but when it comes to the assertion of their emerging individuality, "never say never." They will find ways to evade you. Any kid can beat any parent at this game! The harsher and more persistent your exercise of authority, the cleverer and more devious their efforts to thwart you. Once it gets this far, both parent and child are in a lot of trouble anyway. One of my adolescent patients says:

> My parents are very strict. They really laid down the law about drugs, sex, friends, you name it. I am afraid of them. Every time I tried to talk to them about how hard it is being different from my friends, they would rant and rave and threaten me. I started keeping vodka in one of the beakers in my chemistry set in my room. Vodka has no real odor and I figured the best place to hide it was in plain sight. They never caught on. I felt bad about sneaking, but it serves them right for never listening or trying to understand.

It may not be terribly clear to many kids and even to some parents why any limits concerning drugs are necessary. Explore how each member of your family feels about the reasons listed below and you will get a better sense of what the limits need to be in your family.

Why Kids Need Limits Around Drug Use

1. Many drugs are illegal, and so is underage drinking. Getting arrested and/or having parents called down to the station house is a real bummer for everyone concerned. No one needs an arrest record following him or her throughout life.
2. Peer pressure is very hard to resist. By laying down limits you help your kids to stay "in bounds." When friends pressure them to drink or drug, they can say things like "If my parents see me with red eyes [or funny-smelling breath, or slurred speech], I am going to be grounded." They may still have to deal with being called "chicken," but no real friend would lay that trip on them.
3. The use of drugs is fraught with danger, and I don't mean just addiction. Lots of adults and kids get into

28

trouble (bad trips, drunkenness, fights, accidents, etc.) in a single episode of intoxification. Limits help reduce the dangers.

4. Drinking, drugging, and driving don't mix, and parents are wise to be most assertive on this issue.

5. Limit setting is part of loving when you are a parent. No limits is as bad as too many limits.

6. Many drugs are adulterated or misrepresented (ersatz speed that is really caffeine, ludes that are really Valium, grass laced with PCP or paraquat), and even your best friend can't tell you if he or she doesn't know about it.

7. Parental limits will help your kids to develop internalized limits (which may be exactly the same or may differ). They need a starting point, which is your job as a parent. Their developing experience and maturity will take over from there.

A Rational Guide to Limit Setting Between Parents and Children

Do:	**Don't:**
Set a time and place for what will probably be a lengthy discussion.	Treat this issue lightly.
State the limits clearly and in objective terms.	Be vague.
Make sure the kids are direct parties to the setting of these limits. Put some faith in them.	Forget that kids resent arbitrary authority and will cooperate more readily if they "own" part of the process.
Give yourself and your kids a sense of trust in their ability to deal with these issues.	Predict doom or expect perfect compliance all of the time.

Do:	Don't:
Realize that the purpose of limits is to guide, not to control.	Think your authority is absolute. You won't be there when they try drugs.
State your fears and concerns as parents and take a position on the issues.	Fail to set some limits. Kids need them, and none is as bad as too many.
Try to get a sense of how kids and parents in your community are dealing with the drug issue.	Worry about keeping up with the Joneses. Set limits that meet your family's needs.
Make any sanction clear.	Say one thing and do another.
Be prepared to change the limits based on actual performance; be flexible.	Set them down in concrete.
Realize that if your kids are in trouble, they need your help.	Give up your authority to any outside agency (police, other parents, etc.).
Advise your kids to say nothing without advice of counsel if they are arrested.	Seek to punish before you know the facts. Believe your kids.
Set reasonable limits based on drug facts.	Lump all drugs together (and remember that alcohol is a drug).

There are kids in some families who will violate limits continuously and otherwise fail to respond to parental authority or standards of reasonable behavior. It is important for all children to learn that their behavior has consequences. When kids rebel and repeated efforts, including professional intervention, prove fruitless, then a more radical approach may be called for. One method for dealing with these most difficult situations is a program called Toughlove. Developed by David and Phyllis York, Toughlove's logo is a heart with a clenched fist, and the program draws a tough line indeed. Problem teens are told to "shape up or ship out," meaning to conform to acceptable standards or literally leave home. That is the tough part about Toughlove: a parent must be prepared to say to the youngster, "You have to choose between living in our family as a decent human being or leaving." Kids are not thrown out on the street; they are given the option of staying with friends, relatives, or other Toughlove parents. An important part of the program is the support given to parents by other parents in the Toughlove network. Before presenting your child with this hard decision, make sure you have tried all other avenues and sought professional counseling and advice. For information on Toughlove, see Appendix C.

ABOUT ALCOHOL

I can't tell you how many times over the years I have heard parents say "Thank God my kid only drinks and doesn't do drugs." *Alcohol is a drug!* It is the most popular social drug in America and it is also the most abused (the National Council on Alcoholism estimates that there are 10–13 million adult alcoholics and problem drinkers in the United States). Alcohol is a sedative, or depressant, drug with many properties and actions similar to the barbiturates (which are also sedatives). One of the worst addictions is a combination of pills and booze since the effects are superadditive. One study showed that, used with alcohol, a nearly 50 percent lower dose of barbiturates was lethal than when the drug was used alone. Alcohol has no nutritional value but loads of "empty" calories.

In case you still don't want to think of alcohol as a drug, let me make a comparison between alcohol (Ethanol or ethyl alcohol) and a substance everyone agrees is a drug—heroin. There is no evidence of any long-term damage to the human body from years and years of heroin use. Oh, of course, you can get hepatitis from dirty needles, die from an overdose of the drug, or get shot trying to steal a television set (heroin addiction is a nasty

31

lifestyle). But the heroin itself does not hurt the body. It is metabolized and completely broken down. Now, what happens when you drink a fair amount of booze (comparable to a daily heroin habit) on a regular basis? Well, you see, ethanol can invade any cell in the human body and cause short- and long-term damage to any organ system. You can go from a fatty liver to alcoholic hepatitis to cirrhosis (where liver cells atrophy and die), or you can go from short-term memory loss (blackouts) all the way to Korsakoff's disease (alcohol amnestic disorder). And that's just the medical side. The psychological and emotional problems associated with alcoholism and alcohol abuse are equally awesome.

People develop a tolerance for alcohol. Scientifically, this occurs because of the brain's adaptation to increasing levels of alcohol. Behaviorally, what it means is that over time it takes more of the drug to get the original effect. People who become physiologically addicted to alcohol experience withdrawal when their supply is suddenly cut off or drastically reduced (the same is true for heroin). This withdrawal reaction is typified by elevated temperature, pulse, and heart rate, plus sweating, nausea, disorientation, and fear. The "d.t.'s"—delirium tremens—are the same as withdrawal, only much more exaggerated. Both conditions need to be treated in a hospital setting. *Alcohol is a drug—a powerful sedative drug which must be treated with respect!*

Here is one sad story that makes the point very clearly:

> We enjoyed an open and honest relationship with our son Michael. He came to us when he was seventeen and said that a lot of the kids were getting into drugs and that he was frightened by this. We suggested that perhaps if he were to limit his own behavior to just alcohol he could deal with the peer pressure. Michael thought this was a good idea and even told us that it worked quite well. He just told his friends he preferred to drink while they smoked marijuana or took other drugs. Around graduation time the kids were partying a lot. Michael asked if he could use the family car to take his date and several other kids to the prom. We happily said yes. After all, he had shown

us that he was a sensible and trustworthy person. The night of the prom, at around two A.M., we received a call from the police. Michael and the other kids were involved in a car accident. One child was dead and the others injured seriously. Miraculously Michael received only minor injuries. When we arrived at the emergency room the police informed us that Michael was being arrested for drunk driving. He had drunk the equivalent of a pint of vodka and a half a bottle of champagne. Celebration turned into tragedy. Six years later he still wakes up screaming in the middle of the night and blames himself for what happened. And we thought we had given him some good advice when we said it was okay to drink. How could we have been so blind? Alcohol is just as dangerous as any other drug!

Here are answers to some frequently asked questions about alcohol that may aid you in discussing this subject within your family.

Q: Alcoholics are those bums on skid row. Why should my family worry about it?
A: Only about 5 percent of the estimated 10–13 million alcoholics and problem drinkers in America can be found on skid row. The rest are people just like you and me.
Q: I heard there are no Jewish alcoholics.
A: This is an excellent example of a powerful but false stereotype. The recent work by the Task Force on Alcoholism and Drug Abuse in the Jewish Community of the Commission on Synagogue Relations of the Federation of Jewish Philanthropies of New York has shown this to be untrue. When Drs. Sheila Blume and Dee Dropkin conducted their study of one hundred Jewish alcoholics, they found one A.A. group in New York City that had forty Jewish members. And that was just 1 out of 1300 meetings held in the greater metropolitan area each week. No one is sure about the actual numbers, but alcoholism occurs among Jews, and the time for denial is over. There are many Jewish people in Pills Anonymous (P.A.) as well.

Q: I heard that alcoholism runs in families. Is that true?

A: Many professionals believe that what we call alcoholism is a disease for which there is no known cause or cure. There is some interesting and compelling evidence that leads us to believe that there may be a genetic component, but there is no real definitive proof. Statistically, we know that if one parent is alcoholic, the offspring have a one-in-four chance of developing alcoholism. If both parents are alcoholic, the odds increase to one chance in two. However, there are alcoholics with no family history of the disease.

Q: What happens if you give some coffee to someone who has had too much to drink at a party?

A: The best you can hope for is a wide-awake drunk! It takes the body 1 to 1½ hours to metabolize one drink (12 ounces of beer, 5 ounces of wine, 1½ ounces of whiskey, one highball or cocktail) to the point where there is no accumulation of alcohol in the blood. The caffeine in the coffee will act as a stimulant but cannot counteract the depressant aspects of the alcohol. Cold showers and walks in the night air don't help either. Only the passage of time—as I said, about 1 to 1½ hours *per drink*—can do the trick.

Q: How much alcohol is too much?

A: An alcoholic is someone whose drinking causes a continuing problem in any department of his or her life. For the chronic disease, the key word in the definition is "continuing." For any single episode of drinking, a person is in trouble when his behavior causes a problem for himself or the people around him. This definition doesn't get hung up with how much, how often, or what form the alcohol comes in. All that matters is that when you drink things go wrong. The most important question you can ask someone for whom you have a concern is, "Has anyone ever spoken to you about your drinking?" A positive answer may indicate a drinking problem, and the matter should be pursued further.

Q: Is it true that it's okay for kids to drink beer or wine? Isn't it the hard stuff that causes problems?

A: Alcohol is alcohol, no matter what form it comes in. Beverages differ in their alcohol content: beer and ale contain 3 to 6 percent, wine contains 12 to 14 percent, and hard liquor contains 40 to 50 percent (80 to 100 proof). Problems are caused by drinking too much alcohol no matter how it is packaged. There are alcoholic beverage products that are marketed to look like anything but alcohol (usually containing a lot of sugar). This is an attempt to capture the youth market. All states have laws that prohibit the sale of any alcoholic beverage to those under a certain age. These laws exist because the use of a powerful drug like alcohol needs to be controlled. The official judgment is that kids under the legal age are not mature enough to handle it.

Q: How does someone know when there is a real problem with alcohol in their life?

A: Here are some questions that can help in making a self-assessment (you can substitute the term "drug" for "drink" to test yourself regarding other drugs):

1. Do you usually drink heavily after a disappointment, a quarrel, or when the boss gives you a hard time?
2. When you have trouble or feel under pressure, do you always drink more heavily than usual?
3. Has a family member or close friend ever talked to you about your drinking behavior?
4. Have you noticed that you are able to handle more liquor than you did when you were first drinking?
5. When drinking with other people, do you try to have a few extra drinks when others will not know it?
6. Are there certain occasions when you feel uncomfortable if alcohol is not available?
7. Have you recently noticed that when you begin drinking you are in more of a hurry to get the first drink than you used to be?
8. Do you sometimes feel a little (or very) guilty about your drinking?
9. Did you ever wake up on the "morning after" and dis-

cover that you could not remember part of the evening before, even though your friends tell you that you did not "pass out"?

10. When you are sober do you often regret things you have done or said while drinking?

11. Are you secretly irritated when your family or friends discuss your drinking?

12. Have you tried switching brands or following different plans for controlling your drinking?

13. Do you often find that you wish to continue drinking after your friends say they have had enough?

14. Have you often failed to keep the promises you have made to yourself about controlling or cutting down on your drinking?

15. Do you lose time from work due to drinking?

16. Do you often have trouble performing sexually after drinking?

17. Have you ever tried to control your drinking by making a change in jobs or moving to a new location?

18. Do you try to avoid family or close friends when you are drinking?

19. Do you eat very little or irregularly when you are drinking?

20. Do you sometimes have "the shakes" in the morning and find it helps to have a little drink?

21. Do you get terribly frightened after you have been drinking heavily?

22. Have you recently noticed that you cannot drink as much as you used to?

23. Do you sometimes stay drunk for several days at a time?

24. Sometimes after periods of drinking, do you see or hear things that aren't there?

25. Have you ever been in a hospital or institution because of drinking?

If you answered "yes" to between one and three of these questions, you should carefully consider whether or not you have a drinking problem. If there were four to seven "yes" answers, you should consult an alcoholism expert and discuss the negative role alcohol is playing in your life and what to do about it. Eight or more "yes" answers indicate that you are in serious trouble and should seek treatment services immediately.

DEFINING A DRUG PROBLEM

One of the difficulties in defining a "drug problem" is that it depends on who's doing the defining. Perceptions differ radically within the same family unit, in much the same way as in the tale of the four blind men examining an elephant—each one declares the part he touches to be the definitive beast. Here are some terms defining levels of drug involvement to help us get started.

Experimentation: The first experience or two with a given drug.

Drug use: Periodic or regular use of a drug. No ill effects to self or loved ones.

Drug abuse: Any frequency of usage which leads to ill effects to self or loved ones.

Drug addiction: Compulsion, negative life consequences, and loss of control define addictive process. Physical and psychological dependence are consequences of chronic drug usage. Physical addiction component defined by establishment of tolerance and appearance of withdrawal symptoms upon cutback or stopping. Preoccupation with drugs as a way of life.

The difficulty arises out of one's effort to further define "ill effect." We tend to be very egocentric about these matters. For example, the answer to "How do you know when you're doing too much drugs or alcohol?" is often "When you're doing more than I do!" "Which drugs tend to cause problems?" "The ones I don't use!" One person's "problem" or "ill effect" is not readily agreed upon by others. I believe that the core of this issue is the denial and other ego defenses that people use to twist and distort what is going on. Here are some examples of how these defenses work:

Denial: "I do not have a drug problem." (But others think you do.)

Rationalization: "Everyone else is doing it. Why shouldn't I?" (Because you can't handle it.)

Compartmentalization: "I know I have blackouts, but I can handle my booze." (Person denies connection between events.)

Projection: "I don't need to use drugs all the time. You do." (Person attributes unacceptable behavior in him- or herself to others.)

Displacement: "It's okay for my husband to smoke pot, but I'll kill my kids if they do it." (Fear of husband causes target to be shifted.)

Sublimation: "Who needs those girls anyway? I'd rather go drinking with my friends." (Sexual motive is denied and replaced by socially acceptable alternative behavior.)

Intellectualization: "I only smoke filtered cigarettes, Mother, so there's nothing to worry about." (Denies feelings in oneself and others, very similar to rationalization.)

Since many of these defenses involve unconscious motives and feelings, do not expect people to see the light just because you bring it to their attention. Remember, they are defenses against disturbing information or insights.

Another important aspect of defining a drug problem is to realize that some problems are acute, that is, have a rapid onset and short duration; while others are chronic, usually building up over time and then persisting over time. Both can be either mild or severe. A person who has been through a "bad trip" on a hallucinogenic drug like marijuana or LSD can tell us a lot about the horrors of an acute drug reaction. A child who suffers from the lifelong effects (chronic) of brain damage caused by sniffing airplane glue has a problem of a very different kind. Some negative effects wear off as soon as the drug is completely metabolized (broken down chemically by the body), while others persist because of the damage done while we were using the drug. A person with a hangover pays some dues for the previous night's drinking, but a man who loses his arm in an industrial accident because his judgment was impaired by alcohol pays dues the rest of his life. Some drugs persist in the body for several days, like the THC in marijuana, while others are more short-lived, like alcohol. (By the way, although the THC remains in the body, the "high" lasts only a few hours at best.) What's interesting about drug storage in the body is the effect it may have when you use the same drug again. Science has a lot more to learn about this aspect of drug use.

Another important distinction must be made between a problem or problems preceding the use of drugs and those ca ·d by the use of drugs. While it is certainly true that most people who use drugs do so to party, there are those who use them for other reasons. (Here I am not referring to the proper medical use of drugs.) Many different drugs have the ability to take us away from ourselves and our physical and emotional upheavals. They transport us, temporarily, to less painful states. The business executive hooked on Valium, the teenage pothead, the hidden-alcoholic housewife, the street junkie, the luded-out party freaks are all trying to flee problems in their lives through the use of drugs. In these cases there are pre-existing problems of loneliness, impotence, damaged egos, rejected loves, poor body image, family upheavals, anxiety, depression, and so on. They all have some-thing else in common: using drugs is not the answer to these problems.

The two human conditions most frequently encountered in drug-abusing and addicted populations are depression and anxiety. For these people, drugs provide a stopgap. At best it is only a temporary haven, for when the drugs wear off, the problems are still there. For many, they now have two problems—the original one and the added drug problem. Drugs are only vehicles or means for traveling. They are not an end in themselves.

Parents often ask me to list for them those special things to look for so they will know when their kids are using drugs. I always give two responses to these inquiries: (1) ask the kids directly, and (2) almost all the symptoms that drugs can cause can be brought about by other situations and events. For example, some people tell parents to look for sudden changes in the kid's behavior, such as the quiet kid who becomes outgoing or the outgoing kid who suddenly becomes withdrawn. Drug use? It could just as easily be a hundred other things besides drugs (mood swings are common in adolescence). Another example: the kid starts spending more time in his or her room. Drug use? Try privacy, homework, phone calls to friends. If your child smells like a six-pack, staggers, has blazing red eyes or slurred speech— these are more likely to be signs of actual drug use. I've heard people say that you should look for needle marks. Well, if things have gone that far then you have been missing a hell of a lot about your kid besides drug use. Do you think that anyone knows your child and his or her behavior patterns better than you? Of course not! Don't look to the "experts" to do your job for you. Talk to your kids; ask them; tell them of your concerns for them. You should have been doing this all along. And not just when you think they are playing around with drugs. You should query your kids about anything in their behavior that confuses or upsets you. Drug problems are *people problems* and should be dealt with as such. Only people can fill that void— not drugs.

A person with a drug problem is someone whose use of drugs (including alcohol) causes either an acute or a chronic difficulty for himself or for the people who care about him. Determining that a problem exists is just the beginning. You may still have a problem in dealing with the defensive posture of the drug user. The main point here is that you should be prepared to confront

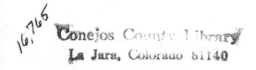

the person directly and honestly with an account of how their drug-taking behavior is affecting you. Also be prepared to state your concerns about what drugs may be doing to them. Stay open to the possibility that the "problem" may be yours and that the two of you may never really agree about the fine distinctions between drug "use" and drug "abuse."

If you want to know how drugs figure in your own life, stop taking them for some significant period of time, like a month or two. (Do *not* stop taking prescription medications without the advice of your physician.) If you are concerned about the effects of stopping nonprescription drugs, check with a knowledgeable professional. See how you do without the drug during this drug holiday. Here are some things to look for:

- Do you miss the drug?
- Are you experiencing any withdrawal effects? (If they get heavy, check with your doctor.)
- Does life seem less full without the drug?
- Are you suddenly aware of problem areas in your life that you had been ignoring?
- Are you having less fun without the drug (in bed, at parties, etc.)?
- Are you feeling tense or anxious?
- Are you feeling depressed?
- Do you feel better without the drug?
- Do you have problems concentrating or meeting goals and deadlines?
- Do you find that you spend a lot of time thinking about the drug?
- Did you put aside a stash just in case you missed it too much?

If your responses to these questions during your drug holiday have caused you some concern, then you should turn back to the section on alcohol and answer the twenty-five questions listed there. Getting more nervous about the drugs in your life? Perhaps the time has come to ask whether you can deal with this issue on your own. If you can't return to the drug with a clear conscience regarding your own health and well-being, then you may have a drug problem. If the conflict is so great that you find the decision weighing heavily in your life, something may be out of balance. Drugs can be used in many ways. Once they become the centerpiece of your existence, there is no doubt that something more vital may be missing from your life. Friends, a good self-image, a decent job—something is missing. You can throw all the drugs you want into that void—it will never be filled. You are probably looking for the right thing (love, respect, belonging, success) but in the wrong place.

HOW TO HELP SOMEONE IN YOUR FAMILY WHO HAS A DRUG PROBLEM

Rule #1: Don't deny the problem. You are in a unique and intimate position to see what is going on with your family member. Avoiding the issue is the worst thing you can do. Very often you can see clearly what the drinking or drugging is doing to the other person, but can you see what it is doing to you? The longer you join in the denial, the worse the problem can become. You are not responsible for the other person's drug use, nor are you responsible for their abstinence. You *are* responsible for your own feelings and reactions. Responsibility can be defined literally as the "ability to respond." Let yourself and the drugging person know that you are affected by their behavior.

Rule #2: Check out how this drug problem is affecting the entire family. Here is a story that makes the point: I once had a staff member who at the age of eleven was sitting on the front stoop of her house with four of her friends on a snowy November day. In the distance the girls could see a man staggering down the street and occasionally falling into the snowbanks. They all found this to be an amusing sight. When the man got closer to where they were sitting, the girls recognized him as the father of my staff member. They picked him up and helped him into the house. He reeked of alcohol. This was the last time she ever had her friends over to her home. The stigma of an alcoholic father led her into isolation and made the family home a taboo place to bring friends. *Everyone* in the family is involved to a greater or lesser extent when someone has a drug problem. The problem is felt in such ways as use of time, space, money, role distribution, arguments, attempts to protect younger members of the family, privacy, power, allocation of family resources and the like. Not sure how the problem is affecting you? Attend a meeting of a self-help group like Alanon or Alateen or Pillanon to hear how people just like yourself have been and are being affected by a drug abuser in the family. It will be an eye-opening experience.

Rule #3: Helping the family to cope is as important as helping the person with the drug problem. I have seen entire families destroyed by one member's serious drug problem. This does not have to be the case. You should hold a family conference without the drug abuser present. Let everyone acknowledge, each in their own way, how the problem is affecting them and how they feel about it. After the initial shock and denial, it is common for feelings of anger and resentment to come to the surface. You will all need each other, and children, including young children, should not be left out. There is more at stake than whether or not the abuser will be able to recover. Younger members of the family will be watching, for example, to see how the parents cope and how they respond to their needs. You must not neglect the rest of the family by pouring all of the family's resources into the abuser.

Rule #4: Realize that feelings are running high and try to come up with a rational plan of action. One approach to the issue which has been helpful in dealing with denial is the process of objective confrontation. At the family conference mentioned above, you can plan to confront the abuser. The rules are: (1) stay calm—emotional exchanges only lead to more defensiveness;

(2) present objective evidence of the abusive behavior (episodes of intoxification, failure to carry out roles, evidence of accidents, broken promises, etc.); (3) ask the abuser to listen patiently and not to defend his or her actions at this time; (4) state how this problem is affecting each of you as a family member; (5) state your willingness to support the abuser; (6) state the limits of this support; and (7) be prepared to offer resources. If you find that this kind of forum cannot be accomplished in your own home, then you can seek the help of an outside professional to guide your family through this process.

Rule #5: Labeling doesn't help. You want the abuser to get to an expert who can help him or her figure out what the problem is. Since denial and the other ego defense mechanisms mentioned earlier are so powerful, you cannot reasonably expect the abuser to buy what you are saying just because you say it (or even present objective evidence). You don't have to label the abuser an alcoholic or an addict (or a head, or a junkie). But you should state your concern and strongly suggest that the individual seek professional advice to sort out the nature of their actual problem. If they refuse, then you have some additional presumptive evidence for the extent of the problem.

Rule #6: Spell out the limits of how far the family is willing to go in supporting the abuser. Make sure the sanctions are clear. I refer you back to the section on limit setting. If the suggestions made there do not work out, then you need to seek outside help to accomplish this. There are growing numbers of family support groups that you can turn to (Alanon, Alateen, Pillanon, Toughlove, to mention a few). Check with local government or private programs to secure referrals of this type. A family has a right not to permit the behavior of one individual to ruin the quality of life for all its members. It really helps to get the support of your own peers to accomplish this difficult task.

Rule #7: You should carefully consider who the actual patient is. It may be the drug abuser or it may be the entire family. One

44

member's drug abuse may be symptomatic of underlying problems within the family as a whole. On the other hand, the abusive behavior may be independent (in the main) of the family dynamics. The best way to tell is to seek out the services of a mental-health professional (psychologist, psychiatrist, clinical social worker) whom you know to be well versed in the area of families and substance abuse. Let this person aid you in forming a plan of action that takes three things into consideration: (1) the needs of the abuser, (2) the needs of the family, and (3) the possibility that the abuser is unwilling to seek treatment. Remember, people use drugs for a reason, and sometimes the reasons reside within the family structure. Whether this is the case or not, the abuser will need family support in his or her recovery, and the family must decide how they wish to accomplish this. Sometimes, in their need to punish the abuser, family members, parents in particular, refuse to consider family-oriented treatment. This is a shame because it means the prognosis will be poor, particularly for young people who must remain at home until they are old enough to leave.

Rule #8: People with drug problems have broken lots of promises. The best way to help is to deal with actual behavior. Action does speak louder than words. Whatever approach is chosen, the acid test (no pun intended) is how everyone actually lives up to their end of the bargain. Progress should be determined by objective criteria (homework done, treatment sessions attended, abstinence accomplished, curfews kept). Other family members will tend to distrust the abuser. The best way to overcome this is for the abuser to win back their trust through realizable goals and actions.

Rule #9: Don't get hung up with your family's image. Helping the abuser and your family are far more important than any stigma and embarrassment you may feel. Once you realize you have a drug problem in the family, you must understand that what is happening to your family is not unique. This problem is occurring all over America. It happens in the best of families

45

and in the worst of families. It is happening to all kinds of folks in a very democratic fashion. Anyone is eligible—the rich and the poor; blacks, whites, Hispanics, Native Americans; educated and uneducated; men and women (boys and girls); families with histories of drug problems and families where there has never been a problem. Use your energies for resolving the problem at hand, not worrying about what your neighbors think. Everyone gossips anyway, so why worry? Your priority is your family. If the stigma is really getting to you, seek out people with similar problems (through self-help groups and drug treatment programs). You will be amazed how many "peers" you have. You need to know you are not alone. And you need to know that these things do happen to "people like us." The harder a family tries to cover up a drug problem, the more exposed they become anyway. Your family, friends, and neighbors are getting hipper all the time. So don't waste valuable energy and time trying to look good by denying the situation. Look good by having the courage to face the problem squarely.

Rule #10: Nothing can be accomplished if the abuser continues to abuse drugs. Drug counseling is the first order of business. When a patient comes to see me (youth or adult) with a drug problem, I consider it my responsibility to marshal resources to help this person stop abusing drugs. Drug abusers do not have the luxury of waiting for the doctor to figure out the answers to the "why?" questions. They could end up dead while the therapist tries to sort out their id, ego, and superego problems. Simply stated, the first order of business is to stop or reduce the drug taking. After this is accomplished, then more insight-oriented types of therapy can be brought to bear. Choose a therapist who has experience with your family member's type of drug problem. Ask lots of questions—it's a right, not a privilege. You don't need arrogant doctors during a drug crisis. Most people can stop abusing drugs without understanding all the reasons why they began or continued to use them. But the treatment must be geared toward this approach. If the prospective therapist or agency thinks months of therapy are needed to understand and deal with the drug problem before drug taking stops, go to another agency or practitioner. The folks in Alcoholics Anonymous (A.A.) have said it best: "First Things First."

SOME COMMON PROBLEMS FACED BY FAMILIES AND HOW TO DEAL WITH THEM

The Great Marijuana Debate

This issue tends to be very divisive. Within families it usually breaks down along generational lines. A lot of things have been attributed to marijuana that scientific research doesn't support. The most objective statement that can be made is that marijuana is not an innocuous drug. Most people use it without ill effect. A few people have a severe negative reaction called a marijuana psychosis, which is a toxic reaction similar to an allergy. Certainly for this minority the drug is anything but innocuous. There are studies that show damage to fertilized mice ova, changes in the brain cells of rhesus monkeys, and a number of similar reactions in a variety of animals. The fact is that no one yet knows the long-term effects of occasional and heavy marijuana use in humans. There is some evidence that there are even more carcinogens (cancer-causing agents) in marijuana smoke than in that of conventional cigarettes.

The definite answers are not yet in, and pro- and antimarijuana forces quote those studies which best support their bias. A 1982 report on marijuana and health released by the National Academy of Sciences states:

Our major conclusion is that what little we know for certain about the effects of marijuana on human health—and all that we have reason to suspect—justifies serious national attention.

In 1982 the American Medical Association and the U.S. Surgeon General warned users of grass that it is not a harmless diversion free of harmful effects. Basing its position on twenty years of

47

published scientific research, the Public Health Service has concluded that marijuana has "a broad range of psychological and biological effects, many of which are dangerous and harmful to health." The harmful effects or suspected effects include:

- Impaired short-term memory and slow learning
- Impaired lung function similar to that found in cigarette smokers
- Decreased sperm count and sperm motility
- Interference with ovulation and prenatal development
- Impaired immune response
- Possible effects on heart function
- By-products of marijuana remaining in the body for several weeks with unknown consequences. The storage of these by-products increases the possibilities for chronic effects as well as residual effects on performance even after the drug has worn off.

It is best to keep in mind that, as I've emphasized before, all drugs have an abuse potential and if mismanaged can cause ill effects. While some drugs carry an outright danger in any amount of use, others may require repeated use before harmful effects are noted. For example, you are far more likely to get sick to your stomach from your first snort of heroin than to experience any ill effects from your first joint of marijuana.

So you see the scientists can't give us definitive enough evidence about grass to tilt the scales in either direction. That means we have to look at it from other perspectives. One of the ills reported to be associated with marijuana use in the young is something psychiatrists have named the "amotivational syndrome." According to this theory, marijuana use causes lethargy and listlessness—the young people neglect their studies, withdraw socially, and lose all ambition. Antimarijuana groups are fond of quoting this one. However, it must be remembered that adolescent drug abuse is a complicated and multidimensional problem. For every kid who may show the signs of this so-called syndrome, there are many thousands who give no evidence of it whatsoever. A teenager who loses all ambition and ceases his studies is indeed going through some kind of crisis. However, rather than the crisis being caused by smoking grass, it is far more likely that it is causing the drug use and the kid is "self-medicating" with grass, which can act as a mild antidepressant. He is using this otherwise recreational drug the same way a psychiatrist would prescribe some antidepressive medication: to counteract feelings of sadness or loss. Again, the problem is not the grass he smokes as much as the situation, internally and externally, that has led him to seek this chemical release. Most kids I've worked with or treated who use grass this way have other nonchemical pressures weighing heavily upon their lives. Once I have helped them to clearly identify the root problems and to face them, the drug abuse diminishes and the school performance (or other educational or vocational choice) improves. The social withdrawal always stems from poor self-image and some actual social rejection. It isn't easy for many of the young to break into the tight cliques that form during the middle and high-school years.

I was on a panel recently where the usual assortment of liberal and conservative viewpoints were being expressed by my co-panelists. When a kid in the audience asked about the apparent hypocrisy surrounding adult use of alcohol versus teenage use of marijuana, one of the speakers said, "Every time you light up a joint the purpose is to get high, while an adult taking a drink has no intention of getting high." He fell right into the trap that the questioner had laid for him. Both marijuana and alcohol are mood-changing drugs. How high you get does depend, in part, on how much of the drug you consume. But it's hypocritical to state that one is taken to alter one's mood while the other is not. Caffeine and nicotine cause changes in mood as well. Ever run out of cigarettes or coffee? So let's at least be honest about the comparisons we make.

The bottom line on the issue of marijuana, as it is for many other drugs, is the effect the drug has on your life and functioning when you take it. Simply taking a toke on a joint is not evidence of drug abuse. Suffering ill effects and wishing to repeat the behavior is drug abuse. Persistence of drug use in the face of serious disruption of functioning is psychological addiction. This can happen with marijuana, but it is still the exception, not the rule.

What is the effect of marijuana (and its chemical sisters—hashish, hash oil, THC extract) on growing minds and bodies? No one is sure. Can marijuana affect unborn fetuses? Again, no one is sure, but it's wise not to smoke *anything* when you are pregnant. We once did not think alcohol could be harmful to unborn children, but we now have clinical evidence of fetal alcohol syndrome (FAS) which shows that drinking during pregnancy can lead to serious problems for the child. Chemicals of all kinds seem to be able to cross the placental barrier. The taking of all drugs carries a calculated risk. In the absence of clear and definitive scientific pronouncements about marijuana, you are well advised to exercise caution and moderation. Millions of people will have no one to blame but themselves if grass turns out to have some as yet unknown negative surprises. There is no intended scare tactic in these statements—just an emphasis on the judicious exercise of common sense and the acceptance of personal responsibility for your own health and the health of your loved ones.

What if It's the Parents Who Are Abusing Drugs?

As adults we usually emphasize the perils of adolescent drug abuse. Here the shoe is on the other foot. For example, there are 13 million adult alcoholics and problem drinkers in America. Many of them have children. In New York it is estimated that 9.4 percent of the state's children have an alcoholic in the family. We do not make nearly enough of an effort in supporting and guiding these children. Here are some ways in which these children are affected and actions they may need to take when their parents are involved in serious drug abuse.

It is not their fault. Kids have a way, when their parents are in trouble, of thinking that somehow they are the cause of the problem. This can occur with marital discord and breakup, child abuse and neglect, and drug abuse. The kid thinks, "If only I had been a better son [or daughter], if only I had behaved better [or done my homework on time, or gotten better grades], or . . ." Kids are not responsible for their parents' drinking and drugging. And they are certainly not responsible for their sobriety. These are choices that adults make for themselves. Kids have to learn to detach themselves from these unfounded guilt feelings and focus on managing their own lives.

Kids must not deny the impact of parental drug abuse. The parents' behavior is probably making them feel scared, helpless, and angry. The parents have probably become unpredictable, making and breaking promises, spending less time with them than before, ranging in their moods from loving attention to callous disregard. There may even be improper sexual attention or advances from parent to child. There may be unexplained beatings or punishment. The kids go through terrible conflicts about their own vacillating feelings of love and hate toward a parent. They begin losing respect for the parent; this is confusing and frightening. These kids need to be brutally honest with themselves about their own feelings, however conflicting or negative they may be. Repressing these natural reactions will only cause more damage. These youngsters are forced to grow up too fast as they ride the emotional roller coaster created by parental drug abuse.

The children need to talk to their parents. One of the reasons that some adults persist in their chemical abuse is that they can fool themselves into believing that they are not harming their families. The children must let the parents know how their behavior is affecting them and how they feel about it. The parents need to know that their children are worried about them. If only one parent is abusing drugs, then the children should speak to the other parent. Kids need to know that you share their perception of what is happening to your partner. They need to understand what is happening to the family. They must not be shut out—drug abuse is a family problem.

Kids must learn not to try to run their parents' lives. It is quite common when one or both parents are in trouble with drugs for the children to seek out a form of role reversal in

51

which they try to care for the hurting adult(s). They begin assuming more responsible roles within the family, plugging gaps and trying to maintain a semblance of normalcy. This tends to bring childhood to a screeching halt and forces kids to grow up too fast. In an effort to hold things together, they may turn into superachievers in school and at home. What the kids really need to do is to lead a parallel existence, in which they take care of their own responsibilities and are not dragged down by the parental behavior. If things get too crazy at home, they need to spend time in the school library or at a friend's house. Seeking out self-help groups like Alateen can be very helpful and supportive in the kids' efforts to keep their own lives together even as their parents may be going to hell in a bottle (or syringe or whatever).

There is a real danger that children may begin using drugs themselves in an effort to punish their parents. The parents have already set an example of "better living through chemistry" and the kids follow in kind. I have worked with families where there has been drug abuse in three generations—children, parents, and grandparents. The real danger is that the kids may find temporary relief from their own bad feelings by using drugs. If this happens they will begin seeking that relief on a regular basis. The fact that the parents may do it with booze while the kids are doing it with other drugs is of no consequence. Getting high is getting high, regardless of what drug is taken.

Kids become isolated and feel terribly embarrassed by their parents. Remember the story of my staff member who, once it became known that her father was an alcoholic, never again invited her friends to her home (she was only eleven years old at the time). Children of drug abusers feel a powerful stigma and are subject to profound feelings of embarrassment. Their own homes become off-limits because they never know when their own parent(s) might do something to cause them to feel ashamed. Even worse, they may stop feeling worthy of their friends and retreat into a lonely world where their only friends exist in their fantasies. These kids are desperately in need of a real friend—

52

someone they can talk to, dump their feelings of fright, anger, and confusion on, and get emotional support from. It is embarrassing to admit that a parent is in trouble with drugs, but it's even harder to go it alone. These kids don't need their friends to have answers, just for them to be there for them when they are hurting.

Even after the kids have done everything in their own power to cope with a bad situation, they may find that they need professional help. It isn't easy to "keep on keeping on" when you are alone and confused. Younger children may approach a favorite teacher or guidance counselor. Older ones may seek out a psychologist, social worker, or psychiatrist. It's a great relief to these kids when they find a confidant who can guide them. They need to know that theirs is not the only family facing this problem. The professional should guide them toward new peers such as those in groups like Alateen or Alanon. The worst thing is for the kids to feel compelled to go it alone and be crushed by the overwhelming pressures of a family in serious trouble.

According to Sharon Wegscheider, who works with the families of alcoholics, the children learn to adopt what are described as "survivor roles." Four of these are described below:

- The family hero. Often the oldest child, he or she works extremely hard at gaining family approval. Usually an overachiever who wants to please, he or she becomes the family's representative to the outside world.
- The scapegoat. Feeling emotionally rejected, this child uses defiance to strike back at the family. A lot of negative energy is focused by the family on this antagonistic child who provides a focus that keeps attention from the drinking parent.
- The lost child. The lost child learns to avoid close relations within the family, spending a lot of time alone or quietly busy. He or she suffers from intense psychological pain and loneliness. The pain is often masked by the apparent self-sufficiency and independence.

- The family mascot. Often the youngest child in the family, he or she is not taken very seriously, mostly due to age. Often hyperactive and may use humor or obnoxious behavior as a means of getting attention.

The Clean Air Act: Smoking at Home

There is growing evidence that exposure to smoke from another person's cigarette may be harmful to the health of nonsmokers (the same holds true for pipe and cigar smoke). There are two kinds of smoke emitted from a burning cigarette. Mainstream smoke is that portion of the smoke drawn directly from the mouthpiece of a tobacco product (pipe stem, cigarette tip with or without a filter, end of a cigar) during active puffing. Sidestream smoke emits from the smoldering tobacco in a steady stream. Smoke particles and various smoke ingredients are found in sidestream smoke in even higher concentrations than in mainstream smoke. Passive inhalation is the involuntary taking in of this sidestream smoke (together with exhaled smoke) by a nonsmoker. People with allergies (including asthma) are more sensitive to this smoke than others. We can't yet definitively state that passive inhalation causes cancer, but future epidemiological studies may prove this to be the case. Here are some nonmedical reactions to parental smoking from a group of fifth-graders I spoke with:

> I don't kiss my father anymore. I can't stand his breath!
>
> My mother's hair and clothes smell like an ashtray full of dead butts.
>
> We stay far away from the family room on football-game days. The smoke makes my eyes water and makes me choke.
>
> It makes me angry that both my parents can smoke in any room in the house. The whole house stinks from cigarettes. Don't I have a right to some clean air?
>
> Last weekend I threw my mother's cigarettes in the garbage. She just went out and bought some more. My father told her that she is addicted and she threw an ashtray at him.

54

I told my mother and father that they are not allowed to smoke in my room anymore.

If you believe that you are actively promoting good health in your home, you had better consider this issue if anyone in your family smokes any tobacco product. At the very least you are polluting the air. At the very worst you may be actively endangering the health of your loved ones.

The Clean Air Manifesto

1. Stop smoking. If you can't, reduce your tobacco intake at home.
2. Keep your smoking limited to as few rooms in the house or apartment as possible.
3. Try to keep your smoking to an absolute minimum when other people are around.
4. Keep the windows open.
5. Make a conscious effort to keep more square footage between yourself and other people (not too effective without proper ventilation).
6. Respect the rights of nonsmokers of all ages.
7. Ask your guests to keep their smoking to a minimum (or if you have stopped, ask them not to smoke at all in your home).
8. Do not smoke at all around infants and toddlers.
9. Do not smoke in your children's rooms.
10. Consider giving it up again. It's for your own health as well as your family's.

By the way, smoking in your car, because it's a smaller space, is even worse. The smell of smoke lingers in a car for many days. Cracking a window open brings in road noise and dirt, so maybe you should not smoke in the car at all. One more good reason: you need both hands to drive. Keeping the pipe, cigar, or cigarette in your mouth means running the risk of having hot smoke go directly into your eyes, obscuring road visibility and possibly leading to an accident. As a matter of fact, statistics show that people who smoke while driving have more accidents than nonsmokers.

Smoking is an addiction to nicotine. Stopping is hard but it *can* be done—30 million people have done it already. While it is true that the vast majority of smokers quit on their own, many people do better in organized programs (with and without group support). For more information, contact your local chapter of the American Cancer Society. However, if you must persist in smoking, remember that nonsmokers have rights too!

Mother's Little Helpers—a Modern-Day Fairy Tale

Once upon a time there was a family—Dad, Mom, and three children. Dad had a rewarding job and often came home late in the evening. All three kids were in school. Mom worked part-time, took care of the house and kids and of course Dad. Mom went to work to help "make ends meet." Mom took care of all the carpools, the family laundry and cleaning, the meals, the social calendar, the PTA and school obligations, and relations with the grandparents. Wow, Mom was really something. Look at the things she could do! But Mom began having trouble sleeping, so off she went to her family doctor. She spent exactly 4½ minutes with the kindly doctor, who told her not to worry and gave her a prescription for a sleeping medication. "These will help you to relax," he said as his nurse ushered in the next patient.

Dad said, "I'll help. I will remind you to take your pills." Mom began sleeping better, but pretty soon she felt that she could not sleep if she didn't take the pills. Dad thought the pills must really be working because not only did Mom sleep but she was hot stuff in bed on most nights. Sometimes Mom and Dad had a glass of wine before going to bed. This made Mom a little spacy, but after all she slept well.

One morning Dad had a lot of trouble waking Mom up. He finally succeeded but Mom said she did not feel well. Dad called the friendly doctor. He did not mention the wine they had drunk. The doctor said she should increase the number of Quāaludes she was taking, but only at night before bedtime. That day Mom did not go to work and had lunch with her friend Sally, who knew a lot about life. She told Sally she had been feeling spacy lately and Sally asked her if she was taking any medication. Mom said, "Yes, I'm taking some Quāaludes to help me to sleep." Mom remembered to mention the wine as well. Sally set Mom straight about mixing a hypnotic sedative like Quāaludes with a liquid sedative called alcohol.

That night Mom gave Dad the word: the "little helpers" she needed did not come in a vial of pills. She said, "Dad, I need you and our three children to be my little helpers. I'll sleep just fine if I can have some more help with all the things I have to do around this family." Dad and the kids loved Mom so they all helped out. Mom slept better than ever before. So did Dad and the kids. And they all lived happily (drug-free) ever after.

CHAPTER TWO

Drugs and School

Our children spend the greater part of their waking hours in school. Beyond the nuclear family, the majority of social and emotional learning occurs within and around the school setting. Some of this learning is adventurous and gratifying. Some of it is painful and confusing. All of it determines the quality of the student's life on a daily basis and acts to mold and shape future practices. Since our kids interact socially as well as academically in school, the use of various drugs has implications for both aspects of their lives.

Parents look to the schools to confront and solve the "drug problem." They blame school officials for not stemming the rising tide of drug use. Teachers and school administrators blame parents for failing to properly guide and raise their children. Everyone blames the police for not stopping the seemingly endless flow of drugs available to kids. Overfocusing on the drugs themselves, parents and educators take crash courses in drug terminology and street slang. They are looking through the wrong end of the telescope. We try to scare the kids, con them with pseudoscientific literature, bully them, tail and arrest them and smear them. The kids take the cues and go underground, drugs in tow.

THE EXTENT OF DRUG USE

What you read in the popular press and magazines and see and hear on television and radio may have already convinced you that school-age children are using a wide assortment of drugs. What you have heard is true.

In 1981 the largest study of its kind, involving 17,000 high school seniors from around the nation, was published by the National Institute on Drug Abuse under the title "Highlights from Student Drug Use in America 1975–1980." Tables 1 through 5 on the following pages are taken from this study conducted by Dr. Lloyd Johnson, Dr. Jerald Bachman, and Dr. Patrick O'Malley of the University of Michigan. The information was collected in 1980. Single copies are available at no charge from the National Clearinghouse for Drug Abuse Information (see Appendix C).

At what grade level does the first use of various drugs occur? Table 1 shows the grade of first use for sixteen types of drugs as reported by the senior class of 1980. Initial experimentation with most illicit drugs occurs during the final three years of high school. Each illegal drug, except marijuana, has been used by less than 7 percent of the class by the time they enter tenth grade. However, with marijuana, alcohol, and cigarettes, most of the initial experimentation takes place earlier. For example, daily cigarette smoking was begun by 16 percent prior to tenth grade, followed by only an additional 10 percent after that. The figures for initial use of alcohol are 55 percent prior to and 38 percent following tenth grade; and for marijuana, 31 percent and 29 percent. The "never used" column is quite revealing. By the time they finish their senior year, only 39.7 percent have not tried marijuana, and only 6.8 percent have not tried alcohol.

The age of first use for many of these drugs points to the need for considerable attention to drug prevention programming, both in the home and in the schools, beginning in the middle years of *elementary school*. By the time the kids have reached the junior high school or middle school, experimentation with various drugs has already begun.

Table 2 shows the prevalence and recency of use of eleven

TABLE 1

Grade of First Use for Sixteen Types of Drugs

Grade in Which Drug Was First Used	Marijuana	Inhalants	Amyl/Butyl Nitrites	Hallucinogens	LSD	PCP	Cocaine	Heroin	Other Opiates	Stimulants	Sedatives	Barbiturates	Methaqualone	Tranquilizers	Alcohol	Cigarettes (Daily)
6th	1.9	1.4	0.1	0.1	0.1	0.2	0.1	0.2	0.4	0.3	0.3	0.2	0.1	0.3	8.0	3.0
7–8th	13.0	2.4	1.2	0.8	0.5	1.0	0.5	0.0	0.5	1.5	0.9	0.7	0.3	1.6	22.2	7.2
9th	16.5	1.9	2.2	2.2	1.4	1.9	1.7	0.2	1.8	4.3	2.5	2.3	1.3	3.0	24.8	5.8
10th	14.7	2.5	2.6	3.5	2.2	2.7	3.3	0.2	2.1	6.6	3.3	3.0	1.8	3.3	19.3	4.7
11th	9.7	2.0	3.2	4.3	3.3	2.6	5.8	0.2	3.4	7.3	4.8	3.2	3.3	4.4	11.9	3.4
12th	4.4	1.7	1.8	2.4	1.7	1.0	4.3	0.4	1.6	6.3	3.2	1.6	2.8	2.6	7.0	1.7
Never used	39.7	88.1	88.9	86.7	90.7	90.4	84.3	98.9	90.2	73.6	85.1	89.0	90.5	84.8	6.8	74.2

60

TABLE 2

**Prevalence and Recency of Use
Eleven Types of Drugs**

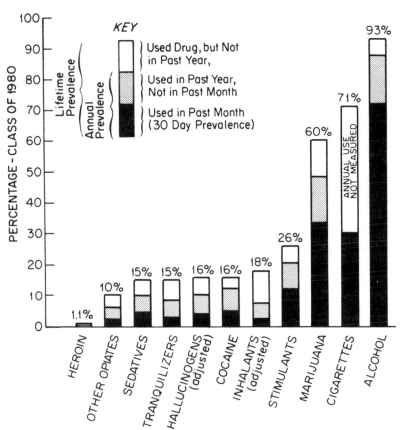

types of drugs as reported by high-school seniors. Before looking at the table, can you guess which drug is the most frequently tried and most regularly and heavily used among youth? If you guessed marijuana or cigarettes you are wrong. Now look at the table.

The answer is *alcohol.* The popularity of this powerful sedative drug warrants equal attention along with all the other drugs of use and potential abuse.

Table 3 shows the trends in annual prevalence of illicit drug use for all seniors who participated in the five years of surveying. In this table, use of "some other illicit drugs" includes any use of hallucinogens, cocaine, and heroin, or any use which is not under a doctor's orders of other opiates, stimulants, sedatives, or tranquilizers.

Table 2 tell us that about two out of every three seniors (65 percent) report illicit drug use at some time in their lives. However, a substantial proportion of them have used only marijuana (28 percent of the sample or 41 percent of all illicit drug users). About four in every ten seniors (39 percent) report using an illicit drug other than marijuana at some time. Marijuana is by far the most widely used illicit drug, with 60 percent reporting some use in their lifetime, 49 percent reporting some use in the past year, and 34 percent use in the past month. The most widely used class of other illicit drugs is stimulants (26 percent lifetime prevalence).

Judging from Table 3, it now appears that 1978 and 1979 may have been the high point in a long and dramatic rise in marijuana use among American high-school students. Until 1978, the proportion of seniors involved in illicit drug use had increased primarily because of the increase in marijuana use. But since 1976 there has been a very gradual, steady increase in the proportion who use some illicit drug other than marijuana, an increase which continued until 1980.

Exposure to drug use by friends is believed to play a pivotal role in initiation into the drug scene. Table 4 shows the proportion of friends using each drug as estimated by seniors in 1980.

If you compare the figures in Table 2 (prevalence and recency of use) and Table 4 (proportion of friends using), you will see how closely personal-use patterns mirror those of friends. The highest levels of exposure involve alcohol and marijuana.

Thirty percent of all seniors say that most or all of their friends get drunk at least once a week! Forty-one percent say they person-

TABLE 3

**Trends in Annual Prevalence of Illicit Drug Use,
All Seniors**

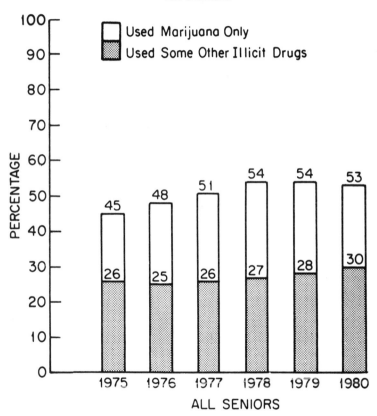

TABLE 4

Proportion of Friends Using Each Drug as Estimated by Seniors in 1980

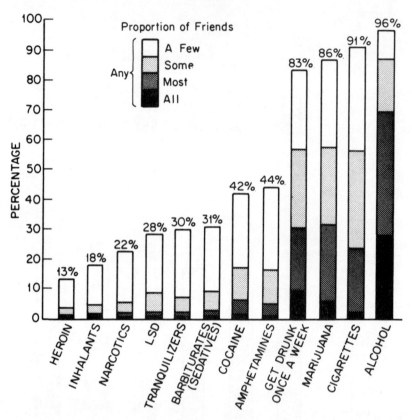

ally had taken five or more drinks in a row during the prior two weeks.

One set of questions in the survey asked for estimates of how difficult it would be to obtain each of a number of different drugs. The answers range across five categories from "probably impossible" to "very easy." Table 5 shows the trends over the five years in perceived availability of drugs.

There are substantial differences in the reported availability of the various drugs. In general, the more widely used drugs

TABLE 5

Trends in Perceived Availability of Drugs

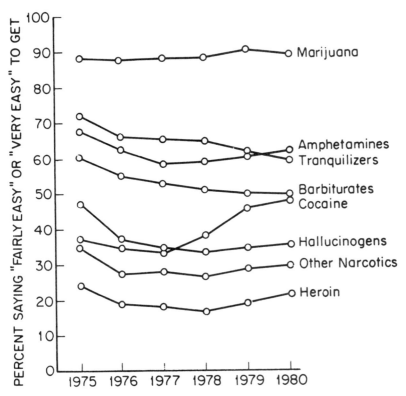

are reported to be the most readily available. Marijuana seems to be almost universally available to high-school seniors; nearly 90 percent report that it would be "very easy" to "fairly easy" for them get it, roughly 30 percent more than the number who report ever having used it. After marijuana, the students indicate that the psychotherapeutic drugs are the most readily available: amphetamines are seen as available by 61 percent, tranquilizers by 59 percent, and barbiturates by 49 percent. Nearly half of the seniors (48 percent) now see cocaine as being available to them.

In 1980 nearly 60 percent of the students said they believed regular marijuana users faced a "great risk" of harming themselves. Three years earlier only 35 percent held that view. In 1978 one in every nine high-school seniors said they were daily users of marijuana. By 1980 the proportion had dropped to one in fourteen. Those who continued to use drugs reported that they now tended to consume smaller amounts and for shorter periods of time. Despite the downward trend, conservative estimates are that, overall, drug use among high-school students remains widespread. Nearly two-thirds of the age group (65 percent) have used an illicit drug, and nearly two out of every five (39 percent) have used an illicit drug other than marijuana. Combined with licit drug use (alcohol, tobacco, etc.), we can see that adolescent drug use is a widespread practice in America.

Just in case you are saying "Thank God my kid only drinks," consider the following information taken from a national study of adolescent drinking behavior involving 5,000 students, age 15 through 17. This study was conducted by the Research Triangle Institute under contract to the National Institute on Alcohol Abuse and Alcoholism and the National Institute on Drug Abuse.[1]

Drinking Levels by Age: 1978 Study

	15	17	18
Abstainer or infrequent	38.6%	29.1%	27.2%
Moderate/heavy or heavier	26.2%	36.3%	36.9%

Moderate/heavy: drank at least once per week with 2 to 4 drinks per occasion, or drank 3 to 4 times per month having more than 5 drinks at a time.
Heavier: drank once a week and had at least 5 drinks per occasion.

1. "Heavier" drinker characterized almost 15 percent of the tenth- to twelfth-graders; 17.3 percent were "moderate/heavy" drinkers; and more than one in four drank at least once a week.
2. By the tenth grade, about seven out of ten students could no longer be called "abstainers." The data show

66

that three out of five kids drank at least once per month. (There are more than 11 million tenth- to twelfth-graders in America.)

3. Three out of ten teenagers in the tenth to twelfth grades could be considered problem drinkers: he or she was drunk at least six times within a year, or experienced negative consequences of drinking two or more times in at least three of six life areas (friends, family, school, dates, police, driving).

4. About one in four reported having driven after having a good bit to drink, and one out of ten reported having done this at least four times within the past year. Car accidents are a leading cause of death among sixteen- to nineteen-year-olds.

5. Comparison data show that the gap between boys and girls is closing. In 1974, 18 percent more girls than boys were moderate drinkers or less. By 1978 this gap had closed to 13 percent. And 19 percent more boys than girls fell into the higher drinking categories in 1974, but in 1978 the difference was just 14 percent.

Young people who drink heavily tend to do less well in school than those who don't drink as much. They also tend to smoke marijuana more and are involved in "unconventional" behavior. While personality and environmental influences are seen as underlying causes, it is reasonable to assert that for teenagers who drink, the chances they will engage in other problem behaviors are greater than for those who don't drink.

College-bound youth report less drug use than those students who are not college bound. Neither of the studies just cited addresses a newer and possibly more dangerous set of practices, namely that of multiple substance use and abuse. Many young people report drug combinations, marijuana and alcohol being the most popular of the mixtures.

A large proportion of youths who become involved in illicit drug use also become multiple drug users. Listed below are the number of additional drugs regularly used by the habitual users

Multiple Drug Use[2]

of those who reported regularly* using:	number of clients	% of the sample	have, on the average, also regularly used the following number of other drugs
marijuana	2,363	86%	3.2
alcohol	2,196	80	3.4
inhalants	525	19	4.5
other drugs	28	1	4.7
amphetamines	890	32	5.3
heroin	215	8	5.4
hashish	754	27	5.5
barbiturates	811	29	5.5
tranquilizers	581	21	5.8
hallucinogens	656	24	5.8
PCP (Phencyclidine)	611	22	5.8
cocaine	263	10	6.0
over-the-counter drugs	136	5	6.2
illegal methadone	49	2	6.2
other opiates	397	14	6.3

* Regular use is defined as weekly or greater use for a period of at least one month.

for each of several drug categories. These figures represent youths twelve to nineteen years of age who were admitted to treatment for drug abuse.

Overwhelming evidence from numerous studies has documented the widespread use of many drugs on college campuses throughout America. You need only to amplify the findings regarding high-school drug use to get some idea of the extent of use in college. College has always served as the setting in which many young people are introduced to alcohol, and many fraternities pride themselves on the ability of their members to put away voluminous amounts of the stuff. A 1982 study[3] of college deans at 181 two-year and four-year colleges and universities in the U.S. found that about 75 percent of students are drinkers. The same study showed that one of six college students drinks excessively and more than one of fifty must leave school ultimately because of drinking problems. The deans classified about half the students as social or experimental drinkers but said 16 percent drank excessively. Colleges have become alarmed at the large amount of drinking on campus and consequent vandalism (as much as 80 percent may be alcohol related). And in traffic accident deaths, half of the 13,370 deaths of people aged eighteen to twenty-four in 1981 were alcohol related. The general perception held by faculty and students is that drinking cannot be stopped, so more and more schools are trying to encourage moderation and responsible drinking behavior. Colleges are employing many measures toward this goal: weekend pickup services for students too drunk to drive, alcohol awareness classes, encouraging drinking within walking distance of living areas (some schools have bars right on campus), student-to-student breathylizer tests to keep blood alcohol levels within legal limits, serving of nonalcoholic beverages at parties. Age limits are being raised for alcohol use. New Jersey, New York, and Connecticut are just a few states that have recently raised the legal drinking age. Students are bitter, claiming that if they are old enough to fight for their country and vote, they are old enough to drink. Most don't believe that changing the laws will actually lower the incidence of young adult drinking. As one college freshman pointed out, "There's plenty of phony identification papers for sale and you can always get a senior to buy booze for you. Bartenders may laugh at phony papers but they will serve you anyway."

Drugs have joined alcohol on the college campus, leading to new patterns of multiple substance use. Parents have wondered what factors tend to place their children at risk before and during the college years. One study,[4] which focused on religiosity and drug use, helped to identify historical (precollege) and current characteristics of high-risk undergraduates.

The study further shows that among frequent users, Jewish students were more likely to be involved in multiple use of drugs other than alcohol; non-Jewish students were more inclined to report heavy use of alcoholic beverages. "Traditionally, Jews have

Drug Abuse Risk Factors for College Students

Past-History Factors	Current Risk Factors
1. History of regular cigarette smoking	1. Poor academic performance
2. History of trouble with the law	2. Dissatisfaction with school
3. Lack of close relationships with parents	3. Widespread peer-group drug usage
4. Never attended religious services	4. No current religious preference
	5. Lack of a strong sense of purpose in life
	6. Tendency to minimize the importance of material accomplishments and to emphasize the importance of values such as freedom and equality

placed great emphasis on academic and professional achievement. It is therefore not surprising to find that, among Jewish students, underachievers in school and those who perceived their college studies to be unrelated to career and life goals were likely to be frequent drug users." The study helps us to see how movement away from traditional values—a history of not attending religious services or no current religious preference—is often associated with drug use. Other studies point to the fact that when young adults escalate their drug use beyond alcohol and marijuana, their academic performance tends to go down.

Drug-use trends are rarely static in nature. They have a way of changing in terms of drug popularity, drug combinations, amount of use, and frequency of use. Let's trace the natural history of one contemporary drug to make this point. Acid (LSD) was first synthesized in 1938, but its hallucinogenic effects were not discovered until 1943 when Dr. Albert Hoffman accidentally ingested some of the drug and recorded the first acid trip. Drs. Timothy Leary and Richard Alpert began studies of the drug in the early 1960s at Harvard's Center for Research in Personality. Students in the Cambridge area began "turning on and tuning in" to the psychedelic (mind-expanding) effects of LSD. The Harvard establishment put the kibosh on student tripping and the experimenters moved their research efforts to the International Federation for Internal Freedom (IFIF) at Cambridge and Zihuatanejo, Mexico. The media picked up on the early reports of acid's ability to induce powerful hallucinations and to tickle and enhance sexual fancies; it became the new drug of rebellion. Between 1963 and 1965 the scientific and popular accounts of the drug stressed pleasure and exploration of consciousness. As a consequence the drug's popularity grew, especially on college campuses. It was not until 1967 that reports of abuse, bad trips, and flashbacks led to the drug's first bad press—again initially in scientific papers and then in the popular media. Use began to wane by the early 1970s and with it the "death" of the peace and love movement. New times demanded new drugs and the search for the safe mind-altering drug continues unabated. Acid seems to be making a comeback, particularly on the west coast, as earlier reports of chromosome damage remain unproven. While acid use flowed and then ebbed, a sister psychedelic drug (albeit far less potent) continued to grow and has virtually been institutionalized in the America drug scene—namely marijuana.

One of the raging controversies of the drug scene for many years has been the "stepping stone" theory that experimentation with and use of one drug can lead to curiosity about other drugs. Some studies point to an association between the use of one substance and future use of other substances. However, there is no evidence that once you use one drug you are locked into a pattern of automatically escalating drug abuse. We have already mentioned some risk factors which seem to predispose young people to drug use and/or abuse. However, as no evidence has established the existence of an "addictive" personality, we must understand that the issue is far more complicated than some of the antidrug forces would have us believe. Certain practical associations do exist. For example, it is known that people who smoke cigarettes are more likely to try marijuana, which is commonly smoked (but can also be eaten). Influences to try alcohol and marijuana usually come from best friends. But the risk factors that can lead to other drug use and abuse are combinations of peer and parental influence, age of first use (the younger you are when you start, the greater the chances of future problems), quality of adolescent/parent relationships, the behavioral model parents provide, parental expectations, and the degree to which deviance is tolerated in the household. It isn't as simple as some would have us believe, i.e., if you smoke pot you will become a heroin addict! Nonsense, despite the fact that most heroin addicts have smoked pot. Again, the relationships as determined by careful study show that there are many overlapping causes of drug use and drug abuse.

There has been a lot of alarm recently about adolescent drinking. We must learn to pay close attention to the terminology employed to describe the use of alcohol. The media often speak about teenage "alcoholism" in their attempts to try to sell newspapers or TV advertising time. Television news coverage focuses primarily on tragedy and gossip. The more sensational, the better. However, the actual number of teenage alcoholics is not known, and while a serious problem for these young people and their families, it is not the pattern of alcohol use that most of us need fear in our young. Alcoholism is out-of-control drinking; it is an inability to use alcohol the way most other people do. The alcoholic usually cannot predict in any episode of drinking how much he or she will consume or what the effects will be. Most adolescent drinkers do not fit this description. Our primary concern must be with the dangers associated with a single episode of drinking in which judgment is impaired. One need not be an "alcoholic" to get into a fight, become pregnant, wreck a car, or commit vandalism. Fifty-five percent of alcohol experimentation occurs before entrance into high school. Helping our kids to deal with this reality and all that it may imply at such a young age is the greater task.

72

The drug problem is not a drug problem as much as it is a people problem. Therefore, alcohol-specific programs of prevention are probably worthless. It is common to find other problems in the lives of young people with drinking problems (other drug use, family discord, deviant behavior), and a more general syndrome of behavior requires something more than an understanding of a specific chemical or drug. Problem drinkers don't live the same kinds of lives as social drinkers. More is at issue than the alcohol. We must work with issues such as family life, self-image, multiple substance abuse, social acceptance, and adolescent sexuality. There are ways that we can help:

- Recognize that young people and adults use drugs for certain reasons and be open to a discussion of the reasons without lecturing.
- At least half the young lie to their parents about illicit drug use (such as marijuana). They do so because they fear punishment and don't want their parents to think badly of them. We must respect forthrightness in our young people but also understand their need for privacy.
- Keep channels of communication open. Drugs, sex, rejection, body image—these are difficult things to discuss, especially with parents. We must encourage kids to state their feelings and ideas even when they differ radically from our own.
- Adults have the right and responsibility to state their opinions and feelings as well. Young people need us to be there for them with our knowledge and experience. They don't appreciate wishy-washy adults. At least agree to disagree.
- Adults should get active in school boards and parents' associations. Make sure your children's schools are addressing social and emotional needs, not just intellectual needs. Make sure school-based drug programs are focusing on the context and issues within the life of adolescents and not just on the pharmacology of drugs.
- When dealing with a young person with a drinking prob-

lem, be on the alert for parental alcohol abuse or alcoholism (if one parent is an alcoholic there is a one-in-four chance of the offspring being alcoholic; if both parents are alcoholics there is a one-in-two chance).

• Many kids get high (on various drugs) because they can't handle their own emerging sexuality. Provide them with factual information and emotional support about human sexuality.

DRUGS AND STUDYING

Over the generations students have learned to use a variety of drugs, both licit and illicit, as study aids. Much of this activity is associated with periods of intensive studying usually referred to as "cramming." Although most students, including those who keep up with the work all semester long, tend to cram just before exams, many are trying to play catch-up in a very risky way. The drugs people use to stay awake during cramming can have some bad side effects and aftereffects. We live in an "instant" society. We want everything to happen fast and easy. Here are several vignettes which show how things can go wrong.

When I was working nights as a nursing student, I could never get used to sleeping during the day. I guess my biological clocks did not want to change. So I started taking amphetamines [very powerful stimulants]. I used the spansules. Throughout the night I would be given to sudden bursts of frenetic energy during which time I was racing up and down the hallways. When the night shift ended I was so wired I had to take some barbiturates [sedatives] to calm me down enough to fall asleep. I got off that roller coaster after just one week.

Back when I was a freshman in college I took an urban planning course. There was no midterm and we had to absorb a lot of material for the final exam. Jeff had been taking incredible amounts of No-Doz [primary ingredient is caf-

74

feine, a stimulant] and drinking pots of coffee [more caffeine]. He stayed up for forty-eight hours straight, studying. On the day of the final he sat in front of me. Five minutes into the exam he fell asleep. I tried to wake him. I poked him in the ribs, pinched him, talked right into his ear— nothing worked. It was very weird. As soon as the exam ended he woke up, staggered back to his room, and slept for twenty-three hours. He flunked the course.

Sheila was really uptight about the big examination in chemistry. She had found that smoking grass relaxed her at other times. So she figured right before the test should help. She got relaxed all right. She was so blissed out that she found the chemistry formulas and equations floating around in one big sea of symbols and numbers in her head. She knew the stuff but could not seem to concentrate and put it all together. She also kept losing track of time. She should have gotten at least a B but ended up with a low C.

By the time I reached my junior year of college I had been drinking pretty steadily. At first I just drank at parties on weekends but I started to party during the week as well. There was always an ample supply of grass and booze in the dorm. My grades stayed up so I did not think I had a problem. It got to the point where I was drinking daily. At the end of the fall semester I studied real hard to prepare for finals. When I sat down to take my math final I ended up staring at a blank page for two hours. I knew I knew the material but could simply not recall any of it. I later learned that I had been having blackouts, which are periods in which short-term memory is disrupted by alcohol.

While it is true that stimulant drugs will keep you awake, they have sometimes been known to play nasty tricks with memory circuits. They do provide a sense of energy but also make it difficult not to fidget, and one can become distracted easily. Time perceptions may be slightly altered and feelings of fear can be intensified. Symptoms of caffeinism closely mirror those of an anxiety condition (see Chapter 3 for details), some of which can hamper rather than enhance test-taking ability. Tranquilizers, on the other hand, can remove that competitive edge. A little test anxiety seems to improve test performance. Too much test anxiety can overwhelm us. If we take drugs in addition to being anxious about the material to be absorbed, the results can be disastrous. Drugs that speed up or slow down the electrochemical processes involved in memory and concentration can be risky. People have walked out of exams feeling, in their drug-induced state, that they had done marvelously well, only to discover they had failed miserably. There is a thin line between the advantage to be gained and the edge to be lost when using drugs to aid in studying and exam taking. Proper study regimens and good health are far more helpful than the unpredictable interactions between the stress of exams and the physical and mental effects of the drugs. The whole idea of waiting until the last moment to study almost guarantees this volatile combination of events.

It is becoming a real goof for more and more kids to go to school high on either grass or alcohol. Kids like to get a big kick out of fooling their teachers. They brag about how naive their teachers are and how hip they are. Most kids believe that alcohol can interfere with schoolwork more than grass can. Common reasons for getting high before class are wanting to feel relaxed, getting through a boring class, and imitating friends. Interestingly, some students can learn while high, while others get too confused or disoriented to do so. It's a risky business at best, and doesn't really make a boring lecture any more interesting. There is always the chance of being caught by school officials, having one's parents brought in, and being suspended. Any student who uses drugs too often, specifically drugs which inhibit memory function and concentration, can end up with poor grades even if everything else in his or her life is okay.

It is not easy to sit down and discuss drugs with your kids. One major study showed that 55 percent of parents never discuss drugs with their children. Clearly the time has come for all parents to face the issue squarely. Here are some questions that can guide you into a frank discussion of the relationship between your youngster's drug and study habits. These questions can be presented in a rhetorical fashion to let your kids know you care. They don't necessarily have to answer them in front of you. It may be better to let them give oblique responses. They'll get the message that you have legitimate concerns without your accusing them of having done anything wrong.

- Have they ever noticed that their grades have suffered when using drugs?
- Have they ever gone to school high?
- Have they ever had trouble concentrating on schoolwork when using drugs?
- Do they get high and party when they should be studying?
- Do they use drugs to help them study?
- Have their teachers ever expressed concern to them about drug use?
- Do all of their friends use drugs?
- Do they cut class to get high?
- Are they using lunch money to buy drugs?
- Is cramming their only method of studying?

These questions are loaded! Again, your child does not have to answer them directly. They are really just a listing of important concerns for both child and adult. The challenge to any student is to seek a balance between studies and pleasure. Those students who value education will find a way not to allow partying to interfere with the work of learning. Most young people I have known who do well in school and also use drugs for recreational purposes (only) have applied the following practices:

1. Drugs do not play a central role in their lives.
2. They are knowledgeable about the drugs they use and are very careful about their drug sources.
3. They never traffic in drugs; they get drugs only from close friends.
4. They don't use drugs as study aids. They watch their health around exam time.

77

5. They don't care what kids deeper into the drug culture think of them.
6. When they use drugs they do so in moderation.
7. They study hard all week, reserving the weekends for partying.

The unmotivated or failing student is most at risk for drug use and abuse. As parents, we must stay on top of our children's school performance so that we may assist them if they get into academic difficulties. To fail to do so increases the risks of drug abuse and makes communication increasingly difficult.

PEER-GROUP PRESSURE

There is an important relationship between peer-group pressure and drug use. Although peer pressure is widely thought to be an issue primarily with young people, the pressure on adults is just as strong. Of course, no one factor can totally account for a person's becoming involved with drugs. There is almost always more than one reason:

1. Drugs make me feel good—I like to get high.
2. Self-medication against feelings of tension, anxiety, and depression.
3. The individual's attitude toward society and the "establishment."
4. Poor family relationships.
5. Boredom.
6. Parental drug-taking behavior.
7. A search for altered states of consciousness.
8. Age: the earlier one is exposed to drug experimentation, the greater the likelihood of continued experimentation and use.
9. Lack of religious affiliation (religiosity).
10. Availability of drugs.

11. Lack of interest in academic life.

12. Absence of goal orientation.

13. Disregard of the law (illicit drugs).

Several of these factors can interrelate and have at least some bearing on peer relations. For young people drugs and alcohol have become an integral part of the youth scene. Their social and cultural world interacts with the larger society in which drugs have become common. Movie plots, television programs, rock and folk music, tee shirts, jewelry—all reflect the drug aspects of the youth and adult cultures. Using drugs as an adolescent is a rite of passage into adulthood. It is a way to grow up, be hip, and leave childhood and parental control behind. Drugs such as alcohol and marijuana have been "institutionalized" as part of the youth scene.

Peer relations start with a single friend, not with the large group. In one study of marijuana and other drug use, it was found that marijuana use by a best friend was the factor which correlated most strongly with the probability and frequency of marijuana use among high-school students, outranking personal, family, or sociodemographic factors. When the study looked at drug use beyond marijuana to other illicit drugs, however, parental and personal attributes were found to increase while peer influences decreased in importance. For these young people, factors such as depression, school performance, educational aspirations, closeness to parents, and reported parental drug use were more important than peer influences.

Experimentation with marijuana and alcohol depends strongly on what close friends and the broader peer group are into. Kids who get into heavier drug usage become members of other and ever-dwindling circles of kids, who usually have drug and nondrug problems coming down on them. This is certainly true of young people and adults who use drugs habitually and compulsively. It is a fact of adolescent life that kids who use drugs and alcohol have more friends who also use drugs and alcohol than "straight" friends. This excerpt of a conversation among a group of tenth-graders (sophomore year of high school, age fifteen) makes the point very clearly.

> JOHN: Most kids have tried booze or grass. I only know a few who haven't.
> BETH: I think it depends on who your friends are. I would never have dreamed of smoking dope if my two best friends weren't doing it.
> PEGGY: You know those kids who hang around the mall near the rear parking lot? They're into some heavy drugs. I don't even see them at school anymore.
> JOHN: Yeah, Charlie ——— hangs out with them. He's really messed up. I heard he got caught trying to sell some pills to an eighth-grader.
> SUSAN: Most kids don't get into that scene. You know, they just party a little on the weekends. Like us.
> PEGGY: That's true, Susan. You can't do drugs during the week and expect to handle all that homework.

In many ways, this conversation typifies the drug experience for most kids. They accept drugs (including alcohol) as part of their world, they speak nonchalantly about them (most of the time), they see real differences between occasional use and regular use, they don't let drugs interfere with other activities (like school or athletics), and they either look down on or worry about kids who are into heavy drug use.

However, what if other kids' opinions and other factors have led your child into this smaller circle of regular drug users? Then everything is inverted. Drugs are a central part of life, kids who don't do what they are doing are "square" or "out of it," sports and academic success are downplayed or ridiculed, and so on. Either way the social milieu is a powerful factor.

Dealing and coping with peer-group pressure can be a difficult experience for all of us. However, with the increasing emphasis on assertiveness in American life, some valuable lessons can be taken from that experience. For most of us it comes down to not saying yes when we really want to say no. Here are some thoughts that may help you and your kids work out your own attitudes toward that very real pressure when it comes along— and it will.

1. Realize that your children will be subjected to these pressures from time to time and that they will have important decisions to make. Help them to understand that these are their own decisions, and that they, not their friends, are the ones who will have to live with the consequences.

2. Explain to them that good, caring friends will want to share experiences with them that they regard as positive (this includes getting high). Also explain that good friends may enthusiastically suggest, but will not ram it down their throats or deride them when they say no. A good friend may try to talk them into it but won't really dump on them for continuing to refuse. Anyone who does is no friend.

3. Tell your kids that from time to time they will not wish to do something they may have done previously with friends. "I'm not in the mood" is all they should have to say. If their friends come down on them, it's the friends' problem, not their own.

4. Help them to understand that many times we begin acting and dressing a certain way because we wish to be accepted by a certain group. Help them to ask themselves if belonging to a group by adopting the group's "image" is what they are after, or do they want genuine friendship with members of that group?

5. Tell them to be prepared to get their feelings hurt. Saying no can lead to rejection. There is no way to avoid hurt feelings if they are going to become their own person. But these feelings will pass a lot quicker than the guilt of going against their own values (selling out).

6. Advise them to keep in mind that, when they do use drugs, they don't have to simply mimic the other kids.

Encourage them to get to know their own limits and to stick with them. Let the next person show off. How much is not the same as how good.

7. Sometimes a white lie can get your child out of the pressure cooker. One of my favorites is "The doctor has me on medication and I can't mix it with anything else," or try "I'm into abstinence this month." The idea is not to say yes when you really want to say no.

8. Encourage them not to fear saying "Let me think about that for a while." After all, it's their health, physical and mental, that is at stake.

9. Ask them to take a hard look at the group of kids they wish to identify with. If using drugs is the only way in, then they ought to think long and hard about why that is. The group may be more interested in conformity to their norms than in your child as an individual. Tell your children to check out other groups who will accept them for what they are already and not what the group wants them to become.

CLIQUES AND POPULARITY

Adolescence is a time when kids actively try on various identities in their search for their own. "Who am I?" is a vital question some people spend a lifetime pursuing. It becomes a particularly acute question in the middle-school and high-school years.

We, as adults, often accuse young people of being conformists when they are usually only playing a game we invented. In their school years, kids tend to separate into various cliques. It is still the exceptional child who is a loner. These cliques go under various names in different parts of the country. Here are a few:

Hitters: used to be called "rocks" in my old neighborhood. These are the tough kids. They are into physical power. They get their kicks by bullying and intimidating other kids. Often called "rowdies" by other kids.

Eggheads: sometimes called "squares." These are the kids who excel academically in school. They are college-bound and serious about their studies. They evoke a lot of envy on the part of other kids.

Heads: These are the kids who are really into drugs. They are often blatant in their drug use. Their lives seem to center around anything to do with drugs and getting high.

Jocks: In any neck of the woods these are the kids who are into athletics and varsity sports. They are often into body building as well.

Lovers: These are the kids who really get into dating and relationships. They never seem to be without a partner but change them quite often. Usually hang around with other kids who are into their scene.

Rockers: not to be confused with hitters. These kids are into rock music and styles in a big way. Most recently they are into "punk" and "new wave." You can catch some strange hair colors in this group.

Goody-Goodies: Harder to stereotype. Usually refers to school leaders, religious kids, school club members, and those perceived as "teacher's pets."

What images do these stereotypes conjure up in your own mind? The mere fact that you can probably elaborate on any one of these shows how powerful they are. Kids want desperately to belong to one or more of these groups. They often go from one to the other, seeing where they can make friends, be accepted, and get comfortable. Sometimes the groups overlap.

Which of these groups use drugs? To some extent they all do. At least they tend to experiment. Some of them, like the heads, the rockers, and the hitters, are better known for their prominent use of drugs. Have you ever heard stories about how much beer the jocks can consume or the steroids they sometimes take or the amphetamines that get them up for the big game? How about the wide assortment of drugs that the lovers prefer (cocaine, marijuana, Quāaludes, amyl and butyl nitrates)? And of course everybody likes to drink. You see the point. All kinds of kids use drugs for all kinds of reasons.

All groups develop norms over time, that is, a common set of beliefs and behaviors. It is important to know the norms of the different cliques. Your kid will have to measure his or her own emerging values against those of the group. But loneliness and a strong desire to belong are powerful motives. So kids join various cliques to get a sense of relatedness and to get into the social scene. As parents you should know who your kids' friends are, where and how they spend their time, and such things as when they are coming home. You can make your feelings known about the people they associate with, but then stand back and allow them to sort things out on their own. Sometimes strongly objecting to their friends guarantees that they will spend more time with them. You must discuss with your kids where to draw the line (for example, establish that you don't want them hanging around with kids who are experimenting with hard drugs or getting into vandalism). Again, short of forbidding certain associations, you must allow them to experiment with new social connections, making and breaking them as *they* see fit. The best you can hope for is that they will seek out your advice and bounce their feelings off you.

Many parents allow themselves to believe that kids who use drugs don't go out for athletics. It's true that the kids who end up in drug treatment programs usually shy away from academic and athletic competition. But this has led to the creation of a myth, that athletes don't use drugs. You have just read about the major ways in which sports and drugs have mixed. If your youngsters wish to enter into competitive athletics (no matter what sport—don't think golfers or tennis players don't get high), then be sure you and the kids do so with your eyes wide open. Here are some guidelines to help keep sports and drugs separate and not equal.

- Find out the coach's policies and attitudes regarding the use of drugs. Some coaches take a very hard line about party drugs and sports, and kids have been kicked off teams for breaking the rules.
- Find out if the team has a "play at all costs—win at all costs" mentality. This is where kids tend to misuse painkillers, whether prescribed by team physicians or family doctors. Misuse of painkillers can lead to a "medical addiction." Remember, pain is a symptom; the underlying cause should be diagnosed (through examination and x-ray procedures). "Toughing it out" can lead to permanent physical disabilities.
- State your position about the use of stimulants. Let your son or daughter know that they have to make it with natural ability. Drugs can ruin concentration and only make athletes "feel" more powerful. They don't actually create power or strength.
- High-school athletes who celebrate after the big game often drive cars. Drugging, drinking, and driving don't mix. A local athlete in my community had a full football scholarship nipped in the bud when he mixed booze, pills, and fast driving. His kidney was punctured in the resulting crash.
- Another risk to budding young athletes' dreams of college scholarships is getting busted for possessing or selling drugs. Colleges don't draft ball players with criminal records.
- There are no chemical shortcuts to hard workouts, proper diet, healthful sleep, and a keen mental edge.

Kids and adults often tell us that getting high can be a pleasant experience, bringing people closer together. Chemicals can break the ice and help us to get rid of some of our social inhibitions, but I do not believe that drugs help people get closer. Drugs can make you "feel" closer, but a close relationship, whether it's between lovers, friends, or relatives, requires hard work. The transient bliss that drugs can produce is no substitute for hard-won affection and respect. Relationships are supposed to have ups and downs. If you or your kids are using drugs to smooth out the rough spots, then you are only deluding yourselves. You may find, in time, that the rough spots can become the reason for losing someone, because you used drugs to ignore them. Here are some pointers that can help your family understand whether your social relationships are being helped or hurt by drugs. The questions are reflective, that is, they are designed to help you ask yourselves some tough questions as a family. Adults can start by volunteering information about themselves.

1. Do you and your friends always get high when you are together?
2. Do drugs seem to dominate the conversations?
3. Do your friends give you grief if you choose not to join them in using drugs?
4. Do you ever get the feeling (in relationships with the opposite sex) that your partner needs to get high in order to enjoy being with you?
5. Does everything you do with your friends have to be experienced through drugs (music, sex, movies, rapping, dancing)?
6. Do your friends keep telling you, in so many words, that their motto in life is "Better living through chemistry"?
7. Do you really know your friends as people? Do they know you?
8. Are your social relationships better when you are high?

If you are unhappy with your answers to these questions, then it is time for you to take a hard look at how you are relating to the friends in your life. If drugs seem to be central to these relationships, maybe you got stoned and missed the intimacy of real friendship. Life is a study in contrasts. People who never try drugs may be missing something, but people who use drugs a lot are usually hiding from others and/or themselves.

SCHOOL-BASED PREVENTION PROGRAMS

Parents too often leave it entirely up to the schools to educate their children about drugs. Chapter 1 has suggested some specific ways of addressing this issue in your own family. Your interest in educating young people should not stop within the confines of your own family. Parents have a strong and positive role to play in supporting and aiding school-based prevention programs. This can be accomplished by being active on school boards and parents associations, and by playing a direct role in the school drug prevention program by speaking with other parents and assisting staff and students.

Administrative support: Everything flows from the top in bureaucracies like schools. Therefore it is essential that the top administrators of your kids' school back the program from its very inception. They control the important logistical supports which are needed for a good program: space allocation; released time for teachers and students for training and program operation/participation; budget for educational materials; communications with students, teachers, and parents. Administrators need to hear from parents. So let them know that you demand quality prevention programs for your kids.

Faculty support: In most schools today teachers are fairly well aware of the impact of drug use and abuse on the student body and on themselves as educators. They will usually give tacit approval to any reasonable approach and more explicit support for programs that they can believe in (based on sound educational principles). Parents should not be alarmed when only a handful of teachers volunteer for prevention programs. You want to involve only those teachers who are really motivated. Ask the kids; they will tell you which teachers they can talk to and really respect.

Parental support: Often the most neglected and yet the most concerned group in the school universe, parents must become

87

directly involved in school prevention programming. You need to know that your kids' school is doing something in the area of drug abuse prevention. Parents should be involved from the earliest stages of such programs. Even if you are not clear as to what roles can be played by parents, you can promote the program through the school board, parents' associations, and meetings with school administrators. Confidentiality issues may prevent parents from getting involved in counseling aspects of your school's program. However, there are many things you can do such as organizing and leading parent discussion groups, reaching out to parents of kids in trouble, clerical support, trips, dramatics, help with phone work, and so on.

Drug education materials: All materials should be scientifically accurate and free of the half-truths, emotional biases, and scare tactics that have, in the past, caused young people to reject them out of hand. I have never been able to compete (in the public-relations sense) with the law-enforcement officers on the panels on which I have served. They come armed with suitcases filled with drugs and drug paraphernalia and horror stories of addiction, overdose, and painful withdrawal. This "bread and circuses" approach always pulls the adults and kids away from considering issues of personal responsibility to ogling gaudy displays of homemade hypodermic needles, hash pipes, glassine envelopes (filled with adulterated heroin), and marijuana joints. Fortunately the police always stop short of showing the audience how to cook and shoot up the dope. A screening committee of students, teachers, and parents can review all proposed books, tapes, films, pamphlets, and speakers before allowing their general distribution.

Role of students: It is a real pitfall to conceive of the students solely in the role of passive recipients of such programs. In order to work, the program must actively belong to them. The programs most acceptable to the student body are those which are student-run and faculty-advised. The greater the role of a select group of well-motivated students in the planning and running of the program, the greater the chances of general student acceptance. The kids who do well in such program involvement:

1. are doing well in school,
2. are liked by other kids,
3. want to work with (not "treat") other kids,
4. have nonrigid attitudes about drug use but generally aren't into drugs, and
5. are plugged into nonchemical ways of having fun.

Kids who used to do drugs should not be excluded if they meet the other criteria. Students are your best bet for creating counter-peer-group pressure. Kids in trouble with drugs don't have non-drug-using friends. The students running your school program can reach out to them, providing new circles of "straight" friends.

The planning committee: This should be composed of faculty, students, administrators, and parents. At the beginning, everyone should feel free to brainstorm. This will help to set the goals for the program. Be realistic here, as change is difficult and success feeds upon itself. Setting modest aims and getting people used to the idea of a new program is enough of a task to keep you all busy for a while.

One of the most difficult and important decisions you will have to make is how to spell out the nature of the program. Will it be identified as and limited to issues of drug use? Or will it have a broader context, dealing with issues concerning all school-age kids, drugs being only one among them? In middle- and high-school settings, when you give the program a drug identity you almost always ensure its failure. This is where you must work out your program philosophy. If you think the drug problem is simply limited to the drugs themselves, then you will miss the single most important lesson of the last two decades: drugs are a people issue! When seeking to mount a program you must create a context in which the many causes of drug experimentation, use, abuse, and addiction are considered. Drug-information-only programs have proven to be ineffective, incomplete, possibly even dangerous, and have generally failed to have the needed impact of a genuinely preventive program. Listen to one of our teachers after two years of involvement:

> When we started out I thought this was going to be an easy job. All I would have to do is memorize all the drug names and effects and warn kids about the dangers. After my first lecture to the kids I found out that they knew more than I did anyway. So I had to realize that the kids had as many and often the same reasons for using drugs as adults I know had for drinking alcohol. From that point on I stopped focusing on the drugs and started trying to get to know the kids. This is when the whole thing came alive for me. I got closer to the kids, started listening more and talking less, and together we struggled toward a prevention program.

Curriculum: There are any number of published curricula which one can learn about by contacting your state drug authority and the National Institute on Drug Abuse (NIDA). You must make sure that the outlined approach will meet the needs of your school. The best curricula are those which are graduated by students' ages. The curriculum must be dynamic, not static. Curricula are only guidelines, not a rehash of the Ten Commandments. There must be a built-in give-and-take. Kids are tired of lectures. Affective education, values clarification, rap groups, habit management—these are the ways to bring across the material. Kids pick up on these formats and really get into them. The only approaches which rigorous research has been able to support in primary prevention are these "new generation" strategies: affective, peer-oriented, and multidimensional approaches.

Physical setting: The program can be run in any number of settings. It is a good idea to set aside a particular schoolroom as a "rap room." This is the kind of place that students can decorate according to their own tastes and feel comfortable in.

90

The room has to ensure privacy and should be away from the main flow of traffic.

Confidentiality: This can be a tricky business. On the one hand you want the kids who are abusing drugs to come to the program, but you are afraid that they won't if the program can't ensure their anonymity. In many states, children are the property (chattel) of their parents, and the parents have a right to know what is happening. Drugs do kill and harm people. The program must abide by various federal, state, and local laws. A general rule of thumb is that the kid must be able to come to the program in confidence. Once he or she has revealed a personal drug problem, the staff must make a determination. If the student can get it together (stop abusing drugs) by joining a program, fine. But if the student is out of control, then the program administrators have a moral (if not legal) obligation to inform the child's family. Parents should lobby for this, and school programs should be "neutral" territory. This is a program policy issue that must be worked out very carefully. There is no room for confusion when people's well-being and the long arm of the law are involved. Some kids are really afraid of terrible consequences at home if their folks find out they are using drugs. Programs must help them to understand that they only contribute to their continued drug abuse by keeping it a secret. The time has come for us to consider a family component to our school prevention programs. When dealing with drug abusers I have found it very useful to introduce the child's parents to other parents I know who have lived through the same experience.

Integrated approach: Schools should be just as interested in issues such as adolescent social and emotional growth and health as they are in academic performance. We should all be upset by the fact that most school administrators take for granted that these issues are addressed in traditional educational approaches. At best, they are by-products of a sound curriculum; at worst, they are totally ignored. We like to talk about preparing the students for the "real" world they will face after graduation.

What about the reality of their daily lives, in and out of school? Schools are wonderful places for kids to learn about the changes their bodies are going through, the realities of competition and cooperation, conformity behavior, responsibility for one's self, human psychology, family dynamics, and so much more. Should these things be taught instead of the three R's? Of course not! These issues should be the context in which the fundamentals are taught. And they all tie in to our concern here: the kids' ability to deal with the drug culture in a responsible way.

Prevention of what? If the major goal of drug prevention programs to date has been primary prevention—stopping young people from experimenting with drugs—we have failed miserably. It may even be that by paying so much attention to the informational approach and letting media hype serve as our main vehicle, we have created the very monster we thought we were slaying. For example, made-for-television movies and docudramas seem to deal only with the horrors of teenage addiction or alcoholism. Think about this the next time you see a TV movie about a twelve-year-old girl, strung out on dope and selling her body. What did you learn? Probably nothing of value. You were titillated. We need to be clear about what we are trying to say to our young people. These programs only create more curiosity and morbid interest.

Secondary prevention programs are those geared toward helping young people already experimenting with drugs to avoid developing drug-related problems resulting from ignorance, arrogance, or immoderate behavior. Kids need our help so they don't:

- get pregnant while high,
- get in cars when the driver has been drinking or drugging,
- ingest dangerous drug combinations,
- freak out on volatile drugs like PCP,
- start dealing drugs.

The key elements of a secondary prevention program are:

1. Sharing of factual drug information
2. Teaching about what drugs do and don't do

3. Exploration of risk factors that lead to drug abuse
4. Frank discussions about peer pressure and conformity
5. Establishing the difference between moderation and abuse
6. Demonstrating ways to handle an emergency situation
7. Exploring alternatives to drugs—nonchemical ways of "turning on" to life and pursuing altered states
8. Creative forums where the kids can talk openly
9. Reaching out to youths in trouble with drugs and other problems
10. Allowing a celebration of youth
11. Developing an ethos of responsibility for one's own body and mind
12. Promoting lifelong practices in good health

The best way to achieve this is for parents and school to work together. In some families these types of issues can be discussed easily; in other families these issues are too hot to handle and need to be addressed in the school setting. That's one reason for making sure the program planning council is comprised of teachers, administrators, students, and parents.

Prevention Program Ideas

Drug Information Library: Available to all students and faculty.

Drug Information Hotline: Gives factual information only. Not a counseling service.

Crisis Intervention Hotline: Gives out drug information and refers callers to available agencies and services.

School Health Fair: Substance misuse is one among other health topics.

Big Brother/Big Sister Program: Kids need healthy role models; older kids befriend and guide younger kids.

Psychodrama and Role Playing: People are growing tired of lectures. Theater using family and adolescent life themes can generate a lot of interest and discussion.

Communication Skills Workshops: Help kids and parents to talk to one another.

Values Clarification Exercises: Stop preaching and help people to creatively formulate and articulate their own values.

Affective Education: Help students to see the powerful role that emotions play in our daily lives.

Sex Education Program: A lot of drug use and misuse occurs around ignorance of our bodies and the relationship between sex and self-image.

Nondrug Ways of Exploring Altered States of Consciousness: This one may take you further than the drug issue. Meditation, running, religious mysticism, yoga—are all fascinating.

Family Life Education Course: Open to parents and students. Can combine didactic (factual) and experiential (exercises) format.

Film Program: Show some good ones and some bad ones and have your audience critique them. Remember, films are only meant to be "triggers" to discussion, not an end in themselves.

Smoking Cessation Program: This is the one that always seems to elude the school setting. You can help kids stop smoking before it becomes a lifelong habit.

Nutrition and Exercise Program: Most kids find "gym" is a drag. Make it more upbeat by helping kids stay trim and eat right through action, not lectures. Junk food may be as harmful as drug abuse.

SOME REALITIES ABOUT DEALING DRUGS

The sale of licit drugs which are controlled substances (can't be obtained without a doctor's prescription—such as Valium) or illicit drugs (illegal by definition—such as heroin) is against the law. That means federal, state, and local ordinances. Laws

94

vary greatly from one part of the country to another, and you need to check this out for your locality. The state police and the local district attorney's office are reliable sources of such information. Even if you think the laws on the books represent "cruel and unusual" punishment or are scientifically inaccurate (how did a hallucinogen like marijuana end up in the same category as heroin or morphine?), your local law-enforcement officials have an obligation to enforce these laws. Some of them do it with relish. In some parts of the country kids and adults end up doing time in jail or prison for a drug offense which would net them only a slap on the wrist in another locale. (See Appendix D for a state-by-state listing of marijuana laws.) Possession of up to seven-eighths of an ounce of marijuana in New York State can only lead to a citation (analogous to a traffic summons) and no criminal record. Try holding that much grass in some southern states and you can end up behind bars and be subject to a stiff fine. However, possess a full ounce or more in New York State and the criminal penalties begin, ranging from misdemeanor to felony depending on the amount and whether or not there was intent to sell. This greater quantity (usually a pound or more of grass, less for other drugs) is called "dealing in weight." Dealing in weight can get you into serious trouble in any state in the Union.

Money or the allure of "free drugs" is the hook that can lead to some big-time headaches for small-time dealers. How do you get free drugs? Consider this from a seventeen-year-old high-school senior:

> It's really easy to keep yourself in free dope, man. Say I buy half a pound of weed [marijuana] for $500. That's eight ounces, right? If I sell seven ounces at $75 per, I take in $525 and I keep one ounce for free and make $25 profit to boot. If I sell the whole eight, I make $100 profit. But I'm not greedy, I just want to keep myself in drugs.

In case someone you know is considering setting up a dealership, consider the sequel:

Things were going along fine for a whole year. I was only selling drugs to people I knew first-hand. I never sold bad stuff. Only quality merchandise—grass and some pills, mostly Quaaludes. You'll never believe what did me in! The cops caught a couple of kids committing vandalism. They were high on beer and ludes. One of the kids, who bought the pills from me, panicked. The cops said if he would tell them where he bought the drugs they would go easy on him. He ratted me out [informed] and the cops nailed me with enough pills in my pocket to get me some heavy time. Some friend!

Drug dealing is big business in America. According to Attorney General William French Smith, gross drug sales nationwide approached $79 billion in 1980, "about equal to the combined profits of America's 500 largest industrial corporations." The illicit marijuana crop in California alone is estimated to be worth in excess of $5 billion. Even lookouts for drug dealers can earn weekly incomes of four to five hundred dollars. The temptations are very real, but it must be kept in mind that the lower down the organizational ladder the drug dealer is, the more vulnerable he is. Middle-class small-time drug dealers don't often appreciate the risks they take when dealing with professional dealers. The *New York Times*[5] told the sad story of Barry S. Weinbaum, a campus drug dealer at Bennington College, whose life was ended at age twenty-two on the Lower East Side of Manhattan; his body was found in a green plastic bag jammed between two decaying buildings. He was dressed in the collegiate clothes that had been his trademark at Bennington. Barry had put himself through school with his earnings from dealing cocaine. The former editor of the college newspaper, captain of the softball team, student of Shakespeare, and proofreader of psychiatric texts met his death traveling in a lethal world of drug dealing in an urban ghetto. Barry wasn't as street-wise as he thought.

Young people rarely understand how frightening it can be to deal with the police. Even when the officers are simply doing their job and not using techniques like entrapment, getting arrested is a real drag. Having their rights read to them, being photographed and fingerprinted, and then having the police call their parents is a shot of reality that anyone can live without.

The police and society in general reserve a special kind of outrage for drug dealers. People are aware that the more drugs are available, the more readily they will be purchased and consumed. Many communities have mounted strong efforts to cut off the supply of drugs coming in. It is certainly true that the really big drug dealers are rarely caught or prosecuted because they hire expensive "dope" lawyers and have some pretty nasty ways of dealing with people who might testify against them. But your local police may be very content to apprehend the small-time dealer. There are several good reasons for this:

1. the law requires them to do so,
2. they are easier to catch and prosecute,
3. the officers may reside in the town where they work and wish to keep drug dealers away from their own families, and
4. arrests lead to promotions.

I have worked with a lot of kids who have been in trouble with the law. Most of them thought the police were "dummies" who busted people only so they could smoke their dope. Experienced officers are very good at this kind of police work and they have some very sophisticated equipment at their disposal. Arresting officers often look like long-distance truck drivers, not cops. These cops are street-wise and love to nail the kid who thinks he can outsmart them.

The trend toward relaxing drug laws so popular during the late 1970s has been halted and may even be reversed. President Carter was seriously considering the decriminalization of marijuana. The Reagan administration shows no similar inclination. With the First Lady's strong interest in the misuse of drugs by the young, it is highly unlikely that any liberalizing trends will be promoted under the present administration in Washington.

Police officers and judges may have a somewhat lenient attitude toward first offenders when the charge involves only simple drug possession. However, they tend to take a much tougher stance when the charge is "possession with the intent to sell" or actual sales. The defendant can forget about saying he was holding it for a friend. No one believes that line anymore. Even if you don't do time or pay a fine (if you are lucky), you will still have a criminal record. If this record includes a felony conviction, it can hurt later on in life. One may find oneself banned from certain professional practices such as law and medicine (the AMA and the ABA have boards of ethics), unable to get bonded, unable to pass security clearances for sensitive positions, and so on. As police records become computerized, it will be easier to keep track of these things, and the likelihood of being haunted forever will increase.

When I was in college I tried just about every drug known on campus including heroin. As an adult I only do grass and coke. I was the finalist for a very lucrative job with a Fortune 100 firm. They made me take a lie detector test as part of the final phase of interviewing. As soon as the tester asked me "Have you ever used . . . ?" and then went down a long list of drugs, I knew I was doomed. Sure enough, he stopped the test and called in someone from the personnel department who explained that the job was no longer mine.

If you or someone close to you is arrested, remember that you have certain rights under the law. As a general rule, you should say nothing without advice of counsel. Anything you say may be held against you in a court of law. Getting arrested can really shake you up, but you must be indicted and found guilty before the penalty of the law can be brought to bear. If your child is arrested, he or she will need your help. Don't assume guilt until you have heard their side of things—no matter what the arresting officer says. The main object is to get them home and to consult an attorney. Letting them sit in jail overnight to "teach them a lesson" presumes guilt.

The wisest approach is to keep Baretta's warning in mind:

"Don't do the crime if you can't do the time." Stay far away from trafficking in drugs.

HELPING KIDS TO HELP THEMSELVES

The youth drug scene is like a net with large holes. Those kids who experiment with drugs, for the most part, will pass safely through the holes of the net, not experiencing any difficulties with the drugs. Then there are those kids who get caught in the net, turning experimentation into use, into abuse, into addiction. Parents and other adults are usually the last to know. This places young people in a unique position to try to come to the aid of their friends. Now this is a tricky business, and there are no rules. Perhaps by getting away from the notion of everyone "doing their own thing," we as adults can aid our young people, including our own children, to develop a higher sense of social responsibility. Kids try on new fads and friends like clothes. They are doing this at the very same time that they are developing a sense of idealism. Kids have a way of reaching out to one another and caring for their peers. By the time most of us became adults we had successfully learned to turn inward, ignoring the needs of others. The kids today see this and shy away from us as jaded and selfish. But if we come to our children with a sense of caring for their greater community as well as our own, we can place drugs in the context of broader and more enduring issues.

In the following pages you'll find some suggestions for your kids to try out when they want to help their friends. By discussing this advice with your children, you can accomplish a number of important goals:

1. show your kids you realize that drug use occurs in a complicated social context,
2. show them that you care about their friends,
3. model the kind of communication skills you wish to impart to them, and

4. show them you realize that the drug issue is about people, not statistics. (These suggestions, by the way, apply to adult friendships as well.)

Modeling moderation or abstinence: People tend to play follow-the-leader. In many situations kids will be afraid to seem "unhip" and will drink or use drugs even when they don't really want to. This is classic conformity behavior (something we worried about a lot in the 1960s). Help your kids to understand this, and to see that groups need models for abstinence and moderation as well as drunkenness and macho drinking bouts. Doing what you really want requires more maturity and assertiveness than simply aping others' behavior. If just one person says "No" or "Enough for me," this can keep a whole group's drinking or drugging from sinking to the lowest common denominator (usually the person who doesn't know when to stop).

Stating concerns: Parents are often better at this than kids. However, kids do it with fewer games. If someone you know is starting to get into trouble when they drink or drug, what do you do? What would you advise your kids to do? One of the most important questions you can ask someone when trying to diagnose a drug problem is, "Has anyone ever spoken to you about your drug taking?" Often the answer is no. By ignoring people in trouble we enable them to get worse. People who con themselves into believing that they are not in trouble with drugs will only get worse if someone doesn't speak up. It's certainly easy enough to ignore them. If you have any real regard for the person in question, you should state your concern without being judgmental or putting them down. *Say:* "I really worry about you when you have been drinking. Last night everyone was laughing at you and putting you down." *Don't say:* "You are really a fool when you drink. Why don't you wise up and stop drinking!"

What needs to be communicated is responsible concern, the heart of which is this: "I love you but sometimes you do dangerous or silly things. And when you do I will tell you about it because

I care." Help your kids to understand how defensive most adolescents are. ("Don't kick a door down when you can use a key.") On the other hand, if you aren't being heard, you can escalate into a more assertive and hard-hitting statement such as: "I have been trying to reach you and you don't seem to want to hear me. If drinking or drugging is more important to you than honest feedback from a friend, you have a problem. If you want to talk about it I'll be around." This approach requires a lot of patience and can be very frustrating. However, keep these two things in mind:

1. No one is responsible for anyone else's drugging or drinking.
2. You are responsible only for sending the message. The other person is responsible for hearing or not hearing.

Using the "horse" concept. This approach takes stating your concerns a step further. The horse concept goes like this:

If you meet a man on the street and he says, "You are a horse," you scratch your head and wonder if he's nuts. If you continue on and meet a friend who says, "You are a horse," you begin to wonder what is going on. If when you arrive home your sister says, "You are a horse," then you might consider having some hay for dinner.

If the person with the drug problem can't hear you alone, then get some more people who share your perception and concern and speak to him or her in a group. Don't "rat pack" or gang up on your friend with everyone being righteous and talking at the same time. Each person should calmly but firmly state his or her concerns and let your friend know that they wish to help.

Taking a position about your friendship: If your friend is letting drugs come between you, then you have an important choice to make. Kids used to complain to me a lot about what a drag it is to deal with "acid heads" and "Jesus freaks." Their basic complaint is that these kids were capable of relating to people

101

only through drugs or their own brand of Christianity. People want to have a direct relatedness to one another. They don't want any third party getting in the way. If your friends are relating to you only via drugs, then they are not valuing you as a person. You may have to ask them to choose between a meaningful relationship with you and getting high (at least when they are with you). The focus here is on persistent drug use. If the drugs mean that much to them, they aren't ready to have you for a friend. This hurts, but it happens quite often when young people and adults start substituting drugs for people.

Seeking advice: When someone you care about is in trouble with drugs and won't listen to your sound advice, it can be very upsetting to you. Maybe someone else needs to be consulted. Where young people are involved there are two ways to go. One way is to keep your friend's identity hidden. The other is to reveal his or her name. As a parent you would like to feel that your own kids can approach you when they have a concern about themselves or a close friend. You will have to help them to see that sometimes professional help is required. If your own child approaches you about a friend, it is not really necessary for you to know the other child's name. If the drug abuse becomes life-threatening, however, the whole equation may shift radically. How long should anyone wait before volunteering a name? There is no simple answer, but it is clear that most people wait too long. You may have to be willing to put the friendship on the line. To ignore a serious situation which then turns ugly or tragic can lead to a lifetime of guilt. It is commendable that kids will seek advice and then try to use that advice with their friend. But kids have to know that when their best efforts fail, other people must be brought into the picture. If "squealing" saves a life, then it certainly is worthwhile.

Lending an ear: A friend is someone who listens. Sometimes just being a good passive listener can be a release and comfort to a friend. Sometimes we have to be active listeners. Many people use drugs to mask unpleasant or painful feelings or life situations.

Try to be there for them when they are not high. If they seem blue or angry or just plain upset, try to get them to talk it out with you. If they do it while they are high, try to get them to talk about it later when they are straight. The task here is to be not a drug counselor but a hearing and caring friend. A good tool to use in these situations is called "reflecting feelings." Instead of making value judgments or giving direct advice, you can say things like "That must be hard to deal with" or "I'll bet that makes you feel real sad." These kinds of statements make it possible for people to open up even more. You can then go on to share your own feelings and thoughts on the subject.

Drawing the line: One of the toughest things we ever have to do with people we really care about, like family members or close friends, is to take a strong position. For example, if you see someone close to you about to snort some heroin, you will be right in letting them know what a dumb and dangerous thing they are about to do and that you want nothing further to do with them if they must persist in using heroin. And no one who values their life will travel in a car when the driver is drunk or stoned—it could end in tragedy. You would be wise to flatly refuse the ride (and even wiser not to permit that person to drive at all). Or if you find out that your friend is spending all his or her money on cocaine and wants to borrow some from you, you would be wise to turn them down.

Turning on to life (without drugs): Happiness is a lull between disasters. Even the most powerful feelings of ecstasy are usually quite short-lived. We keep trying to make "sense out of nonsense." All of us are born with a wonderful capacity to experience life emotionally. Sense is the use of the central nervous system for rational thought. Why do we prohibit using that same mechanism for feeling our emotions (nonsense)? People keep using drugs to get to various states of feeling because we are uptight about expressing and sharing our emotions. Almost all the drug addicts and alcoholics I have known have problems in the area of feelings. Only when they are able to learn to handle these feelings is a drug-free life possible. This means that prevention efforts must address themselves to the social and emotional life of young people if they are to work. Teaching young people to express and talk out their feelings is the ounce of prevention we should be pursuing, instead of lectures on pharmacology. Want to get high without drugs? Try some of the following:

- run across an open field or along a beach
- ask one of your grandparents what life is about
- play with a baby
- give a friend a gift that you made with your own hands
- work hard at something and see it through to completion
- learn to meditate
- stop eating junk food
- write some poetry for yourself (it doesn't have to rhyme)
- climb a mountain
- say thank you more often
- beat the shit out of a pillow the next time you are really angry
- stop biting your nails (or shed another bad habit)
- read a good book (later for the comic books or video games)
- give someone a real long hug
- call your father at work and tell him you love him
- have a good cry about that thing you have been hiding for too long

Feels good just thinking about some of these things, right? The next time you want to get high just ask yourself if the drugs are really necessary. But drugs or not, don't expect to hold on to the feeling for very long. That's how emotions are. They run like a river—from streams to oceans. Don't push the river, flow with it!

Our society is the play-it-safe crowd. We don't seem to want to get involved anymore. We don't want to be hurt. But this is unrealistic—having your feelings hurt is part of living. Like stress, it is unavoidable. If you want to have friends and be intimate with people, you have to take chances. This is the message we must give our young people if we are going to teach them to help others. Showing responsible concern to friends is not easy, but it makes for enduring and more meaningful relationships. The best way to teach your kids is to be a good model yourself. By following the suggestions made in this chapter in the context of school life and combining them with material from the chapter on the family, you will have a good, constructive link between the two places where children spend most of their time.

CHAPTER THREE

Drugs and the Workplace

I was using speed to wake me up and keep me going during the workday. I used downs [barbiturates] and alcohol to get me to sleep at night. The diet pills I took had some more speed in them. I liked to smoke grass and do some cocaine on the weekends. Once in a while I would drop a lude to mellow me out. It got to be a real hassle at work. I have a responsible job and the drugs were getting in the way. It's a full-time job just balancing all the drugs. Sometimes I would forget things and really get disorganized. Eventually I could not keep it all together. So I took a holiday from drugs and everything has been a lot calmer.

—VICE PRESIDENT, *Fortune 500 company*

The kids who came up through the counterculture of the 1960s and early '70s have entered the work force. Whether introduced to drugs during the days of campus protest or in the rice paddies of Vietnam, a whole generation of young people have grown into their maturity for whom drugs were very much a part of that maturing process. Drugs that used to be found among students, musicians, street people, and other fringe groups within society have made their way into the workplace. Mainstream America is turning on. The sweet smell of marijuana is now emanating from corporate boardrooms, typing pools, assembly lines, and union meeting halls. Drugs have become a fact of life in working America. There are many reasons why people use drugs at work:

- to counteract boredom
- to counteract fatigue
- to energize themselves
- to deal with pressure and tension
- to tune out on work
- to get through the workday
- to tranquilize and calm themselves
- to facilitate business deals
- to make extra money selling drugs at work
- to put themselves in a creative frame of mind
- to show off (especially status drugs like cocaine)
- to counteract "burnout"
- to self-medicate against depression and anxiety
- to be more outgoing
- to stay awake
- to shut off nonwork stimuli
- to forget about troubles

This is only a partial list. There are almost as many reasons as there are people using drugs. Some people take drugs as a planned act. Others take drugs without conceiving of their actions as "drug taking"; examples of this are smoking cigarettes, drinking coffee, and the use of alcohol. Some people actively seek to get high while at work. Others take medications, both prescription and OTC (over the counter), to deal with any number of physical symptoms and maladies. (Over $500 million a year is spent on cold remedies alone, and $5 billion a year in wages and productivity are lost due to the common cold.) Few people realize that food acts as a mood changer and happily eat their way through millions of business breakfasts, lunches, and dinners each year, altering their emotional states at work.

There are powerful emotional biases at work when people discuss drugs. Very few people have a neutral attitude. They tend to be defensive, judgmental, argumentative, condescending, proselytizing, grandiose, all-knowing, righteous. People who use drugs all have their own drug(s) of choice and tend to look askance at the next person's choices. In the words of one college student:

> My grandfather had his home-grown wine, my father likes his Scotch, my mother digs martinis and I like grass and hash. It's all the same shit. Man, we are all just trying to get high. It seems when I try to talk about this with my folks that one person's drug is another person's poison. I wish everyone would be a little more honest about what's really going down.

And in the words of a middle-management insurance executive:

> The big bosses down a lot of booze during lunch and after hours. The girls in the secretarial pool like to smoke pot. My colleagues and I enjoy a little coke after work and sometimes we do it when we have to work long hours and meet a deadline. God only knows what drugs the file clerks are doing.

None of these people are addicted. They manage to use drugs in a manner they feel is safe and fun and even productive (at work). They are quick to defend their drugs of choice and can rhapsodize about them for hours. Alcohol has not had to give way to the newer drugs, which have simply been added to the list. Whether your preference is for a brandy alexander or a line of coke, you are chemically altering your consciousness.

The United States Armed Forces constitutes a significant proportion of the American work force, with some 3 million active-duty soldiers and another 3 million military dependents. The military estimates that the equivalent of four battalions of infantry a year are unavailable for duty because of drug-related problems (the soldiers are in jail or in treatment). A Department of Defense worldwide survey[1] of active-duty personnel reported that about 83 percent drank occasionally and 21 percent indicated a heavy beer-drinking pattern (eight or more drinks in a single day at least monthly during the past twelve months). The same survey reported that although the highest prevalence of drinking any alcohol was recorded by senior officers, heavy drinking was reported almost exclusively by enlisted personnel. It is estimated that the cost of lost production to the military due to alcohol abuse is $410 million annually. When a jet plane crashed on the deck of the *USS Nimitz* it was discovered that six out of ten crew members had evidence of recent marijuana use in their bodies. While teaching a course on alcoholism counseling to a group of noncommissioned officers at West Point, I was told:

> Whether you drink or drug has a lot to do with where you are stationed. A tour in Korea is viewed as a drinking man's tour, as the Korean government takes a hard line against drug use. A tour in Europe, especially West Germany, means easy access to a wide variety of drugs including hashish and heroin. I've been all over the world in this man's army and I've seen just about every form of drug use and abuse imaginable.

Vietnam-era veterans strongly resent the stereotype that they are all either drug addicts or alcoholics or walking time bombs ready to commit violent acts against civilians. These men know that a lot of heavy-duty drinking and drugging went on in Vietnam and that some of them came home with a drug problem that required active treatment. But they also know that most of the troops who drank and drugged in Vietnam did not bring the problem home. Studies have shown a surprisingly high remission rate even for heroin addiction, without benefit of treatment. This is true despite the fact that some vets suffer from post-traumatic delayed-stress syndrome and use drugs and alcohol as a self-administered form of relief. One soldier put it this way:

When you are in an insane place like 'Nam you do insane things just to get from day to day. Getting stoned was just another way of counting off the days and passing time between missions until you finished your tour and went back to the world [home].

A practical problem faced by many veterans has been that prospective employers fear they may be undependable because they served in a war that has left them psychological casualties. If there is one thing that a person recovering from addiction needs to ensure that recovery, it is a job. It is essential for a sense of personal and family dignity, as well as for paying the bills.

There are some 13 million alcoholics and problem drinkers in America. Only about 5 percent of these men and women can be found on skid row. The other 12,350,000 are people just like you and me. A $450 million private (profit-making) alcoholism treatment network has grown up to serve the 10 percent of corporate America who can't handle their alcohol. It is also estimated that two-thirds of the drug and alcohol abuse in business and industry is suppressed. Traditionally the drug alcohol has had the greatest degree of acceptance in American society, and therefore in the commerce and industry of that society. It was once common for workers to have a drink on the job (the "4 o'clock dram"). To the extent that the captains of industry tend to predate the newer drugs, they tend to frown upon them. To the extent that your boss is young enough or "hip" enough to have been exposed to coke, grass, and hashish, he or she will probably use them in secret (public espousal would spell condemnation). But the other drugs are coming up from the underground in offices and factories all over America. Workers at all levels, including supervisors, are developing an "emotional radar system" with which they seek out kindred souls in drug use. Most of the cues are subtle, but a certain word used here or there or a phrase unique to the drug culture is a real clue to who is using and who isn't. Don't be fooled by traditional stereotypes. Drug use, just like alcohol use, is becoming very democratic. You don't need long hair or dark glasses or to speak in street slang to appreciate the effects of many drugs. The fellow in the vested suit and rep tie is just as likely to be getting high as the more obvious counterculture types.

As much as 10 percent of the national work force is suffering from alcoholism or problem drinking. The most current official estimates are that alcoholism and problem drinking are causing a loss to American society of $50–60 billion a year. Alcohol abuse and alcoholism feature prominently in lost productivity and sales, health and medical costs, industrial accidents, absenteeism, lateness, grievances, training, and termination costs. Alcoholism also figures prominently in rape, assault, murder, child molesting, child abuse and neglect, spouse abuse and other domestic violence, suicide, automobile accidents, and automobile accident deaths.

More on the Impact of Alcoholism in Industry

1. Nationally, an average of 6 percent of all employees suffer from alcoholism and 4 percent from problem drinking, causing a majority of labor-management problems such as:
   - The alcoholic employee is absent two to four times more often than the nonalcoholic employee.
   - On-the-job accidents to alcoholic employees are two to four times more frequent than among nonalcoholic employees. Off-the-job accidents are four to six times more frequent.
   - Sickness and accident benefits paid out for alcoholic employees are three times greater than for the average nonalcoholic employee.
   - In one assembly plant, out of 746 grievances filed during one year, 48.6 percent were alcohol related.
2. It is conservatively estimated that each alcoholic employee costs a company the equivalent of 25 percent of his or her salary.
3. The annual cost to American industry is in excess of $11 billion.
4. An undetermined percentage of employees are seriously affected by an alcoholism problem in their family.

Drugs in the workplace cost businesses in increased absentee-ism, poor work performance, thefts, accidents, wasted time, and higher insurance rates. Negative consequences to the employee include industrial accidents, failure to be promoted, lost time and pay, bad references, loss of job, and a criminal record (if arrested on the job for illicit drug possession or sale). The American work force is involved in significant rates of regular drug use in all occupational groups except farming.

Heroin addicts can and do hold down paying jobs, are hard to detect, and commit a wide variety of crimes at the work site. Here are some of the "scams" that addicts run in the work setting:[2]

auto mechanic	steals parts and tools
clothing machine operator	steals coats by placing them in the garbage and picking them up after hours
phone installer	falsifies installation orders and sells phones to customers at one-half price
stock clerk	steals negotiable bonds, forges an I.D. and cashes bonds at local bank
medical assistant	steals drugs and syringes
credit collector	steals cash payments
air conditioning installer	steals tools and parts, burgles customers' apartments
steel-mill worker	wholesales large quantities of marijuana in an abandoned section of the plant
pharmacy clerk	steals prescriptions

dry-cleaning-store worker	gives customer receipts to friends who claim the customers' clothing
secretary	steals money from co-workers' purses
supermarket worker	steals meat ("cattle rustling") and sells it in the neighborhood at half-price
truck driver	steals from workers' lockers
nurse's aide	steals syringes and other medical supplies
messenger	steals cash from employer

I have worked with a number of corporate officers who used far more elaborate and sophisticated schemes to steal money from their companies, all to feed a drug habit (heroin or cocaine). I treated a young man who sold both stocks and drugs on the floor of the New York Stock Exchange. I also treated a college registrar who used a computer terminal to secure student loans for fictitious students, all to support his cocaine use. Working addicts are more similar to other workers than they are to nonworking addicts. For example, they tend to be older, better educated, more often married, and are more likely to be white than nonworking addicts. Despite their heroin habits, more than half hold their jobs for a year or more.

RISE AND SHINE

Can you guess what drug these people are talking about?

I can't get started without it. I'm no good to anyone until I have some!

113

Every time I need a lift I take some; it really energizes me.

Some times when I've had too much I really feel wired and a little crazy. Like I can't sit still, or stop talking, and I'm constantly running to the bathroom.

The more I have in the morning, the less I feel like having lunch.

I would never have gotten through my final exams in college without it.

Have you guessed yet? Symptoms of usage in many people are virtually indistinguishable from an anxiety condition. Here is some more information that may help.[3]

MYSTERY-DRUG SYMPTOMS:

irritability

nervousness

nausea

vomiting

diarrhea

epigastric pain (*in region over the pit of the stomach*)

diuresis (*abnormal secretion of urine*)

flushing

arrhythmias (*irregular heartbeat*)

sensory disturbance

insomnia

tremulousness

agitation

palpitations

headaches

ringing in the ears

visual flashes of light

delayed sleep onset

frequent sleep interruption

SIGNS THAT DOCTORS LOOK FOR:
tachypnea (*abnormal rapidity of breathing*)
reflex hyperexcitability
muscle twitching
hyperesthesia (*increased sensitivity to touch*)
extrasystoles (*premature contractions of one of the parts of the heart*)
tachycardia (*abnormal rapidity of the heart*)
arrhythmias (*irregular heartbeat*)

WITHDRAWAL SIGNS INCLUDE:
headache
nervousness
irritability
lethargy
restlessness
drowsiness and excessive yawning
dysphoria (*opposite of euphoria*)
disinclination to work
inability to concentrate
nausea
runny nose

Answer: The drug is *caffeine!* You have just read a description of the symptoms and signs of caffeinism, or "coffee-drinker's syndrome," the name given to chronic caffeine intoxification. People who suffer from caffeinism have a history of drinking a lot of coffee (five to ten cups a day) or other products containing caffeine.

Sixty percent of American adults drink an average of more than two cups of coffee per day; 25 percent drink five or more cups a day; and 10 percent drink seven or more cups a day. It takes about 50 to 100 milligrams of caffeine to produce the characteristic pharmacologic action of the drug. Many people consume enough caffeine each day to produce symptoms of caffeinism with-

Caffeine Found in Foods and Drugs

Source	Caffeine (milligrams)
BEVERAGES	
Coffee (*5 ounces*)	
Drip method	146
Percolated	110
Instant regular	53
Decaffeinated	2
Tea (*5 ounces*) (*loose or in tea bags*)	
1-minute brew	9–33
3-minute brew	20–46
5-minute brew	20–50
Iced tea, can (12 ounces)	22–36
Cocoa and Chocolate	
Cocoa (made from mix), 6 ounces	10
Milk chocolate, 1 ounce	6
Baking chocolate, 1 ounce	35
Soda (*12-ounce cans*)*	
Diet Mr. Pibb	52
Mountain Dew	52
Mello Yellow	51
Tab	44
Shasta Cola	42
Dr Pepper	38
Diet Dr Pepper	37
Pepsi Cola	37
Royal Crown Cola	36
Diet Rite Cola	34
Diet Pepsi	34
Coca-Cola	34
Mr. Pibb	33
Cragmore Cola	Trace
7-Up	0
Sprite	0
Diet 7-Up	0
RC-100	0

Source	Caffeine (milligrams)
BEVERAGES	
Diet Sunkist Orange	0
Sunkist Orange	0
Patio Orange	0
Fanta Orange	0
Fresca	0
Hires Root Beer	0
NONPRESCRIPTION DRUGS (STANDARD DOSE)	
Stimulants	
Caffedrine capsules	200
NoDoz tablets	200
Vivarin tablets	200
Pain Relievers	
Anacin	64
Excedrin	130
Midol	65
Plain aspirin	0
Tylenol	0
Diuretics	
Aqua-Ban	200
Permathene H_2Off	200
Pre-Mens Forte	100
Cold Remedies	
Coryban-D	30
Dristan	32
Triaminicin	30
Weight-control aids	
Dexatrim	200
Dietac	200
Promaline	280

* As tested by Consumers Union for October 1981 issue of *Consumer Reports;* formulations may change.
Source: Consumer Reports, October 1981, © Consumers Union of the United States, Inc.

out consciously realizing it. A child who consumes a lot of chocolate (there are about 25 milligrams per small bar) and cola soft drinks (or others containing caffeine—see the table) runs the same risks of caffeinism due to his lower body weight.

Caffeine belongs to a class of drugs called methylxanthines. The three main drugs found in this class are caffeine, theobromine (found in chocolate milk and cocoa), and theophylline. Decaffeinated coffee contains a small amount of caffeine (about 2 milligrams) and some theobromine and theophylline.

Among heavy users, the drug caffeine causes physical dependence, with withdrawal symptoms and craving. Heroin addicts in both drug-free and methadone-maintenance treatment programs drink an inordinate amount of coffee, up to twenty cups per day. And they will add 3 to 5 teaspoons of sugar to each cup of coffee. This looks like symptom substitution to many in the field who are concerned about switched addictions. These addicts were barely detoxified from heroin before they had already adopted a new drug habit. When I directed the Alcoholism Treatment Program at Beth Israel Medical Center in New York City, we served only decaffeinated coffee to our patients. This was done to eliminate the mood-altering effects of coffee and to prevent gastritis and stomach ulcers so often found in alcoholics.

Caffeine has no nutritional value and only about 5 calories per cup. However, when you add a teaspoon of sugar (15 to 25 calories) and a teaspoon of cream (another 30 calories), you can see how coffee drinking can add to your waistline.

There is a growing controversy about the relative safety of caffeine. There exist a number of presumptive links, based on several studies, between caffeine and a number of serious health problems. Everyone agrees that caffeine stimulates the central nervous system, can constrict blood vessels and speed up the heart, and stimulates the brain, stomach, kidneys, ovaries, and testes. For many people caffeine's action is similar to another stimulant drug—methamphetamine, known as "speed." It first lifts you up and then sets you down, sometimes with depressed feelings. As caffeine causes a rise and fall of blood sugar levels it can lead to symptoms commonly found in hypoglycemia (low blood sugar) such as fatigue, lethargy, and depression.

Joan's Story

Joan had been in and out of psychotherapy over a period of seven years. Diagnosed as suffering from an "anxiety neurosis" by other therapists, she could not understand why all the money she had spent on therapy had not brought her some significant relief. Her family doctor gave her a clean bill of health and suggested she was suffering from "nerves," which led to her first therapy referral. Although the doctor asked her about drinking and drugs it never occurred to him to ask her about her coffee drinking. Fortunately for Joan, she gave herself away in our first session together. She had brought a thermos full of steaming hot coffee! She complained to me of chronic nervousness, periodic bouts of depression, and years of sleep disturbance. All this despite her happy marriage, a rewarding job, and two lovely children. Her doctor had, of course, prescribed a tranquilizer for her "nerves." On workdays Joan drank about twelve to fifteen cups of coffee, and twenty per day on weekends. She had no idea that she had a serious drug problem. I asked her why she brought the thermos of coffee, and she answered that she was nervous and that the coffee helped to relax her. When I explained to her about caffein addiction, it took only two sessions for her to understand and accept what had been happening to her. She did taper off slowly and then switched to decaffeinated coffee. About a month later she had a "slip" and began sneaking more regular coffee. A referral to Pills Anonymous (P.A.) gave Joan the added group support she needed to deal with her drug craving. Today she drinks only drug-free herbal tea and feels much better. This time the total cost of therapy was $250 (P.A. is free). The previous missed diagnosis had cost Joan thousands of dollars in unnecessary therapy.

According to Dr. Sanford Miller, director of the Food and Drug Administration's Bureau of Foods, caffeine is "a potent biologically active material." The FDA is seriously considering two actions at this time: one is the removal of caffeine from its list of "Generally Recognized as Safe (GRAS)" list of food additives, and the second is to eliminate the present requirement that cola drinks contain caffeine. The FDA is taking the position that more needs to be known. Dr. Miller states the agency's position on caffeine (April 1982): "We are not saying it's unsafe, we're just not saying it's safe." Our current concern over caffeine began in 1978 when an advisory committee to the FDA reported that too much caffeine might have a deleterious effect on central-nervous-system development. Since then several studies have linked the drug with birth defects, fibrocystic breast disease (a nonmalignant disorder), and pancreatic cancer.

Researchers from the Boston Collaborative Drug Surveillance Program surveyed hospital patients who had had a coronary and those who had been admitted for other conditions. They found that men and women who drank more than four cups of coffee a day were twice as likely to have a heart attack as those who abstained from it. The fly in the ointment may be the variable of cigarette smoking. According to Dr. Jean Mayer, president of Tufts University and one of America's leading nutrition experts: "While there is a correlation between coffee drinking and cigarette smoking, the reasons for the relationship between coffee drinking and heart attacks remain a mystery." Other studies have suggested an association between coffee drinking and bladder cancer. Again, the villain here may be the association between coffee drinking and cigarette smoking, as a causal relationship between smoking and bladder cancer has been established.

Children who consume six cans of cola per day or the equivalent (in chocolate candy, for instance) become jumpy and speak faster than normal. Adults who consume the same amount of caffeine (about 300 milligrams) have more subjective reactions, such as mood changes.

Because of the possibility of birth defects, more and more doctors are advising abstinence and certainly moderation (no more than two cups or equivalent per day) for pregnant women. In September 1980 Dr. Jere Goyan, then FDA commissioner, said that a pregnant woman should "put caffeine on her list of unnecessary substances which she should avoid." Scientists at Harvard

University studied the effects of coffee drinking in more than 12,000 women and reported their results in the January 1982 issue of the *New England Journal of Medicine.* They found no detectable ill effects on the unborn babies caused by caffeine, but they did find defects caused by cigarette smoking.

In 1981 an editorial appeared in the medical journal *Lancet,* which said that *moderate* coffee drinking had not been definitively shown to cause any harm and recommended that those who enjoyed it should probably continue. According to the *Book of Health,* published by the American Health Foundation, "Used in *moderation* [emphasis added], it [coffee] is not harmful to most people." Dr. Mayer states:

> In the meantime, what is the coffee drinker to do? The answer, I think, is *moderation* [emphasis added]. Coffee drinking can become excessive—up to ten or fifteen cups a day. And if all that coffee contains cream and sugar, the caloric intake can be substantial. It is not unreasonable to set five cups as an upper limit.

Doses are usually described for the "average" person. "Average" or "normal" is a statistical concept and many of us deviate from the norm. Don't worry about your friends who can consume lots of coffee or cola without negative effects. If you are experiencing negative effects from caffeine, all it means is that your body can't handle that drug. Your body is trying to tell you something important and you should be listening.

The next time the coffee wagon comes around in your office, stop and ask yourself, How is this drug affecting me? Do I want the effect? Do I need the effect? Should I modify my intake of caffeine? One way to find out if you are addicted to caffeine is to stop using it for two full days. If you experience any of the withdrawal symptoms listed earlier, then you will know that you are hooked. If you can continue cold turkey, fine, but some of you may find you need to taper off more slowly. The withdrawal symptoms usually come on eighteen hours after your last dose of the drug. They can last from a few days to several weeks.

All that is required to make the symptoms disappear is another dose of caffeine. But then you'd be hooked again.

The choice is yours. There are four alternatives available to you when it comes to caffeine: abstinence, moderation, heavy use, or addiction.

How to Reduce Your Caffeine Habit

1. First try the two-day no-caffeine test to see if you need to cut back. Or you may decide without going through withdrawal that it's time to cut back or quit.

2. Do *not* use tranquilizers to deal with the jitters of withdrawal, or you may end up with another kind of drug problem. They'll pass when the withdrawal is completed. Stay away from sleeping pills as well.

3. Avoid medications, either prescription or OTC, that contain caffeine. (The label on OTC drugs will tell you if caffeine is an ingredient.) If you want to cut out all stimulants, be sure to avoid all the methylxanthines (theobromine and theophylline). Some prescription drugs that contain caffeine are Cafergot, Migralam, Migral tablets, Fiorinal, Eggic, Apectol, Soma Compound and Darvon Compound.

4. Stay away from sodas that contain caffeine (see the table for a list of some that don't).

5. Start cutting back on the amount of coffee you drink. You may want to switch to decaffeinated coffee right away. You can also mix Decaf with regular coffee, gradually reducing the proportions until it's all Decaf. Coffees blended with grain or chicory have less caffeine.

6. Avoid that second cup of coffee. If you are thirsty, drink something else.

7. Switch to drug-free herbal teas. If diet isn't a big concern, switch to low-fat milk, fruit juices, or just plain water. One of my patients does very nicely with club soda with a twist of lemon.

8. Coffee drinkers find they miss that early-morning lift. Do your body and your mind a big favor: get into some good cardiovas-

---

cular exercise instead—jogging, aerobics, calisthenics. Some people use meditation to achieve a state of "relaxed energy" first thing in the a.m.

9. You will experience some craving. This is due to both physical and psychological dependency. Talk it out with someone and don't give in to it. If no one is around, call someone and have them keep you straight until the desire wanes.

AMERICA'S NICOTINE BLUES

Ivan's story

He had been smoking cigarettes since his late teens. At age thirty-four he discovered that he had coronary artery disease. It had advanced so far that triple-bypass surgery was necessary to save his life. The operation was a success, and his mother, his wife, his two sons, and other relatives and friends were relieved. Despite warnings from his surgeon and his cardiologist, he returned to cigarette smoking as soon as the postoperative pain had passed. He has all the insight in the world about his smoking problem. He says he can't shake the addiction. His wife isn't much help, as she smokes too. He knows that smoking is one of the major risk factors in the development of coronary artery disease. His prognosis could turn out to be grim.

Cigarette smokers have something in common with heroin addicts, speed freaks, garbage heads, and alcoholics: their addiction is a way of life. Smokers overdose (burning in the chest, extreme dizziness, vomiting, loss of appetite), they go through some heavy-duty withdrawal (extreme irritability, intense craving, sleeplessness, distractibility, obsessive talking about smoking), and generally tend to adopt behaviors that go along with any addiction: protecting their supply, borrowing money or cigarettes, sneaking cigarettes, lying to themselves and others about stopping, feeling they can't enjoy life without their drug, and using all the other rationalizations and defenses needed to explain away a dangerous and life-threatening habit. Smokers learn to ignore the pleas of loved ones, they learn to deny their own objective medical symptoms, blaming them on other causes, they learn to lie and manipulate, they often invade other people's (nonsmokers') space and rights, they avoid medical checkups for fear of hearing bad news (often missing an opportunity to deal with various illnesses in their earliest stages), and so on.

Tobacco use has been around for centuries. First discovered by explorers among the natives in the Americas, it was brought to England around 1592 by Sir Walter Raleigh. Sailors and traders planted tobacco seeds along their trade routes to ensure ample supplies (you see, they knew about craving even back then).

In the United States, the annual per capita consumption of cigarettes was just under 100 in 1910, up to 400 by 1920, and up to 1,000 by 1930. During World War II, cigarette smoking became extremely popular, particularly among men. This was due in part to the mass manufacturing of cigarettes, which brought the price down. By the 1970s, men and women together smoked a per capita average of 4,100 cigarettes a year. Many male smokers have stopped, while many women have just started. Today the proportion of adult smokers is about the same in both sexes—about 36 percent of both men and women. That's about 60 million smokers! In dollars, retail expenditures for cigarettes increased from an estimated $7.2 billion in 1964 (the year the surgeon general's first warnings on the dangers of smoking came out) to an estimated $10.5 billion in 1970—an increase of 45 percent.

We commonly think of nicotine—the primary hazardous and addicting ingredient in cigarettes, cigars, pipe tobacco, and snuff—as a stimulant. However, it can act as a depressant or tranquilizer as well. Pharmacologically speaking, nicotine is a liquid alkaloid, freely soluble in water. It turns brown on exposure to air and is the chief alkaloid found in tobacco. It has no therapeutic use and has been discarded by modern medicine. Nicotine can stimulate the central nervous system, especially the medullary centers (respiratory, emetic, and vasomotor). This stimulation is followed by depression, and repeated administration of nicotine causes tolerance (you need more of the drug to get the original effect).

The litany of physical damage wrought by smoking is awesome. Here are some of the facts, according to the American Cancer Society.

Fact: Smokers subject themselves to a much greater risk of death or disability at a young age. The death rate of cigarette smokers at all ages is higher than that of nonsmokers. It climbs in proportion to the number of cigarettes smoked, the number of years the person has smoked, and the earlier the age at which they started. Smoking will cause about 130,000 deaths from cancer this year. It is the major cause of cancers of the lung, larynx, oral cavity, and esophagus, and a contributory factor to cancers of the bladder, kidneys, and pancreas. Quitting smoking reduces the risk of cancer.

Fact: Men who smoke less than half a pack a day have a death rate about 60 percent higher than that of nonsmokers; a pack to two packs a day, about 90 percent higher; and two or more packs a day, 120 percent higher.

Fact: Cigarette smoking is one of the major risk factors in heart attacks (others include high blood pressure, obesity, and high blood cholesterol). Cigarette smokers have 70 percent more heart attacks than nonsmokers. When other risk factors are also present, the risk goes up greatly. Cigarette smokers have an abnormally high number of strokes.

Fact: Lung cancer is rare among nonsmokers but is the most frequent cause of death among cigarette smokers after heart attacks and strokes, and is directly related to the number of cigarettes smoked. It is estimated that 85 percent of lung cancers are caused by smoking, causing some 100,000 deaths per year in the United States.

Fact: Deaths from emphysema and chronic bronchitis—lingering diseases which cause suffering for years—increased by 550 percent in the thirty years from 1945 to 1975. Most of those who died were smokers. The more cigarettes smoked, the greater the likelihood of disease. The smoker's risk of death from emphysema and chronic bronchitis is from 6½ to 15 times that of the nonsmoker.

Fact: Male cigarette smokers have about five times the normal risk of dying of mouth cancer. Larynx cancer is six to nine times as frequent among cigarette smokers as among nonsmokers; a smoker's chance of dying from this cancer is four to five times that of a nonsmoker. Deaths from urinary bladder cancer are two to three times as numerous among cigarette smokers as among nonsmokers. Smokers are also more likely to get pancreatic cancer.

Fact: The lung cancer rate of women has doubled in ten years and will eventually equal that of men. Pregnant women who smoke have a greater number of stillbirths than nonsmoking women; and their infants are more likely to die within the first month. Their babies more often weigh less than 5½ pounds—which is considered premature—and are exposed to more risk of disease and death. Women who abstain from smoking while pregnant protect their own health and that of their baby.

Fact: Cigarettes are the cause of more than one-third of all residential fire deaths, according to the United States Fire Administration. In 1981 smoking materials ignited 63,518 homes, caused $305 million in property damage, injured 3,819 people and killed 2,144 others. Congress and a growing number of state legislatures are considering requiring cigarettes that would not burn long enough or hot enough to ignite materials like bedding or upholstery. Cigarette manufacturers are opposing such legislation.

Fact: Sidestream smoke—the smoke inhaled by nonsmokers who are near smokers—is a possible serious health problem.

Fact: Ninety-five percent of those who have quit have done it without organized programs. Stopping "cold turkey" appears to be more effective than cutting down gradually.

Fact: "Brief and simple" advice from a doctor is potentially the most cost-effective way of getting smokers to quit. Smoking prevention programs for young people should stress the social and immediate effects of smoking rather than the long-term medical consequences.

After reading a list like this you can see that addictive behavior is almost completely irrational. Surgeon General C. Everett Koop stated that "cigarette smoking is clearly identified as the chief preventable cause of death in our society," and he declared in 1982 that smoking is "the most important health issue of our time." Denial, rationalization, intellectualization, and other ego defense mechanisms allow smokers to continue smoking with the conviction that these terrible things can "never happen to me."

Are You a Nicotine Junkie?

- Your breath stinks! Do people rarely want to kiss your mouth or stand close to you during conversations?
- Your clothes, hair, fingers, and the drapes and other things in your home or office probably smell pretty awful as well. You can't tell because you became inured to the smell a long time ago.
- You are being perceived by a lot of other people, including your boss, as a compulsive junkie!
- What about your wind? When you play ball or golf or bowl do you find yourself gasping for breath?
- How many people avoid you and your office because they can't stand the smoke? More than you think!
- It's embarrassing when you run out of cigarettes. An otherwise healthy and well-adjusted adult is transformed into a very uptight and nervous person when you have a "nicotine fit."

- What color are your teeth? A close look in the mirror may reveal some strange colors.
- How many times have you burned holes in your clothes or an important document? Ever started a fire in your boss's or a client's ashtray?
- Are your clothes full of ashes? your desk? your bed?
- Do you find that you are running to the bathroom a lot? Nicotine can cause excessive urination and diarrhea.
- Did it ever occur to you that the macho (or macha) image you are trying to project with that cigarette really isn't impressing anyone? It's your own fantasy.

One of the highlights of the 1982 *Surgeon General's Report on Smoking* is the concern regarding sidestream smoke. This is the smoke emitted from smoldering tobacco in a steady stream. Smoke particles and ingredients are found in higher concentrations in sidestream than in mainstream smoke, the smoke drawn directly from the mouthpiece of a tobacco product during active puffing. The authors and sponsors of the 1982 report have urged nonsmokers to avoid inhaling cigarette smoke, even though the link between such passive or involuntary smoking and cancer is still a matter of scientific debate. Two studies, in Greece and Japan, have found an elevated and statistically significant incidence of lung cancer among the nonsmoking wives of smoking husbands. Avoid secondhand smoke whenever possible.

There appear to be special dangers for those who combine cigarette smoking with the consumption of alcohol. A great deal of statistical evidence has been gathered which shows that the risks of cigarette smoking are increased when the smoker also drinks alcoholic beverages. One study analyzed the chemicals in the breath of people while they smoked, while they drank, and while they did both at about the same time. When the subjects both sipped and puffed, a chemical called ethyl nitrite appeared in detectable amounts in the breath. It did not matter whether the drink preceded the smoking or vice versa, as long as they were reasonably close together. Ethyl nitrite is known to produce

mutations in living cells. Such mutagens are often also carcinogenic (cancer causing). Neither smoking alone nor drinking alone
produced detectable amounts of the chemical in the breath. Booze
and smoke appear to be a deadly combination.

In recent years smokers have sought to derive health benefits
by switching to reduced-tar brands of cigarettes. According to
the National Academy of Sciences, smokers who switch to low-
tar, low-nicotine cigarettes are not decreasing their chances of
lung cancer because they tend to puff and inhale more. Therefore
the possible health benefits are doubtful. Smokers of low-tar
brands may unconsciously inhale more deeply and hold the smoke
in their lungs longer to satisfy their craving for nicotine. The
problem is that "most heavy smokers, regardless of brand, tend
to maintain high nicotine levels." Interestingly these findings of
the National Academy of Sciences contradict a similar study
recently released by the American Cancer Society. The ACS study
showed a 26 percent lower mortality rate from lung cancer in
smokers of low-tar, low-nicotine cigarettes when compared with
those who smoked high-tar, high-nicotine brands.

Of course the Tobacco Institute, which represents manufacturers of tobacco products, continues to contend that the question
is "still open" on whether smoking causes cancer. The surgeon
general dismissed that contention, saying, "The evidence is strong
and scientific and we stand by it."

One of the common excuses for continuing to smoke is the
notion that smoking will relax you and get you through times
that are stressful. This can become a deadly rationalization because stress, in its scientific sense, is an unavoidable part of life.
This would then sentence the smoker to a lifetime of carcinogenic
behavior. Let's take a closer look at the real nature of this often
used but poorly understood concept of human stress. According
to Dr. Hans Selye, a leading world expert on the subject:[4]

- Stress is the nonspecific response of the body to any demand made upon it.

- It doesn't matter whether the agent or situation we face is pleasant or unpleasant; what counts is the intensity of the demand for readjustment or adaptation.
- Stress is more than nervous tension.
- Stress is not always the cause of damage. Any amount of normal activity—a game of chess or a passionate embrace—can produce considerable stress without causing harmful effects. Damaging or unpleasant stress is "distress."
- Stress is not always something to be avoided. In fact, it cannot be completely avoided.
- Complete freedom from stress is death.

To be alive is to face stress—each and every day of our lives. How we respond to it and whether or not we are flexible in the face of it is what really matters. According to Dr. Selye we react to all stress through a biological mechanism which he calls the "general adaptation syndrome." It consists of three stages: an alarm reaction (the stimulus grabs our attention), the stage of resistance (in which we actively contend with the stimulus through either "fight" or "flight"), and a stage of exhaustion (during which we rest and replenish ourselves). You are kidding yourself if you think you can ever reach a point where you won't be under stress and therefore not "need" a cigarette to "calm you down." By using smoking to contend with stress you are probably failing to identify the real causes of "distress" in your home or office (and hence are not dealing with them). Stress is a natural part of life—smoking is not! The general adaptation syndrome guarantees the survival of the species—cigarette, pipe, and cigar smoking do not! Smoking stimulates your circulatory and nervous systems, which increases your heart rate, blood pressure, blood sugar levels, and general cardiac output. In essence, you are turning inward by stimulating your system and trying to protect yourself against the outside stimulus. Your body needs to be in good working order to cope with the stresses of everyday life. Smoking directly limits your body's ability to do this. The guilt and shame that accompany addiction to nicotine lead to a vicious cycle: the very cigarette you light up to cope with stress then becomes another stress in your life!

Coping with stress affects eating behavior as well. During the stress response the body stops digesting food as it prepares for fight or flight. Nothing can lead to a postmeal disaster as readily as being uptight while eating. Ever eat a really fine meal and wonder why you have a stomachache, headache, or just feel in a lousy mood? The answer, in a word, is stress. If you are going to lunch with the boss and you're really nervous, eat lightly. If possible get the business dispensed with before you start eating. Ever notice that in the movies real emotional upheaval in a restaurant scene is portrayed as an uneaten meal? So when uptight eat light or even skip a meal.

Stopping Smoking

Thirty million Americans have given up cigarette smoking. Another 55 million Americans are involved in physical exercise. The nation is into fitness and health. Some corporations are providing incentives and educational programs for their employees to encourage a healthy approach to living. More and more, people who indulge in addictive behaviors like smoking are being viewed in a negative light by superiors, peers, and subordinates in the work setting. Those who persist in smoking are viewed with greatly reduced esteem and may find themselves operating in reduced corridors of power and decision making. People will not sit next to you, may fail to invite you to certain meetings, will stand away from you during a conversation, and will generally begin subtle or overt forms of avoidance of you and your office. Worst of all, your superiors may view you as an example of poor health and lacking in self-control. You may be skipped over when it's time for promotions, and a healthier, better-controlled man or woman may move ahead of you. One way to find out how dependent you are on smoking at work is to see how uncomfortable you become when forced to abstain.

Here are some suggestions for quitting successfully.

- Most people do it on their own. Don't be afraid to try—even if you have to try many times. Every cigarette you don't smoke contributes to your health. It takes years for a smoker to catch up with a nonsmoker in terms of the reduced incidence of diseases like lung cancer.

- Consciously cut down on the amount you smoke each day until you reach zero. Not everyone can do it cold turkey. Tapering off slowly will make withdrawal a little easier. You can increase the time interval between cigarettes and the amount of time it takes to smoke a single cigarette—this will automatically reduce the number of cigarettes consumed in a single day. Keep a written record on a small card you can place in the cellophane liner of your cigarette pack. Remember, you are heading for zero!

- Try quitting with a partner. This need not be a spouse. Pair up with another smoker and support each other's commitment to stop completely. Call each other on the phone if you feel the urge to light up—even in the middle of the night. This is the approach called "phone therapy" developed by Alcoholics Anonymous, and it works for many people.

- Smoking behavior is often cued by certain internal states, external events, places, or people. Become familiar with the cues that trigger your smoking behavior. Avoid those that you can and stay mentally vigilant in the face of those that are unavoidable. Anticipate them and use phone therapy if needed.

- Try keeping dead butts in a jar with a little water in it. Visualizing and smelling what tobacco is really about will help to turn off the habit. Inhale some smoke and then blow it through a clean tissue. This is what is going into your lungs!

- For oral types, chew sugarless gum or munch on toothpicks.

- If you need to keep your hands busy, get some worry beads.

132

- Find more direct ways to deal with stress; get into stress avoidance and stress coping at the source of the problem.
- If you find you can't manage quitting on your own, join a mutual support program. You will be among kindred souls who will help reinforce your desire to quit.

WHICH APPETITES ARE WE FEEDING?

Eating behavior can be of a compulsive nature just as drug consumption often is. Immediately some of you may say, "So what! Let people who like to eat enjoy themselves. Does it really matter if we put on a few extra pounds? Everyone can't look like a fashion model! We need some 'love handles' to grab on to. I like my men [women] on the big side!"

Obesity and its associated health risks can't be sloughed off. Those who are overweight are prone to a wide variety of illnesses, including high blood pressure with its attendant risks of stroke and heart attack. The heart attack risk is enhanced by high levels of blood cholesterol and fat and low levels of the protective high-density-lipoprotein (HDL) cholesterol. Obese people are at greater risk of diabetes, certain forms of cancer, gallstones, arthritis, venous thrombosis, chronic bronchitis, accidents including those which are fatal, and surgical complications. And if the people in your company who make decisions about hiring, firing, raises, and promotions look askance at obesity, the results can hurt your career and your income. Although Americans generally have been getting fatter over the last eighty years, people are actually eating less and getting fewer calories than they did in 1900. The explanation is in the change in activity levels. Our modern technological advances have drastically reduced the amount of physical exercise we get. We walk less, lift less; in fact, we do everything less except sit. When we were more physically active we ate more to keep up our energy stores. So now we eat less, but the severe decline in physical exercise has allowed that amount of food we do not burn to turn into fat.

The ideal is regular exercise and a diet that cuts down on

the quantity of food consumed without lessening too much the intake of required nutrients. The best way to lose weight is to adopt a pattern of eating that maintains balanced nutrition while reducing calorie intake sensibly. If any of the fad diets really worked over the long haul, there would be no need for new ones! In my local paper the other night there were six ads for "diet centers." One is the biggest, one is the oldest, one guarantees no pills, another no dangerous diets, and all have testimonials with "before and after" photographs.

Every year millions of pounds are shed and every year the same millions of pounds are put back on. The basic problem seems to be that we want someone else to do it for us. We want instant magic—instant long-lasting magic. What is really required is a basic change in patterns of eating. While diets of all kinds may have a temporary effect, permanent changes in eating habits are the key to long-range success. This means the burden of responsibility falls right back into our own laps. And that is exactly where it belongs. The true bottom line on the issue of obesity is that we must reassume the responsibility for our own lifestyles. If you are concerned about your weight, then recognize that you can do something about it. You have to want to, and you have to face the fact that your eating behavior may resemble a chemical addiction. How? Addiction can be defined as (1) compulsion, followed by (2) negative consequences and (3) loss of control. This is why I am stressing regaining control over your own lifestyle and eating behavior. Too busy making a living to work into an active exercise routine? Did you ever stop to think that your acquisitive years may be cut short by what you are *not* doing *now?*

A pound of fat is the equivalent of about 3,500 calories. A surplus of just 100 calories a day will turn into ten pounds in a year. A brisk twenty-minute walk will use up these same calories. Look at it this way: every time you eat 3,500 calories less than you expend, you use up a pound of fatty tissue. A deficit of 500 calories a day (eating 2,000 and using up 2,500) will lead to a loss of one pound a week (that adds up to fifty-two pounds a year).

For many adults, eating has become the classic example of "looking for the right thing in the wrong place." If being fed in the earliest stages of life is associated with alleviation of hunger, the receiving of love and affection, and a sense of everything being right with the world, then it is easy to see how eating serves the same functions for the adult. However, eating can only *symbolize* these other forms of gratification. Food cannot replace love. Eating oneself through loneliness or anxiety does not address the root of the problem. Yes, it is a primitive method for returning to a better emotional state, but it is a most indirect route for having the other needs met. This type of eating is symbolic pleasure and always leaves one "hungry." Frustrated people who overeat only amplify the frustration, which leads to more eating, which leads to obesity. It can become a vicious cycle. It should be clear by now that whatever model you use to examine the phenomenon (analytic or behavioral), eating has come to mean many things in our society. Food acts as a tranquilizer for some people; it is a reward for others; while many just hurry through meals as if they are nothing more than a necessary nuisance. Once you stop and examine what role—other than plain survival—eating plays in your life, you can begin to make the necessary changes in your eating behavior. Some recent research at UCLA indicates that eating the right nutrients but drastically reduced calories may increase the human life span.

Nutritionists counsel us to eat a healthful breakfast that will fuel us for a morning's work, then a small lunch and a small dinner. The majority of Americans have sedentary jobs. Our bodies do not require the kind of refueling (in terms of calories) that our ancestors needed in 1900 for a job like lumberjacking. We seem to have this mental set which says that if we put in a hard day's work at the office we deserve to eat a "hearty" meal. If we skip breakfast and eat large lunches as well, we are headed for a caloric disaster and our waistlines will show it.

Watch out for food additives too. They can alter mood as quickly as any other drug. Additives are used to color food, lengthen shelf life, enhance taste, and make food look more attractive. Even dog food is manufactured to look appealing to the

135

human eye. Additives are non-nutrient chemicals, most of which are innocuous. There are some 2,800 substances which are intentionally added to the foods we eat. Some additives like red dye #2 or DDT are dangerous. Two food additives are worthy of special mention because they figure so prominently in the American diet: salt and sugar.

Both sugar and salt are added in voluminous amounts to a wide variety of foodstuffs. We know they can be found in such items as sweetened cereals and pretzels. But have you checked the labels of other food items, such as the salt content in tomato juice or soup or bread, or the sugar in granola or ketchup or peanut butter? These are the "hidden" food additives. The average American eats around 128 pounds of sugar a year, which makes sugar our leading food additive. Salt comes in second; Americans eat an average of 15 pounds of salt a year. That comes to about 3 teaspoons of salt a day, far more than our body requires to stay healthy. Both sugar and salt tastes are acquired and are,

Problems Associated With:

Sugar	Salt
Tooth decay: worst when sweets are consumed between meals.	*Hypertension* (high blood pressure): salt is believed to be the main precipitant.
Obesity: sugar adds to the intake of more calories than we use up, which turn into fat.	*Kidney disease:* continuous dumping of excess sodium can lead to kidney malfunction.
Aggravates diabetes: obesity is the highest risk factor for diabetics; they must restrict their overall calories and sugar intake.	*Edema:* excess sodium can increase water in and around body tissues, leading to swelling. Figures in premenstrual tension.
Heart disease: sugar contributes to risk because it releases insulin, which directs the conversion of blood glucose into fatty acids and triglycerides, which promote the development of atherosclerosis.	*Heart disease and stroke:* excess sodium increases likelihood of both.

therefore, subject to change once we decide to do so. Listed below are some hints on how to change salt and sugar eating habits.

Sugar	Salt
Do your own baking and cut down on the amount of sugar you use.	Study food package ingredients carefully.
Don't reward kids or adults with sweets.	Cut out soft drinks with salt added. Switch from club soda to plain seltzer.
Cut out soft drinks. This change alone can bring about a 50% reduction in your sugar intake.	Be on the lookout for high-sodium vegetables like grits, spinach, and sauerkraut.
Reduce sugar in coffee and tea.	Don't add any salt at the dinner table.
Serve fruit. Fresh is best. If you use canned or frozen, look for those packed in water instead of sweet syrup.	Gradually cut back on the amount of salt you are already using.
Eat unsugared cereals for breakfast.	Try other herbs, condiments, and spices.
Stop buying candy or other sweets for the home or office.	Purchase a low-salt cookbook.
Study ingredients on package labels carefully.	Look for foods marked "low-salt" or "low-sodium" when you shop.
Don't use sweets for an energy lift—only diabetics benefit from this. The lift lasts only minutes for the rest of us.	Avoid fast-food restaurants—they use a lot of salt.
	Cut down on processed foods—you will avoid salt and many other additives. Buy fresh food whenever possible

Diet can have both subtle and dramatic effects on our mood and behavior. Consider the following examples:

- Dr. Richard Wurtman of MIT states, "It's likely that early in life people make associations between the consumption of certain foods and changes in how they feel. Then, later on, they unconsciously turn to these foods to re-create the desired feelings."

• The eating of sugars and starches (carbohydrates) can raise the level of a brain chemical called serotonin. Serotonin is associated with feeling relaxed, calm, sleepy, less depressed, and less sensitive to pain. According to Dr. Judith Wurtman of MIT, this may be the reason why so many people binge on carbohydrates when feeling anxious or depressed. She states, "It may also explain why high-protein, low-carbohydrate weight-reduction diets usually fail. These diets cause a serotonin deficiency in the brain which in turn could trigger carbohydrate craving to correct the imbalance."

• Neurotransmitters are brain chemicals that transmit messages between nerve cells. Certain nutrients alter brain levels of these chemicals that regulate a wide variety of brain functions and have a direct effect on mood and performance. One example of such a nutrient is tryptophan, an amino acid found in protein foods like meat, chicken, and fish. Eating such foods raises blood levels of tryptophan, which causes increases in brain levels of serotonin.

• Similarly, another amino acid from protein foods called tyrosine is associated with increased levels of another neurotransmitter called norepinephrine. Norepinephrine and serotonin are viewed by psychiatry as playing major roles in mental depression. Nearly all psychiatric drugs used to treat depression increase brain transmission by one or both of these chemicals.

• Dr. Judith Rapoport of the National Institute of Mental Health reports that children who are high consumers of caffeine (in soft drinks and iced tea) were described as more nervous, more hyperactive, and more easily frustrated and angered than were children who typically consumed less caffeine. She also reported that, contrary to popular impression, sugar had a calming effect on the children in her study. This finding is consistent with the known effects of carbohydrates on serotonin levels in the brain.

As more is learned about the effects of many nutrients on human behavior we will be better able to control our own mood and performance through dietary means. This could ultimately mean less introduction of manufactured drugs into our systems and the return to more natural forms of "self-medication." These studies bring new meaning to the notion "You are what you eat."

Some Hints for Eating Right at Work

- Start with a good breakfast. It will help you be more efficient in the mornings and help you eat smaller lunches.
- Coffee and tea during the workday are fine as long as you don't experience caffeinism. You may want to intersperse fruit juices and other beverages.
- Large business lunches can make you feel stuffed and lethargic and make it difficult to get back to work. Light lunches are good for health and business.
- Alcoholic drinks have "empty" calories and can alter your mood, motor coordination, and ability to think clearly. Go easy on booze, especially at business lunches. People tend to play follow-the-leader with alcohol. Decide what you will do before you get to the restaurant.
- Do not depend on sweets for "instant energy." The lift is elusive. Try a piece of fresh fruit, which contains fructose, a sugar that has fewer calories.
- If you need something in your mouth, try sugarless gum.
- When dining out with customers, pick a restaurant that is not noisy or crowded. The setting is as important as the food in terms of pleasure and digestion.
- Rich desserts are hard to resist. But why spoil a nice meal with a lot of guilt and empty calories? Don't say yes when you want to say no.

- Get out for lunch. Don't make a habit of eating at your desk. Take a break from the work routine. Celebrate your lunch hour. Try to take a walk after eating. Let lunch be a total experience, not just a break from working.
- Bad news and food don't mix. Reading about tragedy in the daily paper while eating is not a good idea. Remember when the Vietnam war poured out of TV sets during dinner? It's an unhealthy combination (stress again).
- Don't wolf down your food. The antacid manufacturers are already making a fortune.
- When you've had a good day, reward yourself with a nutritious and tasty meal, not a big one.
- Plan enough time for meals during the workday.
- If you eat at your desk often enough, just sitting at your desk can become a cue to eat.
- If a busy schedule or deadline necessitates eating while you work, eat lightly, avoid spicy foods, have light snacks handy, and go easy on caffeine.

Common sense can allow you to enjoy the pleasures of eating without the guilt that interferes. Recognize the central role that food and eating play in your life. Then keep the ideal in mind: regular exercise and a diet that cuts down on quantity without sacrificing nutrition.

DRUGS AND SPORTS

In 1982 reports of widespread use of cocaine in the National Football League made front-page news in the *New York Times* and in *Sports Illustrated* magazine. Don Reese, a former defensive lineman with several NFL teams, made the following claim on the cover page of *Sports Illustrated:*[5]

Cocaine can be found in quantity throughout the NFL. It's pushed on players, often from the edge of the practice field.

Sometimes it's pushed by players. Prominent players. Just as it controlled me, it now controls and corrupts the game, because so many players are on it. To ignore this fact is to be short-sighted and stupid.

Other famous players have admitted to the use of this drug. There have been reports of cocaine use by players of other professional sports including baseball, basketball, and boxing. Estimates of the actual incidence of drugs in professional sports are hard to come by. Like other aspects of the drug scene, it depends on whom you are speaking with. The media tend to hype this kind of sensational phenomenon, and sports management tends to cover it up or play it down. The players with a drug problem are the ones who suffer. But they aren't the only ones. Entire teams, players' families, the good name of a school, the reputation of coaches—all are casualties of the athletic drug wars. And the problem is not restricted to professional or even college sports. Competitive athletics start in the junior-high-school or middle-school years, and this is where we must focus our attention to understand the roots of the multiple relationship between sports and drugs.

Leo Durocher said it many years ago: "Nice guys finish last!" The name of the game in competitive athletics is winning. Sometimes that means winning at all costs. The costs are most often paid by the athletes themselves. There are many diet and exercise regimens used for building the powerful bodies that are required in many sports—most notably weight lifting, wrestling, boxing, football and most other contact sports. The enhancement of regular nutrition may start with megadoses of vitamins (which remain unproven in developing athletic prowess). Powerful drugs like anabolic steroids are sometimes used to develop large muscles. Soviet-bloc athletes have been challenged a number of times during world Olympic meets as to their use of such drugs in body building. Even some female athletes use them, and have also been known to take male hormones in an effort to build bulk. The use of hormones and steroids can be very dangerous and involves a whole host of side effects and adverse reactions, which is why most coaches and sports-medicine professionals shun them.

A variety of anesthetic and analgesic drugs are used in sports. These are the chemicals that deaden the sensation of pain and allow injured players to return to the playing field. Some are short acting and are applied topically, like Lidocaine. Others are longer acting and are taken internally, like Demerol. The hotter the competition and the more that is riding on the outcome of a game, the more likely it is that these drugs will be used to keep the better players on the field. Pain is a symptom of an injury or trauma and helps in the diagnosis of such problems. When pain is masked, the player is not aware of the extent or seriousness of the injury. And in sports like football, you go out and play even if you are in pain. Winning is everything and the player is supposed to bear pain like a "real man." But in the eighth grade, at age thirteen or fourteen? It's hard to sit on the bench when family, friends, and schoolmates are cheering your team on. So sometimes the players themselves ask for the drugs so they can get back into the action. And sometimes coaches push the kids to take the drugs. And the parents either ignore or deny the whole thing.

Another facet of drugs and sports is the social side. The reward for many athletes, including the younger ones, after a game well played (or even not so well played) is often a drug. Whether it's a surreptitious can of beer or a marijuana joint or a snort of cocaine, many young athletes look forward to getting high after the big game or meet. Certainly this is not true of all school-age athletes, some of whom shun drugs in any form as part of their caring for their bodies. But it's awfully hard to resist peer-group pressure in a setting where being one of the boys or girls is all-important. It's easy to see how quickly the use of pleasure drugs can spread within a tightly knit social group like an athletic team. Coaches have very little influence against this kind of pressure. Beer drinking in particular is seen as cute and part of the macho trip, so parents tend to make light of such drug use. It is not uncommon these days for girls who want to get closer to athletes socially to use drugs to attract them. This is a game played with a vengeance at the college and professional level, but it begins much earlier. More and more parents are beginning to ask where the team and the cheerleaders are, late on a Saturday night, and why it is so hard for these kids to get up on Sunday mornings. Could be they are hung over. Losers get high too—it's called relief drinking (winning is called celebration drinking).

When I attended a Big Ten college in the midwest in 1960, I roomed with a second-string fullback on the football team. He took me to several team parties and I have never seen such heavy drinking in my life—replete with drunkenness, fights, sexual antics, throwing up, chugalug contests, and drag racing. The ethic was "play hard–party hard" and never miss a practice (no matter how rotten you feel). Looking back, I now recognize some of these high-spirited antics as alcoholic drinking by at least several of the team members. My roommate summed up the whole thing very succinctly: "You practice hard all week, do whatever you're told by the coaches, kick ass and play your heart out on Saturday afternoon and then . . . drink, screw and raise holy hell on Saturday night!"

But he also opened my eyes to something else. Some of the guys were taking some "pep" pills to get up for the big game. The pills, otherwise known as amphetamines, create the feeling of tremendous physical and mental prowess. There were several "speed" scandals in professional football during the 1960s and '70s. Cocaine serves the same function. These stimulant drugs create a powerful elevation of mood, extreme euphoria, and feelings of power and grandeur. One of the things about many sports events that attracts young athletes is that they can find a natural high on the playing field. Some learn to use stimulant drugs to intensify these feelings. Others look for the drugs to duplicate this same exhilaration off the playing field. Once it gets to the point of regular drug use, like daily snorting of cocaine or freebasing (smoking the pure essence of cocaine), the drug takes over and the athletics go right down the tube. Some wealthy pro athletes have lost their fortunes and their playing ability because of drugs like cocaine.

HEALTH PROMOTION IN THE WORKPLACE

My drinking got out of hand to the point where it was interfering with my job. I was missing deadlines, missing important meetings, and calling in sick a lot. It took a couple of years for this to happen, and when it got bad enough my supervisor called me in and told me to shape up or ship out. He also told me about the company psychologist whom I could go see in confidence. At first I thought he was off the wall. Why would I want to talk to a "shrink"? I wasn't crazy. But I was so afraid of losing my job that I went anyway. He helped me to see that the bulk of my problems stemmed from my inability to handle alcohol. He sent me to A.A. and a therapist. I have been sober for just over a year now. My job and my marriage have both improved since I stopped drinking. Thank goodness my company had an employee assistance program or I would have been out of work and out of luck.

—Insurance salesman

Too often people talk about the world of work and the private life of a person as if they were totally separate realities. Certainly there are profound differences, but the essential person remains unchanged in both settings. The problems that affect someone at home are carried into the workplace just as work-related problems are often brought into the home. Most wives can tell what kind of day their husbands have had at work by just looking at their faces when they come through the door. The whole range of human problems and ills have a direct impact upon the work site. Divorces, marital squabbles, problems with kids, poor health, financial troubles, drug abuse, spouse abuse, alcohol abuse and alcoholism, sexual dysfunction—all have a way of eroding productivity and efficiency at work. Over 20 million people—15 percent of the American population—need mental-health services at any time, according to the President's Commission on Mental Health, and 25 percent of the population "is under the kind of emotional stress that results in symptoms of depression and anxi-

144

ety." Most of these people work, and when they arrive at the office or plant their problems arrive with them. The impact of alcoholism alone is staggering. Drug misuse and abuse account for an untold percentage of problems as well.

More than 400 companies have set up preventive programs for their employees over the past decade. These companies must feel that one way or another they will pay for employees' mental

Company	Type of Program
Hospital Corporation of America	Pays its employees by the mile for staying healthy by swimming, jogging, or cycling.
Dow Chemical Company (Texas Division)	Pays cash incentives for their employees to stop smoking.
Mendocino County (California) Office of Education	Cash credit is offered to employees who file medical claims of less than $500 in a year.
New York Telephone Company	A staff of 40 physicians, covering 80,000 employees in more than 1,000 locations. Boasts a 90% success rate in treating hypertension; offers courses in smoking cessation, stress and hypertension control.
International Business Machines	Offers voluntary health screening exam, which has revealed more than 322,000 health problems in 13 years (35% of them previously unknown).
Kimberly-Clark Corporation	Employees fill out a 40-page medical history, submit to a battery of lab tests, and run through a treadmill exercise test during which their heart rate is monitored. Has an EAP and a $2.5 million fitness facility.
Pepsico, Inc.	Maintains a fitness center with a full-time director. Top management has a separate facility. Center can monitor via a computer the amount of calories burned by an employee over a week's time.

and physical problems. Linda B. Nielson, Director of Counseling Services for Insight, the employee assistance program (EAP) at the Kennecott Corporation's Utah Copper Division, says of companies: "They may pay in supervisory time spent trying to improve job performance, or in exorbitant medical costs, or the costs of absenteeism and turnover. Or they can pay for preventive services like Insight."

In New York State in 1982 only 12 percent of the work force had access to an EAP. Listed above are some examples of company "wellness" programs.[6] These companies and others like them have taken the position that problems such as alcoholism, drug addiction, smoking, overuse of sugar and salt, and poor dental hygiene are preventable.

The lever of the job is what makes EAPs successful. You may not want to admit you are crazy or that you have a drinking or drugging problem, but the last thing you want to do is lose

---

How to Recognize a Good Employee Assistance Program

- Program is well advertised, so that all levels of management and labor know about it and how to use it.
- Supervisors are trained to make referrals to the program.
- Employees can gain access to the EAP counselor in privacy, and all communications are held in the strictest confidence.
- Corporate health benefits provide coverage for physical and mental problems, including alcohol and drug abuse.
- EAP counselor has a good list of resources for services for which the benefit package provides coverage.
- Referrals include self-help groups like Alcoholics Anonymous and women's support groups as well as professional practitioners.
- Benefit package includes both in-patient and out-patient treatment of chemical dependencies.
- Supervisors need never know the nature of the personal problem. Their only concern is job-related functioning by the worker.

your job. Besides the financial aspect, Americans have a lot of self-esteem tied up in their work. The pressure of the EAP is strictly job-related, but by getting the employee (and in some cases employer) to proper diagnosis and needed treatment, the whole man or woman benefits right along with the company.

YOU AND DRUGS AT WORK—
A SELF-RATING QUESTIONNAIRE

Take a few minutes to fill out this questionnaire as honestly as possible. Place a check mark next to the alternative that best answers the question.

It's hard enough getting through the average workday. If you find that you are balancing a drug act along with your work responsibilities, you are walking a thin line toward disaster. Whatever your reasons for using drugs at work, you will want to exercise some real caution. Remember the three hallmarks of addiction: (1) a compulsion to use the drug, (2) negative consequences due to use of the drug, and (3) loss of control over the drug (and your life). The damage done by alcohol, caffeine, nicotine, and overeating are far more subtle than the drugs we perceive as more overt tools of abuse. But they take their toll over time, eroding the quality of our lives at work and at home. You are in charge of what goes into your body.

Often	Some-times	Seldom	Never	
____	____	____	____	1. Do you drink more than 5 cups of coffee during a workday?
____	____	____	____	2. Do you use pleasure drugs during working hours?

Often	Some-times	Seldom	Never	
―――	―――	―――	―――	3. Do you feel that drugs help you to work better?
―――	―――	―――	―――	4. Do you smoke cigarettes at work?
―――	―――	―――	―――	5. Is alcohol a part of your business lunches?
―――	―――	―――	―――	6. Do you depend on food with a lot of sugar to give you a lift at work?
―――	―――	―――	―――	7. Do you take tranquilizers to deal with the stress of your job?
―――	―――	―――	―――	8. Do any drugs that you take interfere with your ability to do your job?
―――	―――	―――	―――	9. Has anyone at work ever talked to you about your drinking or drug taking?
―――	―――	―――	―――	10. Do you miss work because of drug or alcohol use?
―――	―――	―――	―――	11. Are you late or do you leave early because of drug or alcohol use?
―――	―――	―――	―――	12. Do people at work hassle you about your smoking?

Often	Some-times	Seldon	Never	
_____	_____	_____	_____	13. Is your job so boring that you need to get high just to get through the day?
_____	_____	_____	_____	14. Do you ever drink or drug before going to work?
_____	_____	_____	_____	15. Have drugs ever interfered with memory function at work?
_____	_____	_____	_____	16. Do you arrange your workday around your drug taking?

How to score: 3 points for every "often" response
2 points for every "occasionally" response
1 point for every "seldom" response
0 points for every "never" response

0–16: Zero indicates no problem at all. The closer you get to 16, the more you must start thinking about how drugs affect you at work.

17–32: Yellow Alert. Drugs are too much a part of your work life and perhaps your private life as well. Cut down and be careful.

33–48: Red Alert. You are in real trouble. It's time to seek professional help for your drug problem!

CHAPTER FOUR

Drugs as Medicine

People have been searching for relief from pain and suffering for thousands of years. The practice of modern medicine is an art that draws upon many sciences, including pharmacology. Our ancestors explored the flora and fauna in their environment for aids to health as well as relief from pain. The technological explosion of the last hundred years has yielded new medicines and a whole health-care industry. By 1981 the total expense for health care in America had reached 9.8 percent of the gross national product (that's more than $162 billion). As a nation we spend billions each year on the ethical, or prescription, medicines prescribed for us by our doctors and even more billions for nonprescription, or over-the-counter, medications that allow us to "doctor" ourselves.

The medications that we take have a profound effect on our physical, mental, emotional, spiritual, and social selves, although we tend to restrict our thinking about medicine to the purely physical. The blossoming of the concepts of holistic medicine, which germinated with the South African philosopher and statesman Jan Christiaan Smuts in the 1920s, has allowed us to see ourselves as whole persons and not simply the sum of our parts (organs). What we eat, how we live, the quality of our environment, our own health practices or lack of same, are all taken into consideration when considering our state of health. The very term "health" is no longer applied solely to its complement, illness and disease; it now relates to positive practices and feeling good. The use and abuse of drugs as medicine are part and parcel of the concerns of holistic medicine, and as such deserve our serious attention. The time has come for us to assume full responsibility for what we put into our bodies in the name of health and not abdicate that responsibility to others.

YOU AND YOUR DOCTOR

Illness and disease are frightening realities. Children take their cues from adults regarding their attitudes toward being sick, getting well, being well, suffering and enduring pain, taking medicine, and relating to doctors and other health-care professionals. One of the first rude awakenings for children, who tend to see parents as all-knowing and omnipotent, is that parents must often turn to "strangers" (family doctors or pediatricians) for help in alleviating illness and discomfort. How we perceive, talk about, and relate to doctors gives a very powerful message to our children. If adults react to the doctor as a source of good counsel and healthful medicine, then the child will tend to trust and listen to the doctor. If, on the other hand, the doctor and the medicine are viewed with suspicion and caution, then our child will pick up these attitudes. If our children see us caring for our own bodies and thereby acting as partners in health with our doctors, they get one kind of message. If they see us not caring for ourselves and waiting for our bodies to break down so we can take them to a technician (doctor) for repair, much like our automobiles, they get an entirely different message.

Consider how you do, in fact, relate to your doctor(s). Take a few moments to fill out the questionnaire below. Check off either "true" or "false" for each item and answer as honestly as you can.

True False

—— —— 1. When my doctor uses terms I do not understand I ask for a simpler explanation.

—— —— 2. Upon arriving home, if I'm not sure about something my doctor said in the office, I will call and ask questions.

—— —— 3. I have a right, as a patient, to ask as many questions as I need to.

—— —— 4. If my doctor gives me written instructions and I can't read the handwriting, I ask to have it written more clearly.

—— —— 5. If I must wait a long time (more than 15 minutes) to see the doctor I will mention this to him or her.

—— —— 6. I do not hesitate to ask my doctor about medications prescribed for me (side effects, dosage, interactions, etc.).

—— —— 7. I make suggestions to my doctor concerning my health.

—— —— 8. I make sure to tell my doctor about any drugs I am taking (including illicit drugs).

—— —— 9. If I feel a second opinion is in order, I will tell this to my doctor.

—— —— 10. I consider myself an equal partner with my doctor when it comes to caring for my health.

—— —— 11. I will ask my doctor to prescribe generic drugs instead of name brands.

—— —— 12. If the doctor indicates a course of medical or surgical treatment, I ask questions about risks versus benefits.

True   False

_____   _____   13. If my doctor treats me like a child or as if I am incapable of understanding, I challenge this or seek another doctor.

_____   _____   14. I do not hesitate to discuss fees and costs.

_____   _____   15. If my treatment doesn't seem to be working well, I call the doctor to discuss this.

SCORING KEY: 1–4 "false":   Like most people, you are not terribly assertive with your doctor.

5–9 "false":   You are taking too much for granted and not sharing in your own health care.

10 or more "false":   You are reacting like a child to your doctor and have totally placed your health in someone else's hands.

People seem to need to "look good" in front of their doctors; we don't want physicians to look down on us. Yet it is terribly important that we report accurately and unashamedly anything affecting our health status. Denial of drug use is one of the things people get caught up in with doctors. Part of this denial may be outright manipulation, but more often it is a psychological phenomenon called "transference." The patient automatically and unconsciously generalizes and "transfers" from past interpersonal relationships with authority figures (doctors are certainly authority figures in our society). We tend to carry over feelings and needs about our parents to our doctors. We act like children in front of them, almost as if they were our own parents. When you combine this transference with the wish we have to see doctors as omnipotent and infallible, you can get some idea about what is going on, emotionally, when you visit your doctor.

Doctors are aware of this "godlike" pedestal that patients put them on. When they are treated this way they go right along with it because it's easier. They have to answer fewer questions

153

that challenge their expertise, and they don't have to spend as much time working hard to explain medical terminology in terms the lay person can understand. This explains, in part, why some doctors have such large practices. Visits can be kept brief when we fail to actively exercise our responsibility as a partner in the relationship.

Dr. Thomas Preston in his book *The Clay Pedestal* suggests we re-examine the doctor-patient relationship:[1]

> The notion of the consummate physician helping the distressed patient during his or her hour of need is undoubtedly the most enduring attraction for the public in its view of the medical profession. The myth of the selfless physician marshalling the forces of science for the welfare of his patients, however, has come to conceal reality rather than to reflect it, and to deflect inquiry into the true nature of medical practice, which falls far short of this mythical ideal.

Dr. Preston points out that frequently the most serious and consequential criticisms of modern medical practice come from the physicians themselves, working and speaking through conventional medical forums.

Educate your children so that they can learn about their own bodies and health issues. Help them learn to deal with health in its fullest sense—the promotion of good health habits and a sense of personal responsibility for that health. Don't let them think of health as important only when something is wrong. Here are some hints on how to accomplish this.

1. Encourage your children to learn the different parts of their bodies. Teach them correct anatomical names. Make a game of it. Use illustrations.
2. When preparing to visit a doctor be upbeat and positive. The child will pick up any negative vibrations that you give off.
3. When at the doctor's, encourage your child to ask questions about any aspect of his or her health or body.

Set the stage by rehearsing at home, and by asking the doctor a question yourself.

4. Don't shy away from "what if . . . ?" questions about health. If you don't know the answer, look it up, or write the question down and save it for your next visit to the doctor's office.

5. Don't talk about doctors as if they were infallible. Don't talk about medicines as if they were magic potions. Everyone makes mistakes, including doctors. Communicate confidence but not omnipotence regarding the doctor.

6. Don't make it sound as if all of life's ills or pains can be alleviated by medicine or medication.

7. Use real medical terms but define them. Cutesy-poo terms don't teach even if they do amuse.

8. When someone in the family is ill, kids see this as a serious matter. Don't shut them out. Explain things on a level they can understand. Let them help in small ways to make the sick person feel better.

9. Teach your child to care for his or her own health through positive modeling of dental care, accident prevention, not smoking, not abusing drugs, moderation in food and drink, and so on.

10. Realize that childhood is a time when lifelong attitudes and health behaviors are forming. Don't leave it to others to shape positive health habits and attitudes in your children.

11. Remember that kids are sharp. They have a built-in "crap detector." They know when you are lying to them or avoiding an issue. Be straight with them.

Tell it like it is, especially with young children. But don't feel compelled to tell them everything at once.

John is in the second grade. He comes home one afternoon and asks his mother, "Where do I come from?" His mother, wishing to be very contemporary and informative, launches into a fifteen-minute lecture on the birds and the bees (human style). After listening patiently to his mother's lecture on human sexuality, little John looks up at her and states, "Ralph in my class comes from Chicago. Where do I come from?"

It makes a lot of sense to allow the physicians, dentists, nurses, and other health-care professionals to act as educated guides and consultants to us regarding our health. It does not make any sense to allow them to take over and control it. The bottom line is that it is your body and you must ultimately pay for your healthy habits or lack of them. By forming a co-equal and active partnership with these health professionals you are using the best of both worlds: responsible self-care and guidance from your consultants. If you don't like or trust the advice from one consultant, find another. This is one area of your life where failing to be assertive can get you into serious trouble.

Now let's get more specific about the role you play concerning drugs and your relationship with your doctor. Here is a questionnaire to test your knowledge about your use of medications.

True   False

1. I know the names of all the drugs I take (both generic and brand name).
2. I always take the medication as prescribed (both the amount and frequency).
3. I always finish taking the medication even if I feel better.
4. I ask my doctor about side effects when he or she offers me medication.
5. I ask my doctor about the main effects (therapeutic benefit) that I can expect from a medication that he or she is prescribing for me.

DRUGS AS MEDICINE

True   False

_____ _____   6. I naturally assume that brand-name drugs work better.

_____ _____   7. I always tell my doctor, dentist, anesthesiologist, surgeon, about any drugs I am taking (street, prescription, over-the-counter, alcohol).

_____ _____   8. I always ask my doctor if the drug he or she is prescribing can interact with other drugs.

_____ _____   9. I always ask if I should take my medication before or after eating.

_____ _____   10. I would never give a friend one of my prescription medications or take one of his or hers.

_____ _____   11. I always ask my doctor if I should restrict any of my activities when taking a medication.

_____ _____   12. I take the drug advertising I see on television with a very large grain of salt.

_____ _____   13. I always ask if it is okay to drink alcohol when taking a prescribed or OTC medication.

_____ _____   14. I always ask my doctor to write down important drug-taking instructions or cautions.

_____ _____   15. I always ask my doctor or pharmacist about the best way to store my medication.

SCORING KEY: 1–4 "false": You need to learn more about the medications you use and the way you use them.

5–9 "false": You are letting someone else take over your own health care. Better hope they have told you everything you need to know to avoid problems.

10 or more "false": You may have already taken drugs the wrong way and experienced unnecessary side effects or even adverse reactions. You need to regain control over your own body and health.

(Question 6 is the only one to which "false" is the correct answer.)

POSITIVE PRACTICES REGARDING THE USE OF MEDICATIONS

Know what you are taking. Some drugs have very similar-sounding names but are dramatically different in their uses and chemical action. For example, *Orinase* (tolbutamide) is a drug used to correct insulin deficiency, while *Ornade* (main ingredient, phenylpropanolamine) is a drug used for the relief of congestion of the nose, sinuses, and throat.

Have your doctor write down both the generic and the brand names (in legible writing). The generic name, or common name, refers to the active drug ingredient. The brand name is what the drug manufacturer chooses to call its product. For example, when we refer to the tranquilizer as Valium, we are using the brand name; the generic name for this drug is diazepam. In Canada, diazepam is marketed under no fewer than eleven different brand names. A four-state, four-year study released in 1982 by the National Center for Health Services Research revealed that pharmacists are virtually ignoring laws permitting the substitution of less expensive generic formulations. The percentage of substituting generic for brand name drugs was low: 8.6 percent in Vermont, 7.4 percent in Michigan, 5.1 percent in Wisconsin, and 2.6 percent in Rhode Island. Dr. Theodore Goldberg of Wayne State University Medical School, the study director, states: "Although the potential for substitution appears great in each state studied, the actual experience has been disappointing." The American Pharmaceutical Association points out that pharmacists lack financial incentives for dispensing generic drugs and that simplification of state laws together with increased experience by pharmacists in handling generics should lead to a substantial increase over the next five to ten years. All drug sales are increasing at 12 percent annually, but the generic market is moving ahead at 14 percent, according to the Generic Pharmaceutical Association. You should ask both your physician and pharmacist for generic equivalent drugs. You stand to save 25 percent or an average of $1.25 for each prescription.

It is a good idea to keep medicines in their original containers and to take these with you when traveling. In case of an overdose or other adverse reaction, the drug can be quickly identified—this could save your life! It might also be a good idea to purchase a book which contains color illustrations of common prescription pills to help you to identify yours by their color and other markings. Always read the label before taking medicine or you are liable to take the wrong stuff or the wrong dose.

Know why you are taking it. We have all heard so much about side effects that we often fail to focus on the positive reasons for taking a drug. It is vital that you tell your doctor everything that is bothering you so he or she can suggest the best course

Drug Factors[2]	Patient Factors	Physician Factors
dose levels	sex, age	training
multiple effects	body size and weight	diagnostic skill
absorption rate	pregnancy, nursing	therapeutic skill
distribution	pharmacogenetic factors	experience with drugs
metabolism		
excretion	biochemical status	concomitant therapy
duration	nutritional status	attitude toward drug therapy
route of administration	drug metabolism	
	disease (vast multiplicity of factors)	attitude toward patient
habituation		
addiction potential	idiosyncrasy, hypersensitivity	attitude toward disease
tolerance		
side effects	contraindications	
toxicity	precautions	
idiosyncratic reaction	toxicity	
hypersensitivity	margin of safety	
margin of safety	concomitant therapy	
precautions	personality factors	
contraindications	attitude toward disease, drugs, doctors	
pharmaceutical properties		
chemical properties	cost	
drug interactions		

of treatment. If that treatment includes medication, you should know specifically why that particular drug is recommended and what its benefits are. All drugs have what are called multiple actions. You want to know what the principal beneficial action is. You will also want to know about the other actions commonly referred to as side effects. The drug your doctor prescribes should be the "drug of best choice." Many factors go into this decision.

You will want to know if this drug is the best available for your illness or disease. You will want to know if the intended therapeutic actions outweigh any side effects or possible adverse reactions. Do not agree to any course of drug therapy until you thoroughly understand this benefit/risk ratio, the financial commitment involved, and have had all your questions answered. Do not permit any doctor to rush you through a discussion of the medications, as this is the part of your treatment you are in charge of at home.

Take only as prescribed. Some people like to alter dosages and intervals between dosages. "If one is good, two is better" can be just as dangerous as "I feel better so I'll only take half as much." Taking too little of a medication can put insufficient amounts of the drug into your body to bring about the desired therapeutic benefit. Overdosing or putting too much of a drug into your system can bring the drug to toxic (poisonous) levels in the body. People don't OD (overdose) only on drugs like heroin.

Make sure that you understand exactly how to take the drug. You must know the route of administration (oral, injection, topical, nasal, etc.), how often to take it (once a day, twice a day, etc.), what time of day to take it, whether to drink it down with water or something else, before or after mealtimes. Ask questions. Don't leave the doctor's office until you understand. Have the doctor write it out, or his nurse if you can't read his instructions.

Check with your doctor before modifying the amount or the frequency of your drug taking. If you should skip a dose, ask the doctor what to do—don't "double-up" on your own. Very often people stop taking their antibiotics as soon as they feel better. Symptoms may be responding to the medication, but the underlying illness causing these symptoms requires the full course of the medicine. Otherwise the symptoms may re-emerge. If your doctor told you to take the medicine for ten days, take it for the full ten days. Make sure you follow specific instructions given to you about any medication. Exceptions to this occur when there are side effects or adverse reactions (see below).

Dealing with side effects. As mentioned above, the taking of any drug is a delicate balance between risks and benefits. Here is an example. A person suffering the symptoms of a serious depression may be well advised to take a tricyclic antidepressive medication like Elavil (amitriptyline). Physicians and pharmacologists know that drugs like Elavil can significantly reduce (about 80 percent of the time) the depressive symptoms (loss of appetite, lack of energy, diminished interest in sex, sleep disturbance, feelings of hopelessness). They also know that certain side effects such as drowsiness, blurring of vision, dryness of the mouth, constipation, and impaired urination can be expected when this drug is taken. For most people the side effects become reduced over several weeks, but for others they may persist. In the case of the clinically depressed person the risks may be far outweighed by the benefits. The expected and unavoidable side effects may be seen as a small price to pay for a course of drug therapy designed to alleviate the debilitating effects of the depression. This kind of decision should be a joint venture between patient and doctor. If the precipitating events in the patient's environment can be identified, this will help in the treatment. In many cases psychotherapy may be indicated along with or instead of the medication. But if the depression proves unresponsive to talk therapy, the patient should not be denied drug therapy. After the patient has been on the medication for a while the doctor and patient can experiment by putting the patient on a "drug holiday" to see if the depressive symptoms return.

All drugs have multiple actions: the principal action (the benefit) and side effects. Make sure your doctor discusses both types of action when considering any drug therapy. This will help you to more intelligently weigh the risks and the benefits.

Dealing with adverse reactions. There are many patient factors involved in drug taking. Some people have idiosyncratic or hypersensitive reactions to drugs. Your doctor cannot usually predict these types of adverse reactions. The most extreme reactions are allergic in nature (ranging from a rash to anaphylactic shock). You must inform your doctor *immediately* if you suffer any adverse reaction. The doctor can change the dosage or switch to another medication. Remember, side effects can be predicted (and should be discussed with your doctor before taking the drug), but adverse reactions usually cannot. Ask your doctor before taking the drug if he is aware of any possible adverse reactions for that drug. Ask for the major warning symptoms of adverse reactions for that particular drug, or look in one of the many consumer guides to drugs. While it may seem like a good idea to cease taking a drug if you have an adverse reaction, the best thing you can do is speak to the doctor before the next scheduled dose. You should report all side effects, adverse reactions, and overdoses to the doctor. If you can't reach the doctor before your next scheduled dose, find out if he or she has another doctor "on call" and contact that doctor, or call your pharmacist, or contact a physician in the emergency room of a local hospital.

It is a good idea to keep a written record of all adverse reactions. You should note the names (generic and brand), dosage, and the actual reaction. It is important to know the generic name because another doctor might prescribe the same generic drug under a different brand name, which will lead to a repeat of the adverse reaction. Since most people use more than one doctor, it is important to become a full partner in your health-care record-keeping. You will want to keep a note on dosage because sometimes negative effects can be reduced by changing dose levels. You should inform your doctor of any known drug allergies— don't wait to be asked. It's also a good idea to wear a "medical alert" bracelet or necklace which states drug allergies. At the very least carry this information in your wallet (but don't bury it).

Informing the doctor about drugs you are taking. Most people are far too passive in the way they interact with their doctors. You must take responsibility for your end of the partnership. One way to do this is to tell your doctor about any other drugs you may have taken recently or plan to take again soon, as well as those you are presently taking. This includes any "street" or "recreational" drugs (marijuana, cocaine, ludes, amyl nitrate, etc.). Don't forget to include alcohol, nicotine, and caffeine as well. Be sure to tell your regular family doctor about any drugs prescribed by other physicians (even if they were prescribed some time ago, if you are liable to be using them the doctor must know about them). I have known former heroin addicts who were enrolled in methadone (a powerful synthetic narcotic) maintenance programs who did not tell their surgeons that they were on the program. So, naturally, the surgeon wrote a typical medication order for managing postoperative pain. Because these patients' bodies were regularly receiving 80 to 100 milligrams of methadone per day, the amount of postoperative analgesic (painkiller) needed to successfully reduce pain was two to three times the normal dose. It always pays to level with the doctor, up front! After all, it's a confidential doctor-patient relationship. The only thing getting in your way is your image (your need to look "good" in front of your doctor). Be certain to tell not only your doctor but also your surgeon, anesthesiologist, and dentist about all the drugs you are taking. Again, don't forget to include street drugs and OTCs.

During pregnancy and breast feeding. Many drugs pass through the placenta and reach the fetus. Many also find their way into breast milk. In both these ways the drugs can be passed to the fetus or child. You must tell your doctor all the drugs you are taking as soon as you learn that you are pregnant. Now you have two lives to consider, and this dramatically alters the benefit-to-risk ratio. Therefore, a frank discussion with your gyne-

163

cologist/obstetrition is in order to ensure both your health and that of your child. The same wisdom applies to the period when you are breast feeding.

The fetus is most sensitive to drugs during the first trimester (first twelve weeks) of pregnancy, so it's a good idea for women who *think* they are pregnant to exercise the same caution as a woman who knows she is pregnant. Women who are sexually

Drug Use During Pregnancy[3]

Drug Name	Effect on Fetus	Safe Use of Drug
NICOTINE	Heavy smoking can lead to low-birth-weight babies, which means that the baby may have more health problems. Especially harmful during second half of pregnancy.	Should be avoided.
ALCOHOL	Daily drinking of more than 2 glasses of wine or a mixed drink can cause "fetal alcohol syndrome": babies tend to low birth weight, mental retardation, physical deformity, and behavioral problems including hyperactivity, restlessness, and poor attention spans.	Should be avoided.
ASPIRIN	During last 3 months of pregnancy frequent use may cause excessive bleeding at delivery, and may prolong pregnancy and labor.	Under doctor's supervision.

Drug Name	Effect on Fetus	Safe Use of Drug
TRANQUILIZERS	Taken during the first 3 months of pregnancy, may cause cleft lip or palate or other congenital malformations.	Avoid if you might become pregnant and during early pregnancy. Use only under doctor's supervision.
BARBITURATES	Mothers who have taken large doses may have babies who are addicted. Babies may have tremors, restlessness, and irritability.	Only under doctor's supervision.
AMPHETAMINES	May cause birth defects.	Only under doctor's supervision.
MARIJUANA	Unknown.	Should be avoided.

active and may conceive are also wise to be very selective about the drugs they take. A woman who is trying to conceive should exercise the same degree of caution as a woman who is already pregnant. These women should inform any doctor that may prescribe medication that they are trying to conceive and might become pregnant at any time. Don't forget the dentist.

Pregnant women should keep careful records of all drugs taken during that time and make sure to include any OTCs. Remember the thalidomide and DES nightmares in which serious birth defects were caused by these drugs. The effects were not known until years later and officials are still trying to contact some of the mothers who took these drugs. The FDA has noted that "No drugs have been proven 100% safe for the unborn and we can't say there is no risk. Some risks are so small we can't detect them in laboratory or clinical trials." As a result aspirin and hundreds of thousands of other OTCs will have to carry the following warning as of December 3, 1983: "As with any drug, if you are pregnant or nursing a baby, seek the advice of a health professional before using this product." As many as 300,000 products may be affected by this new standard warning. Up until this decision by the FDA, only a limited number of nonprescription drugs had carried warnings to pregnant or nursing women.

Storage and dating. It is vitally important to know how to store medications (prescription and OTC). The first thing to keep in mind is that almost any drug, particularly adult-strength drugs, can act as a poison if taken by a curious young child. Childproof container caps can sometimes be a royal pain, but you should have no doubt about their being responsible for saving young lives. So use them, and do not keep medicine bottles or vials laying around unopened. Although a skull and crossbones is a universally accepted signal of danger among adults, it may serve more as an object of fascination to a young child. Your local poison control center can give you a sticker which in my part of the country is commonly referred to as "Mr. Yuk." The label is green in color and looks like this:

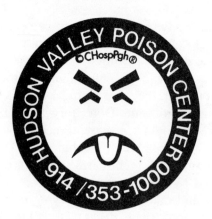

Young children seem to get the message that the stuff inside any container with a picture of Mr. Yuk on it must really taste horrible (yucky) and are less likely to put it in their mouths. You can put Mr. Yuk stickers on cleaning fluids and other poisons as well. Accidental poisoning is the fifth most common cause of death in the United States, with about 80 percent of all poisonings hitting children. Child poisoning is the most common pediatric emergency after trauma. Dr. Daniel Spyker of the University of Virginia's Blue Ridge Poison Center warns that you should not automatically follow antidote instructions on labels. The New York City Poison Control Project examined the labels of more than 1,000 common household products including cleansers, polishes, laundry products, drain openers, OTCs, insecticides, and car-care products. More than 85 percent of the instructions examined proved inadequate, incorrect, or dangerous. While new studies show that water may speed absorption of some poisons, milk will dilute any toxic substance without causing further damage. Keep a supply of ipecac, a syrup that induces vomiting, but it's best not to induce vomiting without the advice of a poison center. Be sure to have the phone number for your local poison control center, emergency squad, police, and hospital where you can read them in a hurry. You don't want to have to start looking up phone numbers in a real emergency. A good place to keep these numbers is pasted right on your phone or next to it. Possible poisoning, by the way, is another very important reason for knowing the names (generic and brand) and dosage strength of all the medications in your home. Those of you who live in rural and suburban areas should become familiar with poisonous plants. Contact your local poison control center for a list (with diagrams) of such plants.

Don't keep any medications in the bathroom medicine cabinet. The heat and humidity from showers, baths, and sink water cause drugs to deteriorate and spoil faster. The heat and humidity can even get inside those childproof containers. They tend to be airtight but not airproof, and spoilage does occur. Most drugs will do fine in a cool, dry place. Be sure to ask your doctor and/or pharmacist for storage instructions for every medication (including OTCs).

Some drugs remain chemically "pure" and effective over considerable periods of time. Others may deteriorate and spoil a lot sooner. It is important to know the "shelf life" of all medica-

167

tions. Some products are dated and read "Do not use after ———[date]." Others do not have such label instructions. Ask your doctor and/or pharmacist for this information. Throw out all drugs that have expired (flush them down the toilet). When in doubt, it is safer to discard the medication than to hold on to it. Look in your medicine cabinet. If you have drugs that are out-of-date, or have no label (so you are not sure what they are), or you really never use—throw them away. Most of us tend to hold on to every drug we ever bought. It doesn't make sense to hoard drugs that may be ineffective. Ask your doctor for some guidance as to what constitutes a sound family medicine cabinet. The odds are that you are overstocked with unnecessary and outdated drugs. No matter where you store your medications, *keep them out of the reach and view of young children!*

Contraindications. There are existing conditions or diseases that will not permit the use of certain drugs. The term used to warn the doctor, pharmacist, and consumer is *contra* (against) *indication* (to point out). Another way of stating this is: any symptom or circumstance indicating the inappropriateness of a form of treatment which is otherwise advisable. Some contraindications are stern in their warnings and are called "absolute." These absolute warnings are given to prevent the use of a drug that would expose the patient to extreme hazard. Other contraindications are milder and are called "relative." A relative warning does not completely forbid the use of the drug but certainly requires that special consideration be given to the decision to use it. This is a good example of how the benefits and risks need to be weighed together. Let's use oral contraceptives as an example of the two types of contraindications. There are more than twenty-five brand-name oral contraceptives sold in the United States. A phrase that is commonly used to indicate an absolute contraindication is "This drug should not be taken if. . . ." In the case of the oral contraceptives, this drug should not be taken if

- you have ever had or are now experiencing any form of phlebitis, embolism, stroke, angina, or heart attack;

- you have either impaired liver function or active liver disease (common in alcoholism);
- you have ever had cancer of the breast or reproductive organs;
- you suffer from abnormal and unexplained vaginal bleeding;
- you are allergic to either of the drugs (estrogen and progestin) contained in the brand you wish to purchase (check the label).

The phrase associated with relative contraindications is "Inform your doctor before taking this drug if. . . ." In the case of the oral contraceptives, inform your doctor before taking this drug if

- you have ever had an unfavorable reaction of any kind to any oral contraceptive;
- you have high blood pressure;
- you have a history of asthma or heart disease;
- you have epilepsy;
- you have cystic disease of the breasts;
- you have fibroid tumors of the uterus;
- you have a history of migraine headaches;
- you have diabetes or a tendency to diabetes;
- you smoke more than fifteen cigarettes a day;
- you have a history of endometriosis;
- you plan to have surgery within one month or less.

As you can see, contraindications are an important part of the decision-making process regarding whether or not to use a specific drug or entire drug family. (In fairness to the pill, it now appears that it may protect many women against two forms of cancer and other ailments.)

Food and drink while taking drugs. Just as some drugs don't mix well together, certain foods and drinks don't mix well either when you are undergoing drug therapy. Let's start with the simple stuff.

When you are given a prescription (or an OTC product is recommended by your physician or pharmacist), ask what liquid should be used to swallow that pill or wash down that elixir. Plain water is usually okay, but it's a good idea to know if other liquids (juice, soda or pop, milk) can be used safely. Some drugs should be washed down with a lot of water (like antibiotics, as a rule), while others require just a sip or two. The next thing you will want to know is whether the drug should be taken before, during, or after a meal. If it's before or after, find out how long before or how long after. Food helps some drugs to be absorbed into the body, while it does not help others. Doctor doesn't seem to know? Then ask him or her to find out, or ask your pharmacist. Don't leave it to chance!

The next thing you need to know is whether or not there are any restrictions to your diet during the drug therapy. For example, when the more commonly used tricyclic antidepressants don't work, doctors (psychiatrists in particular) will often make use of the MAO (monoamine oxidase) inhibitors. Included among the MAO inhibitors are Nardil (phenelzine), Marplan (isocarboxazid), and Parnate (tranylcypromine). All of these drugs must be combined with a carefully restricted diet. The reason is that the MAO inhibitors must not be allowed to combine with a substance called tyramine. The combination causes a severe elevation in blood pressure which can lead to very strong hypertensive headaches and stroke. Some of the foods and drinks containing tyramine are chicken liver, pickled herring, cheddar cheese, coffee, figs, chocolate, yogurt, beer, sherry, and Chianti wine.

Combining alcohol with many medications can lead to real trouble. The most serious trouble comes from mixing alcohol (a liquid sedative) with solid-state sedative drugs like the barbiturates (Seconal, Tuinal, phenobarbital), hypnotics (Dalmane, Quāālude), and tranquilizers (Miltown, Librium, Valium). These drug combinations quickly lead to overdosing. The main danger is that their effects are additive and can lead to depression (oversedation) of the central nervous system, causing anything from

170

drowsiness to death. Antihistamines (Actifed, Allerest, Benadryl, Dristan, Dimetapp, to name a few) can make you feel drowsy and sedated. If you add alcohol to this, you are increasing the sedative effect. So whether your antihistamine comes in prescribed or OTC form, don't mix it with alcohol if you plan to drive or operate machinery.

Limited activities. Ever catch yourself saying something like this: "I'm too busy to be sick" or "I'll just work my way through this allergy season"? Many people just can't be bothered with being ill or suffering from conditions which tend to slow them down. That's one of the main reasons people use drugs as medicine. Over $500 million are spent by Americans each year on over-the-counter drugs alone to try to counteract the effects and symptoms of the common cold. Each year $5 billion are lost in wages and productivity due to the cold. Most OTC cold remedies (and there are many) contain antihistamines in varying amounts and types. Antihistamines like Benadryl (diphenhydramine hydrochloride) are also hypnotics, or sleep inducers, and allergy sufferers are warned not to drive, operate machinery, or fly a plane while taking this drug. However, since the common cold is caused by a virus (or combination of viruses) and is not an allergy, the cold remedies containing antihistamines are useless.

Some drugs have side effects which can lead to a change in activities. For example, the MAO inhibitors used to treat depression, such as Nardil, Marplan, and Parnate, while they may help with many of the major depressive symptoms, also can put a real damper on your sex life. Some of the sexual dysfunctions associated with these drugs are impotence, problems with urination, impaired ejaculation (men), and delayed orgasm (women). Some sexual dysfunction can occur with the tricyclic antidepression medications as well. Some drugs do not permit people to have much exposure to the sun (such as the phenothiazines used to treat psychosis).

Be sure to ask your doctor if there will be limitations to your usual activity regimen when drugs are being prescribed. If your activities have to be limited, take this as part of your course of treatment. If you are ill you cannot expect to operate at 100 percent of capacity. Admit you are human and take it easy.

Drug interactions. The body is always striving toward an ideal state which doctors call homeostasis (a state of equilibrium of the body's internal environment). A wide variety of biochemicals naturally exist in the human body and work toward that ideal. In recent years scientists have discovered naturally produced opiatelike substances in the central nervous system called endorphins. It is the endorphins that probably bring about a state called the "runner's high." While helping to counteract the pain of distance running, the endorphins produce an interesting "side effect": they cause the runner to feel "high" and exhilarated.

When things go wrong with our bodies (illness or some condition), science seeks to provide what nature often cannot. What is important to understand here is that once you start taking medicine (prescription or OTC) you are already causing a drug interaction. The interaction occurs between naturally existing body chemicals and the drugs you have introduced into your body in the form of medicine. If you take one medical drug (with its multiple actions), the body will accommodate and combine with this drug. The desired effect is relief from suffering. Side effects may have to be tolerated. We hope no adverse reactions occur. Therefore, as a general rule of thumb, the fewer drugs we take the better. The fewer drugs we take simultaneously, the better. This greatly reduces the chance for adverse reactions.

We have already considered food/drug interactions and drink/drug interactions. Now you must consider drug/drug interactions. When you mix drugs together, one and one don't always equal two. In some cases the effects are directly additive, as with booze and barbiturates (both sedatives). In other cases the drug combination produces an effect which neither alone could produce, or an effect may result which is greater than the total effects of each agent acting by itself. If you were to combine diazepam (Valium) with alcohol (two or more drinks), you could get so stoned that it would feel as if you had taken 50 milligrams of the drug instead of only 5, because of the additive sedative

172

effect. In the extreme it can result in coma and death. There are other interactions which can be harmful. If you mix Flagyl (metronidazole), an antimicrobial drug used to treat infections like vaginitis, with alcohol you can expect nausea, stomach cramps, vomiting, and headaches. If you combine aspirin with an anticoagulant like Coumadin (warfarin), you could die from severe hemorrhaging. There are many other interactions, too numerous to mention here.

Keep in mind that nicotine can cause some drugs to break down chemically in the body more quickly. According to the 1979 Surgeon General's Report on Smoking and Health, ". . . Smoking of tobacco should be considered one of the primary sources of drug interaction in man."

Smoking and coffee drinking seem to go together. In one study, it was found that smokers metabolize the caffeine in coffee twice as fast (three hours as opposed to six) as nonsmokers. As smoking can influence the metabolism of many other drugs as well, make sure you inform the doctor that you are a smoker.

How to Avoid Negative Drug-to-Drug Interactions

1. When your doctor prescribes medicine, ask him or her if there are any specific other drugs to avoid. Ask about party drugs, tobacco, alcohol, and OTCs as well.

2. If it becomes necessary to take another medication, call your doctor to make sure that the two can be combined safely.

3. Keep in mind that another good reason to tell your doctor about drugs you are already taking is that they can significantly alter the results of laboratory tests. You don't need drugs masking a problem that is really there or creating the apparent existence of a condition that is not really there.

4. Don't take anyone else's medications on top of your own.

5. Try to keep the number of drugs you take to as few as possible.

6. Create a home reference library of relevant books (see the annotated bibliography for suggestions).

Practicing medicine without a license. The person sitting next to you at work acts just the way you do when you are uptight and nervous. So you offer him one of your Valium tablets. *Wrong!* You are at a party and develop a splitting headache. Your hostess, wishing to relieve your pain, offers you one of her Fiorinal with codeine (main ingredient, butalbital). You have taken Fiorinal *without* codeine (main ingredient, phenacetin) before for a headache, so you figure "Why not?" and you take it. *Wrong!* You could be in for a real surprise when the codeine mixes with the alcohol you consumed just a little while before—codeine increases the effects of sedatives like alcohol.

Only your doctor, together with you, can weigh all the relevant factors to be considered when taking drugs as medicine. Don't give your medicine to anyone else and don't take medicine prescribed for anyone else—the results could be disastrous. Leave the prescribing to the professionals. Your friends may give you drugs you don't need or that can harm you. You should not press your physician to give you drugs you do not need.

Stopping medications. If you want to stop smoking cigarettes on your own, you will be in good company, as 95 percent of those who quit did so on their own. But knowing when and how to stop taking prescription (and even some OTC) medications is something for which you need your doctor's advice. For example, Barbara Gordon describes in her book *I'm Dancing as Fast as I Can* what can happen when a person suddenly stops taking Valium after using it daily for years. The physical and psychological withdrawal effects can be really nasty and dangerous. Many drugs, like Valium, require step-down, or gradually decreasing, doses to ease any possible withdrawal effects. Allow your doctor to establish a detoxification protocol for any drug you are planning on stopping. If your doctor seems uncertain, tactfully ask him or her to get the information from a reliable source.

Do not stop taking a drug on whim—check it out with your doctor first. If you fail to fill a prescription for some reason, tell your doctor.

174

Stocking the medicine cabinet. Overstocking medicine cabinets should be avoided. Your medicine chest should include only those health-care products likely to be used on a regular basis. The *FDA Consumer* and *Consumers' Research Magazine* recommend the following suggested items that will meet the needs of most families:

Nondrug Products

- adhesive bandages of assorted sizes
- sterile gauze in pads and a roll
- absorbent cotton
- adhesive tape
- elastic bandage
- small blunt-end scissors
- tweezers
- fever thermometer
- hot water bottle
- heating pad
- eye cup for flushing objects out of the eye
- ice bag
- dosage spoon (common household teaspoons are rarely the correct dosage size)
- vaporizer or humidifier
- first aid manual

Drug Items

- analgesic-aspirin and/or acetaminophen. Both reduce fever and relieve pain, but only aspirin can reduce inflammation.
- emetic syrup of ipecac to induce vomiting. Read the instructions on how to use these products.
- antacid

- antiseptic solution
- hydrocortisone creams for skin problems
- calamine for poison ivy and other skin irritations
- petroleum jelly as a lubricant
- antidiarrhetic
- cough syrup—nonsuppressant type
- decongestant
- burn ointment
- antibacterial topical ointment

They further recommend antinausea medication if any family member is prone to motion sickness, a laxative, and some liniment. Seasonal items, such as insect repellents and sunscreens, round out the list.

Drugs and your children. While most illnesses in childhood are far from life-threatening and can be easily diagnosed and treated, most parents feel helpless when childhood illness occurs. One of the best ways to alleviate this parental anxiety is to become educated about responsible care for the sick child. As far as medication goes, the first guiding principle is that parents must assume responsibility for the use of all medicines that their children take! You will find helpful consultants in your doctors (pediatrician, internist, pediatric specialists) and your pharmacist, but as parent you take the direct role:

- to act as the facilitator of information between the child and the doctor.
- to teach your child the correct ways to use medicine.
- to make sure the medicine is taken properly and on time.
- to carefully monitor therapeutic progress and/or side effects.
- to prevent adverse reactions due to under- and overdosing (and other causes).
- to protect your child from ineffective and even dangerous medications (including OTCs). There are special dangers

176

to guard against for drugs that may impair normal development.

- to make sure that your children take their medicine, following the doctor's orders, even when extremely reluctant or when they are feeling better.
- to report any side effects, adverse reactions, overdoses and paradoxical effects to the doctor immediately. Paradoxical effects occur when a drug acts in a manner opposite to the one intended, such as a sedative acting as a stimulant.
- to ensure that contraindications are observed (there are many for children under twelve years of age).

There are drugs that represent a clear and present danger to children, and yet they are still on the market and some doctors are still prescribing them. Tetracycline belongs to the antibiotic family of drugs. Even though warnings have been accompanying all tetracycline preparations since 1972, some doctors are still prescribing them for children. Here is what the warning says:

The use of drugs of the tetracycline class during tooth development (last half of pregnancy, infancy, and childhood to the age of 8 years) may cause permanent discoloration of the teeth (yellow-gray-brown). This adverse reaction is more common during long-term use of the drugs but has been observed following repeated short-term courses. Enamel hypoplasia (malformation of teeth) has also been reported. Tetracyclines, therefore, should not be used in this age group unless other drugs are not likely to be effective or are contraindicated.

This class of drugs also has a long list of mild and serious adverse reactions. Side effects may include infections, often due to yeast organisms which can occur in the mouth, intestinal tract, rectum, and/or vagina, resulting in rectal and vaginal itching. Clearly for children under nine years of age, the risks far outweigh the benefits.

Brand-Name Antibiotics Containing Tetracycline

Achromycin	Sumycin
Mysteclin-F	Tetracycline HCL
Panmycin	Tetracycline syrup
Robitet	Tetracyn
SK-Tetracycline syrup	Tetrastatin
and capsules	Topicycline

This is just one example of drugs which are clearly contraindicated for younger children. Children also should not take cold remedies containing alcohol or antihistamines without specific directions from your doctor. It is a good idea for children to avoid combination-ingredient OTCs in general: (1) the doses may be wrong for children, (2) the ingredients may be ineffective, (3) the ingredients may mask symptoms which can warn you of a more serious health problem, and (4) the more ingredients, the greater the chances of side effects and adverse reactions. At least check with your pharmacist before purchasing OTCs for your child. If he or she is not sure about its safety or effectiveness for a child, *don't buy it!*

Remember, most illnesses run their course and disappear without any help from medication. More often than not it is your desire to provide instant relief to the suffering child that leads to the taking of too many or unnecessary drugs. Many pediatricians have "phone hours" which can save you the cost of an office visit.

When the dosage instructions tell you to administer a "teaspoon" of medicine, be careful! The common household teaspoon can vary in size from 2.5 to 9 milliliters. The recommended medical teaspoon is 5 milliliters. Ask your pharmacist to provide you with one of these accurate measuring instruments to ensure accuracy of dosage. It's a good idea to shake the bottle when the medication comes in liquid form to ensure mixing of all the ingredients. When pouring medications into measuring cups, do it at eye level and put a fingernail on the level you wish to fill to—both aid in accuracy.

Children vary greatly in size and weight. Two children may be the same age but one can be small and thin while the other is tall and heavy. The most accurate dosages are those that are computed by body-weight equivalents. Ask your doctor how your child's physique affects medication dosages.

Keep a written record of all side effects and adverse reactions that your child has to any drug, both prescription and OTC. Report these to your doctor as well. When it is time for a new medication, you can help by reminding your doctor of any of these negative effects.

Drugs taken by infants and young children must be monitored carefully for any possible impairment of normal growth and development. As mentioned previously, you should find out what food and drink is to be avoided while your child is undergoing drug therapy.

Let's take a look at the human side of administering medicine to your child.

1. Be matter-of-fact. Don't make a big deal out of it. There is no reason to apologize. Act as though you expect your child to be both courageous and cooperative.

2. Be honest. Don't tell them it tastes good when it really does not. Tell them it is medicine (even if it tastes like candy). Kids often ask if "it tastes bad." It helps if you know how it actually tastes. One response can be "It tastes like black cherry to me; how do you think it tastes?"

3. If physical restraint becomes necessary, don't display angry feelings, and get it over with as quickly as possible.

4. When mixing medicines in a drink, it's a good idea not to use things which your child drinks often. They may then resist that item in the future, even when it doesn't contain medicine.

5. Kids have a right to explanations that are geared to their age and comprehension. Keep it simple.

179

6. Tears are part of illness and sometimes of taking medicine. A little reassurance and love can go a long way.
Guilt does not help a parent who is doing exactly what
should be done to alleviate the illness.

7. If you react negatively to the medicines that you as
an adult have to take, don't be surprised if your kids
have the same reaction to their medicine.

8. If you combine the medicine with some food (like apple-
sauce), don't give the child too much food. Illness usually causes a diminished appetite (and you want them
to swallow all the medicine).

9. If you can crush the pill or capsule and mix it with
food, this will help. It takes time to learn how to swallow
a whole pill.

10. If the child gives you a hard time, lengthy negotiations
are not a good idea. The medicine is for the child's
health and well-being and therefore is not negotiable.
If it becomes a real ordeal, consult your pediatrician
for advice.

Sometimes our children are introduced in very innocent ways
to the "high" that drugs can produce. One evening as we were
seated around the dinner table, my son began describing his experiences with "space breath." When we all reacted with "What
is space breath?" he reminded us of how, when seven years old,
he was introduced to a new dentist who made a game of "astro-
nauts" out of his initial visit. The office became a space ship,
the chair became a couch in the rocket, and the mask which
dispensed the nitrous oxide (laughing gas) became (in my son's
imagination) "space breath." My daughter reacted to this hilari-
ous story by stating how much she enjoyed using the "sweet
air," as the dentist calls it. Nitrous oxide is a general-acting inhal-
ant anesthetic and works by helping the central nervous system
block the perception of pain (while drilling or cleaning). It leads
to an altered state of consciousness, not unlike marijuana, causing
feelings of giddiness, lightheadedness, and mild hallucinations.
Its effects wear off very quickly, and as used by dentists it is a

safe drug. But if you don't want your kids to get stoned at the dentist's office, then you may want to ask him or her to skip the "space breath" and use Novocain instead.

Drugs and older people. Homeostatis is the body's attempt to operate at a "steady state," or a state in which everything is in balance. As we grow older it becomes more difficult for the body to operate in this steady state, and this renders some bodily tissues more susceptible and sensitive to the actions of many drugs. So during the earliest and later years of life we must exercise special cautions in the use of all drugs as medicines— both prescription and OTC. Some of the changes that the body goes through in aging that directly affect the way it handles drugs are: (1) problems in the digestive system which change the way in which drugs are absorbed by the body, (2) reduced functioning of the liver and kidneys which makes it harder for the body to eliminate and metabolize (chemically break down) many drugs, (3) changes in the responsiveness of the nervous and circulatory systems which may mean smaller drug doses are required, to avoid reaching toxic levels, and (4) impairments in mental functioning such as memory which make the proper taking of medicines more problematic.

Retired people make up about 11 percent of the population but receive 25 percent of dispensed prescriptions. Adverse reactions occur three times more frequently in our older population. More than 85 percent of elderly ambulatory patients and 95 percent of elderly institutionalized patients receive drugs, 25 percent of which may be ineffective or unneeded. More than 70 percent of one elderly population study used nonprescription drugs without the knowledge of their primary-care provider.

It is not easy for an older person to shake off side effects and adverse reactions, and the drug therapy can become downright debilitating to an otherwise vital individual. The weighing of risks and benefits must be most carefully considered along with the careful selection of a dosage schedule. Some older people living alone may require assistance in following drug treatment therapies. Also, it is very common to find older persons involved in the use of more than one drug at the same time. The problems associated with this are negative drug interactions, greater risk of side effects and adverse reactions, interference with laboratory tests (possibly masking or delaying accurate diagnosis), and increased cost to the patient (many of whom live on fixed incomes).

Guidelines for Older People Taking Medications

1. Make sure the drug therapy is really indicated. For example, older people need less sleep, and what appears to be insomnia may be quite normal in the developmental sequence of aging.

2. Taking several drugs at a time is not a good idea. Make sure that your regular doctor knows all the drugs you are taking (including caffeine, nicotine and alcohol).

3. Since older people's bodies can't tolerate the same dosage and strength as younger people's, it's a very good idea to establish tolerance by starting with smaller-than-standard doses. Some doctors may even provide a free sample to test for side effects before putting you through the expense of a filled prescription.

4. Use easy-off caps and lids. Avoid childproof containers, as arthritis can make opening a medicine container a painful ordeal or even impossible.

5. Don't take drugs in a dimly lit room. Read the label carefully, and make sure you are taking what you are supposed to and in the right amount.

6. If you have trouble with your vision, ask the pharmacist to type the labels in all capital letters. Make sure the drug name and instructions are readable.

7. Ask your doctor for simple dosage instructions. Whenever possible, a single daily dose is preferable. As you grow older dosages usually need to be changed. Ask your doctor about this. Take nothing for granted. Ask lots of questions.

8. Many medications can be prepared in liquid form. Avoid large pills (tablets and capsules) if simpler dosage forms are available.

9. Sometimes people forget what they have taken or when they took it. The only drugs that should be kept at a bedside are emergency drugs like nitroglycerine. To avoid these problems, read labels carefully and keep a daily written record of what you took and when you took it.

10. Know the expiration dates of your drugs. It is important to discard outdated drugs.

11. Do not be embarrassed to discuss costs with your doctor and pharmacist. Generic drugs can often be substituted for the more expensive brand names. Different drugstores charge different amounts for drugs (of all kinds), so a little comparison shopping is in order. Pick pharmacies where you can get questions answered as well.

One of the problems faced by older people is loneliness. Another is boredom. People seek to counteract these unpleasant realities through an altered state of consciousness, i.e., by getting stoned. Older people use alcohol and prescription medications as well as OTCs to alter their moods. Some even use recreational and street drugs when they can get them. This is a risky business at best, often leading to dangerous and deadly drug combinations. Drug abuse and habituation are not only problems of the young.

If you care about your older relatives and friends, then you can possibly do them a big favor by having a serious discussion with them about the drugs in their life. By following your own common sense and the guidelines listed here you may help someone to (1) avoid unnecessary and harmful or ineffective drugs, (2) find a doctor and pharmacist who are cooperative in answering patients' questions about their medications, (3) avoid abusing drugs, (4) keep drugs from ruining the quality of their lives, and (5) learn to accept the realities of growing older without seeking "magic" from pills.

THE PHARMACIST

So far our emphasis has been on responsible self-care coupled with a good working relationship with your doctor(s). A modern-day partnership around drugs as medicine must include a third, equally important, member: the pharmacist. When you make use of both consultants as advisers on drugs, you are taking advantage of the best of both worlds—medicine and pharmacology. Many of you will remember, sometimes with a good deal of affection and nostalgia, the friendly and helpful neighborhood druggist. He knew your whole family and everyone else in the neighborhood. People often approached him with intimate concerns about health, in some cases instead of the doctor. He was someone you trusted with your health and felt a certain closeness with. Contrast that with the modern pharmacy. Often it is part of a large chain; the store sells many things besides medications; the pharmacists are hidden behind a bullet-proof barrier or on a raised platform (both of which diminish any chance for private conversation); you don't know their names and they don't know yours; in short, the whole arrangement has changed for the worse. Hospital pharmacy, interestingly enough, has been moving in the opposite direction. Pharmacists have come out from behind their cages, participate in rounds with the doctors, meet with patients, and are a more involved part of the hospital treatment team. The more doctors in hospitals interact with pharmacists, the more they come to value their input into the patient's total care plan.

The pharmacist who owns or works in a profit-making drugstore has an inherent conflict. He is a trained professional with a good working knowledge of the latest in drug effectiveness and safety. But he has to choose between his profit motive and his ethical sense of what's good for the consumer. For example, he is often forced to choose between selling you a more expensive name-brand product and a less expensive but equally effective generic drug. Or he may have to choose between selling you an ineffective over-the-counter product and suggesting that you not purchase that item. He is also under a lot of pressure from drug manufacturers to purchase, stock, and prominently display their products. The manufacturer's representative is more interested in products that sell than in their therapeutic benefits. (Drug companies routinely sell products not approved in the United

States to other nations where less rigorous standards permit their sale. One manufacturer marketed to an African nation infant formula that American officials would not permit to be used by babies in this country!) Drug manufacturers provide only the minimum required information about side effects and adverse reactions on their packaging, while the pharmacist may know much more that the patient should be told. The pharmacist finds himself faced by many ethical dilemmas, but many have solved these in favor of the consumer without hurting their profits. Shop around for the ethical pharmacist. You should choose him or her with the same care as you do your doctor, in terms of both competence and morality.

Choosing a Pharmacist

1. You want someone you can talk to. The pharmacist should be patient and understanding. If he or she is too busy to talk with you, find someone who will.

2. Pharmacists should be a source of expert information concerning types of drugs, side effects, adverse reactions, contraindications, efficacy of products, etc. And they should be willing to share this information with you both verbally and in writing. They should be happy to answer your questions—no matter how silly or naive you think they sound.

3. Keep this ideal in mind when choosing a pharmacist: "Your pharmacist should provide you with safe and effective medications at the lowest rate of cost."

4. Good pharmacists don't stock really lousy products in their stores.

5. Good pharmacists will steer you away from a product they feel is not good for you, even if it means losing a sale.

6. One of the best ways that pharmacists can be of help to an individual patient is to keep a record or profile on each of their customers. The profile should include both prescription and OTC information.

7. A good pharmacist will attend to you personally, giving you information about how to take the medicine and side effects

to watch out for. Some pharmacies even provide this information in writing.

8. If the pharmacist has any questions about what the doctor has prescribed, he or she should not hesitate to contact the doctor.

9. An ethical business person tempers the need to make a living with a careful guarding of their professional reputation.

Drug prices vary considerably, not only between generic and brand-name drugs, but also between pharmacies. As drug prices are presently increasing at the rate of about 7 to 10 percent a year, this can become an important part of your budget. However, price alone does not make a good pharmacy. It is definitely worth a few extra dollars a year to find a pharmacist who really meets the criteria we've defined.

The best approach to drug therapy is a situation where:

1. The doctor is clear and explicit in advising the patient about the drug to be used—intended benefits, known side effects, dosage instructions, and so on.

2. The pharmacist assists and reinforces the directions given by the doctor and answers any questions the patient has.

3. The patient has used both consultants and clearly understands the intentions of the therapy and what to do if problems arise.

If any of the ingredients are missing, problems can occur. If you are a hospital patient and a regimen of drug therapy is being prescribed, ask lots of questions and don't hesitate to ask that a pharmacist be made available to speak with you if you so desire. For example, many patients in hospitals are routinely given orders for sleep medication before anyone (including the doctor) knows if they will have trouble sleeping. If you don't want or need a medication, discuss it with the doctor and the pharmacist. Some hospital pharmacies are now providing both in-patients and out-patients with "patient package inserts," which patients can read and thereby learn more about what they are taking and how to take it. This is particularly useful when patients leave the hospital. Some hospital pharmacies operate telephone services which give out drug information, and some operate poison hotlines. These are valuable services and you should have their phone numbers within easy reach in case of emergency. Your neighborhood pharmacist should be willing to answer phone inquiries as well. If he won't, find one who will.

THE "DATED" PHYSICIAN

"Drug mills" are operated by unscrupulous doctors who only want to make money at the expense of the practice of good medicine. "Doctor Feelgoods" supply their patients (for a handsome fee) with stimulants, sedatives, narcotics, tranquilizers, hypnotics, ad nauseam. My wife, a registered nurse, had occasion to act as a private-duty nurse for a wealthy couple in their late sixties whose rear ends were completely shot out by four decades of Demerol (a powerful synthetic narcotic) addiction. The drug and hypodermic needles had been faithfully supplied by their doctor during this entire time period. The two patients whined like street junkies when their medication was late in coming.

Psychiatrists appear to be overrepresented among impaired (chemically dependent) physicians for both alcoholism and drug addiction. State medical societies are working on legislation and guidelines to protect the physician and the patient when impairment occurs. Doctors, just like the rest of society, have come to see drugs as quick and easy solutions for our ills. We are all brainwashed into believing that there is a "pill for every ill." Doctors are continuously having drugs of every conceivable description pushed at them by drug manufacturers' sales representatives. It's no wonder they succumb to the same drug maladies as the rest of us. If you have reason to suspect that your doctor is either impaired or indiscriminately pushing drugs, it's time to seek out a new doctor.

It is far easier to avoid drug mills and impaired physicians than it is to avoid a far more common phenomenon—the dated physician. It is important to understand that many different subjects must be covered in medical school curricula and that different disciplines and departments compete actively to get a piece of the action. Most medical students and physicians-in-training are exposed to a minimum of material on pharmacology—the study of drugs, their origin, nature, properties, and their effects on living organisms. They may be exposed to clinical pharmacology, which is the actual use of drugs on live patients, during their internship and residency. But few doctors learn much during the four years of medical school about the basic science of pharmacology which will enable them to keep apace of the information explosion in the field. The pharmacology they do study is sandwiched between so many other courses that it is certainly fair to assume that this subject matter does not receive a high priority in medical training. This is a shame, because the prescription of various medicines is most doctors' stock-in-trade.

How then do doctors keep up with the new drugs that are constantly coming into the marketplace? One way is through a publication called the *Physicians' Desk Reference* (*PDR*). This large volume is the doctor's main source of information regarding drugs, including side effects, main actions, adverse reactions, contraindications, cautions, and the like. How do the various drugs get listed in this tome? The manufacturers pay to have their products listed in the *PDR*. The *PDR* is actually one large advertising venture. How else do doctors learn about drugs? They read the pharmaceutical companies' advertisements in a wide variety of medical journals. And finally, the major source of information for the practicing physician is the sales force of the drug manufacturers, called "detail people."

The main thrust of the *PDR*, the journal ads, and the detail persons is to sell drugs to the doctor. The detail people know how busy most doctors are and are only too happy to provide them with promotional materials lauding the purported benefits of their products (not to mention the free samples). Doctors prove to be just as gullible as the layman when it comes to some of the seductive claims and slick advertising coming at them from the drug companies. Dr. Richard Burack, author of *The New Handbook of Prescription Drugs,* comments:

> It is time to remind medical students, doctors-in-training, and all of the concerned public that the aims of the drug manufacturers are different from the aims of good doctors. The manufacturers wish to maximize their profits by encouraging doctors to write as many prescriptions as possible for the most expensive drugs. Manifestly, good doctors should minimize writing prescriptions and, as purchasing agents for patients, should do all they can to keep the cost of necessary medications as low as possible.[4]

A related problem is that doctors may fail to consider that non-medicinal remedies may work as well as or better than those employing medicine. In 1979, an article in the *Journal of the American Medical Association* stated that:

> Although a complete picture of prescribing practices is not at hand, the conclusions of two influential groups of physicians and researchers who have studied the matter are that the average physician is insufficiently educated in clinical pharmacology, often misled by industry advertising and "detail men," and inadequately informed of the alternatives to pharmacological therapy.[5]

The discovery of a number of drugs and drug families has been of great value to the practice of modern biomedicine and surgery. But the simple truth is that there are very few breakthroughs. An awful lot of the so-called new drugs are in fact "me-too" products. When a drug company does discover a new drug, that drug may be patented, and the patent is good for seventeen years before its generic equivalent can be marketed and sold. Many of the me-too drugs have the exact same generic chemical ingredients in the same dosages but with different filler substances (used to bind the product). However, each company markets this drug under its own unique brand name and prices vary considerably. Where do doctors learn about these me-too drugs? From the same *Physicians' Desk Reference,* professional-journal ads, and detail people as all the other prescription drugs.

Do drug manufacturers always tell the truth in their advertisements? Consider the following examples regarding commonly used OTC products in the analgesic (pain-killing) family of drugs. The analgesic market represents approximately $1 billion per year.

Claim: Bufferin (manufactured by Bristol-Myers Co.) is "twice as fast as aspirin."

Fact: The only pain reliever in Bufferin is aspirin. Despite the fact that Bristol-Myers claims that Bufferin enters the bloodstream faster than plain or unbuffered aspirin, the company couldn't furnish the Federal Trade Commission with any significant medical evidence that the speed of aspirin absorption has anything to do with the speed of pain relief.

Claim: "New, improved" Bayer (manufactured by Sterling Drug Co.) is "better-tolerated than regular aspirin" and "There's never been an aspirin like it. Ever."

Fact: Bayer is nothing but regular aspirin. The coating on the product may make it easier to swallow, but that's all.

The FTC recently issued a cease-and-desist order against the American Home Products Corporation and its advertisement for Anacin and Arthritis Pain Formula. The order was upheld, upon appeal, by the federal courts. Michael Pertschuk, a member of the FTC, said, "I'm not going to say they're liars, but I am sure going to say they engaged in deception and created false impressions." Anacin ads have used phrasing like:

Claim: "Two Anacin tablets have more of the one pain reliever doctors recommend most than four of the other leading extra-strength tablets."

Claim: "Anacin starts with as much pain reliever as the leading aspirin tablet, then adds an extra core of this specific fast-acting ingredient against pain."

Claim: "Doctors know Anacin contains more of the specific medication they recommend for pain than the leading aspirin, buffered aspirin, or extra-strength tablet."

Fact: The extra level of pain reliever is more aspirin. According to FTC testimony, extra aspirin has no proven effect on the speed or quality of pain relief. The only thing that separates Anacin from store-brand aspirin is a pinch of caffeine, which has no pain-relieving qualities.

Why are the aspirin manufacturers so reluctant to disclose that the product they are selling is aspirin? According to Samuel Murphy, Jr., the lawyer who argued American Home Products' case before the court: "I don't think it's a question of being reluctant to disclose. Most people know what's in the product. What you're trying to do in advertising is to get people's attention in a very short span of time." The FTC notes that aspirin "is so commonplace that a maker of one aspirin-based pain reliever seeking to differentiate its product from the rest faces a formidable marketing task. What better way to meet this challenge than to establish a new identity for the product dissociated from ordinary aspirin, and then to represent it as special and more effective than its competitors?" Caveat emptor—let the buyer beware!

Ours is a drug-taking society. The drug-seeking behavior is so ingrained in us that we are disappointed if we leave the doctor's office without at least one prescription for medicine to "cure" us. The physician's prescription writing is often a knee-jerk response, but so is our eagerness to be the recipients of the drugs (even to the extent that people can experience effects not caused by the pharmacologic agent—this is called the placebo effect). There are many cogs in the wheel that produces the dated physician. They are: (1) minimal training in basic and clinical pharmacology, (2) pressure from pushy and persuasive detail people,

(3) proliferation of me-too drugs and combination drugs, (4) pressure from pill-hungry patients, (5) lax enforcement of standards and guidelines by the Food and Drug Administration, (6) equally lax enforcement by the Federal Trade Commission regarding outrageous advertising claims, and (7) the information explosion in the pharmaceutical field. So we end up with a doctor with a threadbare start in pharmacology relying on profit-oriented sales people to provide you, the overanxious public, with a seemingly endless variety of medicines, only some of which are helpful.

Consumers and doctors alike look to federal regulatory agencies like the FDA to protect us from drugs that fall below established standards of effectiveness and safety. Yet one out of every eight prescriptions filled in the United States—169 million prescriptions, costing over $1.1 billion, in 1979—is for a drug not considered effective by the government's own standards. This lack of effectiveness means you are exposing yourself to risks that carry no benefits! In their revealing book *Pills That Don't Work,* Dr. Sidney Wolfe, Christopher M. Coley, and the Health Research Group (founded by Ralph Nader) report on 607 drugs considered ineffective by the FDA that, as of August 1980, were still on the market and still being prescribed by doctors. About two-thirds of these products are combinations, which means that while the risk of side effects increases proportionately, the benefits of these ineffective drugs does not increase at all. The reasons for their continued use: "Governmental inefficiency, lethargy and timidity, orchestrated by heavy pressure from drug companies to keep these drugs on the market." Even after the National Academy of Sciences National Research Council had ruled on the effectiveness of all prescription drugs approved for marketing between 1938 and 1962 (the year the drug laws were amended), it took a lawsuit by the American Public Health Association and the National Council of Senior Citizens to get the FDA to expedite the removal of these less-than-effective drugs from the marketplace.

What is the answer to this dilemma, of which the dated physician is only the tip of the iceberg? Nothing less than a massive campaign of drug education. The campaign must be mounted by a consortium of doctors, pharmacologists, consumers, pharmacists, and researchers. None of these people should be on the payroll of drug manufacturers! It is a requirement of most doctors that they participate in continuing educational programs in order to ensure continuing licensure. Drug updates must be part of a nationwide mandated curriculum for physicians. If the FDA were not so subject to budget cutting and political pressuring, perhaps it could meet its own mandate and help give us the protection we need. FDA guidelines on patient package inserts (PPIs) are now undergoing the same kind of foot-dragging that has characterized the removal of ineffective drugs. Some people are more interested in their own profits than in other people's health.

In January 1982 ABC News covered OTC cold remedies on their program *20/20*. Every year Americans spend millions of dollars seeking relief from cold symptoms. According to the experts interviewed by correspondent John Stossel, the only things that can help your cold are: (1) aspirin or a Tylenol-type substitute for pain, (2) a spray for your nose (watch out for "rebound"— the need to keep using them, leading to a functional addiction), and (3) dextromethorphan for a dry cough. Nothing else seems to work on a cold. This means that the manufacturers' claims for their products (particularly combination products) are all bunk! The claims are either exaggerated, patently false, suggest unneeded ingredients, or are otherwise misleading. Until the day that this massive educational campaign for doctors and the public is launched, and until the FDA and the FTC get their acts together, here are some questions you can ask your doctor to avoid the problem:

1. Have you prescribed this medication before? for my illness or condition? with what results?
2. Has the manufacturer made any claims for this drug which in your experience are unwarranted?
3. What is the research evidence that this drug is effective?
4. What reference materials (besides the *PDR*) do you use to keep abreast of the latest drug developments?

5. Would you mind if I consulted my pharmacist about this drug?

6. When was the last time you took an update course on drugs?

7. Do you subscribe to any drug publications not produced by drug manufacturers (newsletters, bulletins, etc.)?

Be assertive. Doctors don't like these kinds of questions, but you can help your doctor to realize that as an informed patient you want him or her to be an informed doctor.

Another reason for being assertive with doctors and pharmacists to secure needed drug information is the way the federal government has been dragging its feet about patient package inserts (PPIs). Under the Carter administration the FDA had announced plans to require PPIs for 375 prescription drugs. Met with a furious uproar from the American Medical Association and the drug industry, the FDA reduced their plans to a pilot program involving only ten drugs. The Reagan administration suspended the pilot program in January 1981 and formally buried it in September 1982. In October 1982, with great fanfare the AMA in cooperation with a group called the United States Pharmacopeial Convention began a voluntary drive to provide instruction sheets written in plain language on twenty widely used medicines including tranquilizers, insulin, oral penicillin, and nitroglycerin. The program is costing $2.7 million, $1.8 million being donated by drug companies and the rest by the 240,000-member AMA. The Carter plan had been scuttled because the AMA claimed the language in some leaflets might frighten some patients into not taking the medicine. The new sheets are being touted as "honest, accurate, reflective of fact and yet not frightening."

WOMEN BEWARE!

I am a female alcoholic and I've been getting over on doctors for years. I've been diagnosed as schizophrenic, severely depressed, and a hysterical personality. I have suffered from neuritis, ulcers, gastritis, and a fatty liver. Over the years I have been given prescriptions for Thorazine, Compazine, Mellaril, Valium, Librium and God knows how many drugs for my physical problems. I have seen no less than eighteen doctors over a period of fifteen years and not a single one of them knew I was an alcoholic. Not one ever took an alcohol or drug history. Of course I wasn't going to volunteer my "drinking problem" to them, but damn it, they never asked, either! You know what these doctors did do for me? They got me cross-addicted!

When I first met Martha (not her real name) she was really strung out on booze and tranquilizers. After getting her detoxified from both drugs, I took her to an internist who knows about alcoholism and drug abuse, and I took her to her first meeting of Alcoholics Anonymous. I read her old medical records very carefully and could find plenty of evidence of alcoholism (hidden between the lines) and very little of major mental disorder that fit her behavior while dry and clean. Psychotherapy consisted of her making a long hard climb back to self-respect while going to A.A. almost daily for a year (she still is quite active). Her old doctors had mistaken a toxic psychosis caused directly by the alcohol and sedative pills for an actual schizophrenic break. Her depressions were understandable in terms of her heavy drinking and remorse over this drinking. Her hysteria was simply a cry of pain and a plea for help. Male physicians were too ready to see her as a weak and sick woman who just needed some medicine to make her all right. They gave her neither the time nor the respect she deserved and needed. What they did give her was prescriptions, sexist attitudes, and the short end of the medical stick. I wish Martha's story were the exception. I'm afraid it's much closer to being the rule. Looking at the way women are treated by various health-care professionals is a real eye-opener.

Item: A group of doctors in California wanted to know how male physicians would respond to five common medical complaints: back pain, headaches, dizziness, chest pain, and fatigue. What they found is that workups for these complaints were significantly more extensive for male than for female patients. The conclusion: male physicians tend to take illness more seriously in men than women.

Item: The House Select Committee on Narcotics Abuse and Control held hearings to discover why so many women were taking mood-altering drugs. They found that "thirty-two million (42%) women compared to 19 million (26%) men have used tranquilizers prescribed by a doctor. Sixteen million (21%) women as compared to 12 million (17%) men have used physician-prescribed sedatives and 12 million (17%) women as compared to 5 million (8%) men have used amphetamines ordered by a doctor. An estimated 9 million women use tranquilizers, 3 million women use sedatives, and 1 million women take their first stimulants prescribed by a doctor in any given year."

Item: A nationwide survey of more than 15,000 A.A. members showed that 29 percent of the women but only 15 percent of the men were addicted to other drugs besides alcohol. Of new A.A. members age thirty or younger, 55 percent of women were cross-addicted, compared to 36 percent of men.

Item: A landmark study in mental health asked a group of psychotherapists to define, respectively, a mature healthy man, a mature healthy woman, and a mature healthy adult. With a high degree of agreement the therapists defined a healthy mature woman as more submissive, less independent, less adventurous, less competitive, more excitable in minor crises, more easily hurt, and more emotional than a mature healthy man. A mature healthy adult was described in a manner remarkably similar to a man. The study results demonstrated a pervasive sexist attitude among therapists.

Item: In a study of staff and patient attitudes toward women in a drug-free therapeutic community treatment agency, staff viewed women as more emotional, more sensitive, limited by their biology, needing to please men, and implicitly "sicker" than men. Staff also placed greater emphasis on interpersonal relationships being uniquely female addict problems. A stable relationship with a man was thought by staff to be more important to success in treatment for a woman, while realistic job plans were considered more important to a man.

Item: In a study of attitudes toward women in a methadone maintenance program, the staff greatly underestimated the extent to which female clients felt unable to express their feelings, have bad feelings about their bodies, feel they are not smart, and feel they need more education. In brief, staff had more trouble perceiving the problems of their female clients than of their male clients. This was surprising considering the disproportionate number of women on the clinic staff.

Item: A number of separate studies have come to similar conclusions regarding drug advertising and women. Many of the drug ads suggest the use of mood-altering drugs as the best treatment for problems that are often beyond traditional medical and psychiatric concepts of illness. Many of the "problems" targeted in the drug ads are everyday life problems that could better be dealt with by psychotherapy, social action, or closer ties between people. Many ads portray women who supposedly can't cope with their "role" and women who "bother" their husbands and doctors. Rather than suggesting coping with or learning to handle these problems, the drug industry promotes the use of drugs to ease "anxiety."

Item: An examination of statistics on drug overdoses maintained by the National Institute on Drug Abuse shows that women continue to predominate over men. The highest percentage is found among white women and the lowest among white men. Most prominent among the drugs involved in emergency-room drug episodes are Valium, aspirin, Dalmane, Darvon, Elavil, and Librium.

Sexism has permeated the practice of medicine, pharmacotherapy, psychotherapy, and the treatment of drug and alcohol problems. Eighty-eight percent of all doctors are men. The number of women presently in medical school is increasing significantly (some 30 to 40 percent) but it will be some years before they join the ranks of practicing physicians.

Evaluating Mental-Health Programs and Therapists

Almost 90 percent of psychoactive medications are prescribed by doctors other than psychiatrists, mostly "general practitioners." The general practitioner relies on the prescription pad and has little training in mental health and quality-of-life issues, which leads to overprescribing, especially for women.

- Many doctors are "too busy" to give women patients the time needed to really hear the full context of the problems they are experiencing. Note the actual amount of time that you spend with the doctor on your next visit. Bet it doesn't take more than a few minutes for a cursory exam and a real quick chat, and you probably emerge with at least one prescription.
- Many doctors harbor a wide range of sexist attitudes, and because of this tend to see many problems in terms of women resisting the roles they ought to be content to fill. It goes something like this: "If you would just stay home and care for your husband and kids, everything would be fine. In the meantime here is a prescription for something to calm your nerves."
- Many doctors derive much of their perceived power from being able to provide instant relief through medication. It also keeps them from having to get involved in underlying issues. Thus, very often they tend to be ignorant of or otherwise ignore nondrug remedies to the problem.

A balance needs to be struck between the use of psychoactive medications and the use of other approaches and therapies that do not include drugs, such as psychotherapy, self-help, mutual support groups, anonymous societies such as Alcoholics Anonymous, and herbal, natural, and folk medicines.

Here are some general guidelines to help you in choosing practitioners and agencies that (a) may use drug therapy and (b) claim they can help you with an existing drug problem.

1. Problems exist in a context. Is the helper interested in hearing about your general situation? Willing to try to understand your problem within the context of your lifestyle? The problem may be personal, interpersonal, or impersonal in nature. Can the helper assist you in pinpointing sources of problems outside of yourself as well as within you?

2. What attitudes does he harbor about women in general? Does he believe that the rights and roles of women in society are to be restricted or expanded? Does he treat you as a person or a woman? Is he trying to force you into preconceived roles or is he helping you become what you want to be?

3. When considering drug therapy for psychological problems, is the drug therapy part of a total plan of treatment or the only service being offered? As a rule, drugs alone deal with symptoms. You will probably want to get to the underlying cause(s) and should therefore ask for more than a prescription for medication.

4. Is the helper willing to seriously consider nondrug alternatives? For example, many people have found that proper diet and exercise help with anxiety and stress in place of drugs. Does the helper respect your right not to take drugs?

Some specific considerations if drug therapy is being proposed:

1. Does your doctor give you adequate information about benefits and risks so that you feel you can make an informed decision?

2. Can the doctor suggest some relevant reading material on the drug before you make your decision? Can he

199

or she introduce you to anyone who has taken this drug and been helped?

3. How long will you have to take the drug? Will the doctor consider a "drug holiday" when the crisis is past to see how you manage on your own?

4. Is counseling or psychotherapy being recommended along with the medication, or is the drug being touted as a cure-all?

5. Is the doctor really familiar with your unique problem? Has he or she dealt with many cases like yours? Is the drug being recommended specific to your problem or is it a general "psychic panacea" for "nerves" and "uptight ladies"?

Choosing a drug treatment program:

1. Are there women on staff in clinical and administrative policy-making positions? Remember, everything falls from the top in organizations.

2. What is their track record in working with female clients? Can you talk with some of their women clients before enrolling?

3. If you wish, can your therapist or counselor be a woman?

4. Does your therapist respect your individual needs as opposed to treating you as just another woman with a drug problem?

5. If you want help with educational or vocational concerns, can they provide it? The ability to earn a living is a vital part of recovery for men and women.

6. Are they knowledgeable about your drug(s) of abuse? Some programs try to be all things to all people. Some do better with drug problems while others do better with alcoholism.

7. Is there an end point in treatment? Can you graduate into less intense treatment as you progress in your recovery?

8. Do they provide services for physical, psychological, and spiritual recovery? Do they understand the special needs of women and relate to them as an essential part of treatment?

Some problems do not need to be put into diagnostic categories and placed in the hands of professionals or paraprofessionals. Have you considered your own personal network of friends and associates? Many people are able to work things out or to get through a crisis by turning to a friend who will listen and care. Sisterhood can be very powerful indeed. You should explore self-help and support groups in your community like Alcoholics Anonymous (A.A.), Pills Anonymous (P.A.), consciousness-raising groups, Parents Anonymous (for child-abuse problems), Toughlove (for serious problems with adolescent children), programs sponsored by the National Organization for Women (NOW), and many others. The psychology committee of NOW's New York chapter has put together an informative guide entitled "A Consumer's Guide to Nonsexist Therapy," which deals with choosing a therapist and the rights of clients in therapy. You may also wish to contact local feminist organizations for listings of self-help and support groups in your area.

The task force on sex bias and sex role stereotyping in psychotherapeutic practice of the American Psychological Association has provided some excellent guidelines for therapy with women:

1. The conduct of therapy should be free of constrictions based on sex roles, and the options explored between you and the practitioner should be free of sex role stereotypes.
2. Your therapist should recognize the reality, variety, and implications of sex-discriminatory practices in society and should facilitate your examination of options in dealing with such practices.
3. Your therapist should be knowledgeable about current scientific findings on sex roles, sexism, and individual differences resulting from sex-defined identity.

4. The theoretical concepts employed by your therapist should be free of sex bias and sex role stereotypes.

5. Your therapist should demonstrate acceptance of women as equal to men by using language free of derogatory labels.

6. Your therapist should avoid establishing the source of personal problems within you when they are more properly attributable to situational or cultural factors.

7. Your therapist and you should mutually agree upon aspects of the therapy relationship such as treatment modality, time factors, and fee arrangements.

8. While the importance of the availability of accurate information to your family is recognized, the privilege of communication about diagnosis, prognosis, and progress ultimately resides with you, not with the therapist.

9. If authoritarian processes are employed as a technique, the therapy should not have the effect of maintaining or reinforcing stereotyped dependence of women.

10. Your assertive behaviors should be respected.

11. The therapist whose female clients are subjected to violence in the form of physical abuse or rape should recognize and acknowledge that the client is the victim of a crime.

12. Your therapist should recognize and encourage exploration of your sexuality and should recognize your right to define your own sexual preferences.

13. The therapist should not have sexual relations with a woman client nor treat her as a sex object.

When you are satisfied that you are in the hands of a competent nonsexist doctor who takes the time to understand your needs and situation, you should consider drug therapy as one of the resources available to you. Aside from the blatantly ineffective drugs, some medications can be a definite aid in some cases. Don't throw the baby out with the bath water. But make sure that you are an equal partner to the decision to enter into drug therapy with a full understanding of all the risks and benefits. Stand up for your rights as a woman and a consumer.

WARNING: THIS DRUG MAY BE HABIT FORMING!

Most people associate drug dependency and addiction with illegal street drugs. The legal status of a drug does not have a thing to do with its potential for becoming habit forming. Many prescription and OTC drugs have a potential for physical and psychological dependence. To understand addiction, we must start with some clearly defined terminology.

Tolerance: As your body adapts to drugs over time, certain tissues react less vigorously to the drug's presence. This cumulative resistance to the pharmacological effects of a drug is called tolerance. It occurs when the repeated use of a given dose produces a decreased effect. This means that the person will have to take increased doses to get the original effect.

Withdrawal: The cluster of characteristic reactions and behavior unique to the stopping (or severe reduction) of a specific drug. Different drugs create different withdrawal syndromes. Depending upon the drug, amount taken, and frequency of usage, withdrawal can range from mild to life-threatening. Physical addiction is required for withdrawal to occur.

Physical addiction: Physical addiction is evidenced by either tolerance or withdrawal symptoms. Since tolerance is actually brain tissue getting "used" to certain levels of a drug being present, withdrawal is the body's way of making a statement, which we commonly call craving. Withdrawal symptoms are caused by the body's trying to cope with a sudden upheaval in body chemistry.

Psychological addiction: This is the belief that one can't function properly or cope with the stresses of daily living without the drug in question. It is a compulsive need for a drug's mental effects; the user feels his or her well-being is threatened without it. Sometimes referred to as habituation, it may exist alone or with physical addiction.

Functional addiction: This is what is sometimes called a "medical" addiction. It happens when a drug effectively relieves an annoying or distressing condition and the body becomes increasingly dependent upon the action of that drug to maintain well-being. These drugs usually act on symptoms and do not involve the brain in creating altered states of mood or consciousness. Functional addiction is different from physical and psychological addiction.

According to the General Accounting Office, the investigative arm of Congress, the abuse of prescription drugs causes far more deaths than use of illegal drugs. "Millions of Americans abuse prescription drugs, often with tragic results," stated their report released in November of 1982. The federal Drug Abuse Warning Network showed that prescription drugs "dominate the statistics" on drug related deaths and emergencies. In 1980, prescription

Drug-Abuse Warning Network
Top 20 Controlled Drugs Abused
(Calendar Year 1980)

| | | | Drug mentions reported by | |
| | | | --- | --- |
Drug	Type	Controlled Substances Act Schedule	EMER-GENCY ROOMS Number	MEDICAL EXAM-INERS Number
Diazepam (Valium)	P	4	16,603	346
Heroin	I	1	8,487	885
Methaqualone	PT	2	5,958	137
Flurazepam (Dalmane)	P	4	4,538	92

Drug	Type	Controlled Substances Act Schedule	Drug mentions reported by	
			EMER-GENCY ROOMS Number	MEDICAL EXAM-INERS Number
Marijuana	I	1	4,513	10
PCP	I	2	4,441	43
Cocaine	I	2	4,153	265
D-Propoxyphene (Darvon)	P	4	2,964	326
Phenobarbital	P	4	2,861	225
Amphetamine	PT	2	2,658	37
Chlordiazepox-ide (Librium)	P	4	2,602	48
Methadone	P	2	2,500	376
Secobarbital/ amobarbital	P	2	2,183	144
Acetaminophen w/codeine	P	3	1,980	5
Pentazocine (Talwin)	P	4	1,914	66
Ethchlorvynol (Placidyl)	P	4	1,834	103
Speed	PT	2	1,808	0
Chlorazepate (Tranxene)	P	4	1,719	5
Oxycodone (Percodan)	P	2	1,498	3
LSD	I	1	1,452	2
Total P & PT			53,620	1,913
Total I			23,046	1,205
Total			76,666	3,118

P—Prescription drug; normally found in the legitimate market
PT—Prescription-type drug; significant origins outside legitimate domestic market
I—Illegal drug
Drugs are listed by generic name (example, brand names are in parentheses)

drugs were identified in 3,535, or 74 percent, of 4,747 deaths attributed to drugs by medical examiners. In the same year hospital emergency room reports showed that 71,431, or 75 percent, of 95,502 drug emergencies were due to the misuse of prescription drugs. In that year, fifteen of the twenty drugs most frequently mentioned were prescription as opposed to illegal drugs. The table above shows the distribution of these drugs as recorded by the federal government's Drug Abuse Warning Network (DAWN).[6]

In 1978 and again in 1979, the House Select Committee on Narcotics Abuse and Control held public hearings on prescription drug abuse, and their conclusion was that these drugs were being overprescribed by physicians and diverted into the illegal market. A 1979 national survey conducted by the National Institute on Drug Abuse showed that the nonmedical use of prescription drugs was second only to the use of marijuana/hashish.

Many of the drugs that are addicting belong to that broad class of drugs called "painkillers." Americans spend over $1 billion a year on OTC painkillers alone. People are determined to use chemicals to avoid or alleviate pain. The nostrums of the great American medicine show during the 1800s brought more narcotics like opium and morphine into American homes than all the modern-day hard drug dealers combined. In 1900, for example, it has been estimated that 3,300,000 doses of opium were sold every month in the state of Vermont alone. That was enough to give every man, woman, and child in that state a continuous daily supply of one and one-half doses. Reports from this period suggested that the national population of those who became physically dependent on opium well exceeded 200,000. How could this have happened when people were partaking of such innocent-sounding concoctions as "Ayer's Cherry Pectoral," "Dover's Powder," "McMunn's Elixir of Opium," "Godfrey's Cordial," or "Mrs. Winslow's Soothing Syrup"? Their manufacturers made extraordinary claims for this wide assortment of compounds and elixirs, covering every malady from diarrhea to "women's troubles" to "consumption cures."

What was really going on was that people were either relieving pain getting high, or were "blissed out" (as with tranquilizers) by these opium-containing "medicines." Morphine was even used by some doctors to treat alcoholism. The result was that many of the alcoholics switched over and became morphine addicts.

In 1906 the Pure Food and Drug Act was passed. This act required that medicines containing opiates and certain other drugs had to say so on their labels, along with drug quantity and purity. But it wasn't until the passing of the Harrison Narcotics Act of 1914 that all opiates were removed from the open market and made available only through a doctor's prescription.

Analgesics are painkilling drugs. Opiates like morphine began the widespread use of such drugs over a hundred years ago. Many soldiers during the Civil War were treated with morphine and then spent many postwar years with a "medical addiction," that is, an unintentional addiction caused by the administration of the drug for pain relief. In order to be an ideal painkiller an analgesic drug would have to:

1. be potent enough to afford maximum pain relief;
2. be nonaddicting;
3. exhibit a minimum of side effects such as constipation, nausea, vomiting, and respiratory depression;
4. not cause tolerance to develop;
5. act promptly and over a long period of time with a minimum amount of sedation;
6. be relatively inexpensive.

One might ask whether the fact that opiates cause feelings of euphoria is a beneficial effect. It would certainly seem so, but part of our Puritan heritage is the Protestant prohibition against pleasure. Although pharmaceutical manufacturers are sparing no resources in the search for the ideal analgesic, it continues to elude them. Many products were once promoted as nonaddicting narcotics but usage over time inevitably led to physical and psychological dependency. Included among these drugs are heroin (which has no current medical usage in the United States), Demerol (meperidine), Dilaudid (hydromorphone), and the latest contestant, Talwin (pentazocine). When pentazocine was first introduced in 1967 it was believed that it came close to the ideal. However, it was soon learned that the drug can produce both physical and psychological dependence if used in large doses for an extended period of time, thus making it useful only for short-term management of pain.

Chronic pain is often a major feature in terminal illness. Recurring or persistent pain is most often accompanied by anxiety, depression, loss of appetite, and the inability to sleep. The hospice movement which began in England and spread to the United States has developed a compassionate and humanistic approach to pain management. In 1975 at St. Christopher's hospice in London an oral medication known as Brompton's Mixture provided patients with significant relief from the pain and distress associated with terminal cancer. Brompton's mixture, or "cocktail," consisted of:

diamorphine HCL	5–10 mg
cocaine	10 mg
alcohol (90%)	1.25 ml
syrup	2.5 ml
chloroform water to	10 ml

A phenothiazine was also given to potentiate, or boost, the effect of diamorphine (heroin), and to act as an antinausea drug and tranquilizer. Brompton's cocktail has been replaced in the United States by a morphine-alcohol solution commonly known as "hospice mix." This combination of ingredients is morphine sulfate in a 20 percent alcohol solution, to which flavoring agents and sugar are usually added. The side effect of sedation from the administration of morphine every four hours tends to disappear after a few days. Constipation can be treated with a combination of diet and stool softeners. This treatment can also be used at home in cases of similar life-threatening illness. (Consult your physician regarding the medical and legal aspects of such treatment.)

It is not only the narcotic or analgesic drugs that can cause any one of the three types of addiction. Let's consider two natural bodily functions: bowel movements and clear nasal passages. From time to time we all experience constipation. If you take a laxative you may come to depend upon that laxative to obtain normal bowel movements. Once this happens (and remember, there is no mood alteration or getting high with this kind of drug), you are in trouble. If constipation persists it may be because the constipation is a symptom of an underlying disorder and you should consult your doctor. When there is no pathological condition existing, it is better to find nonchemical ways to treat the problem of constipation—such as proper diet. The "rebound effect," which occurs when the desired state brought about by a drug leads to a dependency upon the drug, has been known to happen with nasal sprays as well. The spray clears up your nasal congestion for a while and then you find yourself stuffed up again or maybe feeling even worse, so it's back to the spray. This is a growing problem among cocaine sniffers, who use nasal sprays to deal with their chronically runny noses. It doesn't take long for the functional addiction to develop. Both of these are examples of functional addictions and rarely are conceived of as drug dependencies. But they are addictions just as real as the psychological and physical ones.

There are OTCs that can lead to physical dependencies and worse. The FDA has been warning people about a painkiller called phenacetin (acetophenetidin) since 1977, stating that it "is not safe for OTC use because of the high potential for abuse, the high potential for harm to the kidney . . . and the lack of compensating benefits of the drug." The FDA has concluded that this drug has high abuse potential, giving the user a slight euphoric feeling along with mild stimulation. But it's still on the market in a variety of OTCs. According to the 1982 *Physicians' Desk Reference,* the following medications still contain phenacetin:

A.P.C. tablets	Emprazil-C tablets
A.P.C. with Butalbital	Fiorinal
A.P.C. with Codeine	Fiorinal with Codeine
Apectol tablets	SK-65 Compound Capsules
Butalbital with APC tablets	Soma Compound
Emprazil tablets	Soma Compound with Codeine

Check the label on *all* OTCs to see if they contain this drug as well.

There are drugs like diazepam (Valium) which can be physically or psychologically addictive or both. Some physicians are easily manipulated by "street wise" drug users for these types of drugs. Hypnotic sedatives like Quāālude, Parest, and Sopor are popular with these manipulators. Large doses of these cause physical and psychological dependency. One has to take care with cross-addicting drugs as well. For example, a person who takes barbiturates and also drinks alcohol, both in subaddicting amounts, may find himself developing a tolerance, as both are sedatives with very similar chemical actions.

Because so many drugs have side effects, adverse reactions, contraindications, addiction potential, and the like, it has become very important to know as much as possible about the drugs we take. The drug manufacturers and the doctors don't seem to want us to know too much about the drugs they produce and prescribe. Why else are they fighting the institution of patient package inserts, and why else is the FDA dragging its feet on this issue? Like so many issues involving drugs, there are two sides to the coin. You already know the "down side" about how patients are treated as ignorant children by drug companies and many doctors. The other side of the coin, at least from the doctor's point of view, is that there really are patients who, if told about a certain potential drug effect, will be certain to experience that effect. People are very open to suggestion, especially when they are sick, and doctors are afraid that telling us what might happen when we take a drug, particularly side effects and adverse reactions, will guarantee that it will happen. Perhaps many of us deserve to be viewed this way by our doctors. By abdicating personal responsibility for drug taking and placing it all in the hands of someone we perceive as being the right hand of God, we have brought this grief down on our own heads. When we take back this personal responsibility, then we can say to the doctor, "I want to know everything that is important in making a benefit/risk decision about this drug!" And that includes information about habit-forming drugs. We must know whether or not medicines contain ingredients that risk any of the three types of drug addiction. This has implications for:

- deciding whether or not to take the drug.
- avoiding the addictive potential.
- respecting the importance of taking it only as prescribed.
- planning for discontinuation of the drug so that none of its potential for dependence and tolerance, and therefore withdrawal syndrome effects, are realized.
- checking out your desire to use this drug for purposes other than it was intended.
- avoiding tolerance and the need for escalating doses.

Many people have become addicted to OTC and prescription medications through ignorance. Educate yourself and know what you are taking!

ALTERNATIVES

As you have just read, all is not well in our modern world of standard medicine. After reading about the many risks and dangers involved in contemporary drug therapy, it is only natural for the question to arise, Are there alternatives? The answer is yes, but you must be willing to greatly expand your awareness of approaches that fall outside of standard medicine. Once you have done this you are in a far better position to choose from a broader range of remedies. The central idea is to view "traditional" and "contemporary" methods of healing not as antagonistic, but rather as points along a broad continuum of possible remedies. I commend to you the holistic view as an organizing principle around which to make these important choices. Here I mean that holistic medicine is a model rather than just a series of techniques that define its practice. Here are the elements that are central to this model.[7]

1. Holistic medicine addresses itself to the physical, mental, and spiritual aspects of those who come for care.

2. Although it appreciates the predictive value of data which are based on statistical models, holistic medicine emphasizes each patient's genetic, biological, and psychosocial uniqueness as well as the importance of tailoring treatment to meet each individual's needs.

3. A holistic approach to medicine and health care includes understanding and treating people in the context of their culture, their family, and their community.

4. Holistic medicine views health as a positive state, not as the absence of disease.

5. Holistic medicine emphasizes the responsibility of each individual for his or her health.

6. Holistic medicine emphasizes the promotion of health and the prevention of disease.

7. Holistic medicine uses therapeutic approaches that mobilize the individual's innate capacity for self-healing.

8. Though none would deny the occasional necessity for swift and authoritative medical or surgical intervention, the emphasis in holistic medicine is on helping people to understand and to help themselves, on education and self-care rather than treatment and dependence.

9. Holistic medicine makes use of a variety of diagnostic methods and systems in addition to and sometimes in place of the standard laboratory examinations.

10. Physical contact between practitioner and patient is an important element of holistic medicine.

11. Good health depends on good nutrition and regular exercise.

12. Holistic medicine includes an appreciation of and attention to sensuousness and sexuality.

13. Holistic medicine views illness as an opportunity for discovery as well as misfortune.

14. Holism includes an appreciation of the quality of life in each of its stages and an interest in improving it as

well as acknowledgment of the illnesses that are common to it.

15. Holistic medicine emphasizes the potential therapeutic value of the setting in which health care takes place.

16. An understanding of and a commitment to change those social and economic conditions that perpetuate ill health are as much a part of holistic medicine as its emphasis on individual responsibility.

17. Holistic medicine transforms its practitioners as well as its patients.

The kind of active partnership between patient/consumer and practitioner implied in this model makes you far more responsible for your own state of health and well-being. To participate in this model means giving up the notion of "instant" relief and dependence on practitioners as the sole dispensers of relief and comfort. The good news is that a willingness to embrace this model can often mean a real decrease in reliance on drug therapies for many maladies. It means moving from being the passive recipient of pills and elixirs to being the active promoter of your own relatively drug-free health. Listed below are some of the techniques and therapies which have become an active part of holistic medical practice in the United States and other countries.

Biofeedback: With the aid of electronically enhanced biological feedback, physiological mechanisms, previously believed to be outside of voluntary control, can be controlled by the individual after brief training periods. Biofeedback has positive effects on such problems as tension headaches, migraine, essential hypertension, insomnia, Raynaud's disease, sinus, tachycardia, bronchial asthma, functional colitis, stuttering, urinary retention, sexual dysfunctions, drug abuse, hyperactivity, anxiety, and phobias.

Autogenic Training: A highly systematized technique designed to generate a state of psychophysiological relaxation, the opposite of the state of stress. Specific practices and exercises are taught that allow the individual to achieve a state of deep relaxation, enabling the body and mind to carry out their own recuperative and healing processes.

Meditation: Meditation is a whole family of techniques that have in common a conscious attempt to focus attention. It is used to achieve altered states of consciousness and as a system of self-regulation. It can induce powerful subjective changes in one's view of one's self, of nature, and of other people. It can lead to altered states similar to those brought about by hypnosis and deep muscle relaxation exercises.

Hypnosis: Hypnosis may be many things but is generally agreed upon as some sort of altered awareness and behavior as compared with the presumably normal awake state. It can be used as posthypnotic suggestion to directly relieve symptoms and to override any unconscious resistance, or as a medium for substituting good physical responses for disturbed ones, and can gain access to selective memory to reveal cause-and-effect relationships in physical and emotional problems. It is used to help manage pain, as a technique of anesthesia, in obstetrics and gynecology, and as a means of communicating with unconscious or critically ill patients.

Chiropractic: Chiropractic involves manipulation of the spine and joints and views the nervous system as the crucial element in proper bodily functioning. Recently chiropractors have begun to include diet and exercise regimens and healing modalities such as acupuncture, massage, and homeopathy. Chiropractic is seen as an alternative to surgical and pharmacologic remedies. As research efforts increase, more objective evidence of the value and importance of alteration in musculoskeletal structures to bodily functioning may be demonstrated. For the moment, most testimonials are individual. Most of you know someone who swears by their chiropractor.

Acupuncture: Chinese medicine seeks to maintain or restore a balance between yang and yin much as our concept of homeostasis, which refers to a balance of opposite forces to insure proper functioning of physiological systems. Tiny hair-thin needles are painlessly inserted and removed, and while in place they create a tingling or heavy sensation. Modern research shows that acupuncture is most effective as an alternative to analgesic drugs in the management of certain kinds of pain: musculoskeletal pain, muscle contraction, migraine headaches, and various neuralgias. It is used as an alternative to surgical or pharmacologic management of pain and for some patients is an extremely effective technique.

Homeopathic Medicine: From the Greek *homois,* meaning similar, and *pathos,* meaning suffering or sickness. The basic law of homeopathy is based on the law of similars, or "like is cured by like." The law of similars states that a remedy or medicine can cure a disease if it produces in a healthy person symptoms similar to that of the disease. This stimulates the body's own healing powers. Homeopaths do not prescribe combination drugs, preferring to work with one symptom and one medicine at a time. They also stress minimum dosage. They also believe that much chronic disease is due to the incorrect treatment of prior acute illness, leading to its suppression and eventual emergence in a chronic form.

There are other techniques and therapies too numerous to describe here, such as herbalism, natural medicine (naturopathy), exercise, food and nutrition, light and sound in health, psychic healing, touch, etc. For further readings on the subject consult the bibliography.

CHAPTER FIVE

Getting High

In this chapter we will take a look at the risks and benefits that accompany the use of pleasure drugs. You may hear people refer to them by a variety of names—recreational, pleasure, street, leisure, good times drugs. They all refer to the assortment of drugs that are used in the pursuit of pleasurable states. Regardless of what drug we are talking about—a martini, a fine wine, a cold beer, a joint (marijuana cigarette), a line of cocaine, a handful of ludes (methaqualone)—the end result of drug use is the same: a change in our mood and consciousness. Is the desire to alter consciousness periodically an innate, normal drive analagous to hunger or the sex drive? Seventy percent of adult America drinks alcoholic beverages; over 15 million people have tried cocaine; over 40 million people have tried marijuana and some 12 million use it regularly; and so it goes for many other drugs as well. The National Institute on Drug Abuse recently estimated that Americans spend at least $120 billion a year on controlled substances and their consequences.

DON'T PUT IT INTO YOUR SYSTEM UNLESS YOU KNOW WHAT IT'LL DO TO YOU

Remember when you were a little kid and your mother warned about what could happen if you placed foreign objects in your mouth? She was concerned about your health and did not want you to get sick. The same warning still holds true today and can easily be applied to drug usage. But it isn't just your mouth that you need to exercise caution about. There are many ways to take drugs: you can inject them into your body (skin popping just under the surface or mainlining, heading straight for a vein); you can smoke them (using rolling papers, bongs, carburetors, pipes, and other smoking paraphernalia); you can ingest them through the mucous membranes of your nose (sniffing and snorting); you can drink them (and not just alcohol: people who are into reggae music and the Jamaican culture enjoy drinking concoctions made with cannabis extracts); and you can eat them (anything from hash brownies to psychedelic mushrooms like peyote and psilocybin). Pill takers, particularly fans of barbiturates and hypnotics like Quaaludes (methaqualone), often speak of "eating" their pills. There are a lot of ways to get high.

How do you really know what you are putting into your system? Let's say you are at a party and drugs are offered. This is the time to remember your mother's warning. Once you are high, it may be too late. Everybody is so busy being hip, bragging about their "reliable" connections and the good "shit" that they were able to "cop."

When you go into a liquor store or supermarket and purchase a bottle of spirits or wine or beer, you believe you are getting what it says on the label, including type of spirits and alcohol content. You assume purity and quantity of dose because your experience has taught you that these things are uniform from purchase to purchase. The same holds true, in general, for prescription drugs and over-the-counter medications. But have you ever stopped to consider what really is in alcoholic drinks? One researcher, Hebe B. Greizerstein, of the New York State Division of Alcoholism and Alcohol Abuse, has found that, along with the principal active ingredient, ethanol, most alcoholic beverages contain such items as lead, iron, cobalt, histamines, tannins, phenols, and trace amounts of a large number of other organic and inorganic compounds.[1] The Center for Science in the Public Interest claims that over a million people may be allergic to substances in beer, wine, and liquor. They cite, as one example, the common preservative sulfur dioxide as causing allergic reactions, and further claim that yellow dye no. 5, allowed in beer and spirits, has brought problems to "tens of thousands" of aspirin-sensitive people. The beverage industry has fought against labeling requirements, claiming they are expensive and unnecessary, and that consumers would not understand them. Is it safe to assume these ingredients carry no health risks? One class of chemical compounds added to alcoholic beverages, called cogeners, are already suspected of being largely responsible for variety in the severity of hangovers. The answer to this question should probably be the same as the cautions regarding marijuana use, namely that in the absence of conclusive scientific evidence, if you must drink alcohol or smoke grass, judicious moderation and an alertness to new discoveries are in order. In the interim it would certainly be helpful to consumers in calculating risks and benefits of alcoholic beverage consumption if the products carried labels that disclose all the ingredients.

Having considered alcohol products that you had previously taken for granted, consider the fact that once you step into the world of illicit or pleasure drugs, all bets are off concerning acts of faith! This same act of faith applied to drugs bought "on the street" can lead to serious trouble. The products are not labeled, there are no assurances of quality control, many substances resemble each other in color and consistency, price varies greatly, and the seller does not have to comply with any licensing or regulatory requirements. To put it mildly, appearances can be very deceptive, and you won't find any warnings from the surgeon general's office either. And yet millions of people are making drug-taking an act of faith every day. Very few stop to consider the psychology of drug taking as an act of faith.

In the partying situation we tend to assume that:

- the drug is what people say it is;
- our friends and acquaintances would not give us anything harmful;
- if we are told this is "good stuff," there is no need to question it;
- the dose is reliable;
- we are going to get high in ways we have previously experienced.

Taking these kinds of things for granted has gotten people into serious trouble.

It is much safer to ask questions than to make this act of faith. Check it out! Be skeptical. Don't let anyone else assume your responsibility for something that you are going to put into your body. Ask questions about the drugs you are offered, and if you don't like the tone or content of the answers, *don't take the drug!* Remember, if you decide to take the drug you must be prepared to live with the consequences, good and bad.

Jim's story

Jim always thought of himself as a pretty hip drug user. He had never been beat in a drug deal, and always got what he paid for. He prided himself on his ability to score good stuff and enjoyed turning on his friends. When his usual marijuana connection got busted he heard about a new one from a "friend." He bought a dime bag ($10) of what he was told was high-quality grass and proceeded to share it with three friends. They all smoked, expecting to get a nice marijuana high. Within twenty minutes two of his friends were acting very weird and Jim was starting to experience feelings of paranoia. Realizing that something was terribly wrong, they had the good sense to go to a hospital emergency room. One of his friends became violent and had to be restrained. Fortunately, the doctor in the ER knew his street drugs. The boys had smoked some very low-grade grass which had been laced with angel dust (PCP or phencyclidine), a volatile and powerful animal tranquilizer with hallucinatory effects. Neither Jim nor his friends thought he was very hip after that experience.

Phencyclidine (PCP, hog, angel dust) was formerly used to sedate large animals like jungle cats and elephants, but it made them so agitated and disoriented before putting them under that it has been abandoned by veterinarians. Kids picked up on it as a drug which causes a strong high and certain psychedelic effects (similar to marijuana). However, it carries some awesome unwanted side effects like severe disorientation, paranoia, violent behavior, depression, and confusion, so that its risks far outweigh any apparent user benefits. It rarely affects the same person the same way upon subsequent use and is therefore very unpredictable. It's a real bummer and should be avoided altogether. Take a lesson from Jim and his friends. This is one of those "I dare you to try it" drugs. Stay away from it!

Drug dealing is a very lucrative and a virtually uncontrollable business. Unscrupulous dealers find plenty of ways to cut corners and increase profits—all at your expense. Here are some examples of how they do it.

Ways to Get Beat in the Illicit Drug Market

What it's supposed to be	What it often turns out to be
High-grade marijuana	Low-grade (very little THC and other mind-altering ingredients)
	Oregano (sometimes laced with PCP)
	A mixture of a small amount of high-grade grass with a lot of low-grade stuff
Dexedrin, Eskabarb, Dalmane, Valium	Mild stimulants like ephedrin, caffeine, phenylpropanolamine, called "look-alike" drugs; sold in

What it's supposed to be	What it often turns out to be
	health stores and on the street. Danger is that you get a bogus reaction and are in trouble when you take the real thing because it's much stronger (false sense of being able to handle the drugs).
Amphetamines	Caffeine. You'll get a fraction of the lift at top-market prices.
Methaqualone (ludes)	Valium or phenobarbital (both very dangerous at high dose levels).
Cocaine	You get very little or no coke. Coke is cut with lactose (milk sugar), powered milk, Epsom salts, caffeine, talcum powder, sucrose, glucose, quinine, strychnine, aspirin, vitamins, cornstarch, menita, inositol, mannitol, and flour.
	You get coke substitutes like lidocaine, procaine, benzocaine, and tetracaine, which can collapse blood vessels, reduce heart muscle strength, and cause low blood pressure. A person who can handle coke could go into shock if he is allergic to coke substitutes.
Heroin	Low doses (1% to 4%) cut with a lot of quinine or milk sugar.
Assorted pills in capsule form	Dealer removes active ingredients and substitutes cheaper and sometimes dangerous ingredients.

Amphetamines are stimulant drugs which have been used by medicine for appetite suppression, abnormal hyperactivity disorders, and narcolepsy (sleep disorder). Picked up by the drug scene because of their boost to psychic and physical energy levels, they became the object of one of the few street prevention programs ever launched in this country. "Speed Kills" buttons were found in the East Village and the Haight-Ashbury areas during the late 1960s. Speed is making a comeback, but most of the stuff you buy on the street is not the genuine article. Dr. John Morgan reported in the *Journal of Psychoactive Drugs* that 90 percent of the street speed is look-alikes containing caffeine, phenylpropanolamine (a nasal decongestant and appetite suppressant), and ephedrine (a decongestant).[2] These clever look-alikes resemble the real thing, but actually give you very little bang for the buck and can be downright dangerous because of additives and impurities.

Methaqualone (Quaalude, Sopor, Parest) is a hypnotic (sleep inducer). Drug scene people like the alcohol-like high and tout the drug as giving a good "body high" somewhat like an aphrodisiac. In the case of ludes the unscrupulous dealer has several ways to cheat the consumer. It is rare to find the genuine article on the street. The counterfeits are referred to as bootlegs; the biggest item in this category is the Lemmon 714 (Lemmon manufactures legitimate Quaalude). The bootleg looks like the real McCoy, right down to the scoring and crispy edges. Sometimes these bootlegs are not made from raw methaqualone. Valium is substituted in high doses, leading to nasty and dangerous highs with vomiting and even the danger of coma, usually followed by a two-day hangover. The other common substitute is phenobarbital, which is a slow-acting, long-lasting barbiturate. Because it takes longer to experience the high than with real ludes, the user may take another. This is extremely dangerous because one lude-size dose of phenobarbital is greater than the therapeutic dose for a twenty-four-hour period; two is greater than the minimum lethal dose. Phenobarbital is very dangerous when mixed with alcohol because both are sedatives and the effects are additive.

Once you have decided to take a drug, it is a good idea to

titrate the dose in direct proportion to the information available about purity and dose. Titration is the chemist's process for determining the concentration of a substance in solution. The layman's version of this is as follows: the less you know about a drug, the more caution you want to exercise when taking it. By first taking a small amount and then waiting to experience the actual effects, you can save yourself some unwanted effects or at least minimize bad ones. Once you feel comfortable with what is actually happening to you, then you may opt to take a little more and again see how it actually works on your body and mind. Don't be a pig—it could lead to a real bad trip. You can also lose some of the more subtle effects of the drug. What's the hurry? There is one major caution here: many drugs alter the way in which we perceive the passage of time. Use a clock or watch, not your subjective senses (which are now altered), to check the time. You may wish to titrate known doses to make the effects last a little longer and to avoid the building-up of a tolerance to the drug (needing more to get the original effect) (this is how addiction begins). This "take a little and wait" approach is used by seasoned pleasure seekers.

This caution can save your life, particularly when mixing drugs. The following story shows what can happen, even to street-wise drug users, when perceptions are altered by drugs.

Dino's Story

Dino did drugs between the ages of fourteen and eighteen. His life was out of control, and he spent two years in a drug-free residential treatment program to do some growing up. Five years out of treatment, he slipped back into heroin addiction. He began using methadone he purchased in the street to slowly detoxify himself from the heroin. Withdrawal from opiates is often accompanied by sleep disturbance. After forty-eight hours of not sleeping, Dino added one more element to his home remedy. He got hold of some barbiturates to help him to sleep, but he had absolutely no experience with this type of drug (preferring opiates and hallucinogens). He took two "goofballs" (phenobarbital), and after what he thought was one hour (actually only ten minutes), he took two more. The next thing I knew, Dino had me on the phone; he was very drowsy but in a definite state of confusion and panic. I used every tactic I could think of (including having him put an ice pack on his testicles) to keep him walking and talking, while I called the emergency squad on the other phone. He was okay, but the ambulance driver told me that if he had fallen asleep he would probably never have regained consciousness.

People like to share drugs, and this means that they will also share the various equipment used to get high. Passing joints, pipes, bongs, hookahs (water pipes), carburetors, and other smoking apparatus is quite common. However, so are colds, flu, and herpes (simplex and not so simplex). The same holds true for devices used to sniff cocaine, which are usually inserted into one's nostrils. Dirty needles transmit hepatitis and other communicable diseases. Air bubbles in syringes can kill you. Sharing equipment is another act of faith that can get you in trouble. No one's naked eye can see the microbes that can cause the trouble. Remember that we are in the midst of a venereal disease epidemic and some really nice hip people are transmitting these diseases through an act of love! The same cautions apply to the "loving sharing" of drugs. So keep your act clean, exercise a little caution, and your drug experiences won't cost you.

COCAINE—THE HIGH PRICE OF GETTING HIGH

Cocaine is an alkaloid derived from the leaves of the *Erythroxylon coca* (a shrub which is cultivated in, among other places, Peru, Chile, Bolivia, and Mexico). It starts as a residue extracted from the leaves ($200 to $300 a pound), and when refined and cut with various products costs anywhere from $1800 to $2500 per ounce (for high-quality, relatively pure coke). Current street prices put the final adulterated product (12 percent cocaine) at about $100 to $150 per gram (the amount most commonly purchased by users). The American public used to have easy and legal access to cocaine in the form of such innocent-sounding nostrums as "Agnew's Powder," "Anglo-American Catarrh Powder," and "Ryno's Hay Fever and Catarrh Remedy." Many of what we now call over-the-counter (OTC) drugs contained cocaine and sold like hotcakes between the 1890s and 1914, the year the Harrison Narcotics Act was passed. Although cocaine is a stimulant drug with no narcotic features, in 1922 Congress prohibited most importation of coca leaves and officially defined it as a narcotic (a designation that still applies today). Cocaine used to be an ingredient in the original Coca-Cola formula (dropped in 1903) and was advertised "to cure your headache" and "relieve fatigue" for only 5 cents. Émile Gautier's Vin Mariani was celebrated by many famous people during that same time. Popes Leo XIII and Pius X, Sarah Bernhardt, Émile Zola, Jules Verne, and H. G. Wells all endorsed this rather plebeian wine which contained a tiny proportion of coca extract. Bernhardt said, "Vin Mariani is indispensable to dramatic and lyric artists. I would be unable to go on without it." Enrico Caruso stated of Vin Mariani, "I found it excellent for the voice. It gives particular energy to the artist when fatigued." It sold well in Europe and to a lesser extent in America before Gautier's death and the Harrison Act put it out of business. The most famous of cocaine's proponents was a Viennese neurologist named Sigmund Freud. In writing of his personal experiences with the drug to his fiancée, Martha Bernays, Freud stated:

> Woe to you, my Princess, when I come. I will kiss you quite red and feed you till you are plump. And if you are froward you shall see who is the stronger, a gentle little girl who doesn't eat enough or a big wild man who has cocaine in his body. In my last severe depression I took coca again and a small dose lifted me to the heights in a wonderful fashion. I am now busy collecting the literature for a song of praise to this magical substance.[3]

Sounds like great stuff when you read these accounts! Here is a more up-to-date account of what can happen when you play with cocaine.

Arthur's story

I started out snorting a little in my friends' homes. It hit me immediately what a nice drug I had discovered. Sure it cost a lot of money but I was always into showing off anyway. Addicting? I thought not—after all, this wasn't heroin or speed. So I began buying it by the gram at first and then by the ounce, telling myself I was actually saving money by buying it in larger quantities. I was able to make love longer, rap longer, and everything was so crystal clear and beautiful. At first I could stay high for about fifteen or twenty minutes after a few blows [snorts], but later on I would only stay up for about ten minutes. The trips got shorter and the drug bills got higher. What I did not realize is that I was becoming obsessed with coke. I reached the point where all I wanted to do was get high. People were always hitting on me for coke or money to buy coke. I experienced some real bad depressions after coming down so I dedicated my life to staying "up." People started telling me that I was acting increasingly paranoid and weird but I just said "that's the drug" and kept right on going. At the point at which I finally stopped I was spending about $4,000 a month on coke and had completely lost my perspective on my work, my friends, sex, everything!

Cocaine is not physically addicting, but psychological dependency (the desire to bring about this altered state repeatedly) is very real. This psychic dependency stems from the drug's powerful euphoric reaction. Even laboratory animals love it. One report states that rats would press a bar 250 times to obtain caffeine, 4000 consecutive times to obtain heroin, and 10,000 times in a row to obtain cocaine. That's a pretty powerful positive reinforcer. Richard Pryor, who knows how enticing the drug can be, stated in his film *Live on the Sunset Strip:* "You've been doing it more than two weeks—you're a junkie. You won't be able to stop." Pryor reportedly almost burned to death as a result of freebasing cocaine. Freebasing is a method of processing cocaine hydrochloride down to its most powerful essence and then smoking it;

the ether used in the process is highly flammable. Most users snort it sharply up into their nostrils using rolled bills, straws, or coke spoons. Some people inject it into their veins. This method of administration leads to a euphoric "rush" and feelings of elation which have often been compared to a sexual orgasm (this is probably due to the greater amount taken into the body this way), but it causes a loss of subtle effects, and the euphoria is shorter-lived. Therefore the peak experience and the "comedown" occur more rapidly. The addiction liability increases as the user moves from snorting to freebasing to injection. Most researchers do not report a tolerance effect with cocaine, but more and more chronic users are reporting that the trips on coke get shorter and less intense, requiring larger quantities of purer dose to achieve the original euphoric effect. This may be a "temporary tolerance," which is experienced only by chronic users and not by periodic pleasure seekers. Some users mix the coke with heroin (called a speedball) to prolong the pleasant effects and produce a "roller coaster effect." The catch is that the roller coaster can make you feel "like you're tearing your body in half." This is how John Belushi is reported to have ended his life. It's hard to know, as Belushi was reported to have been into coke, heroin, and alcohol. Cocaine may potentiate the lethal nature of heroin.

There is no doubt that cocaine is increasing in popularity. Over 15 million people have used it in the United States, and it has made the cover of *Time* magazine. Although the number of primary cocaine abusers is low (about 2 percent) in federally funded drug treatment programs, the number has tripled in the past several years. Cocaine-related deaths are relatively few in number (19.1 deaths per 10,000 medical-examiner reports), but they have also been reported on the increase (up from 4.5 deaths per 10,000). One of the main problems with drug-related statistics is that we don't know how many such deaths went undetected because of ignorance or because the drug was metabolized completely before death (this takes about six hours for coke). Doctors also often fail to list drugs or alcohol as the cause to save the family any "embarassment."

One of the reasons for cocaine's popularity is its purported role as an aphrodisiac. Some users claim it actually causes sexual arousal, while others state that it enhances the sexual experience. Since cocaine is a topical anesthetic (it can deaden sensation), it has been rubbed on the head of the penis or on the clitoris to prolong intercourse. Many of coke's sexual claims are dose-related (use too much and you blow it). With doses of a gram or less per day, coke may enhance sexuality, delay ejaculation, and produce more intense and satisfying orgasms. At higher doses users often report a decreased interest in sexuality. In fact, sex can't compete with coke at higher levels of regular use.

So why a special caution about cocaine? There are several reasons. The first is that people con themselves into believing that coke is "safe" and nonaddicting and refuse to exercise the respect the drug should command from everyone. The euphoric effects of the drug are powerfully reinforcing, and users want to repeat the experience again and again. The gradual building up of psychic dependence leading to a compulsion is slow and insidious. People who have found that marijuana has caused them no problems believe that they will have the same experience with coke. Drugs are like coins—they have two sides. If coke has a side that is a powerful reinforcer, it also has its dark side. If you feel increased mental and physical strength while using coke, how might you feel when the coke wears off? You are borrowing future energy and, like a bank loan, it has to be paid back. You feel let down, ordinary, maybe a little depressed. Either you let this feeling pass or you decide to get back up, which means you have to do some more coke. This is how the craving for the drug can insidiously creep into your life. You like the high so much that everything else feels like a "low." If you are freebasing, mainlining, or snorting regularly (daily), you run the risk of "crashing." This crashing is somewhat comparable to what happens after a speed "run" (many hours or even days of shooting amphetamines). Crashing involves profound feelings of the opposite of euphoria—dysphoria. One way to describe dysphoria is as the inability to create and hold good feelings. As chronic use increases and/or dosage goes up, the user runs the risk of going beyond dysphoria into a full-blown cocaine psychosis with para-noid delusions and hallucinations. The main reaction to the stop-ping of coke use is a feeling of depression. This reactive depression (in reaction to the absence of the drug) is accompanied by intense craving, represented by an overpowering compulsion to continue using the drug.

Another problem associated with cocaine is its price. It's the status drug—the one that lets everybody know you are a person of means. In the drug scene it's the ultimate ego trip. If you have enough to turn on your friends, you get the oohs and aahs that go with all conspicuous consumption (until you run out of coke). Prices keep going up (supply and demand) and potency generally goes down (more adulterant, less coke). People who become psychologically dependent upon the drug spend incredible amounts of money on it. When you factor it out, it comes to something on the order of about $200 per hour of being high. Coke becomes more important than anything else. In 1980 alone street sales of cocaine reached an estimated $30 billion.

Cocaine, like many other stimulants including caffeine, acts as an appetite supressant. But before you run out to score some coke as a diet aid, remember the price, both in dollars and in possible problems. Cocaine is a powerful seducer. Your money, your sex life, your friendships, your job—all may be replaced by that fine white powder. This is one drug that means business.

Less is known about the physical problems. One often hears reports of heavy users having nasal problems. However, the num-ber of users suffering the worst of these problems—the perforation of the nasal septum (the membrane dividing the two halves of the nose)—is rare but on the increase. The major adverse physical reactions involving cocaine are reported to be inflammation of the nasal mucosa, nasal sores, and nasal bleeding. These problems are caused by particles of the drug that become lodged in the small hair follicles of the nose. If they get caught in the sinus cavities, they can cause headaches and congestion. This leads to the characteristic runny nose seen in many regular coke users. To avoid this, users chop up the larger flakes or crystals with a razor blade to make it into as fine a powder as possible (more absorption of coke and fewer particles to clog). Users will also "snort" water or nasal sprays to keep the mucosa clear of particles. Again, as cocaine is a topical anesthetic it causes feelings of numbness in the nose, throat, and sinuses. Freebasing is probably dangerous to the respiratory system because it constricts the blood vessels of the lungs. Cocaine users who inject the drug run all the risks that heroin addicts, speed freaks, and all so-called needle freaks (people who do drugs with syringes) run. These include abscesses and sores, overdosing, hepatitis, tetanus, pneumonia, and lung abscesses.

Addiction can be defined as having three elements: (1) compulsion (repetitive urge), (2) negative consequences, and (3) loss of control (the drug takes over). This definition can help you to see that people can get "strung out" on coke just as with many other drugs. You must weigh the risks and the benefits. Any drug that can promise as much pleasure and excitement as cocaine requires thoughtfulness and caution when used. If you must do coke:

- do it infrequently;
- don't mess with needles;
- take proper care of your nose;
- make sure you can afford it;
- remember that it's a felony bust if you get caught;
- remember it can lead to heavy-duty psychic dependence;
- remember it can lift you up real high and set you down hard;
- don't freebase—it's a much quicker route to dependency;
- make sure it's the "real thing" and not an adulterant or substitute.

The National Institute on Drug Abuse has found no health problems associated with "recreational use" defined as one to two grams a week or less taken nasally. "Most coke users don't get into trouble," says Dr. Robert C. Peterson, NIDA's director of research. "Even regular users probably just snort up on weekends like in Woody Allen movies." Sticking to this pattern of use requires vigilance and self honesty on the part of the user or the dangers listed above will become part of your cocaine experience.

The use of cocaine has become so pervasive in areas of the country like Hollywood, California, that new treatment approaches are springing up to meet the problem. Modeled after Alcoholics Anonymous, Pills Anonymous, and Smoke Enders, programs vary in cost and effectiveness. "Coke Enders" meets at Wilbur Hot Springs Health Sanctuary, a health farm in Williams, north of San Francisco. Another program is run by the Beverly Glen Hospital in Los Angeles. One group that meets on the West Coast boasts so many celebrities that one person says, "On a good night it's like walking in Ma Maison [a prominent Beverly Hills restaurant] or Elaine's." Most people attempting to stop the compulsive use of cocaine will require a great deal of group support to achieve their goal. This is particularly true when they develop a dual addiction, to alcohol or other sedatives used to ease the "crashing" after a coke run. These people must learn to be abstinent from both the uppers and the downers.

LUDES

Methaqualone was introduced in 1965 as a sedative-hypnotic (it will calm you and induce sleep) that was touted as being safer and less addicting than barbiturates (Seconal, Tuinal, Nembutal, Butisol, Amytal). It is manufactured in the United States as Parest (Parke-Davis), Quaalude (Lemmon), and Sopor (Arnar-Stone). Some of the street names for methaqualone are ludes, love drug, Qs, quas, quads, 714s, sopers, wallbangers, and disco biscuits. Ludes were intended to provide relief of mild to moderate anxiety or tension (sedative effect), and at higher doses taken at bedtime to relieve insomnia (hypnotic effect). Some of the side effects are lightheadedness in the upright position, weakness, and unsteadiness in stance and gait. Users are warned by doctors prescribing methaqualone not to take it for more than three months continuously. Ludes took off like a rocket, becoming the sixth most frequently prescribed drug in this country. In some sections of the country "lude doctors" began to prescribe the drug for anyone with vague complaints of being tense or suffering from sleeplessness (and willing to pay the price of an office visit, ranging anywhere from $25 to $150). Lude users exchange names of these doctors and end up with multiple prescriptions, usually selling many of the pills for $8 to $10 apiece. One of my patients in New York City tells the following story:

> It's getting real hard to cop authentic ludes on the street. So your best bet is to tie into two or three lude docs. All you have to do is talk about how uptight you are and how you can't sleep, and you've got yourself a prescription— no other questions asked. This way you get a legal script, go to your local pharmacy, get your pills, and you're in business. I usually keep a few bottles for myself and sell the rest at $9 apiece.

Remember the warning about adulterants? The Drug Enforcement Administration found a shipment of raw methaqualone in Florida in April 1982 that could have given hepatitis to thousands. Ludes are rarely prescribed by conscientious doctors. A sharp drop has been reported in prescriptions by New York doctors, and the decline has been attributed to prosecutions of "stress-relief centers" which used licensed physicians for the mass prescribing of the drug. The drop was also aided by better controls on its distribution by the manufacturers.

You may have noticed that ludes are called the "love drug." That's because part of the lore on ludes is that they are the aphrodisiac-of-choice for people who are into sex and drugs. *High Times* magazine said that "methaqualone did for seduction what McDonald's did for hamburgers." One or two ludes make the user feel a tingling relaxation of the body's muscles, a warm feeling, a sense of disinhibition and recklessness, and a flaring of sexual desire. It induces feelings of closeness and intimacy between relative strangers and artificially transposes a mild attraction into a "deep understanding." That certainly explains why someone might be tempted to drop a few pills. But this drug carries with it some real dangers that fans are not likely to tell you about. There is real addiction liability—both physical and psychological. After a couple of weeks of steady use, inexperienced users find themselves eating ludes like candy. Tolerance sets in very quickly and you need more and more to get the original desired effect. This leads the user to believe that the drug is relatively safe. But with escalating use, the difference between a dose that can get you high and one that can kill you gets smaller and smaller. More than ten tablets and you can suffer a fatal overdose.

Ludes in combination with alcohol can produce stupor, coma, and respiratory depression. This is called "luding out." The main danger of luding out is that methaqualone (like many tranquilizers) suppresses the gag reflex. A passed-out person who vomits may breathe in the vomit, leading to brain damage or death from oxygen loss.

Watching someone who is really stoned on ludes is like watching a drunk. Large doses cause a numbness in the arms, neck, and skull; minor injuries will not be felt until the drug wears off. Flaccid arms and spastic legs are not uncommon, and the person is quite disoriented. Speech is slurred and often incoherent. Suddenly stopping the drug can lead to withdrawal with convulsions. All detoxification should be done in a hospital setting. Ludes can also lead to some nasty hangovers, particularly when combined with alcohol. As sedatives usually mess up sexual performance, the so-called aphrodisiac effect is probably nothing more than the releasing of inhibitions (similar to the effect of relatively small amounts of alcohol). Once you have experienced "better sex" with ludes, you run the risk of not striving for sexual enjoyment without the drug. So if you must use this risky drug you are well advised to use it infrequently and in small amounts.

HEROIN

The word "heroin" derived from the German word *heroisch,* which means heroic or powerful. The drug is aptly named, because as one junkie I know puts it: "Man, it's the greatest feeling

233

in the world 'cause it's the feeling of nonfeeling. Nothing gets through—no physical pain and no mental pain. The biggest loser feels like a winner when he's high on smack." There are basically three ways to use heroin: snort it like cocaine; "skin-pop" it by injecting it just under the surface of the skin (like an allergist's scratch test); "mainline" it by injecting it right into a vein. Middle-class people not driven to blotting out the harsh realities of daily life at the bottom of the social heap have tended to shy away from needle drugs like heroin and methamphetamine. But heroin can be snorted like cocaine, and a new form of heroin has been available since 1977 which can be used in other ways. This is Persian heroin, which has street names like Persian brown, dava (the Iranian word for medicine), Persian, lemon dope (it requires an acid solution like lemon juice to make it soluble enough for injection), rufus, and Southwest Asian heroin. This Persian heroin can be snorted or smoked, which are the two most common forms of use. It can be smoked by mixing it with conventional tobacco or marijuana. It can also be heated up in powder form and the vapor inhaled through a straw. This method is called "chasing the dragon," something that used to be done only with opium. It can also be eaten. This Persian heroin has created some serious problems, because people who previously ran like hell when opiates like heroin were mentioned are now being seduced into using the drug since they don't have to use needles like "real junkies."

On the street, the common white heroin used by addicts runs about 2 to 6 percent pure. Persian, which is marketed on the street as a dark reddish brown granular powder, tends to run as high as 90 percent pure. The expense of the drug gives it the same snob appeal as cocaine among the more affluent drug users and thus contributes to its reputation as a very hip drug. A tenth of a gram will cost you about $75, while a comparable dose of white heroin will cost about one-third that amount. Some people use it as an "antidote" for coming down from cocaine (particularly if one is freebasing).

Another part of the heroin mystique is generated by addicts' frequent references to the orgasmic rush (initial subjective feelings after taking the drug) brought on by high-quality heroin. The addict quoted above says, "It's like your whole body comes." It is also common to hear people describe the warm feeling that bathes the whole body, creating intense feelings of well-being. This feeling has been compared by many to the sensations surrounding fellatio (oral sex performed on the male). Once addicted, the addict loses interest in actual sex—the drug suffices—unless it's related to getting more heroin (prostitution).

There has been a significant upsurge in heroin abuse among middle-class whites, mainly because people kid themselves into thinking they don't run the same risks as mainlining heroin addicts run. They do! Remember, the Persian heroin is available in much greater purity, and therefore potency. Daily use for about thirty days leads to physical addiction, and withdrawal pains are severe—again, it is strong, high-quality dope. The higher the euphoria, the higher the cost of withdrawal. The same applies to its potential for overdose, which can be life-threatening.

As more and more kids and adults get into trying heroin,

Dangers of Heroin Usage

1. The drug takes over your life. Working, loving, playing, all go down the drain. One becomes totally obsessed with the drug.

2. Physical addiction does not require needle injections of the drug. Smoking Persian heroin can lead to physical and psychological addiction. You can crave the drug and develop a narcotics hunger before you are physically hooked.

3. The death rate associated with 90-percent-pure heroin is much higher than with the low-grade white heroin.

4. Addiction to heroin is damn difficult to shake. Whether it's methadone maintenance or drug-free treatment, the ability to remain heroin-free is a crap shoot at best. You end up either taking methadone for the rest of your life or hoping you are part of the small percentage of people who make it after drug-free treatment.

---

the peer pressure that used to guarantee that heroin be avoided at all costs is seriously eroding. An article in *High Times* magazine states: "Heroin has become mass hip. Like black leather pants and imported French cigarettes, it confers a special status to its user. With an armful of tracks underneath a Giorgio Armani sports jacket, this year's junkie is no sleazy social leper—ne's suddenly fashionable." Treatment programs have been reporting an upsurge in middle-class white addicts since 1977, with no signs of decrease in sight.

Heroin carries a very high benefit/risk ratio with the deck stacked on the side of the risks. The cost of attempting to achieve the special oblivion possible with heroin is the obliteration of your present lifestyle. An addiction to heroin, particularly high-grade heroin, is a nightmare—a nightmare that is happening to nice white middle- and upper-class kids and adults.

SUPER POT

In 1964 two Israeli chemists, Gaoni and Mechoulam, isolated the major psychoactive substance in marijuana, 1-delta-9-trans-tetrahydrocannabinol, more commonly referred to as THC. Research is underway involving other cannabinoids with names like cannabicyclol, cannabichromene, cannabigerol, cannabivarol, and cannabidivarol to learn what role they play in intoxification and related phenomena like the "munchies," the insatiable eating behavior sometimes associated with pot smoking. What is known is that the more THC, the stronger the high. The three main strains of cannabis are *Cannabis sativa,* with its familiar star-shaped leaf, native to North America; *Cannabis indicta,* an import from Asia, more potent than *sativa; Cannabis ruderalis,* an import from the Soviet Union, now being referred to as the latest "super-strain." As a rule *sativa* contains the least THC, *indicta* more, and *ruderalis* the most. Thanks to Yankee ingenuity all three strains have been cultivated as sinsemilla. Sinsemilla is Spanish for "without seeds." Cannabis is remarkable for being able to change its sex. Under certain conditions, male plants can turn

236

into female plants and vice versa. Plants grown from seeds from far-flung corners of the world will take on characteristics of the local strain after three generations. These are hearty and versatile plants. Sinsemilla is marijuana without the male plants. Growers cull out the males the moment their sex characteristics are spotted. Female plants put out more resins and therefore more THC. According to one aficionado, "You get high on sinsemilla and you get stoned on Colombian." Sinsemilla is the pot smoker's plant of choice and sells for $250 to $300 per ounce. A lot of it is grown in California, making certain parts of that state a veritable marijuana farmers' market.

There are other super pot strains around and most of them are imports. They go under such names as Puna Butter, Maui Wowie, Thai Sticks, Panama Red, Acapulco Gold, Kuna Gold, and ganja (Jamaica). The main point is that due to the greatly increased THC content, this super pot should command a great deal of respect and cautionary warnings, particularly for novices. The *sativa* that America grew up on in the 1960s is far less potent than the super pot of the '80s. Even experienced *sativa* users find that the *indicta* and sinsemilla plants will get them "very, very stoned" and that the high will last for many hours. Users of super pot, sometimes called "exotic," have reported going to sleep stoned and waking up stoned the next morning. One used to hear stories about many people failing to get high the first few times they smoked. This happened mostly with *sativa* and is far less likely to occur with the newer, more powerful strains. First-time users of the new stuff are getting extremely stoned. Motor coordination, concentration, balance, speech, clear thinking are all profoundly affected. If you have an opportunity to try these forms of marijuana, take one toke, at the most two, and then wait a while. Failure to titrate the dose in this manner can lead to very lengthy and intense drug experiences. Again, moderation and common sense are the hallmarks of judicious drug use. Failure to use them could lead to some very bad trips, even for experienced smokers. Many smokers report a tolerance effect in which once used to the stronger strains they cannot go back to the less potent stuff. While this type of tolerance may not lead to dependence, it can lead you into more expensive purchases than you can handle. Once you are spending money on drugs that should be going for other things like rent and food, you have a drug problem. You can't necessarily trust someone else's "head" to guide your pot experiences. Not only do strains differ in potency, but the placebo effect (realizing drug effects because they are expected) can cause one smoker to differ greatly in the subjective drug experience from any other smoker.

COMBINING DRUGS

A new word has entered into our vocabulary: polypharmacy. It means using more than one drug, sometimes at the same time, sometimes separately.

The use of any drug involves a fine balance between benefits and risks. When you put two drugs together, this equation becomes a lot more complicated and dangerous. While many drug combinations are possible, the one most prevalent in the studies done by treatment people and researchers is alcohol in combination with other drugs. An educated physician (up-to-date on drug interactions) or pharmacist will warn you about the potential hazards of mixing alcohol with certain prescription and over-the-counter (OTC) medications. Who will warn you about combining alcohol with street drugs, or street drugs with licit drugs? You will need to know some terminology to proceed with your education.

Tolerance: As your body adapts to drugs over time, certain tissues react less vigorously to the drug's presence. This cumulative resistance to the pharmacological effects of a drug is called tolerance. It has occurred when the repeated use of a given dose produces a decreased effect. This means that the person will have to take increased doses to get the original effect.

Cross-tolerance: After tolerance to a specific drug has developed, tolerance to others in the same or a related drug class

238

will also be present. Example: someone tolerant to a barbiturate will also be tolerant to other barbiturates, other sedatives, alcohol, and the minor tranquilizers.

Synergism: When two drugs act similarly, they are said to be synergistic.

Antagonism: When two drugs have opposing effects, they are said to be antagonists. An example would be Narcan (naloxone), a narcotic that is antagonistic when combined with heroin.

Additive: When two drugs acting similarly are used together and the result is a simple summation of effect, they are said to be additive. An example is combining Scotch and wine.

Supra-additive: Also called *potentiation.* When the effect of two synergistic drugs is greater than the sum of their doses, they are said to be supra-additive. An example is combining alcohol and sedatives like the barbiturates.

In order to see how the kinds of chemical interactions listed above actually work, let us use one type of mixture: alcohol and another drug. Alcohol (ethanol is what the chemists call it) is a central nervous system (CNS) depressant and a general anesthetic. It has the capacity, like other anesthetics, to cause an initial depression of the inhibitory control mechanism. That's why we feel free and loose when we first drink. However, as more alcohol is added to the human body the CNS gets further depressed and sedated. The chemical interactions listed below occur at a cellular level and are not under conscious control. The only thing you can really control is what and how much goes into your body—after that, involuntary systems take over.

Many people are ignorant about the negative effects of combining drugs; others deliberately combine drugs to get a "better" high. It is known that the majority of drug-dependent persons, some 80 percent, abused alcohol before becoming addicted to other drugs. The literature also reflects the fact that about 30 percent of drug-dependent people use alcohol as a substitute for

Alcohol and Other Drug Combinations

If a person drinks and also uses:	This is what can happen:
Narcotics (heroin, morphine, methadone, etc.)	Effect is additive. Addicts are very vulnerable to liver disease. This combination is a frequent cause of death in addicts. Darvon (propoxyphene) users should exercise great care as this drug closely resembles methadone in its chemical structure.
Sedatives (barbiturates, hypnotics, hypnotic-sedatives)	Effects are supra-additive. Sedatives and alcohol both produce tolerance and cross-tolerance. Both are addicting and the withdrawal syndrome is identical. Combination has a powerful effect on mental and motor tasks: it worsens performance. This can lead to accidental suicide because of supra-additive aspect.
Minor tranquilizers (Valium, Librium, Miltown, Equanil, etc.)	Effects are additive. Combination causes increased sedation and can interfere with both concentration and coordination. In high enough amounts it can be lethal.
Marijuana	The THC (delta-9-tetrahydro-cannabinol) in grass has a sedative effect, and combined with alcohol the effects are additive. Cross-tolerance has not been established. Motor skills and coordination worsen with this combo.
Stimulants (amphetamines, Ritalin, caffeine, etc.)	The initial excitability and disinhibition of alcohol can be synergistic with amphetamines, leading to overactivity and in-

240

GETTING HIGH

If a person drinks and also uses:	This is what can happen:
	ducement of increased hostility and paranoia. Blood alcohol levels are unaffected by caffeine, even though some people report feeling more "wide awake." Coffee does not sober anyone up.
Antidepressants (Elavil, Nardil, Marplan, Sinequan, Parnate, Tofranil, Vivactyl, Norpramin, etc.)	Antidepressants are not stimulants. They have a sedative quality. Depending on which antidepressants and what kind of alcoholic beverage, the reactions can include excess sedation, incoordination, stomach upset, dangerously high blood pressure, and death.
Antihistamines (Benadryl, Chlor-Trimeton, etc.)	Effects are additive in terms of sedation. Antihistamines are present in many OTCs, so read the ingredients on the label. Interaction impairs motor and mental coordination.

their preferred drug of abuse, as well as a means of boosting, balancing, counteracting, and sustaining the effects of other drugs. People who use psychotropic (mind-altering) drugs indiscriminately are called "garbage heads" and run a high risk of dangerous interactions. Alcohol abuse and alcoholism are significant problems for former drug abusers who have gone through drug-free rehabilitation programs, as well as those on methadone maintenance programs. In one major study of over 1000 alcoholics in treatment it was found that 44 percent of them used drugs (mainly tranquilizers and barbiturates) before treatment of their alcoholism and 30 percent after treatment. Treatment programs in the fields of both alcoholism and drug abuse report that the multiple (sometimes called polydrug) abuser suffers from more problems than the single-substance abuser. The polydrug patients have more significant medical, psychological, and adjustment problems and have poorer prognoses than the users of one drug. Their histories read like waking nightmares, with a great deal of family pathology in their backgrounds.

Many drugs alter time perception so that you think a lot of time has passed when in fact only minutes have gone by. When drugs are combined, this distortion of time perception is even greater. Better make sure you use a watch or clock to judge time. And remember to titrate the dose(s); otherwise, combining drugs can lead to the hospital emergency room, the psychiatric ward, or even the cemetery!

SEX AND DRUGS

SALLY: Sex is sooooo nice when you drop a lude!

RALPH: Ludes slow me down too much. Have you ever tried poppers [amyl or butyl nitrate] just before orgasm? That will really blow your mind.

SUSAN: Poppers make me dizzy and give me a headache but the orgasm is real nice.

JOE: You're all crazy. The only drug to take when you're having sex is cocaine. You feel so intense that everything seems to explode. Don't waste your time with that other shit!

PHIL: My wife and I prefer some good grass or a little hash oil. We really get into some long and lazy loving when we are high.

JANE: I think you're all very silly and have missed the point. Sex is so much fun, why does anyone need drugs to get off? Okay, once in a while you might want to ball when you are stoned, but only once in a while.

This conversation took place among upper-middle-class adults. No junkies in the group. They all use drugs in a way they consider fun and safe. They are quick to defend their drug(s) of choice and can rhapsodize for hours about the virtues of getting high.

Some people will find these practices amusing; others will find them sad, still others will find them alarming, or interesting, or informative. People have plenty of opinions about the use of drugs and plenty of opinions about human sexuality. When you ask them about both together, you'd better stand back because no one can remain neutral about a topic like this. There are a lot of myths, folklore, old wives' tales, and just plain nonsense surrounding the use of drugs and human sexuality. Pro- and antidrug groups both tend to mislead us about these complicated human behaviors. In their extreme rigidities, each tends to over-simplify and generalize. Somewhere in between lies the truth.

The first step in unraveling the mystery is to have a clear understanding of just what mechanism controls human sexuality. Here is one woman's opinion:

> My sexuality is many different things about me. The way I wear my hair, my clothes, my perfume, the way I speak. I think it may come out more in the attitudes that I project than the way I actually look. The way I come on to people can be very sexual or asexual. The jokes I tell are the easiest way for me to talk about sex. I am aware of my sexual self even when I am not engaged in overt sexual activity. My imagination can fire up my body. I guess the easiest way to say it is that my whole being is involved in my sexuality.

The most powerful sex organ in the human body is the brain! The brain and central nervous system make up the command center for all human functioning, including sex. It's the brain, with its marvelous ability to remember past delights and project future ones, that stands at the center of our sexual lives and functioning.

Sex is used to sell just about every imaginable product. Cosmetics, clothing, alcohol, cars, cigarettes, motorcycles, hair-care products, and on and on. Sex is used to sell drugs too. Many drugs, both licit and illicit, promise enhanced sexuality. Look at all those happy couples sensuously sipping beer, wine, and hard liquor. Check out some of the sex publications and see what products they are advertising—everything from placebo sex aids to vitamin E. Let's take a closer look at the concept of a placebo, because it is central to the sex and drugs issue. A placebo effect is any effect attributed to a drug that is not actually a consequence of the pharmacological properties of the drug. Mental set is what determines that a placebo will work. I once witnessed three out of four people claim to be stoned after smoking what they thought was marijuana. It was actually conventional tobacco and some dried leaves (all four were regular cigarette smokers). Medical research is full of dramatic examples of the placebo effect. If your mental set is that the drug is going to turn you on sexually and the setting is conducive to expressing your sexuality, then your wish will probably come true. People have an amazing ability to fool themselves. We fill our heads with illusions about what drugs will do for our sex lives, and then someone will come along who can profit from that illusion. Voilà—the drug is purchased, and then taken, and . . . Sometimes it works and sometimes it doesn't. Sometimes our heads fool our bodies and sometimes they don't.

Many people are inhibited and uptight when it comes to such things as joyfully acknowledging their sexual selves, exploring their own bodies, sharing fantasies with partners, enjoying sex without guilt, enjoying sex without the fear of not performing well, coming on to someone sexually, and speaking freely about the subject. Part of that inhibition and tension is also the failure to take proper care of our health (body and mind). Obesity, cigarette smoking, flaccid muscles, short wind, and the like all impede sexual enjoyment. In addition, the media has us believing that if we are not constantly aroused sexual athletes we have failed! We buy the hype and end up believing that everyone else is having a better time in bed than we are. So off we go into our sexual adventures carrying a lot of anxiety, guilt, self-doubt, fear of failure, and hope for the best. And then someone says "Hey man, sex is better with drugs! Get with it! Turn on and enjoy!"

People have been searching for the perfect aphrodisiac for thousands of years. Spanish Fly is a ground-up beetle called cantharides, which burns the lining of the bladder and urethra and reflexly stimulates the sexual organs. It causes erection of the clitoris, engorgement of the labia, and tingling of the vagina in women, and causes an immense and painful erection in men. It can also cause ulcers throughout the intestinal tract and dysentery. It can cause convulsions and death. How did this dangerous drug earn its reputation as an aphrodisiac? Because people foolishly interpreted the bladder and urethral irritation as sexual arousal.

According to doctors and scientists there is no true aphrodisiac. It's either the placebo effect or a misinterpretation like the one about Spanish Fly. If the drug we take is defined as an aphrodisiac and we expect it to cause sexual arousal, then the odds are that it will.

The word "aphrodisiac" comes from the name of the Greek goddess of love, Aphrodite. It applies to something that increases sexual desire or excitement. Scientists may insist on well-controlled double-blind studies of aphrodisiacs before calling them by that name, but there is no doubt that drugs do indeed affect sexual desire and excitement.

A wide variety of drugs enhance or interfere with sexual functioning. As for pharmaceuticals you can obtain from your doctor, you will probably discover that the doctor is just as uptight when it comes to talking about sex as you are. However, since some drugs are real sexual downers, it is important that you overcome your timidity and ask if any of the prescribed drugs or OTCs you are taking can adversely affect your sex life. (Do not start or stop taking a drug without first discussing it with your doctor.)

How any drug will affect you sexually depends on how much you take. Shakespeare said it best when it comes to drinking too much alcohol:

. . . it provokes the desire, but it takes away from the performance . . .

Macbeth

In the drug scene this is known as going "one toke over the line." When people get high they often feel amorous, but too

245

Drugs That May Interfere with Sexual Functioning[4]

alcohol (in large enough amounts or used chronically)

alseroxylon (Rau-Tab, Rautensin, Rauwiloid)

amphetamines (high dose or chronic use)

anabolic steroids

atropine (antispasmodic elixir)

barbiturates

belladonna

bethadidine

butaperazine (Repoise)

chlordiazepoxide (Librium)

chlorpromazine (Thorazine)

chlorprothixene (Taractan)

chlorthalidone (Hygroton)

cimetidine (Tagamet)

clofibrate (Atromid-S)

clonidine (Catapres)

cyproterone acetate

debrisoquine

deserpidine (Harmonyl)

desipramine (Norpramin, Pertofrane)

diazepam (Valium)

dicyclomine (Bentyl)

diethylpropion (Tenuate)

diethylstilbestrol (Stilphostrol, Tylosterone)

disopyramide (Norpace)

disulfiram (Antabuse)

doxepin (Adapin, Sinequan)

estrogens

fenfluramine (Pondimin)

fluphenazine (Prolixin)

furosemide (Lasix)

guanethidine (Esimil, Ismelin)

haloperidol (Haldol)

heroin

hydralazine (Apresoline, Lopress)

hydromorphone (Dilaudid)

imipramine (Tofranil)

isocarboxazid (Marplan)

levodopa (Bendopa, Dopar, Levopa)

lithium (Eskalith, Lithane, Lithonate)

mazindol (Sanorex)

mebanazine (Actomol)

meperidine (Demerol)

mesoridazine (Serentil)

methadone

methantheline (Banthine)

methscopolamine (Pamine)

methyldopa (Aldomet, Aldoclor, Aldoril)

morphine

nicotine

nortriptyline (Aventyl, Pamelor)

opium

oral contraceptives

pargyline (Eutonyl)

perphenazine (Trilafon)

phenelzine (Nardil)

phenmetrazine (Preludin)

phenoxybenzamine (Dibenzyline)

prazosin (Minipress)

prochlorperazine (Compazine)

propantheline (Probanthine)	thioridazine (Mellaril)
protriptyline (Vivactyl)	thiothixene (Navane)
rauwolfia (Raudixin,	tranylcypromine (Parnate)
Raupena, Rauserpa)	triamterene (Dyrenium)
rescinnamine (Moderil)	trifluoperazine (Stelazine)
reserpine (Serpasil, Diupres)	tryptophan
scopolamine	
thiazide diuretics (Hydrodi-	
uril)	

much of any drug can mess you up either physically or mentally and make sex less than enjoyable or even impossible.

Alcohol and other drugs alter perception, change moods, block out certain stimuli from within and without, dissolve inhibitions against many things including sex, reduce anxiety, and the like. They do this by intervening in various biochemical processes in the body (many of which are in the central nervous system—

Drugs That May Enhance or Increase Sexuality[4]

alcohol (in small amounts, varies from person to person)	hashish/hash oil
	isobutyl nitrite
	LSD (d-lysergic acid diethyl-
amphetamines (in small amounts)	amide tartrate 25)
	marijuana
amyl nitrite	MDA (methylenedioxy-
androgens (Methyltestoster- one)	amphetamine)
	mescaline
barbiturates (in small amounts, very similar to al- cohol)	methaqualone (Sopor, Parest, Quaalude), (in small amounts)
bromocriptine (Parlodel)	peyote
butyl nitrite	psilocybin
cocaine	STP (2,5-Dimethoxy-4-meth-
DMT (dimethyltryptamine)	ylamphetamine) (DOM)
glutethimide (Doriden)	

the command center). The body undergoes a chemical change brought about by the drug. On a behavioral level we interpret these changes based on expectations, set, and setting. Our drug-taking can influence actual sex at any one of the four phases of the sexual response in men and women.

Excitement: Different things turn on different people, leading to erection, lubrication—initial arousal.

Plateau: Body completes readiness for sexual activity: full erection of penis and clitoris, more lubrication, nipples become erect.

Orgasm: Peak of activity leading to ejaculation and orgasm. Stimulation leads to pleasure and involuntary muscle contractions in both men and women.

Resolution: Rest period after orgasm. Women if aroused again do not require a rest; men, on the other hand, seem to require rest before continuing.

All kinds of claims are made for the drugs that enhance sex. It appears that most impact on the excitement phase. By disinhibiting many of the psychological and emotional blocks to arousal, drugs allow people to "turn on" sexually after turning on with drugs. All those fears and hang-ups about technique, should-I-shouldn't-I, and morality often dissolve in the admixture of natural desires and mind-altering drugs. Since getting high violates social custom and having sex often does the same, it is no wonder that the two activities seem to go hand in hand.

Some people use drugs because they want to block out all thoughts and ideas and experience only feelings. It is probably true that those who indulge in casual sex need drugs like ludes or alcohol to attain an "I just want to ball" attitude. Uncomfortable with the "meat rack" approach to human relations, they have to get stoned first. Many pornographic films portray the seduction of reluctant women by means of marijuana, alcohol, and other drugs. The idea is that social inhibition is the only barrier to unfettered sexuality and that women need to be "set free" by men. It's time we laid this ancient stereotype to rest. Some people use drugs to slow down the sexual response so that they may savor it longer. This often applies to foreplay and afterplay—or to actual intercourse. Afterplay is one of the most neglected aspects of sexuality. Real time may not change, but in a stoned condition people may feel as if they are spending more time in sex play. Sometimes real time is prolonged, as with the topical application of cocaine to the sexual organs.

Others may use drugs to gain a sense of potency and sexual energy or to intensify orgasm. The inhalants, which go under many different names (Aroma of Man, Locker Room, Oz, Rush, Bolt, Heart On, Hi Baller, to name just a few), are available without prescription. These volatile inhalants are actually amyl nitrite, butyl nitrite, and isobutyl nitrite. Only amyl nitrite requires a prescription. Commonly called poppers or snappers because you have to break the ampule (hence the popping sound), these drugs are said to give a powerful lift to orgasm if sniffed just before you reach that state. This will require you to stop what you are doing to break the ampule and inhale the drug. While users report various pleasurable effects, the drugs do have a rather pungent odor and can cause dizziness and headaches. Kids like to sniff this stuff to get high even if they are not having sex.

Some people in the drug scene use sex as a commodity. Most of us are familiar with the stories about women heroin addicts who sell their bodies to support their habits. Heroin inhibits the achievement of orgasm and ejaculation in men but does not inhibit the ability to achieve and maintain an erection. A particularly handsome fellow whose current girlfriend was a former beauty queen had an interesting quid pro quo going. He kept her in lengthy love-making sessions and she kept him in drugs.

Many drug-using people remain convinced that the drugs are creating and not merely enhancing their sexuality. Actually, all the drugs are really doing is releasing something that already exists within us. Drugs create a temporary illusion during which we are no longer alienated from our bodies, where guilt, sin, and shame dissolve, and where we are freed from the "tyranny of the orgasm." It is easier to stop worrying about technique and the mechanics of sexuality when you are stoned.

Perhaps more than anything else, the drugs help people to relax. When we are relaxed we are much freer to enjoy sex. It seems that millions of Americans have a problem being able to relax enough to really enjoy sex. Sexuality is a combination of the mind, the body, and the spirit all bound up in the joyful act of giving and receiving. Drugs can become unnecessary for many when they find nonchemical ways to freer sexual expression.

SEX AND DRUGS QUESTIONNAIRE

True   False

1. Do you and your partner(s) often get high before making love?

2. Is sex better when you use drugs than when you don't?

3. Do you, when planning a night of love-making, make sure that you have a supply of drugs (including alcohol)?

4. When combining sex and drugs, do you ever have trouble remembering what happened the night before?

5. Do you have trouble relaxing sexually without drugs?

6. Have drugs ever messed up your sexual performance?

7. Do you stop in the middle of lovemaking to get high?

8. Do you use drugs to "seduce" your partner(s)?

250

True   **False**

_____   _____   9. Do you have difficulty achieving orgasm without drugs?

_____   _____   10. Do you have a hard time remembering the last time you made love without being high?

Scoring key: 1–3 "true": Drugs are playing a role in your sex life. Is that what you really want?

4–6 "true": You have come to rely quite heavily on drugs to ensure feeling states that can be achieved without them.

7–10 "true": Your sex life is totally dependent upon the use of drugs. You have a problem with drugs that requires treatment. Better check out your sexual functioning after you are drug-free for a while to see if you have a problem in that area as well.

Everything exists in contrast to something else. Sex and drugs are nicer when sex without drugs is good. If you can get it on only with drugs, then something is wrong. Ninety percent of sex therapy is psychotherapy; it is often our emotional selves that need sorting out in order to find sexual fulfillment. Drugs can achieve this, but it is strictly short-term. Why? Because it's "state-dependent" sexuality; you'll have to get high to get back to that "state" each time. You can end up with a functional addiction—believing that good sex without the drugs is impossible. It is better to get there without the drugs and then perhaps choose to use them once in a while for variety. I have treated many drug-related sexual burnouts. In most cases there is nothing physically wrong. The problems are more in the areas of body image, guilt, clumsiness, and fear of rejection. These people ended up trading their lovers for a drug habit. It happens without their realizing what is happening.

It happens in adolescence in two distinctly polarized ways. One way is for kids to get into the drug scene to the exclusion of all else—thereby successfully avoiding (at least for the moment) any confrontation with their own sexuality. Then there are the "lovers," who get into drugs and sex but who really exchange nothing of emotional value with their partners.

Sex and Drugs

- Your date may not want or need any drugs to be interested in sex. Some folks get insulted if they think you need to get high to enjoy their company.
- Titrate the dose.
- Remember, it's your brains that are in charge—so be careful how you feed your head.
- Everybody is different in how they enjoy sex. Stay loose and be open.
- Getting stoned is a good way to end up pregnant. Take care of business in the birth control department before getting high.
- If you need drugs to enjoy sex, it's time to seek some professional help.
- Drugs or no drugs, don't say yes when you want to say no.
- Sex talk and shared fantasies are a great turn-on.
- Good sex is not the exclusive playground of the young and the beautiful.
- Don't get hung up with technique. Let it flow and enjoy the giving and receiving of pleasure. Guide your lover. Tell him or her what you like.
- Variety is the spice of life. Make love at different hours, in new places. Surprise each other. Try different things.
- It's very helpful to realize that if you take care of your body, your body will take care of you. Keep in shape and stay healthy.

ETIQUETTE

Like few other images, the character of the pusher stirs up deep-seated emotions. There is a special kind of revulsion for the person who sells drugs. Many people say, "If we just clean

252

up the pushers, everything will be all right!" Aside from the fact that consumer demand is what so dramatically affects supplies, our definition of pusher has been too narrow. Many people "push" drugs, if we define the term to mean the sale, promotion, and use of mind-altering substances. Besides the street drug dealer, the list includes doctors, pharmacists, patients, liquor stores, grocery stores selling beer, advertising agencies, sellers and manufacturers of prescription and OTC drugs—and family members, friends, cultural gurus, trend setters, and party hosts and hostesses. Modern-day party throwers can and do supply their guests with the widest assortment of drinkables, smokables, popables, snortables, and eatables (food is a mood changer and reinforcer). Where once an adequately supplied bar would suffice, many party givers now feel compelled to offer good grass or cocaine.

Social competition is fast and furious in some sets, and finding a good connection (pusher) isn't all that easy. Some catering houses now ask if the revelers will require a "smoking room" set aside from the general festivities.

Bars in the home have become a status symbol among the middle class. According to the *Summary of the 3rd Annual Report on Alcohol and Health* submitted to the U.S. Congress by the Secretary of Health, Education and Welfare (1978):

> The nation's per capita consumption of alcoholic beverages increased during the 1960s, in a trend generally attributed to more liberal alcohol control laws, to an increased proportion of young people in the population, and to a higher number of women drinking. Per capita consumption, based on sales data, has risen little since 1971, ranging from 2.63 to 2.69 gallons of absolute ethanol (ethyl alcohol) per person 14 years of age and older. This consumption level is the highest recorded since 1850.

As a host or hostess you must use some wisdom in your role as "drug pusher" at your parties. You will provide the chemicals, the setting in which they will be used, and you may in fact set the tone for the use of these chemicals. You are not responsible for what your guests do—that is their own affair—but you must accept responsibility for the setting, and you should be prepared to aid your guests if they get into trouble. Attention to these matters can mean the difference between a good time and a disaster.

A new variable is creeping into the selection process when guest lists for parties are drawn up: knowing who does and does not use a variety of drugs. If getting high is a central theme of the party, then you would not want to put nonusers in the embarrassing position of feeling like oddballs. They may become hostile and defensive, say things like "I don't need that to have a good time," and make an early exit. If drugs define part of the good time at your party, then some thoughtfulness about heterogeneous and homogeneous crowds is in order.

Another thing to keep in mind is the physical setting. Most of us don't enjoy crowded quarters; crowding breeds aggression. Many people when faced with crowds drift into other parts of the house where you may not want them to go. So attention to space is important. If you don't want people openly using drugs like grass or cocaine, you should provide a room for this separate purpose—otherwise you may notice some funny odors emanating from the bathroom. If, on the other hand, you don't wish people to do this in your home, do not assume they know that. A discreet comment away from the hearing of others is in order. Don't be surprised if they get high anyway.

Having a bartender who can exercise some discretion is a good idea. Volunteers often turn out to be unintentional pushers, pouring with a heavy hand. It's a good idea to make use of a shot glass rather than guesstimates of how much one is pouring. It is not necessary to pour doubles, either. People can always come back for more. Don't feel compelled to constantly foist drinks or other chemicals on your guests. Wait until drink glasses are empty, and check out your guests' behavior. If someone says "No thanks," don't feel that you must keep offering. If you are providing other drugs, then reasonable amounts are indicated, especially if you are providing high-grade stuff.

One of the more difficult things you may be called upon to deal with is setting limits for your guests. When someone has had too much drink, drug, or food (overeating or eating chemically altered foods), you should directly express your concern for them. How much is too much? This is tricky, but things like being overly boisterous, stuporous, hostile, or intimidating, being sick to one's stomach, slurring speech, bumping into things, spilling food or drinks all qualify as danger signs. Your own common sense and your expectation that people should respect your property and other guests is a good rule of thumb. You are not obligated, in any sense of the term, to provide another drink or toke or whatever to a guest who can't handle it. It's better to risk their ire on the spot, followed by a sober conversation the next day. If they can't "forgive" you, it's their problem, not yours. If they are experiencing a real problem with drugs, then at least you did not add to it.

It's a good idea to serve nonalcoholic drinks in addition to the beer, wine, and liquor. Some people don't drink alcohol. Those getting high on other chemicals may not wish to combine them with alcohol (generally a wise thing not to do). Serving snacks will slow down the rate at which alcohol is absorbed into the bloodstream. If people pig down a lot of drugs and booze and end up stoned out of their minds, you may begin to wonder just what the original intent of the party was anyway. You will be right to be concerned if the chemicals seem to be the sole source of fun at your party.

If you are into herbal cooking (as in marijuana, hashish, mescaline, psilocybin) or esoterica from the bar, give your guests fair warning about the special ingredients. As a rule, drugs that are eaten take longer to be absorbed through the stomach lining (as compared with the lungs or nasal mucosa), and there is a "delayed" reaction. However, when the high registers it tends to be strong and last quite a while. So don't get carried away with psychoactive ingredients. If using potent potables like overproof rum (151 proof) or strong tequila (the one with the fermentation worms at the bottom), be sure to tell your guests to expect an extra jolt, and to watch how many drinks they consume.

For those of you who have planned a whole evening of food and drink, let your guests know so that they can plan their drug use accordingly. Cannabis products (marijuana, hashish, hash oil) with a lot of 9-delta-THC (researchers think this is what causes "the munchies") have a tendency to cause overeating. Cocaine is a powerful appetite suppressant, so it's best served after dinner. (Some diet clinics do a heavy underground business in cocaine and amphetamines.)

If you are serving different alcoholic beverages before, during, and after the meal, let your guests know this so they can choose between your yummy cooking and their mood changers. Many hosts and hostesses have learned the hard way to bring out the nonalcoholic chemicals after the meal.

Be very careful with leftovers of herbal cooking. Some Alice B. Toklas brownies (brownies cooked with marijuana or hashish) stashed in a friend's refrigerator were discovered by the babysitter. This fifteen-year-old girl ate a whole brownie and then started to feel very weird. Her mother had to take over the babysitting chores while she went home and fell asleep. This created a moral dilemma for the owner of the brownies, who ultimately decided to tell the sitter's parents the truth. The girl was fine and the parents took it in stride, but sometimes things do not work out so well.

John's story

> John did not know the punch had been spiked with LSD. He ate a lot of pretzels and potato chips and drank a lot of punch to deal with his thirst. When he began tripping it seemed pleasant at first. Then things got very scary. John felt like he was going crazy. His father came to the party and drove John to the nearest emergency room. No one told either John or his father about the acid. John was admitted to the psychiatric unit suffering from what appeared to be paranoid schizophrenia, the worst of all the mental illnesses. It took two days on the unit plus the knowledge that John had ingested LSD (thanks to an anonymous phone call) for everything to return to normal.

DRINKING, DRUGGING, AND DRIVING: A PRESCRIPTION FOR DEATH

On average, alcohol is metabolized by the human body at the rate of one ounce per hour. That's the equivalent of one shot glass of distilled spirits, one can of beer, or one glass of wine. This amount of alcohol will yield a .02 percent level of blood alcohol content (BAC). The chart listed below will help you to determine your blood alcohol content based on your body weight and the number of drinks you have consumed over a given period of time. This chart is based upon New York State law where over .05 percent BAC is considered driving while impaired and .10 percent and up is considered driving while intoxicated (DWI).

Body Weight	DRINKS (Two hour period)											
100	1	2	3	4	5	6	7	8	9	10	11	12
120	1	2	3	4	5	6	7	8	9	10	11	12
140	1	2	3	4	5	6	7	8	9	10	11	12
160	1	2	3	4	5	6	7	8	9	10	11	12
180	1	2	3	4	5	6	7	8	9	10	11	12
200	1	2	3	4	5	6	7	8	9	10	11	12
220	1	2	3	4	5	6	7	8	9	10	11	12
240	1	2	3	4	5	6	7	8	9	10	11	12

BAC= Blood Alcohol Content	Caution. . . Keep your BAC under .04%	Driving While Impaired above .05%	Driving While Intoxicated (DWI) .10% and up
	You're playing it safe	First offense • $250 fine • up to 15 days in jail • 90-day loss of license	First conviction: • $350–500 fine • Up to one year in jail • Possible three-year probation • Minimum six-months loss of license

Most states use the .10 percent to determine the DWI standard. Check your own state laws.

No amount of coffee, cold showers, fresh air, or food will increase the rate of metabolism. What coffee and food will do is give the person more nondrinking time and allow for the alcohol already in the system to be metabolized (broken down chemically and excreted through urine or sweating). All you get when you give coffee to someone who has had too much to drink is a wide-awake drunk! The Food and Drug Administration (FDA) has issued a warning against products that purportedly sober people up, stating that there is no scientific proof that anything can minimize inebriation and stressing that no drug has been approved for that purpose. "The FDA is unaware of adequate and well-controlled scientific studies which demonstrate that any product or ingredient can prevent or minimize inebriation. There is an obvious danger if motorists, in particular, rely on a product's claims that it will sober them up unless such claims are substantiated."

A common problem at parties is the person who has had too much to drink or drug. The central issue becomes what to do after you have shared your polite concern, you have closed the bar, you have stopped passing out other drugs, and someone is in trouble. You have already taken the first important step by seeing to it that this person does not put any more drugs into his or her system. Your second concern must be to see that he or she gets home safely. If this is impossible, be prepared to let the person sleep it off at your place. Under no circumstances should you allow this person to drive a car! Let me share some awesome statistics with you in the hope that none of your guests will ever be counted among these chilling numbers.

- Drunk drivers kill 25,000 men, women, children, and babies each year on American highways. They injure another 750,000. That is nearly 70 persons killed and 2,054 seriously injured each and every day.
- In New York State, between one-third and one-half of all fatal accidents involve a driver who has been drinking.

Over 1,000 persons were killed by drunk drivers in 1980; another 20,000 persons were seriously injured.

- Drunk driving is the leading killer of our youth, those age fifteen to twenty-four, in New York. Motor vehicle accidents harm more than three times as many New Yorkers as do cancer, heart disease, and stroke combined.
- Added to this horrifying human toll is the economic cost of alcohol-involved car crashes—a total of $702 million in 1979 alone resulting from:

$562 million in lost work or productivity
$4.3 million in increased insurance costs
$60 million in medical costs
$9.7 million in legal and court costs
$54 million in vehicle and property damage
$12 million in a combination of funeral costs, accident investigations, and traffic delays.

In a study conducted by the Eagleton Institute of Politics at Rutgers University in 1982, it was found that one in four New Jersey drivers (27 percent) admitted to drinking alcoholic beverages while driving. Of those who were between eighteen and twenty-nine years old, 43 percent said they drank while driving, and 38 percent of all the men questioned admitted doing so. In addition, two-thirds of the men thirty and older and half of all the men interviewed (a total of 503) said they had been at the wheel when passengers were drinking.

Grass-roots activity has begun a ground swell of popular support for tougher drunk driving laws. Spearheaded by a California-based organization known as Mothers Against Drunk Drivers (MADD), the outcry for changes in the law is getting results. In April of 1982 President Reagan created a special commission to combat drunken driving. "Americans are outraged that such slaughter can take place on our highways. The mood of the nation is ripe to make headway to solving the problem," the President said. The commission's first recommendation urges all states to raise the drinking age to twenty-one, as Maryland and New Jersey did recently. Congress has approved grants to states that tighten their drunk driving laws as has been done in New York and seventeen other states. For example, as indicated in the blood alcohol level chart, a drunk driver (DWI) in New York State pays a minimum fine of $350 and loses his or her license for six months. For information on how to contact MADD and similar organizations consult Appendix C: Where to Find Help. Legal limits have not been established for drugs other than alcohol, and there are no incidence and prevalence statistics for the relationship between them and highway accidents and fatalities. This is an area that requires more research. Alcohol in combination with other drugs probably accounts for a significant number of vehicular problems.

Back to our stoned party guest. If he or she came with someone and can get a ride home, that's fine. But if the intoxicated person insists on driving, you must find a way to prevent this. Offer to drive the person home, or have someone else do it. Offer to let him stay over at your home. Stay with him, give him something to eat and some coffee or tea, and don't let him drive until he has sobered up or gotten straight, in the case of drugs. If a person persists in wanting to drive, you can:

1. Take away the car keys and pretend that they are lost.
2. Ask others to help you convince him that it is not safe for him to drive (don't put him down, just state your concern for his safety).
3. Get others to help you if he gets physical. Use restraint only if really necessary.
4. Speak calmly and rationally. People who are loaded are quick to think they are being challenged.

There are things you can do to protect yourself and others from drunk drivers. Wear seat belts and shoulder straps at all times, and ask your passengers to buckle up. Restraints could cut highway casualties in half. Minimize nighttime driving, particularly on weekends. About 80 percent of drunk driving occurs between the hours of 8 P.M. and 8 A.M. Report any suspicious or erratic driving to police.

DEALING WITH ADVERSE DRUG REACTIONS

Denial that anything can happen to us or our friends is responsible for more deaths in the drug scene than anyone cares to acknowledge. The attitude "it can't happen to me" can be a real killer. We tend to see the dangers associated with drugs as happening only to that skid-row wino or that strung-out junkie nodding on the street corner. There are many things that can go wrong in a single administration of a drug. One need not be a junkie to get into trouble. A college student chugalugs a fifth of gin and dies on the spot. Another college student chokes to death on his own vomit after doing a combination of opium and barbiturates. A famous entertainer's daughter walks out of a window on LSD because she thinks she can fly. What about Natalie Wood and William Holden? And Janis Joplin, Jimi Hendrix, John Belushi, Marilyn Monroe, Elvis Presley, and many, many others? Richard Pryor is reported to have almost burned to death while freebasing cocaine. Many of these tragedies could have been prevented.

At large gatherings like rock concerts, there are usually trained medical staff and volunteers to help people who drink or drug too much. It isn't unusual to hear the doctor ask the person who brought the comatose kid into the emergency area, "What did he take?" Too often the answer is, "A red one, a blue one, and a green one." Specific information is needed to treat drug overdoses. When seeking help for someone, you must try to establish what he or she took, how much, and when. This type of information can save lives. Thorazine (chlorpromazine) is a major tranquilizer that is often used to ease the panic reaction which can be part of a "bad trip" on LSD. However, if the person took a different hallucinogenic drug like STP (2,5-dimethoxy-4-methylamphetamine), the use of Thorazine could spell grim news:

261

Thorazine may potentiate the effects of the STP, which often contains belladonnalike adulterants. Mixing a hallucinogenic drug like DMT (dimethyltryptamine) with chlorpromazine could result in death. Most emergency rooms are using Valium (diazepam) to deal with panic attacks. The adulterants in street drugs and the volatile combinations of multiple drug use make it terribly important that you have factual information. Do not attempt to administer any drugs on your own. Call a doctor or poison control center to find out what to do. If you are stoned your time sense will probably be altered, so use a clock or watch to establish the passage of time. In a party situation it's usually a good idea for the host and/or hostess not to get too loaded. By staying fairly straight you can act as a "shepherd" over your flock. If you find that you have to call for medical assistance, find out what prescription or OTC drugs the person in trouble may have taken, in addition to drugs consumed while partying.

Drinking and drugging can cause or aggravate life-threatening circumstances. Examples are choking, inability to breathe, stroke, and cardiac arrest. If you know basic life support you can save a life. The ABCs of cardiopulmonary resuscitation (CPR) are:

- opening and maintaining an airway (A);
- providing ventilation through rescue breathing (B);
- providing artificial circulation (C) through the use of external cardiac compression.

Basic life support is a two-part emergency first aid procedure. First recognizing the problems: obstructed airway, arrested breathing, and cardiac arrest; and second, properly applying CPR until a victim recovers sufficiently to be transported or until advanced life support is available. Advanced life support is basic life support plus the use of specialized equipment to monitor and drugs to stabilize the patient. Advanced life support is done only by specially trained emergency medical personnel. Courses on CPR are available to all interested persons; you can get more information by contacting the American Heart Association, your family physician, or the cardiology department of your local hospital.

It is estimated that over 650,000 people die from heart attacks every year, with about 350,000 of these deaths occurring outside a hospital, most commonly within two hours after the onset of symptoms. Many other victims die from stroke, automobile accidents, drowning, electrocution, suffocation, and drug intoxication. The more people who know CPR, the more lives can be saved. Listed below are some of the things to look for that might require the application of CPR. These are general guidelines and are not meant as a substitute for taking the formal course.

Warning signs of a heart attack:

1. Pain or discomfort, usually pressure and a burning sensation in the lower chest or upper abdomen. May be a squeezing in the center of the chest which can be severe. People often report that it feels like someone is standing on their chest.

2. These sensations may come and go. The pain can also be felt in the back or shoulder and may spread or radiate into the arms (most often the left arm) or into the jaw or upper abdomen.

3. This type of pain lasting two minutes or more can indicate that a person is having a heart attack.

4. Other symptoms may include sweating, nausea, palpitations (awareness of a fluttering or irregular heartbeat), and shortness of breath.

5. The victim may be pale, or feel faint or dizzy with a sense of impending disaster.

The early warning signs of a heart attack are sometimes confused with indigestion (a risk at all parties). Most people will deny that they are having a heart attack, writing the symptoms off to indigestion, anxiety, or even a passing reaction to drugs taken at the party. The delay in seeking medical attention brought about by this denial can cause the loss of life. It is far better to have the medical experts rule out a coronary event than to let a lay person make this fatal misjudgment.

Warning signs of a stroke:

1. The primary sign is a feeling of sudden, temporary weakness or numbness of the face, arm, and/or leg on one side of the body.
2. Other symptoms include temporary dimness or loss of sight, especially in one eye, and unexplained dizziness, loss of balance, and falls.

When a victim is unconscious, you cannot get him to respond to normal noise, touch, feeling, or pain. This can result from the victim's airway being obstructed, his breathing actually being arrested, or his heart having arrested. Timing is critical: the sooner you reach the victim and determine what procedure to apply, the greater the likelihood of saving a life. It takes only six to ten minutes after the heart stops for permanent brain damage to occur. You must ascertain which of the possible life-threatening conditions prevails. Again, in order to properly learn these steps, you should enroll in a CPR course, where you can learn and practice what to do in an emergency.

Information on assisting a person who is choking is outlined on the following pages.

Some drugs can induce seizures (also referred to as convulsions), particularly in people who are habituated to alcohol and other sedative drugs.

Warning signs of seizures

1. Neck movements, facial twitching, and eyelid blinking.
2. These may progress to include movements of the upper extremities, shoulder, and chest and may also affect the lower extremities. These movements tend to be brief and explosive.
3. Person may make explosive involuntary utterances which can include repetitive obscenities.

When faced with a person having seizures, there are only a limited number of things to do. In the majority of cases the

Choking on food is the sixth leading cause of accidental death—killing more Americans than airplane crashes or firearms. Older people are the most frequent victims of choking, but it can happen to anyone.

Choking most often occurs when
- meat is not cut into small enough pieces
- someone is laughing or talking while chewing
- reflexes are dulled by alcohol
- children are running or playing with food or foreign objects in their mouths

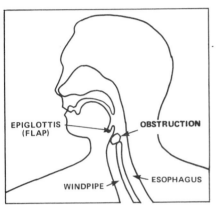

How to recognize choking

Persons who are choking
- suddenly cannot speak, breathe or cough
- may frantically toss their heads or run from the room in panic
- turn blue and finally collapse

SINCE DEATH FROM CHOKING CAN OCCUR WITHIN MINUTES, *SPEED IN REMOVING THE OBJECT WHICH IS BLOCKING THE WINDPIPE IS CRUCIAL.*

First aid for choking

Stand by but **DO NOT INTERFERE WITH A PERSON WHO CAN SPEAK, COUGH OR BREATHE.** If the victim cannot speak, cough or breathe, immediately have someone call for emergency medical help while you take the following action:

FOR A CONSCIOUS VICTIM STANDING OR SITTING

❶ 4 back blows

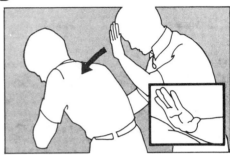

- Stand just behind and to the side of the victim. If necessary, provide support by placing one of your hands on the victim's breast bone. The victim's head should be lower than the victim's chest.
- With the heel of your other hand, give 4 quick, sharp blows between the shoulder blades. If unsuccessful, try...

❷ 4 abdominal thrusts

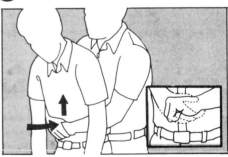

- Stand behind the victim and wrap your arms around his or her waist. Allow the victim's head and upper body to hang forward.
- Make a fist with one hand. Grasp the fist with your other hand, placing the thumb side of the clenched fist against the victim's abdomen—slightly above the navel and below the rib cage.

265

CAUTION: Make certain your fist is below the rib cage or you may injure the victim!

- With a quick inward and upward thrust, press your fist into the victim's abdomen. Repeat this action 4 times if necessary. (The abdominal thrust is often called "the Heimlich Maneuver" because it was originated by Dr. Henry J. Heimlich, a Cincinnati surgeon.)

REPEAT 4 BACK BLOWS AND 4 QUICK THRUSTS UNTIL THE VICTIM IS NO LONGER CHOKING OR BECOMES UNCONSCIOUS.

FOR A VICTIM LYING DOWN OR UNCONSCIOUS

NOTE: Persons trained in mouth-to-mouth resuscitation may attempt to ventilate an unconscious victim. If ventilation is not immediately successful, begin the following sequence:

 ## 4 back blows

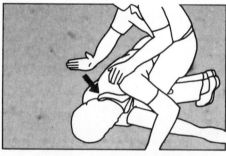

- Roll the victim onto his or her side, facing you, with the victim's chest against your knee.
- With the heel of your hand, give 4 quick, sharp blows between the shoulder blades. If unsuccessful, try...

 ## 4 abdominal thrusts

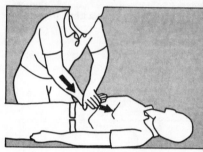

- Roll the victim onto his or her back and take position alongside the victim's hips.
- Place one of your hands on top of the other with the heel of the bottom hand on the victim's abdomen between the navel and the rib cage. Push in and upward 4 times. Your shoulders should be directly over the victim abdomen.

 ## clear mouth

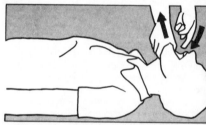

- Check to see if food or object has been dislodged into mouth. Open the victim's mouth by grasping both the tongue and lower jaw between the thumb and fingers and then gently lift the jaw upward.
- Insert the index finger of the other hand down along the inside of the cheek and into the throat as far as the base of the tongue.
- Then use a hooking action to dislodge and remove the food or foreign body. Be careful not to push food back into windpipe.

REPEAT EACH STEP OF THE SEQUENCE UNTIL SUCCESSFUL, STOPPING AS SOON AS THE VICTIM BEGINS BREATHING.

CHOKING FIRST AID FOR INFANTS AND CHILDREN

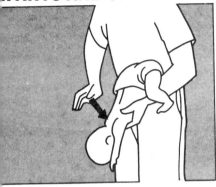

Place the victim face down on your forearm so that the head is lower than the body. Deliver several sharp blows with the heel of your hand to the child's back between the shoulder blades.

SELF HELP

If you're alone, make a fist with one hand and place thumb side against your abdomen. With the other hand, grasp your fist and press your fist in and upward in sharp, thrusting moves. Another method is to press your abdomen forcefully against the back of a chair or a railing, so air is forced out of your lungs to expel the object.

OBTAIN IMMEDIATE MEDICAL CARE

- All choking victims should seek medical care—even if they seem fully recovered. While complications can result from the use of abdominal thrusts on a pregnant woman or someone with a pre-existing medical disorder, first aid for choking should still be used if the victim is in danger of death by choking.

A UNIVERSAL SIGN

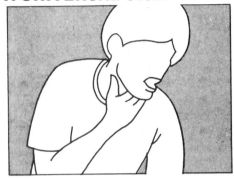

- Efforts have been started to teach a universal sign to use if choking. Signal for help by grasping the neck between the thumb and index finger of one hand.

Source: State of New York, Office of Health Promotion, Department of Health

---

attacks terminate harmlessly by themselves, regardless of what you do or don't do. People accustomed to dealing with seizures make little of them and do not become excited—this is important for you to keep in mind. *Do not panic!* What you can do is:

- Keep the shirt or blouse collar loose.
- Keep the person away from furniture and other objects which can cause injury.
- If you can, before the teeth are clenched, try to put a soft item between the teeth. Do *not* put your finger in the person's mouth.

Do not make a big fuss when the seizures have passed. Let the victim regain his composure in a separate room and give him something to drink (no alcohol). If this is his first seizure, or if he seems very upset, or if seizures repeat, get him to a hospital or call his doctor. If the recovering victim is too out of it for you to get any relevant information, then medical intervention is in order.

In an Emergency

- Have emergency phone numbers where you can read them quickly.
- Don't panic. Stay calm and think things out carefully.
- Don't hesitate to ask for help from others.
- Don't let denial ("It can't happen to me") stop you from being prepared to deal with an emergency.
- Learn what to do for a choking victim.
- Seriously consider taking a course in CPR.
- Remember the importance of accurate and reliable information about drugs taken (all kinds of drugs).
- Don't try to be a doctor—be an informed and responsive lay person.

Dealing with a bad trip: As a final consideration, let's take a serious look at the psychologically untoward drug reaction. Holistic medicine does not separate the mind, the body, and the spirit. Psychological states influence the body and vice versa. Keep this in mind when dealing with someone who is "freaking out" on drugs.

Anxiety and "blues and blahs" are part of our modern age. The difference between these states of feeling and a reaction to drugs is the intensity of the experience and/or the fact that the victim's condition may be quite upsetting to those nearby. Freaking out or having a bad psychological reaction to a drug (often called a bad trip) has many features:

- severe fright or panic
- extreme anxiety (specific or diffuse)
- profound feelings of sadness
- very distorted body image
- confusion and disorientation
- paranoid ideation
- hallucinations (visual, auditory, or tactile)
- seriously impaired judgment or reasoning ability
- depersonalization
- extreme distractibility
- fear of death
- fear of losing one's mind

The main thing to keep in mind is that the person who is freaking out is temporarily in a lot of trouble and needs some human kindness and reassurance.

1. Put the person in a quiet room away from disturbing noises and lights and curious people. The victim is extremely sensitive to stimulus input and is easily distracted.

2. Feeling that one is losing one's mind is quite common. Reassure the person that this is the drug working and that the feeling will pass when the drug wears off.

3. Depending on what the person took and how strong the dose, you may have to stay with him or her for a few hours. If you go to an emergency room, be prepared to stay the whole time.

4. Do not be judgmental or berate the victim. Speak in a calm and soothing voice. The person who stays with the victim should be someone the victim trusts.

5. Sometimes physical contact can be very important. Holding hands or holding or even gently rocking the victim in your arms can be very reassuring. However, if he is going through some paranoid feelings, he may not want anyone to touch him. Go with the flow.

6. Make the person physically as comfortable as possible—lots of pillows, a blanket, a comfortable chair. Try to restrict the person to that one room. However, as paranoid feelings sometimes include fear of being trapped, you may have to move around the house or apartment with him.
7. Light snacks and beverages are okay. No booze or drugs!
8. Do not leave the victim alone at any time. Stay there and give continuous psychological support.
9. Orient the victim often as to time and place.
10. If it gets rough, have someone help you. You can take turns staying in the room with the victim. Assure the victim that someone will be there at all times.

The pursuit of pleasure by means of drugs can be a risky business. Perhaps someday we will have safer compounds with which to pursue what Carlos Castaneda has called "separate realities." If you are open and honest with yourself about both risks and benefits of drug taking, you can draw your own line between drug use and drug abuse. The difference between short-term pleasures and long-term nightmares is sometimes only a snort, toke, or shot. Remember that most of what you experience while high is simply another aspect of yourself. Drugs may show us things about our inner selves and exaggerate or emphasize them, but they never can put something there that did not already exist. Drugs can delight and instruct or frighten and harm us. The difference depends on how much responsibility you are willing to take about what goes into your body.

APPENDIX A:

Summary of Drug Information

TYPE OF DRUG: STIMULANTS

Amphetaminelike Drugs

Generic names: Amphetamine, benzphetamine, dextroamphetamine, diethylpropion, levamphetamine, methamphetamine, methylphenidate, phendimetrazine, phenmetrazine, phentermine

Brand names: Amodril, Bamadex, Benzedrine, Biphetamine, Desoxyn, Dexedrine, Didrex, Eskatrol, Fastin, Fetamin, Ionamin, Obotan, Obetrol, Plegine, Preludin, Ritalin, Tenuate, Tepanil, Tora, Wilpo

Street names: Bennies, black beauties, copilots, dexies, hearts, meth, pep pills, speed, uppers, ups

Indications: Appetite suppression (anorexics), hyperactivity, fatigue, narcolepsy

Contraindications: During or within 14 days following the administration of monoamine oxidase (MAO) inhibitors (antidepressants). Patients with a history of drug abuse. Patients suffering from severe anxiety or who are in an agitated state. Hyperthyroidism (overactive thyroid disorder). Many of these drugs are also contraindicated for persons with symptomatic cardiovascular disease, glaucoma, advanced arteriosclerosis (hardening of the arteries), being treated for high blood pressure.

Possible side effects and/or adverse reactions: Nervousness, increased heart rate, insomnia, dizziness, headache, tremor, euphoria, dysphoria,

271

dryness of the mouth, unpleasant taste, heart palpitations, rapid or irregular heartbeat. Some serious adverse reactions include alteration of insulin in the management of diabetes, increased blood pressure, changes in libido, sexual impotence, behavioral disturbances, and amphetamine psychosis.

Physical dependency: Yes

Psychological dependency: Yes

Other information: The *PDR* contains the following warning: "Amphetamines have a high potential for abuse. They should thus be tried only in weight reduction programs for patients in whom alternative therapy has not been effective. Administration of amphetamines for prolonged periods of time in obesity may lead to drug dependence and must be avoided. Particular attention should be paid to the possibility of subjects obtaining amphetamines for non-therapeutic use or distribution to others, and the drugs should be prescribed or dispensed sparingly." Safety in pregnancy has not been established. Do not use during breast feeding without discussion with your doctor. Should not be used for more than two weeks for appetite control. Sudden stoppage of the drug can lead to extreme fatigue, mental depression, and sleep disturbance (at high doses). Most of the drugs sold on the street as amphetamines are caffeine or other drug substitutes.

Cocaine

Generic name: Cocaine

Brand name: None. No medical use today. Derived in illicit drug factories from the leaves of *Erythroxylon coca.*

Street names: Bernice, coke, flake, girl, happy dust, lady, snow

Indications: No medical indications. Cocaine stimulates the central nervous system, leading to euphoria, excitation, restlessness, and a feeling of heightened mental and physical power. One of the pleasure drugs associated with sex.

Possible side effects and/or adverse reactions: As dosage increases tremors and convulsions can occur. Overdose is characterized by anxiety, depression, headache, confusion, dry throat, dizziness, and fainting. Although deaths are rare, they can occur from cardiovascular or respiratory collapse. Inflammation of the nasal mucosa, nasal sores, and nasal bleeding are not uncommon when coke is snorted. Cocaine psychosis can occur and is very similar to amphetamine psychosis.

Physical dependency: No

Psychological dependency: Yes

272

Other information: There is no evidence for physical dependency, but chronic users report a "temporary tolerance" with the high getting shorter. When use is heavy or continuous, a strong psychic dependency occurs. This danger is increased when coke is freebased or injected. Frequent users go through some nasty depressions and craving when they stop. The price can put you into debt rather easily.

Nicotine

Generic name: Nicotine
Brand name: None as such. Found in all tobacco products.
Street name: None
Indications: None. It has been discarded as a therapeutic agent by modern medicine.
Contraindications: Should not be used by anyone with respiratory problems. Smoking increases metabolism in the human body. There is evidence that smoking increases the metabolism of painkillers like Talwin (pentazocine) and Darvon (propoxyphene, phenacetin, etc.) and the asthma medication theophylline (found in Bronkaid, Bronkotabs, Elixophyllin, Marax, Tedral, Quadrinal, etc.). The result is that smokers probably get diminished therapeutic benefits of these drugs.
Possible side effects and/or adverse reactions: Nicotine acts as a stimulant on the heart and nervous system. When tobacco smoke is inhaled, the immediate effects on the body are a faster heartbeat and elevated blood pressure. It also causes users to urinate more frequently. The tars and carbon monoxide cause a long list of serious health problems, including cancer and cardiovascular and respiratory ailments, some of which can result in death.
Physical dependency: Yes
Psychological dependency: Yes
Other information: The risks greatly outweigh the supposed benefits. It's caveat emptor all the way.

Xanthines

Generic names: Caffeine, theobromine, theophylline
Brand names: Caffeine: in coffee, tea, colas (check ingredients), cocoa and chocolate products, and the following prescription medications and OTCs:
APC, Apectol, Buff-A Comp tablets, Butalbital with APC tablets, Cafamine T.D. capsules, Cafergot, Cafergot P-B, Cetased, Efed II, Emprazil,

273

Esgic, Excedrin, Fiorinal, G-1 capsules, Medigesic Plus, Migral, Migralam, No Doz, Pacaps, Repan, Rogesic, SK-65 Compound, Soma Compound, Synalgos, Synalgos-DC, T-Gesic, Vanquish, Vivarin, Caffedrine capsules, Anacin, Midol, Aqua-ban, Permathene H₂O Off, Pre-Mens Forte, Coryban-D, Dristan, Triaminicin, Dexatrim, Dietac, Promaline

Theobromine: in Anthemol, Anthemol-N

Theophyllin: in Accurbron, Aerolate, Aquaphyllin, Azma-Aid, Bronkodyl, Bronkolixir, Bronkotabs, Constant-T, Elixicon, Elixophyllin, Isofil T.D., Isuprel Hydrochloride, LāBID 100 & 250, Marax, Mudrane GG, Physpan, Pulm, Quibron, Respbid, Slo-Phyllin, Somophyllin, Sustaire, Synophylate, TEH, Tedral, Theobid, Theobid Jr., Theoclear L.A., Theo-Dur, Theofedral, Theolair, Theon, Theo-Organidin, Theophedrizine, Theophyl, Theophylline, Theospan, Theostat, Theovent, Quadrinal
Street names: None
Indications: Stimulants, pain relievers, diuretics, cold remedies, weight control aids, asthma relief, arteriosclerosis, etc.
Contraindications: Severe heart disease, active stomach ulcer, allergic reaction to any previous dosage
Possible side effects and/or adverse reactions: nervousness, insomnia, increased urine output, nausea, vomiting, diarrhea, stomach irritation, headaches, heartburn, palpitations, dizziness, confusion, agitation (varies greatly according to dose and individual).
Physical dependency: Caffeine: yes
Psychological dependency: Caffeine: yes
Other information: No stimulant should be substituted for normal sleep where physical alertness is required. The effects of the xanthines are additive and cross-tolerant, when taking medications with xanthines, keep your consumption of such beverages as coffee, tea and colas accordingly low. Experts suggest no more than five cups of coffee per day (as evidence is unclear regarding the safety of caffeine, moderation is the smartest way to go).

TYPE OF DRUG: SEDATIVES

Alcohol

Generic name: Ethyl alcohol or ethanol
Brand names: Many different brands of beer, wine, and liquor. Many people are surprised at the number of medications which contain alcohol.

Some alcohol-containing preparations for coughs, colds, and congestion:

Drug	% of alcohol
Actol Expectorant	1.5
Ambenyl Expectorant	5.0
Calcidrine Syrup	6.0
Chlor-Trimeton Syrup	7.0
Citra Forte Syrup	2.0
Coryban-D Syrup	7.5
Demazin Syrup	7.5
Dilaudid Cough Syrup	5.0
Dimetane Elixir	3.0
Dimetane Expectorant	3.5
Dimetane Expectorant-D.C.	3.5
Dimetapp Elixir	2.3
Hycotuss Expectorant & Syrup	10.0
Lufyllin-GG	17.0
Novahistine DH	5.0
Novahistine DMX	10.0
Novahistine Elixir	5.0
Novahistine Expectorant	7.5
Nyquil Cough Syrup	25.0
Ornacol Liquid	8.0
Periactin Syrup	5.0
Pertussin 8-Hour Syrup	9.5
Phenergan Expectorant, Plain	7.0
Phenergan Expectorant, Codeine	7.0
Phenergan VC Expectorant, Plain	7.0
Phenergan VC Expectorant, Codeine	7.0
Phenergan Expectorant, Pediatric	7.0
Phenergan Syrup Fortis	1.5
Polaramine Expectorant	7.2
Quibron Elixir	15.0
Robitussin	3.5
Robitussin A-C	3.5
Robitussin-PE and -DM	1.4
Robitussin-CF	4.75
Rondec-DM	.6

Drug	% of alcohol
Theo-Organidin Elixir	15.0
Triaminic Expectorant	5.0
Triaminic Expectorant D.H.	5.0
Tussar-2 Syrup	5.0
Tussar SF Syrup	12.0
Tussi-Organidin	15.0
Tuss-Ornade	7.5
Tylenol Elixir	7.0
Tylenol Elixir with Codeine	7.0
Tylenol Drops	7.0
Vicks Formula 44	10.0

Other commonly used drugs containing alcohol:

Drug	% of alcohol
Alurate Elixir	20.0
Anaspaz PB Liquid	15.0
Aromatic Elixir	22.0
Asbron Elixir	15.0
Atarax Syrup	.5
Tincture of Belladonna	67.0
Benadryl Elixir	14.0
Bentyl with Phenobarbitol Syrup	19.0
Cas-Evac	18.0
Carbrital Elixir	18.0
Choledyl Elixir	20.0
Decadron Elixir	5.0
Dexedrine Elixir	10.0
Donnagel	3.8
Donnagel-PG	5.0
Donnatal Elixir	23.0
Dramamine Liquid	5.0
Elixophyllin	20.0
Elixophyllin-KI	10.0
Feosol Elixir	5.0
Gevrabon	18.0
Ipecac Syrup	2.0

SUMMARY OF DRUG INFORMATION

Drug	% of alcohol
Isuprel Comp. Elixir	19.0
Kaochlor S-F	5.0
Kaon Elixir	5.0
Kay Ciel	4.0
Kay Ciel Elixir	4.0
Marax Syrup	5.0
Mellaril Concentrate	3.0
Minocin Syrup	5.0
Modane Liquid	5.0
Nembutal Elixir	18.0
Tincture of Paregoric	45.0
Parelixir	18.0
Parepectolin	.69
Propadrine Elixir	16.0
Serpasil Elixir	12.0
Tedral Elixir	15.0
Temaril Syrup	5.7
Theolixir (Elixir Theophylline)	20.0
Valadol	9.0
Vita-Metrazol Elixir	15.0

Street names: Joy juice, booze, hootch, white lightning, 3.2, vino, and many other localized slang terms

Indications: Ethanol has no specific medical indications. Doctors prefer other sedatives to alcohol. As you can tell from the list above, alcohol is used *in combination* with many drugs. Now you know why some cold remedies give you the rest you need (the sedative effects of the alcohol).

Contraindications: Alcoholics. People with allergic reactions to alcohol. Persons with any number of medical conditions which are aggravated by alcohol—see your physician for further information. Liver disorders top the list. Persons taking disulfiram (Antabuse) must be very alert to alcohol in medicines. So must people taking sedative drugs (effects are additive and supra-additive).

Possible side effects and/or adverse reactions: The headache, upset stomach, and lousy feeling that come with a hangover. Alcohol can

277

dull sensation and impair muscular coordination, memory, and judgment. Taken in larger quantities over a long period of time, alcohol can damage the liver and heart and can cause permanent brain damage. Repeated drinking induces tolerance to the drug's effects and dependence. Withdrawal occurs in dependent persons. Pregnant women should avoid alcohol, as more than 3 ounces per day can lead to fetal alcohol syndrome (FAS).

Physical dependency: Yes

Psychological dependency: Yes

Other information: Alcohol should not be mixed with many other medications. Ask your physician or pharmacist for further information. Driving and operating heavy machinery when drinking can be dangerous.

Barbiturates

Generic names: Amobarbital, butabarbital, phenobarbital, secobarbital, amobarbital with secobarbital

Brand names: Alurate Elixir, Amytal, Buff-A Comp, Buticaps, Butisol, Carbrital, Gustase-Plus, Levsin/Phenobarbital, Levsinex/Phenobarbital Timecaps, Mebaral, Nembutal, Pentobarbitol, Pentothal, Phenobarbital, Plexonal, Secobarbital, Seconal, Sedapap-10, Solfoton, T-Gesic Capsules, Tuinal

Street names: Barbs, goof balls, goofers, bluebirds, blue devils, blue heaven, nimbys, yellow jackets, red devils, reds, double trouble, rainbow, tuies

Indications: Relief of anxiety (benzodiazepine tranquilizers are safer), hypnotic or sleep induction effect (newer nonbarbiturate hypnotics are considered safer), preanesthetic medication, prevention of epileptic seizures

Contraindications: History of porphyria, history of an allergic reaction to any barbiturate drug, drug dependency, marked impairment of liver function, alcoholism

Possible side effects and/or adverse reactions: Drowsiness, lethargy, a sense of mental and physical sluggishness, skin rash, hives, localized swelling of eyelids, face or lips, drug fever, "hangover," dizziness, unsteadiness, nausea, vomiting, diarrhea, paradoxical excitement, respiratory depression, apnea

Physical dependency: Yes

Psychological dependency: Yes

Other information: The use of alcohol or any other sedative drug has an additive effect. Do not plan on doing any mental concentration or driving of a vehicle when using barbiturates. Consult your doctor about drugs which should not be mixed with barbiturates (like coumarin anticoagulants). Some people experience a paradoxical effect when taking barbs as sleep medicine—after 2 to 4 weeks they keep you up instead of putting you to sleep. There is little to recommend barbiturates in the drug scene or in medical circles.

Nonbarbiturates

Generic names: Carbromal, chloral hydrate, ethchlorvynol, ethinamate, flurazepam, glutethimide, methaqualone, methyprylon

Brand names: Ativan injection, Carbrital, Dalmane, Doriden, Dorimide, Equanil, Felsules, Hydroxyzine HCI, Largon, Mepergan Injection, Noctec, Noludar, Parest, Placydil, Phenergan, Quaālude, Remsed, Somnafac, Somnos, Sopor, Unisom Nighttime Sleep-Aid, Valmid

Street names: Ludes, love drug, Qs, quas, quads, 714s, sopers, wallbangers, disco biscuits, CB, Ciba, sleeping pills

Indications: Sleep induction (hypnotic), preoperative sedation, relief of tension or anxiety (low doses)

Contraindications: Pregnancy, nursing, alcoholism, drug abuse history, allergic reaction to any dosage form, patients with hepatic or renal impairment or severe cardiac disease

Possible side effects and/or adverse reactions: Lightheadedness in the upright position, weakness, unsteadiness in stance and gait, headache, "hangover" effect (excessive sedation), numbness and tingling in the arms and legs, indigestion, nausea, vomiting, diarrhea, skin rash

Physical dependency: Yes

Psychological dependency: Yes

Other information: Avoid large doses or continuous use. The nonbarbiturate sedatives may increase the effects of alcohol, other hypnotics, tranquilizers, antihistamines, pain relievers, and narcotic drugs. These drugs can impair mental alertness, reaction time, etc., and should not be taken if you must drive or operate heavy machinery. Sudden stopping can lead to withdrawal—see your doctor about stepping down gradually. Alcohol should be avoided completely for 6 hours before taking these drugs for sleep.

Minor Tranquilizers

Generic names: Chlorazepate, chlordiazepoxide, diazepam, flurazepam, hydroxyzine, lorazepam, meprobamate, oxazepam, prazepam, promazine

Brand names: Tranxene, Librium, Libritabs, SK-Lygen, Librax, Menrium, Valium, Dalmane, Atarax, Vistaril, Equanil, Miltown, Serax, Ativan, Sparine

Street names: The big "V," tranqs, libs, nerve pills, tranks

Indications: Relief of mild to moderate anxiety and nervous tension (without significant sedation), preoperative apprehension, withdrawal symptoms of alcoholism

Contraindications: Known hypersensitivity to these drugs, alcoholism, pregnancy, nursing (speak with your physician), diabetes, glaucoma (narrow-angle type), children under 6 months, psychotic patients

Possible side effects and/or adverse reactions: "Hangover" effect, drowsiness, lethargy, unsteady gait and stance, increase in the blood level of some diabetics, ataxia, changes in libido, tremor, double vision, blurred vision, menstrual irregularities, fainting

Physical dependency: Yes for most

Psychological dependency: Yes

Other information: One of the big problems with tranqs is that they were really intended for periodic management of acute anxiety or tension, but people take them daily—thus developing a functional ("I can't function without the drug") addiction. Tranqs can increase or decrease the effects of many other drugs. For example, Valium can increase the effects of other sedatives, sleep-inducing drugs, tranqs, antidepressants, narcotic drugs, oral anticoagulants of the coumarin family, and antihypertensives. Meprobamate (Dalmane) may decrease the effects of oral anticoagulants, estrogens, and oral contraceptives. Alcohol should be used only with extreme caution. Pregnant women should avoid tranqs. Valium can increase the likelihood of birth defects. Physical dependency can lead to serious withdrawal symptoms if intake is stopped suddenly. Consult your doctor for an appropriate detoxification schedule. As with any other sedative, the operation of a car or heavy machinery may prove dangerous.

Major Tranquilizers (Antipsychotic Drugs)

Generic names: Acetophenazine, butaperazine, chlorpromazine, chlorprothixene, haloperidol, fluphenazine, mesoridazine, perphenazine, prochlorperazine, thiothixene, thioridazine, trifluoperazine, trifluopromazine

Brand names: Tindal, Repoise, Chlor-PZ, Thorazine, Tranzine, Promapar, Taractan, Haldol, Permitil, Prolixin, Lidanar, Serentil, Trilafon, Compazine, Navane, Mellaril, Stelazine, Vesprin

Street names: None

Indications: Restoration of emotional calm, relief of severe anxiety, agitation, and psychotic behavior. Antiemetic (antinausea) effect

Contraindications: Varies from drug to drug and includes: allergic reaction to any dosage form, severe heart disease, Parkinson's disease, mental depression, bone marrow disorder, very young children, comatose states, presence of large amounts of central nervous system depressants (alcohol, barbiturates, narcotics), heavy use of alcohol

Possible side effects and/or adverse reactions: The phenothiazines (e.g., Thorazine) can cause a condition known as tardive dyskinesia with muscle spasms affecting the jaw, neck, back, hands, and feet. Facial twitching, tongue clicking and the like. Discolored urine (may be of no consequence), drowsiness, change in libido, dryness of the mouth, nasal congestion, impaired urination, lethargy, blurred vision, constipation, skin rash

Physical dependency: No

Psychological dependency: Yes

Other information: Although used to combat psychosis, these drugs are taken by many people as major tranquilizers to cope with minor psychological problems. They are used to a great extent in nursing homes. Safety has not been established in pregnancy. Ask your doctor for guidance concerning breast feeding. It is a good idea not to take these drugs over long periods of time. A "drug holiday" is a good way to see how you can cope without the drugs. This should only be done in cooperation with your doctor. These major tranqs can put a real crimp in your sex life. Mixed with alcohol these drugs can quickly lead to oversedation. Withdrawal from these drugs should be gradual.

Phencyclidine

Generic name: Phencyclidine

Brand name: Serynl, Sernylan (these are animal tranquilizers)

Street names: PCP, angel dust, hog, killer weed (KW), dust, TAC, TIC, erth, green, sheets

Indication: None in humans. Used as a veterinary anesthetic and

tranquilizer. Used only as an illicit drug for its mind-altering effects.
Contraindications: None—not used as medicine for humans. However, any illicit use causing an allergic reaction to any dose form should not be repeated.

Possible side effects and/or adverse reactions: Low doses cause loss of inhibition. Higher doses produce an excited, confused intoxification which can include any of the following: muscle rigidity, loss of concentration and memory, visual disturbances, delirium, feelings of isolation and paranoia, convulsions, speech impairment, violent behavior, fear of death, and changes in body perception. The toxic psychosis that can be induced by PCP closely resembles schizophrenia.

Physical dependency: No

Psychological dependency: Yes. Tolerance to psychic effects is reported by chronic users, and psychological dependence described as craving is reported.

Other information: This drug is quite volatile and can affect different users in vastly disparate ways ranging from withdrawal to severe agitation. Even experienced users cannot be certain how it will affect them each time. Often sprinkled over oregano or parsley and smoked, it is also found sprinkled on marijuana or as a bogus marijuana substitute. Cheap and easy to make and sells for less than grass on the street. A derivative of PCP called Ketamine is now becoming popular.

TYPE OF DRUG: OPIATES AND SYNTHETIC NARCOTICS

Generic names: Heroin, hydromorphone, meperidine, methadone, morphine, opium

Brand names: Dilaudid, Demerol, Adanon, Dolophine (no medical use of heroin)

Street names: H, junk, smack, horse, scag, shit, dollies, M, morph, Miss Emma, dreamer, O, Op, black stuff, meth

Indications: Relief of moderate to severe pain, detoxification from opiate drugs, methadone maintenance therapy, preoperative medication, support of anesthesia, obstetrical analgesia

Contraindications: History of opiate drug abuse, hypersensitivity to any of these drugs, patients using MAO inhibitors, using antihypertensive drugs

Possible side effects and/or adverse reactions: All of these drugs are highly addicting, with tolerance and withdrawal syndromes. Respiratory and circulatory depression, lightheadedness, dizziness, nausea, vomiting, sweating, dry mouth, constipation, lowered libido, visual disturbance, uncoordinated muscle movements, weakness, euphoria

Physical dependency: Yes

Psychological dependency: Yes

Other information: Chronic users who inject these drugs run the risks of embolism, hepatitis, sores, abscesses, blood poisoning, inflammation and collapse of veins, congestion of the lungs, and pneumonia. Opiate habits become very expensive and often lead to a criminal lifestyle to support the habit. Heroin and other opiates are a real sexual downer. Use of any of these drugs with other CNS depressants can result in serious oversedation. Science is still searching for an effective nonaddicting painkiller.

TYPE OF DRUG: ANTIDEPRESSANTS

Mono-amine Oxidase (MAO) Inhibitors

Generic names: Flurazolidone, iproniazid, isocarboxazid, mebanazine, nialamide, pargyline, phenelzine, pheniprazine, phenoxypropazine, piohydrazine, tranylcypromine

Brand names: Actomol, Adapin, Catron, Drazine, Eutonyl, Furoxone, Marplan, Marsilid, Nardil, Niamid, Parnate, Tersavid

Street names: None

Indications: Gradual relief of emotional depression and lifting of mood, usually used when depressed patients are not responsive to tricyclic antidepressant drugs.

Contraindications: Ever had an allergic reaction, advanced heart disease, impaired liver function or disease; taking any other antidepressant drugs or sympathomimetic drugs (such as amphetamines, dopamine, epinephrine, etc.); excessive amounts of caffeine, foods containing tryptophan (broad beans) or tyramine (cheese, beers, wines, pickled herring, chicken livers, yeast extract, etc.).

Possible side effects and/or adverse reactions: Vary from drug to drug and include: insomnia, lightheadedness, dizziness, weakness, feeling of impending faint in the upright position (orthostatic hypotension), blurred vision, muscle twitching, vertigo, headache, tremors, impaired memory. Sexual dysfunction including impotence, problems with urination, impaired ejaculation in men, and delayed orgasm in women. Incompatible with many other medications (including many OTCs) and certain foods.

Physical dependency: No

Psychological dependency: Possible

Other information: MAO inhibitor antidepressants are used mainly when the tricyclics are either contraindicated or ineffective. When used carefully with a restricted diet they can help. Tricyclics are preferred because they have milder side effects. Severe dietary restrictions are necessary so that hypertensive episodes, which can lead to a stroke, do not occur. These drugs are real sexual downers.

Tricyclic Antidepressants

Generic names: amitriptyline, clomipramine, desipramine, doxepin, imipramine, nortriptyline, opipramol, protriptyline, trimipramine

Brand names: Anafranil, Aventyl, Elavil, Ensidon, Norpramin, Pertofrane, Presamine, Sinequan, Surmontil, Tofranil, Vivactil, Amitryl, Endep, Etrafon, Limbitrol, Triavil, Antipress, Imavate, Janimine, Pamelor, Adapin

Street names: None

Indication: Gradual improvement of mood and relief of emotional depression

Contraindications: glaucoma (narrow-angle type), ever had an allergic reaction, taking or have taken an MAO inhibitor within the last 14 days, recovering from a recent heart attack, child under 12 years of age

Possible side effects and/or adverse reactions: Dry mouth, blurred vision, constipation, urinary retention, drowsiness, eye pain, irregular heartbeat, fainting, shakiness, increased appetite for sweets

Physical dependency: No

Psychological dependency: Rare

Other information: Drowsiness should disappear after a few weeks but driving can be hazardous during this early period. People find that if they stand up slowly the dizziness is reduced. Patience is required as it may take up to 6 weeks for all benefits to be experienced (about 70% of patients get them).

TYPE OF DRUG: MARIJUANA AND ITS COUSINS

Generic name: Cannabis sativa is the hemp plant, from which marijuana is derived. There are roughly 360-odd chemicals in the cannabis plant. Delta-9-tetrahydrocannabinol (THC) is one of a total of 61 canna-binoids found in the plant and is the one that gets you stoned and probably is responsible for the "munchies" (powerful hunger induced by smoking strong marijuana). There are powerful cousins to marijuana grown in other parts of the world such as ganja (Jamaica) and bhang (India). Marijuana is only one-tenth as strong as hashish, which is the pure resin of the plant.

Brand names: Not commercially marketed. With special permission physicians may prescribe THC for certain conditions.

Street names: Pot, grass, mary jane, weed, smoke, shit, reefer, hemp, herb, thai stick, dope, ganja, hash oil, m.j., stuff

Indication: Used to treat some forms of glaucoma and as an anti-emetic (antinausea) drug for the reaction to cancer treatment.

Contraindications: Allergic reaction to cannabis products, hypersen-sitivity to the drugs contained in marijuana, respiratory ailments (which prevent smoking), history of drug abuse. The effects of marijuana on growing young bodies are not known at this time. Grass may contain carcinogenic elements (this too is not yet known for sure).

Possible side effects and/or adverse reactions: Euphoria, dry mouth and throat, "munchies," disorientation, difficulty in concentration, com-pulsive talking ("motor mouth"), giggling and hysteria, altered sense of time, increased heart rate (usually subsides), reddening of the eyes, altered sense of body image, acute panic anxiety reaction, and very rarely a marijuana-induced psychosis

Physical dependency: No

Psychological dependency: Possible

Other information: Safety in pregnancy has not been established; women are advised not to smoke at all during pregnancy. A lot more research is needed on the long-term effect of marijuana use. Effect of drug will depend on set, setting, and THC content. Beware of adulterants like paraquat, fungal growths, salmonella, and PCP.

TYPE OF DRUG: HALLUCINOGENS

Generic names: Mescaline, psilocybin, lysergic acid diethylamide (LSD), dimethyltriptamine (DMT), 2,5 dimethoxy-4-methylamphet-amine (STP), methylenedioxyamphetamine (MDA)

Brand names: None. Illicit hallucinogens are sold under a wide vari-ety of street names.

Street names: LSD: acid, cubes, "25," Lucy in the Sky with Diamonds (from the song by the Beatles); some street "brands" have included blotter, blue cheer, microdots, sunshine, windowpane, white lightning, chocolate chip, clear light

Mescaline: buttons, divine cactus, peyote

Psilocybin: flesh of the gods, magic mushroom, sacred mushroom

DMT: lunch-hour trip, businessman's trip

STP (DOM): serenity, tranquility and peace

Indications: No medical indications at this time. Research with LSD in the treatment of alcoholism and mental illness has stopped. Some of the hallucinogens (also called psychedelics) such as peyote and ganja are used in religious rituals.

Contraindications: Allergic reactions or hypersensitivity to these drugs, emotional instability, medicines and other drugs that can cause adverse reactions, great fear of these drugs

Possible side effects and/or adverse reactions: The infamous "bad trip" with exaggerated body distortion, fear of death, going insane, or being abandoned—generally any bad reaction to the altered perceptions caused by hallucinogens. Usual effects are changes in sensation, depth perception, passage of time, body image. Wide range of emotional reactions is possible. Some people never return from a trip, spending months or longer in a frightening altered state. Flashbacks—re-experiencing the LSD effects without ingesting more acid—can occur. Watch out for bogus drugs when buying on the street.

Physical dependency: No

Psychological dependency: Possible but rare

Other information: For reasons that are not clear, LSD seems to be making a comeback. Perhaps the kids of today think that they missed something from the '60s. These drugs are not to be taken lightly. If someone is on a bad trip, consult Chapter 5 of this book.

TYPE OF DRUG: THE VOLATILE INHALANTS

Generic names: Amyl nitrite, butyl nitrite, isobutyl nitrite
Brand names: Amyl nitrite (Aspirols and Vaporole)

Butyl and isobutyl nitrite: Aroma of Man, Ban Apple, Black Jac, Bolt, Bullet, Cat's Meow, Cum, Dr. Bananas, Gas, Hardware, Heart On,

Hi Baller, Jac Aroma, Krypt Tonight, Loc-a-Roma, Oz, Rush, Satan's Scent, Shotgun, Toilet Water. Most of these are sold as "room odorizers."
Aroma, Krypt Tonight, Loc-a-Roma, Oz, Rush, Satan's Scent, Shotgun, Toilet Water. Most of these are sold as "room odorizers."

Street names: poppers, snappers

Indications: Amyl nitrite is a vasodilator which relaxes smooth muscle so small blood vessel are expanded and blood pressure is lowered. Relief of heart pains associated with angina pectoris, relaxation of sphincter muscles. Butyl has no medical uses.

Contraindications: Allergic reaction to any dose form. Amyl nitrite is available only upon prescription from your doctor. Not described in the 1982 *PDR*.

Possible side effects and/or adverse reactions: Headache, dizziness, accelerated heart rate, nausea, nasal irritation, cough (only the headache tends to persist). Men can lose erection.

Physical dependency: No

Psychological dependency: Possible

Other information: Kids sniff this stuff to get high. Kids and adults use it to experience intensified orgasms during sex. Butyls smell awful. Effects are very short-lived, lasting only minutes. The problem is that you have to stop sexual activity to use this stuff, which can be a real turn-off, especially for women. Don't be fooled: this foul-smelling stuff is anything but a "room odorizer" (its FDA designation). A wide variety of solvents are also sniffed, particularly by kids, in an effort to get high. The table below lists these solvents and some of their physical effects.

Abused Solvents

Volatile Solvent	Physical Effects
1. aromatic hydrocarbons:	
benzene	bone marrow, liver, heart, adrenal, and kidney impairment
xylene	bone marrow impairment
toluene	bone marrow, liver, kidney, and CNS impairment

Abused Solvents

Volatile Solvent	Physical Effects
2. aliphatic hydrocarbons:	
hexane	polyneuropathy
naphtha	low toxicity
petroleum distillates	low toxicity
3. halogenated hydrocarbons:	
trichloroethylene	cardiac arrhythmia, kidney, and liver impairment
1,1,1-trichloroethane (methylchloroform	CNS, lung, kidney, cardiac, and pancreas impairment
Carbon tetrachloride	lung, liver, kidney, and CNS impairment
ethylene dichloride	spleen, CNS, liver, and kidney impairment
methylene chloride	CNS, liver, and kidney impairment
4. freons:	
trichlorofluoromethane (FC11)	cardiac arrhythmia
dichloroflouromethane (FC114)	cardiac arrhythmia
cyroflurane	cardiac arrhythmia
dichlorotetraflouromethane (FC12)	cardiac arrhythmia
5. ketones:	
acetone	low toxicity
cyclohexanone	
methylethylketone	peripheral neuropathy, pulmonary hypertension
methylisobutylketone	peripheral neuropathy
methylbutylketone	peripheral neuropathy
methylamylketone	peripheral neuropathy
6. esters:	
ethyl acetate	liver and kidney impairment
amyl acetate	low toxicity
butyl acetate	low toxicity

Abused Solvents

Volatile Solvent	Physical Effects
7. alcohols: methyl alcohol isopropyl alcohol	optic atrophy low toxicity
8. glycols: methyl cellulose acetate ethylene glycol	liver and kidney impairment liver, kidney, lung, and CNS impairment
9. gasoline, leaded	lung, bone marrow, liver, CNS, and peripheral nerve impairment

Source: S. Cohen "Inhalants and Solvents," Chapter in *Youth Drug Abuse: Problems, Issues, and Treatment,* ed. G. M. Beschner and A. S. Friedman. Lexington, Mass.: Lexington Books, 1979, p. 287.

APPENDIX B:

Additional Readings

Ernest L. Abel. *Marihuana, The First Twelve Thousand Years.* McGraw-Hill Book Company, New York, 1982.
Well written and fascinating. Compresses a great deal of historical information into a paperback. A must for understanding marijuana from a historical frame of reference. Scholarly but easy to read.

Alcoholics Anonymous World Services, Inc. *Alcoholics Anonymous—the story of how many thousands of men and women have recovered from alcoholism.* New York: Alcoholics Anonymous World Services, Inc., 1976.
Known as the "Big Book," it is the definitive text on A.A. Excellent source book for students and those who are members. For those looking for practical information, the book *Living Sober* published by the same folks is about 450 pages shorter.

American Pharmaceutical Association. *Handbook of Nonprescription Drugs,* 5th ed. Washington, D.C.: American Pharmaceutical Association, 1977.
People who are into OTCs will find this expensive ($20) book quite objective and straightforward. Gives an overview of many medicines and tells you the ingredients in many products. Geared for the pharmacist, but can be read by the layman with a dictionary handy. If Joe Graedon recommends it, it must be good.

Baker, Charles E., Jr. *Physicians' Desk Reference.* 36 ed. Oradell, N.J.: Medical Economics Company, Inc., 1982.
This is the physician's "bible" when it comes to prescribing medication. The drug manufacturers pay to place their product information in this tome. It is over 2000 pages in length and contains information on approximately 2000 products. Contains 38 pages of color plates to help you identify various products. Products are indexed by name, category, generic and chemical name, diagnostic information. Also contains a list of poison control centers and a guide to management of drug overdose. Cost is high, about $19.95 in

most bookstores. For less expensive and easier-to-read books with similar (but not as comprehensive) information see Long, Graedon, and Silverman. This *PDR* deals only with prescription medications. The same publisher also has created a *PDR* for nonprescription drugs and a *PDR* for ophthalmology.

Beschner, George M., and Alfred S. Friedman. *Youth Drug Abuse: Problems, Issues and Treatment.* Lexington, Mass.: Lexington Books, 1979.
This 681-page compendium of writings and research on the youth drug scene is not for the beginner unless you are willing to wade through a lot of statistical material. Excellent reference source for serious students of the subject. Dr. David Smith, Diane Striar, and I wrote a nonstatistical chapter on treatment services for youthful drug users.

Blaine, Rabbi Allan. *Alcoholism and the Jewish Community.* New York: Commission on Synagogue Relations, Federation of Jewish Philanthropies of New York, 1980.
Compendium of writings scratching the surface of a long-denied phenomena: the alcoholic who is a Jew. Contains a general overview, a Jewish historical perspective, studies on Jewish alcoholism, the role of home, family, and community, the role of the rabbi and the synagogue. Ellen Bayer and I wrote a chapter about the first spiritual retreat for Jewish alcoholics. A good source book for the beginner.

Brecher, Edward M., and the Editors of *Consumer Reports. Licit and Illicit Drugs.* Boston: Little, Brown and Company, 1972.
An excellent primer for those who are new to the drug scene. Contains an extensive amount of interesting historical material on a wide variety of drugs—caffeine, narcotics, amphetamines, barbiturates, inhalants, LSD, marijuana, and hashish. The authors arrive at some unique and unorthodox conclusions and make some startling recommendations for policies governing treatment and prevention of drug abuse.

Bush, Patricia J. *Drugs, Alcohol and Sex.* New York: Richard Marek Publishers, 1980.
Pulls together a wide literature into a cohesive text. Examines the effects of many different classes of drugs—street, prescription, OTC. Dr. Bush collected specific data on drugs and sex from 250 people and compares their statements with findings in the literature. Excellent sections of aphrodisiacs and placebo effects.

The Editors of *Consumer Reports. The Medicine Show,* rev. ed. Mount Vernon, N.Y.: Consumers Union, 1979.
The subtitle is "Some plain truths about popular remedies for common ailments." This is a wonderfully objective and informative book which covers a wide range of illnesses, conditions, and drugs. Debunks wonder and miracle drugs. Can be obtained from Consumer Report Books, Dept. AA10, P.O. Box 350, Orangeburg, New York, 10962.

Freudenberger, Herbert J., and Geraldine Richelson. *Burn-Out: the High Cost of High Achievement.* Garden City, N.Y.: Doubleday & Company, Anchor Press, 1980.
Explains one of the major reasons why people try to anesthetize and tranquilize themselves with drugs. Particularly relevant to the subject of drugs in the workplace. Easy reading but extremely thought-provoking.

Gordon, Barbara. *I'm Dancing as Fast as I Can.* New York: Harper & Row, 1979.
One woman's nightmare with the drug Valium. Shows how sudden stopping of a drug can lead to serious withdrawal reactions, including mental breakdown. Moving story of Ms. Gordon's struggle to recover.

Graedon, Joe. *The People's Pharmacy—2.* New York: Avon Books, 1980.
This is the second book in a series (first one was entitled *The People's Pharmacy*). Joe Graedon may be the best friend that the American public has when it comes to prescription and OTC drugs. His informative style is delivered with honesty and humor. He lays all the sacred cows to rest and helps us to understand how our best protection is information, which he supplies in abundance. *The People's Pharmacy* should be in every home in America. Some of the sections in the book include drug interactions, for women only, vitamins, drugs and your head, drugs and children, drugs and older people, and saving money in the pharmacy.

Hastings, Arthur C., James Fadiman, and James S. Gordon, eds. *The Complete Guide to Holistic Medicine—Health for the Whole Person.* New York: Bantam Books, 1980.
Encyclopedic in scope, this paperback is a wonderful introduction to holistic medicine. It serves as an excellent overview to the subject without losing a sense of objectivity. It can help you to see that your own responsibilities for your health are within your grasp. But you will require new ways of looking at yourself. Deals with everything from foods as medicine to death and dying.

Johnson, Lloyd D., Jerald G. Bachman, and Patrick M. O'Malley. *Highlights from Student Drug Use in America, 1975–1980.* The University of Michigan, Institute for Social Research and the National Institute on Drug Abuse. Available from the Alcohol, Drug Abuse, and Mental Health Administration, Printing and Publications Management Branch, 5600 Fishers Lane (Rm.6C–02), Rockville, Maryland 20857.
Excellent source material on student drug use and drug trends during this five-year period. Useful for comparing localities with national trends. Contains a lot of statistics, charts, and graphs.

Knowles, John, ed. *Doing Better and Feeling Worse: Health in the United States.* New York: W. W. Norton, 1977.
Carefully spells out the importance of individual responsibility for our health. Also explores political, technological, and fiscal realities of health care in a time when nearly 10 percent of our GNP is spent on health. Strong emphasis on health maintenance as opposed to "fix it when it breaks down" approach.

Lingeman, Richard R. *Drugs from A to Z: A Dictionary.* 2nd ed. New York: McGraw-Hill Book Company, 1974.
Still timely. A great introduction to the mysterious-sounding jargon of the street drug scene with entries from the world of medicine as well. Now you can learn just what your children are talking about when they use terms like lids, jay, lady, buzz, etc.

Long, James W. *The Essential Guide to Prescription Drugs—What You Need to Know for Safe Drug Use.* New York: Harper and Row, 1980.
Available as a large paperback at half the price of the *PDR*. Well written and easy for the lay person to understand. It contains information on 212 generic drugs (1466 brand names) in the form of drug profiles; many useful tables of drug information such as drug interactions, pregnancy, photosensitivity, sleep, alcohol, mood, etc. Clearly defines drug terminology and uses a very straightforward format. Book is indexed by brand and generic names.

292

ADDITIONAL READINGS

Marin, Peter, and Alan Y. Cohen. *Understanding Drug Use—An Adult's Guide to Drugs and the Young.* New York: Harper & Row, 1971.
The authors provide parents of adolescents with perceptive insights into their children and the drug scene. Has a realistic focus and, unlike many other books on the subject, expresses an affection and respect for adolescents. While some specifics may be out of date, the emphasis on people and not drugs is illuminating.

Martin, James K. and Mark Lender. *Drinking in America.* Free Press-Macmillan, 1982.
A historical review of drinking behavior in America from Colonial times to date. Objective and unbiased, it avoids the emotional traps and gives a vivid and humorous account of the 200 years of warfare between wets and drys.

Rubinstein, Morton K. *A Doctor's Guide to Non-Prescription Drugs.* New York: Signet Books, 1977.
A thought-provoking and extremely practical guide. Book is organized by type of illness or condition, making it easy for you to look up drugs by complaint. Contains a lot of educational material about what to take and not to take. Has loads of information about combination drugs. Inexpensive paperback.

Russianoff, Penelope, ed. *Women in Crisis.* New York: Human Sciences Press, 1981.
The proceedings of the first annual Women in Crisis Conference held in New York City in 1979. Contains seven articles directly on women and drugs, including my own on sexism in drug abuse treatment. Entire book is well done and informative. Must reading for those who act as advocates for women.

Sandmaier, Marian. *The Invisible Alcoholics—Women and Alcohol Abuse in America.* New York: McGraw-Hill Book Company, 1980.
One of the best books available on the subject of women and alcohol. Written by the former Director of Women's Programs for the National Clearinghouse for Alcohol Information and Chair of the National Women's Health Network's Alcoholism Policy Committee.

Scher, Jordan M., ed. *Drug Abuse in Industry: Growing Corporate Dilemma.* Springfield, Ill.: Charles C. Thomas, 1973.
Good introduction to basic concerns of drug use in the workplace. Quality of articles varies greatly but gives an excellent first exposure to a complicated issue. My study of drug-related crime in business and industry appears in this volume.

Selye, Hans. *Stress without Distress.* New York: Signet Books, 1974.
Learn about the scientific nature of human stress. Better than the pop psychology books on the same subject. Selye has an interesting philosophy for living as well as being the expert on stress.

Silverman, Harold, and Gilbert Simon. *The Pill Book—The Illustrated Guide to the Most Prescribed Drugs in the United States.* New York: Bantam Books, 1979.
Contains 21 pages of color illustrations of medications. Deals with the 1000 most commonly prescribed drugs with information about drug properties, dosages, side effects, and adverse effects. Has sections on how drugs work, drugs and food, 20 questions to ask about medicine, and other points to remember for safe drug use. Easy to read, inexpensive paperback.

Spotts, James V., and Franklin C. Shontz. *Cocaine Users—A Representative Case Approach.* New York: The Free Press, 1980.
An intensive study of nine different users of cocaine. Background section provides a good introduction to history, pharmacological and physiological actions, and social usage patterns and effects of the drug. Strong emphasis on context and lifestyle of cocaine use.

Weil, Andrew. *The Natural Mind—A New Way of Looking at Drugs and the Higher Consciousness.* Boston: Houghton Mifflin Company, 1972.
One of the most innovative and exciting books on drug use ever written. Goes beyond many stereotypes to explore drug use as a natural pursuit of altered states of consciousness. Easy to read and understand, it will stimulate your thinking about many establishment blind spots about drug use. Explores an interesting dichotomy between "stoned" and "straight" thinking. Dr. Weil is a Harvard-trained physician who provides new ways of thinking about a problem that has divided our nation.

Wolfe, Sidney M., Christopher M. Coley, and the Health Research Group. *Pills That Don't Work—A Consumers' and Doctors' Guide to Over 600 Prescription Drugs That Lack Evidence of Effectiveness.* Farrar, Straus, Giroux: New York, 1980.
We all need this one because the Food and Drug Administration keeps on dragging its feet. The book carefully explains the various categories of drug effectiveness (or lack of same), and then lists over 600 drugs which have failed to meet these definitions but are still on the market. Fascinating reading about a real rip-off.

APPENDIX C:

Where to Get Help

You can obtain educational materials from the following agencies of the Federal Government:

National Clearinghouse for Drug Abuse Information
5600 Fishers Lane, Room 10A–56
Rockville, Maryland 20857

National Clearinghouse for Alcohol Information
Box 2345
Rockville, Maryland 20850

Technical Information Center
Office on Smoking and Health
5600 Fishers Lane, Room 1–16
Rockville, Maryland 20857

National Clearinghouse for Mental Health Information
National Institute of Mental Health
5600 Fishers Lane, Room 11A–33
Rockville, Maryland 20857

National directories of drug abuse and alcoholism treatment programs are available at a nominal cost from:

Superintendent of Documents
U.S. Government Printing Office
Washington, D.C. 20402

Programs are listed by counties within states. In addition, most states have what the federal government has designated as a Single State Agency responsible for drug and alcohol matters. In some states the two are combined, while in others they are separate agencies. Contact your state government for further information.

Information on alcoholism is also available from:

National Council on Alcoholism (NCA)
733 Third Avenue
New York, New York 10017

There exist local affiliates of NCA in most major cities across America. Contact the central office listed above for further information.

For information on Alcoholics Anonymous meetings in your area as well as a variety of pamphlets on A.A.'s philosophy and program, contact:

Alcoholics Anonymous World Services
P.O. Box 459
Grand Central Station
New York, New York 10017
You can usually find an A.A. office in most major cities; contact them for local meeting information.

Al-Anon sponsors self-help groups for spouses, children and other relatives of alcoholics and also has local offices listed in your phone directory. The address for their central office in New York is:

Al-Anon Family Group Headquarters
P.O. Box 182
Madison Square Station
New York, New York 10010

The National Institute of Mental Health has prepared a fact sheet on mutual self-help groups for consumers. It is available at no charge from:

The Consumer Information Center
Department 609K
Pueblo, Colorado 81009

Directories of mutual-help groups are also available from:

National Self-Help Clearinghouse
33 West 42nd Street
Room 1227
New York, New York 10036

For further information on the Toughlove program write to:

Toughlove
Post Office Box 70
Sellersville, Pennsylvania 18960

To find out more about poisons in the home, send a stamped, self-addressed envelope to:

Mr. Anthony DiMarco
New York City Poison Control Project
Bellevue Hospital Center
27th Street and First Avenue
New York, N.Y. 10016

APPENDIX D:

The Marijuana Laws

State & Statute	Amount	Possession: 1st Offense	Possession: 2nd Offense	Cultivation	Sale
Alabama	Up to 2.2 lbs. for personal use	0–1 yr. & $1000	2–15 yrs. & $25,000	2–15 yrs. & $25,000	2–15 yrs. & $25,000
20-2-2 20-2-23 20-2-70 20-2-80	Up to 2.2 lbs. not for personal use	2–15 yrs. & $25,000	2–30 yrs. & $50,000	2–15 yrs. & $25,000	2–15 yrs. & $25,000
	2.2–2000 lbs.	5–15 yrs. & $25,000	3–30 yrs. & $50,000	3–15 yrs. & $25,000	3–15 yrs. & $25,000
	2000–10,000 lbs.	5–15 yrs. & $50,000	5–30 yrs. & $100,000	5–15 yrs. & $50,000	5–15 yrs. & $50,000
	More than 10,000 lbs.	15 years & $200,000	15–30 yrs. & $400,000	15 yrs. & $200,000	15 yrs. & $200,000
Alaska	Any amount for private personal use in home	Legal	Legal	Legal	n/a
	Any amount for personal use not in a public place	$0–100	$0–100	$0–100	n/a
17.10.010	Up to 1 oz. in public	$0–100	$0–100	$0–100	n/a
	Smoking marijuana in public	$0–1000	$0–1000	n/a	n/a
through 17.12.150	More than 1 oz. in public for personal use	$0–1000	$0–1000	n/a	n/a

State & Statute	Amount	Possession: 1st Offense	Possession: 2nd Offense	Cultivation	Sale
Alaska (cont.)	Any amount for personal use in car or by a person under 18 yrs.	$0–1000	$0–1000	$0–1000	n/a
Arizona 36–1001 36–1002. 05 & 06	More than 1 oz. not for personal use	0–25 yrs. & $20,000	0–life & $25,000	0–25 yrs. & $25,000	0–25 yrs. & $25,000
	Any amount	1½ yrs. & $0–150,000	1½–3 yrs. & $0–150,000	1½ yrs. & $0–150,000	7 yrs. & $150,000
Arkansas 82.2601	Up to 1 oz.	0–1 yr. & $1000	0–5 yrs. & $10,000	2–10 yrs. & $10,000	2–10 yrs. & $10,000
82.2614 82.2617 41.901	Over 1 oz. (Rebuttable presumption of intent to deliver)	2–10 yrs. & $10,000	2–10 yrs. & $10,000	2–10 yrs. & $10,000	2–10 yrs. & $10,000
California Health & Safety Code 11357 thru 11360	Up to 1 oz.	$0–100	$0–100	$0–100	2–4 yrs.
	Over 1 oz.	0–6 mos. & $500	0–6 mos. & $500	16 mos.–3 yrs.	2–4 yrs.
Colorado 12.22.403 12.22.412	Up to 1 oz. not in public	$0–100	$0–100	1–14 yrs. & $1000	1–14 yrs. & $1000

300

Statute	Amount	1st Offense	2nd Offense	Cultivation	Sale
Colorado (cont.)	Up to 1 oz. in public	0–15 days & $100	0–15 days & $100	1–14 yrs. & $1000	1–14 yrs. & $1000
	More than 1 oz.	0–1 yr. & $500	Probation–2 yrs. & $500–1000	1–14 yrs. & $1000	1–14 yrs. & $1000
Connecticut	Less than 4 oz.	0–1 yr. & $1000	0–5 yrs. & $3000	0–2 yrs. & $1000	0–7 yrs. & $1000
19.443 19.480 19.481	Over 4 oz.	0–5 yrs. & $2000	0–10 yrs. & $5000	0–2 yrs. & $1000	0–7 yrs. & $1000
19.480A 19.450A	More than 2.2 lbs.	0–5 yrs. & $2000	0–10 yrs. & $5000	5–20 yrs.	5–20 yrs.
Delaware 16.4701 16.4714 16.4752 through 16.4754	Any amount	0–2 yrs. & $500	0–7 yrs. & $500	0–10 yrs. & $1000–10,000	0–10 yrs. & $1000–10,000
Florida 893.02 893.13 through 16.4754	Up to 20 grams	0–1 yr. & $1000	0–1 yr. & $1000	0–5 yrs. & $5000	0–5 yrs. & $5000
	20 grams–100 lbs.	0–5 yrs. & $5000	0–5 yrs. & $5000	0–5 yrs. & $5000	0–5 yrs. & $5000
	100–2000 lbs.	3–30 yrs. & $25,000	3–30 yrs. & $25,000	3–30 yrs. & $25,000	3–30 yrs. & $25,000
	2000–10,000 lbs.	5–30 yrs. & $50,000	5–30 yrs. & $50,000	5–30 yrs. & $50,000	5–30 yrs. & $50,000

State & Statute	Amount	Possession: 1st Offense	Possession: 2nd Offense	Cultivation	Sale
Florida (cont.)	Over 10,000 lbs.	15–30 yrs. & $200,000	15–30 yrs. & $200,000	15–30 yrs. & $200,000	15–30 yrs. & $200,000
Georgia 79A.802 79A.811	Up to 1 oz.	0–1 yr. & $1000	1–10 yrs.	1–10 yrs.	1–10 yrs.
79A.9917	1 oz.–100 lbs.	1–10 yrs.	1–10 yrs.	1–10 yrs.	1–10 yrs.
	100–2000 lbs.	5–10 yrs. & $25,000	5–10 yrs. & $25,000	5–10 yrs. & $25,000	5–10 yrs. & $25,000
	2000–10,000 lbs.	7–10 yrs. & $50,000	7–10 yrs. & $50,000	7–10 yrs. & $50,000	7–10 yrs. & $50,000
	More than 10,000 lbs.	15 yrs. & $200,000	15 yrs. & $200,000	15 yrs. & $200,000	15 yrs. & $200,000
Hawaii 712.1240 712.1249	Up to 1 oz.	0–30 days & $500	0–30 days & $500	0–30 days & $500	0–1 yr. & $1000
706.640	1–2 oz.	0–1 yr. & $1000	0–1 yr. & $1000	0–1 yr. & $1000	0–1 yr. & $1000
	2 oz.–2.2 lbs.	0–1 yr. & $1000	0–1 yr. & $1000	0–1 yr. & $1000	0–5 yrs. & $5000
	More than 2.2 lbs.	0–5 yrs. & $5000	0–5 yrs. & $5000	0–5 yrs. & $5000	0–5 yrs. & $5000

State & Statute	Amount	Possession: 1st Offense	Possession: 2nd Offense	Cultivation	Sale
Idaho 37.2701 37.2705	Up to 3 oz.	0–1 yr. & $1000	0–2 yrs. & $2000	0–5 yrs. & $15,000	0–5 yrs. & $15,000
37.2732	More than 3 oz.	0–5 yrs. & $10,000	0–10 yrs. & $20,000	0–5 yrs. & $15,000	0–5 yrs. & $15,000
Illinois 56.5.703 through	Up to 2.5 grams	0–30 days & $500	0–30 days & $500	0–6 mos. & $500	0–6 mos. & $500
56.5.705 38.1005 8.1,9.1	2.5–10 grams	0–6 mos. & $500	0–6 mos. & $500	0–1 yr. & $1000	0–1 yr. & $1000
	10–30 grams	0–1 yr. & $1000	1–3 yrs. & $10,000	1–3 yrs. & $10,000	1–3 yrs. & $10,000
	30–500 grams	1–3 yrs. & $10,000	2–5 yrs. & $10,000	2–5 yrs. & $10,000	2–5 yrs. & $10,000
	Over 500 grams	2–5 yrs. & $10,000	2–5 yrs. & $10,000	3–7 yrs. & $10,000	3–7 yrs. & $10,000
Indiana 35.48.1.1 35.48.2.4	Up to 30 grams	0–1 yr. & $5000	0–2 yrs. & $10,000	0–1 yr. & $5000	0–1 yr. & $5000
35.48.4. 10–12	More than 30 grams	0–2 yrs. & $10,000	0–2 yrs. & $10,000	0–2 yrs. & $10,000	0–2 yrs. & $10,000
Iowa 204.101 204.204	Any amount	0–6 mos. & $1000	0–18 mos. & $3000		

State & Statute	Amount	Possession: 1st Offense	Possession: 2nd Offense	Cultivation	Sale
204.401 204.410 204.411	Under 1 oz.			0–6 mos. & $1000	0–6 mos. & $1000
	Over 1 oz.			0–5 yrs. & $1000	0–5 yrs. & $1000
Kansas 65.4101 65.4105 65.4127B 21.4501 through 21.4503	Any amount	0–1 yr. & $2500	1–10 yrs. & $5000	0–1 yr. & $2500	1–20 yrs. & $10,000
Kentucky 218A.010 218A.050 218A.990	Any amount	0–90 days & $250	0–90 days & $250	0–1 yr. & $500	0–1 yr. & $500
Louisiana 40.961 40.964 40.967	Up to 100 lbs.	0–6 mos. & $500	0–5 yrs. & $2000	0–10 yrs. & $15,000	0–10 yrs. & $15,000
	100–2000 lbs.	5–10 yrs. & $25,000	5–10 yrs. & $25,000	5–10 yrs. & $25,000	5–10 yrs. & $25,000
	2000–10,000 lbs.	10–15 yrs. & $50,000	10–15 yrs. & $50,000	10–15 yrs. & $50,000	10–15 yrs. & $50,000
	More than 10,000 lbs.	15–20 yrs. & $200,000	15–20 yrs. & $200,000	15–20 yrs. & $200,000	15–20 yrs. & $200,000

State & Statute	Amount	Possession 1st Offense	Possession 2nd Offense	Cultivation	Sale
Maine 17A.1107 through 17A.1103 17A.1106 22.2383	Up to 1½ oz. for personal use	$0–200	$0–200	$0–200	n/a
	1½ oz.–2 lbs.	(presumed to be for sale)		0–1 yr. & $1000	0–1 yr. & $1000
	2 to 1000 lbs.	(presumed to be for sale)		0–5 yrs. & $2500	0–5 yrs. & $2500
	More than 1000 lbs.	(presumed to be for sale)		0–10 yrs. & $10,000	0–10 yrs. & $10,000
Maryland 27.277 27.279 27.286 27.286A 27.293 27.287	Any amount for personal use	0–1 yr. & $1000	0–2 yrs. & $2000	0–1 yr. & $1000	n/a
	Any amount not for personal use	0–5 yrs. & $15,000	0–10 yrs. & $30,000	0–5 yrs. & $15,000	0–5 yrs. & $15,000
	More than 100 lbs. imported into state	0–25 yrs. & $50,000	0–50 yrs. & $100,000	n/a	0–25 yrs. & $50,000
Massachusetts 94C.1 94C.31	Any amount	Probation	0–6 mos. & $500	0–2 yrs. & $5000	1–2 yrs. & $5000
94C.34 94C.32C.	50–100 lbs.			Mandatory 1 yr. & $500–10,000	Mandatory 1 yr. & $500–10,000

305

State & Statute	Amount	Possession: 1st Offense	Possession: 2nd Offense	Cultivation	Sale
Massachusetts (cont.)	100–2000 lbs.			Mandatory 3 yrs. & $2500–25,000	Mandatory 3 yrs. & $2500–25,000
	2000–10,000 lbs.			Mandatory 5 yrs. & $5000–50,000	Mandatory 5 yrs. & $5000–50,000
	More than 10,000 lbs.			Mandatory 10 yrs. & $20,000–200,000	Mandatory 10 yrs. & $20,000–200,000
Michigan 333.7403	Any amount	0–1 yr. & $1000	0–2 yrs. & $2000	0–4 yrs. & $2000	0–4 yrs. & $2000
Minnesota 152.01 152.02	Up to 1½ oz.	$0–100	0–90 days & $500	0–5 yrs. & $15,000	0–5 yrs. & $15,000
152.15	More than 1½ oz.	0–3 yrs. & $3000	0–6 yrs. & $5000	0–5 yrs. & $15,000	0–5 yrs. & $15,000
Mississippi 41.29.105 41.29.115	Up to 1 oz. (not in vehicle)	$100–250	5–60 days & $250	0–10 yrs. & $15,000	0–20 yrs. & $30,000
41.29.139	Up to 1 oz. (in vehicle)	0–90 days & $500	0–180 days & $1000	0–10 yrs. & $15,000	0–20 yrs. & $30,000
41.29.147	1 oz.–1 kilo (2.2 lbs.)	0–3 yrs. & $3000	0–6 yrs. & $6000	0–10 yrs. & $15,000	0–20 yrs. & $30,000

State & Statute	Amount	Possession: 1st Offense	Possession: 2nd Offense	Cultivation	Sale
Mississippi (cont.)	More than 1 kilo	Mandatory 3 yrs. & $10,000	Mandatory 6 yrs. & $20,000	0–10 yrs. & $15,000	3–20 yrs. & $30,000
Missouri 195.010 195.017	Up to 35 grams	0–1 yr. & $1000	0–5 yrs. & $1000	0–5 yrs. & $1000	5 yrs.–life
195.200	Over 35 grams	0–5 yrs. & $1000	0–5 yrs. & $1000	0–5 yrs. & $1000	5 yrs.–life
Montana 45.9.101 through	Up to 60 grams	0–1 yr. & $1000	0–3 yrs. & $1000	1 yr.–life	1 yr.–life
45.9.103	More than 60 grams	0–5 yrs.	0–5 yrs.	1 yr.–life	1 yr.–life
Nebraska 28.401	Up to 1 oz.	$100	0–5 days & $200	0–5 yrs. & $10,000	0–20 yrs. & $10,000
28.405 28.416	1 oz.–1 lb.	0–7 days & $500	0–7 days & $500	0–5 yrs. & $10,000	0–20 yrs. & $10,000
	More than 1 lb.	0–5 yrs. & $10,000	0–5 yrs. & $10,000	0–5 yrs. & $10,000	0–20 yrs. & $10,000
Nevada 453.096 453.161 453.337	Up to 1 oz. by a person under 21	0–6 yrs. & $1000	1–6 yrs. & $5000	1–15 yrs. & $5000	1–15 yrs. & $5000
453.336	Any amount, all other ages	0–6 yrs. & $5000	1–10 yrs. & $20,000	1–15 yrs. & $5000	1–15 yrs. & $5000
New Hampshire 318B.26	Up to 1 lb.	0–1 yr. & $1000	0–7 yrs. & $2000	0–15 yrs. & $2000	0–15 yrs. & $2000

State & Statute	Amount	Possession: 1st Offense	Possession: 2nd Offense	Cultivation	Sale
New Hampshire (cont.)	More than 1 lb.	0–7 yrs. & $2000	0–15 yrs. & $2000	0–15 yrs. & $2000	0–15 yrs. & $2000
New Jersey 24.21.5	Up to 25 grams	0–6 mos. & $500	0–6 mos. & $500	0–5 yrs. & $15,000	0–5 yrs. & $15,000
24.21.2 24.21.19 24.21.20	More than 25 grams	0–5 yrs. & $15,000	0–5 yrs. & $15,000	0–5 yrs. & $15,000	0–5 yrs. & $15,000
New Mexico 30.31.2	Up to 1 oz.	0–15 days & $50–100	0–1 yr. & $100–1000	9 yrs. & $0–10,000	18 mos. & $0–5000
30.31.6 30.31.22 30.31.23	1–8 oz.	0–1 yr. & $100–1000	0–1 yr. & $100–1000	9 yrs. & $0–10,000	18 mos. & $0–5000
30.31.28	8 oz.–100 lbs.	0–5 yrs. & $5000	1–5 yrs. & $5000	9 yrs. & $0–10,000	18 mos. & $0–5000
31.18.15	Over 100 lbs.	3 yrs. & $0–5000	9 yrs. & $0–10,000	9 yrs. & $0–10,000	18 mos. & $0–5000
New York Penal 221.00 through 221.55	Up to 25 grams in private	$0–100	$0–200	0–1 yr. & $1000	0–1 yr. & $1000
Public Health 3382	25 grams–2 oz., or 2 oz. in public	0–3 mos. & $500	0–3 mos. & $500	0–1 yr. & $1000	0–4 yrs.

Statute	Amount	1st Offense	2nd Offense	Cultivation	Sale
3306	2–4 oz.	0–1 yr. & $1000	0–1 yr. & $1000	0–1 yr. & $1000	0–4 yrs.
3302	4–8 oz.	0–1 yr. & $1000	0–1 yr. & $1000	0–1 yr. & $1000	0–7 yrs.
	8 oz.–1 lb.	0–4 yrs.	0–4 yrs.	0–4 yrs.	0–7 yrs.
	1–10 lbs.	0–7 yrs.	0–7 yrs.	0–7 yrs.	0–15 yrs.
	Over 10 lbs.	0–15 yrs.	0–15 yrs.	0–15 yrs.	0–15 yrs.
North Carolina 90.87	Up to 1 oz.	$100	$100	$100	0–5 yrs. & $5000
90.94	1 oz.–50 lbs.	0–5 yrs. & $5000	0–5 yrs. & $5000	0–5 yrs. & $5000	0–5 yrs. & $5000
90.95 90.95(h)	50–100 lbs.	0–5 yrs. & $5000+	0–5 yrs. & $5000+	0–5 yrs. & $5000+	0–5 yrs. & $5000+
	100–2000 lbs.	7+ yrs. & $25,000+	7+ yrs. & $25,000+	7+ yrs. & $25,000+	7+ yrs. & $25,000+
	2000–10,000 lbs.	14 yrs.+ & $50,000+	14 yrs.+ & $50,000+	14 yrs.+ & $50,000+	14 yrs.+ & $50,000+
	10,000 lbs. or more	35 yrs.+ & $200,000	35 yrs.+ & $200,000	35 yrs.+ & $200,000	35 yrs.+ & $200,000
North Dakota 19.03.1. 01 05	Up to ½ oz. not in vehicle	0–30 days & $500	0–60 days & $1000	0–10 yrs. & $10,000	0–10 yrs. & $10,000
23	½–1 oz., or up to 1 oz. in vehicle	0–1 yr. & $1000	0–2 yrs. & $2000	0–10 yrs. & $10,000	0–10 yrs. & $10,000

State & Statute	Amount	Possession: 1st Offense	Possession: 2nd Offense	Cultivation	Sale
North Dakota (cont.)	More than 1 oz.	0–5 yrs. & $5000	0–5 yrs. & $5000	0–10 yrs. & $10,000	0–10 yrs. & $10,000
Ohio 2925.01 2925.11	Up to 100 grams	$0–100	$0–100	6 mos.–5 yrs. & $2500	6 mos.–5 yrs. & $2500
	100–200 grams	0–30 days & $250	0–30 days & $250	6 mos.–5 yrs. & $2500	6 mos.–5 yrs. & $2500
	200–600 grams	6 mos.–5 yrs. & $2500	1–10 yrs. & $5000	1–10 yrs. & $5000	1–10 yrs. & $5000
	More than 600 grams	1–10 yrs. & $5000	2–15 yrs. & $7500	2–15 yrs. & $7500	2–15 yrs. & $7500
Oklahoma 63.2.101 63.2.201 63.2.401 63.2.402	Any amount	0–1 yr.	2–10 yrs.	2–10 yrs. & $5000	2–10 yrs. & $5000
Oregon 475.005 475.992	Up to 1 oz.	$0–100	$0–100	0–10 yrs. & $2500	0–10 yrs. & $2500
	More than 1 oz.	0–10 yrs. & $2500	0–10 yrs. & $2500	0–10 yrs. & $2500	0–10 yrs. & $2500
Pennsylvania 35.780.	Up to 30 grams	0–30 days & $500	0–30 days & $500	0–5 yrs. & $15,000	0–5 yrs. & $15,000

310

State & Statute	Amount	Possession 1st Offense	Possession 2nd Offense	Cultivation	Sale
113	More than 30 grams	0–1 yr. & $5000	0–3 yrs. & $25,000	0–3 yrs. & $25,000	0–3 yrs. & $25,000
Rhode Island 21.28. 1.02 2.08 4.01 4.11	Any amount	0–1 yr. & $500	0–2 yrs. & $1000	0–30 yrs. & $50,000	0–30 yrs. & $50,000
South Carolina 44.53 370 190 110	Up to 1 oz.	0–30 days & $100–200	0–1 yr. & $200–1000	0–5 yrs. & $5000	0–5 yrs. & $5000
	More than 1 oz.	0–6 mos. & $1000	0–1 yr. & $2000	0–5 yrs. & $5000	0–5 yrs. & $5000
	10–100 lbs. (presumed for sale)			1–10 yrs. & $10,000	1–10 yrs. & $10,000
	100–2000 lbs. (presumed for sale)			5–25 yrs. & $25,000	5–25 yrs. & $25,000
	2000–10,000 lbs. (presumed for sale)			10–25 yrs. & $50,000	10–25 yrs. & $50,000
	Over 10,000 lbs. (presumed for sale)			15–30 yrs. & $200,000	15–30 yrs. & $200,000
South Dakota 22.42.1	Up to 1 oz.	0–30 days & $100	0–30 days & $100	0–30 days & $100	0–1 yr. & $1000

State & Statute	Amount	Possession: 1st Offense	Possession: 2nd Offense	Cultivation	Sale
22.42.6 22.42.7	1–8 oz.	0–1 yr. & $1000	0–1 yr. & $1000	0–1 yr. & $1000	0–2 yrs. & $2000
	8 oz.–1 lb.	0–1 yr. & $1000	0–1 yr. & $1000	0–1 yr. & $1000	0–5 yrs. & $5000
	Over 1 lb.	0–2 yrs. & $2000	0–2 yrs. & $2000	0–2 yrs. & $2000	0–5 yrs. & $5000
Tennessee 52.1409 52.1422 52.1432	Up to ½ oz.	0–1 yr. & $1000	1–2 yrs.	1–5 yrs. & $3000	0–1 yr. & $1000
	More than ½ oz.	0–1 yr. & $1000	1–2 yrs.	1–5 yrs. & $3000	1–5 yrs. & $3000
Texas 4476.15 1.02 2.03 4.05 4.01	Up to 2 oz.	0–180 days & $1000	30–180 days & $1000	0–180 days & $1000	2–10 yrs. & $5000
	2–4 oz.	0–1 yr. & $2000	90 days–1 yr. & $2000	0–1 yr. & $2000	2–10 yrs. & $5000
	4 oz.–50 lbs.	2–10 yrs. & $5000	2–20 yrs. & $10,000	2–10 yrs. & $5000	2–10 yrs. & $5000
	Over 50 lbs.	Up to life & $500,000	Up to life & $500,000	Up to life & $500,000	Up to life & $500,000
Utah 58.37.2 58.37.4 58.37.8	Any amount	0–6 mos. & $299	0–1 yr. & $1000	0–5 yrs. & $5000	0–5 yrs. & $5000

Statute	Amount	1st Offense	2nd Offense	Cultivation	Sale
Vermont T.18 4201	Up to ½ oz.	0–6 mos. & $500	0–2 yrs. & $2000	0–5 yrs. & $5000	0–5 yrs. & $5000
4224	½–2 oz.	0–3 yrs. & $3000	0–3 yrs. & $3000	0–5 yrs. & $5000	0–5 yrs. & $5000
	More than 2 oz.	0–5 yrs. & $5000	0–5 yrs. & $5000	0–5 yrs. & $5000	0–5 yrs. & $5000
Virginia 18.2 247.1	Up to ½ oz.	0–30 days & $500	0–1 yr. & $1000	0–30 days & $500	0–1 yr. & $1000
248.1	½ oz.–2 lbs.	0–30 days & $500	0–1 yr. & $1000	0–30 days & $500	0–10 yrs. & $1000
	More than 2 oz.	0–30 days & $500	0–1 yr. & $1000	5–30 yrs.	5–30 yrs.
Washington 69.50 101	Up to 40 grams	0–90 days & $250	0–90 days & $250	0–5 yrs. & $10,000	0–5 yrs. & $10,000
204	More than 40 grams	0–5 yrs. & $10,000	0–10 yrs. & $10,000	0–5 yrs. & $10,000	0–5 yrs. & $10,000
West Virginia 1.101 2.204	Any amount	3–6 mos. & $1000	3 mos.–1 yr. & $2000	1–5 yrs. & $15,000	1–5 yrs. & $15,000
	(Possession of less than 15 grams: presumption is against intent to distribute. Can get conditional discharge.)				
Wisconsin 161.01 161.14 161.41	Any amount	0–30 days & $500	0–30 days & $500	0–15 yrs. & $15,000	0–5 yrs. & $15,000

State & Statute	Amount	Possession: 1st Offense	Possession: 2nd Offense	Cultivation	Sale
Wyoming 35.7 1002 1014 1031 1038 1040	Any amount	0–6 mos. & $1000	0–1 yr. & $2000	0–6 mos. & $1000	0–10 yrs. & $10,000
District of Columbia 33.401	Any amount	0–1 yr. & $100–1000	0–10 yrs. & $500–5000	0–1 yr. & $100–1000	0–1 yr. & $100–1000
Federal Law 21 USC.841	Any amount	0–1 yr. & $5000	0–2 yrs. & $10,000	0–5 yrs. & $15,000	0–5 yrs. & $15,000

Notes

INTRODUCTION

Knowles, J., Ed. *Doing Better and Feeling Worse: Health in the United States.* New York: W. W. Norton, 1977, page 80.

CHAPTER ONE

1. Adapted from the pamphlet entitled *Drinking Etiquette* printed by the National Institute on Alcoholism and Alcohol Abuse, 1980.
2. Body weight standards taken from *The Book of Health—A Complete Guide to Making Health Last a Lifetime.* E. L. Wynder (Ed.), Franklin Watts, New York, 1981, page 289.
3. Mayer, Jean. *A Diet for Living,* David McKay Company, New York, page 65.
4. Erikson, E. H. *Childhood and Society,* W. W. Norton & Company, New York, 1963, page 80.
5. Freud, S. *A General Introduction to Psychoanalysis,* Washington Square Press, Inc., New York, 1963, page 364.
6. Fuqua, P. *Drug Abuse: Investigation and Control,* Gregg Division, McGraw-Hill Book Company, New York, page 12.

CHAPTER TWO

1. Rachal, V. J. et al. *Adolescent Drinking Behavior, Volume I, The Extent and Nature of Adolescent Alcohol and Drug Use: The 1974 and 1978 National Sample Studies,*

Center for the Study of Social Behavior, Research Triangle Institute, October 1980, adapted from page 52.
2. Farley, E. C., Santo, Y. and Speck, D. W. Multiple Drug Abuse Patterns of Youths in Treatment. Chapter in *Youth Drug Abuse: Problems, Issues, and Treatment,* Beschner, G. M. and Friedman, A. S. (Eds.) Lexington Books, Lexington, Mass., 1979, page 154.
3. Ingalls, Z. Higher Education's Drinking Problem, *The Chronicle of Higher Education,* Volume XXIV, Number 21, July 21, 1982, page 1.
4. Daum, M. and Lavenhar, M. A. *Religiosity and Drug Use: A Study of Jewish and Gentile College Students,* Services Research Report, National Institute on Drug Abuse, U.S. Department of Health, Education and Welfare, 1980, page 20.
5. *New York Times,* Life and Death of a Campus Drug Dealer, Sunday, September 5, 1982, page 1.

CHAPTER THREE

1. National Clearinghouse for Alcohol Information, National Institute on Alcohol Abuse and Alcoholism, *Alcohol and the Military,* Alcohol Topics In Brief, RPO 362, February 1982, page 2.
2. Levy, S. J. A Study of Drug Related Crime in Business and Industry. Chapter in *Drug Abuse in Industry: Growing Corporate Dilemma,* Scher, J. M. (Ed.), Charles C. Thomas, Springfield, Ill., 1973, pages 143–157.
3. Slaby, A. E. et al. *Handbook of Psychiatric Emergencies: A Guide for Emergencies in Psychiatry,* Medical Examination Publishing Company, Flushing, New York, 1975, page 70.
4. Selye, H. *Stress Without Distress,* Signet, 1974.
5. Reese, D. and Underwood, J. I'm Not Worth a Damn, *Sports Illustrated,* Volume 56, No. 24, June 14, 1982, page 1.
6. List adapted from *New York Times* article entitled New Health Plans focus on "Wellness," August 24, 1981, page D7.

CHAPTER FOUR

1. Preston, T. *The Clay Pedestal: A Re-examination of the Doctor Patient Relationship,* Madrona Publishers, Seattle, 1981, back flap.
2. Smith, M. C. and Knapp, D. *Pharmacy, Drugs and Medical Care,* Williams and Wilkins Company, Baltimore, 1972, pages 173 and 174.
3. Task Force on Women, *Deciding About Drugs—A Woman's Choice,* National Institute on Drug Abuse, U.S. Department of Health, Education and Welfare, 1979, page 13.
4. Burack, R. *The New Handbook of Prescription Drugs,* Ballantine, New York, 1976, p. xxii.
5. Medical News. Physician Prescribing Practices Criticized; Solutions in Question. *Journal of the American Medical Association,* 241:2353–2360, 1979.
6. Table adapted from Prescription Drug Abuse, *Consumers' Research Magazine,* January 1983, Volume 65, No. 1, page 25.
7. Hastings, A. C., Fadiman, J. and Gordon, J. S. *Health for the Whole Person—The Complete Guide to Holistic Medicine,* Bantam Books, New York, 1981, pages 17–26.

NOTES

CHAPTER FIVE

1. Mack, R. E. What's Really in Alcoholic Drinks?, *Update: News about Alcoholism and Related Issues,* New York City Affiliate, Inc., National Council on Alcoholism, Vol. III, No. 7, November–December 1982, page 5.
2. Morgan, J. P., and Kagan, D. Street Amphetamine Quality and the Controlled Substance Act of 1970, *Journal of Psychoactive Drugs,* Vol. 10(4), 1978.
3. Jones, E. *The Life and Work of Sigmund Freud,* Anchor Doubleday, Garden City, New York, 1963, page 55.
4. Table adapted from Bush, P. J. *Drugs, Alcohol and Sex,* Marek, New York, 1980, pages 255–258 and Long, J. W. *The Essential Guide to Prescription Drugs,* Harper and Row, New York, 1980, page 809.

Index

Acid (*see* LSD)
Acupuncture, 215
Addictive behavior:
  defenses against, 37–38
  elements of, 230
  terminology of, 203–204
Additive effects, of drug combinations, 239, 240
Aging, medication in, 181–183
Al-Anon, 44, 53, 296
Alateen, 44, 52, 53
Alcohol consumption:
  allergic reactions in, 218
  and automobile accidents (*see* Drunk driving)
  with cigarette smoking, 128–129
  coffee drinking with, 34, 258
  and drug use, 31–32, 56–57, 238, 239–242
    methaqualone, 233
  family influence and, 3–4
    discussion guidelines for, 33–36
  legal age for, 35, 69, 260
  with medications, 170–171, 172, 173

  in pregnancy, 164, 278
  rise in, 253
  in schools and colleges, 59, 60t, 61t, 62, 64t, 66–69, 68t, 72–74
Alcohol content:
  in alcoholic beverages, 34–35
  in medications, 274–277
Alcoholic beverages, contents of, 34–35, 217–218
Alcoholics Anonymous, 296
Alcoholism:
  in army, 109
  defined, 34, 72
    self-assessment test for, 35–37
  drug abuse with, 239, 241
  family history and, 34
  family impact of, 42–43, 53–54
  information sources on, 296
  stereotypes about, 33
  withdrawal reaction in, 32
  in women, 196
  in workforce, 110–111
Alpert, Richard, 71
Amotivational syndrome, 48–49

Amphetamines, 271–272
  with alcohol, 240–241
  dealer substitutions for, 221, 222
  deaths and emergencies from, 205
  and pregnancy, 165
  in schools, 64t, 65t, 68t
  side effects of, 271–272
  in sports, 143
  uses for, 220, 222
  for women, 196
Amyl nitrates, 60t, 286–287
Anacin, 190–191
Analgesic drugs, 207
  advertising claims for, 190–191
  (*See also Specific types*)
Angel dust (*see* PCP)
Anslinger, Harry, 15
Antibiotics, tetracycline in, 178
Antidepressants, 283–284
  with alcohol, 241
  side effects of, 283–284
  tricyclic, 284
Antihistamines:
  activity limitations with, 171
  with alcohol, 241
Antipsychotic drugs, 280–281
Aphrodisiacs:
  drugs as, 242–252
    cocaine, 228
    methaqualone, 232, 233
    placebo effect in, 244
  Spanish Fly, 244–245
Army, U.S., drug use in, 108–110
Aspirin, 175, 193
  drug interactions with, 173
  in pain relief products, 190, 191
  in pregnancy, 164
Athletes, drug use by, 84–85, 140–143
Autogenic training, 213–214
Automobile accidents, alcohol-related, 32–33, 67, 69, 257–261
  (*See also* Drunk driving)

Bachman, Jerald, 59
Barbiturates, 278–279
  with alcohol, 240, 279
  in pregnancy, 165

  in schools, 60t, 64t, 65, 68t
  side effects of, 278
Belushi, John, 227
Bhang, 285
Biofeedback, 213
Bladder cancer, caffeine and, 120
Blood alcohol content (BAC), body weight and, 257
Bootlegs, 222
Brain function, nutrients and, 138
Breast feeding, drug use in, 164, 272, 281
Brompton's Mixture, 208
Bufferin, 190
Burack, Richard, 189
Butyl nitrates, 60t, 286–287

Caffeine:
  with cigarette smoking, 120
  daily consumption of, 115, 118
  in food and drugs, 116–117, 273–274
  health effects of, 118–121, 274
  hyperactivity and, 138
  intake reduction for, 121–123
  intoxification, 75–76, 114–115
  in pregnancy, 120–121
  (*See also* Coffee drinking)
Cancer:
  and cigarette smoking, 125, 126, 129
    passive inhalation in, 54
  coffee drinking and, 120
  marijuana smoking in, 47
Cannabis (*see* Marijuana)
Carbohydrates, craving for, 138
Cardiopulmonary resuscitation (CPR), 262–270
"Chasing the dragon," 234
Childproof container caps, 166
Children:
  accidental poisoning of, 166–167
  alcohol consumption by, 59, 60t, 61t, 62, 64t, 66–67, 68–69, 72–74
  choking first aid for, 267
  of drug abusers, 50–54
  drug free modeling by, 99–103
  drug use by:
    clique membership and, 82–84
    family influence on, 1–4

Children (*cont.*)
  parent relations and (*see* Family(ies), and drug use)
  peer influence on, 62, 63t, 64, 78–82
  in school and college, 59–71
  eating health habits for, 7
  health education for, 151, 154–156
  medications for, 176–181
  administration of, 179–180
  dosage of, 178–179
  tetracycline in, 177–178
Chiropractic, 214
Chlorpromazine (*see* Thorazine)
Chocolate, caffeine content of, 116
Choking, first aid for, 265–267
Cigarette smoking:
  addictive, 123–124, 127–128
  with alcohol consumption, 128–129
  in automobiles, 55–56
  and caffeine, 120, 173
  fire deaths from, 126
  health risks of, 125–126, 129
  in home, 54–56
  incidence of, 124
  of low-tar and nicotine brands, 129
  passive inhalation and, 54, 126, 128
  in pregnancy, 121, 126, 164
  quitting strategies for, 127, 131–133
  in schools, 59, 60t, 61t, 64t
  under stress, 129, 130–131
Clay Pedestal, The (Preston), 154
Cliques, and drug use, 82–84
Coca-Cola, 225
Cocaine (coke), 272–273
  abuse of, 227, 230
  treatment for, 231
  administration of, 227
  as aphrodisiac, 228
  athlete use of, 140–141
  cost of, 224, 229
  crashing from, 228–229
  dealer substitutions for, 221
  deaths and emergencies from, 205, 227
  freebasing, 226–227, 230
  with heroin, 227
  in nostrums, 225
  physical problems with, 229–230
  psychic dependency on, 226, 228
  recreational usage of, 230–231
  in schools, 60t, 61t, 64t, 65, 68t
  side effects of, 272
Cocoa, caffeine content of, 116
Coffee drinking:
  alcohol intoxication and, 34, 241, 258
  caffeine content and, 116
  health effects of, 118, 119, 120
  reduction of, 122
  and smoking interaction, 173
  (*See also* Caffeine)
Congeners, 218
Cold remedies, 107
  alcohol content of, 274–277
  antihistamines in, 171
  caffeine in, 117
  for children, 178
  effectiveness of, 193
Coley, Christopher M., 192
Colleges (*see* Schools and Colleges)
Comprehensive Drug Abuse Prevention and Control Act, 16–18
Contraindications, 168–169
Controlled Substances Act of 1970, 16–18

Dalmane (*see* Flurazepam)
Denial, of drug problem, 38
  objective confrontation in, 43–44
Depression, drug therapy for, 161
Diazepam (*see* Valium)
Diet:
  calorie intake in, 134, 135
  with drug therapy, 170
  food additives and, 135–137
  salt and sugar, 136–137
  mood and behavior and, 137–139
  physical exercise and, 133–134
  for weight loss, 134, 135
  for working people, 139–140
  (*See also* Eating behavior)
Diuretics, caffeine in, 117
DMT (dimethyltriptamine), 285, 286
Doctors:
  chemically dependent, 187
  drug knowledge of, 188–189, 191–192

Doctors (*cont.*)
  as drug pushers, 187
  patient relations with, 151–157, 163
    drug information in, 193–194, 210–211
    women patients, 194–198, 199–203
Dow Chemical Company, 145
Driving while intoxicated (DWI)
  standards, 257–258
Drug(s):
  adverse reactions to, 162–163, 219–220, 223–224, 229, 233, 271–287
    choking, 265–267
    heart attack, 263
    life support procedures in, 261–270
    psychological, 268–270
    seizure, 264, 267–268
    stroke, 264
  alcohol consumption with, 233, 238, 239–242
  body damage from, 31–32
    prescription drugs and, 56–57
  allergies to, 162–163, 278
  combinations of, 67–68, 223–224, 238–242
  dealing in:
    broad definition of, 252–254
    dangers of, 96
    law and, 95–96, 97–99
    profits in, 96
    substitutions in, 220–222
  information sources for, 295–296
  laws, 16, 207
    on drug dealing, 95–96, 97–99
    drug schedules under, 16–18
    on marijuana use, 18, 95, 97
    by state, 299–314
    reform of, 18–19, 97
  look-alike, 221, 222
  prevention programs:
    for employees, 145–147
    in schools, 87–94
  side effects of, 161–162, 185–186, 219–220, 271–287
  withdrawal from, 115, 174, 203
  (*See also Specific types*)

Drug taking behavior:
  at college and university (*see* Schools and colleges, drug use in)
  family and (*see* Family, and drug use)
  image *vs* true self and, 11–12
  levels of, 37
  for medical therapy (*see* Medications)
  for pain avoidance, 8–12
    by athletes, 142
  for pleasure, 13–15, 19–20, 85–86
    at parties, 253–256, 262
    (*See also* Pleasure drugs)
  during pregnancy, 163–166, 280, 281
    aspirin, 164
    marijuana, 285
  problem, 37–47, 49–50
    acute *vs* chronic, 38–39
    of alcoholics, 239, 241
    with cocaine, 227, 230
    deaths and emergencies from, 204–205
    defenses against, 37–38
    depression and anxiety in, 39–40
    family response to, 42–47
    with heroin, 235–236
    with methaqualone, 233
    of parents, 50–54
    self-assessment for, 41–42, 147–149
    support groups for, 44, 52, 53
    therapy in, 46–47
  in schools (*see* Schools and colleges, drug use in)
  stepping stone theory of, 71–72
  at work (*see* Workplace, drug use in)
  by women, 196, 197
Drunk driving:
  blood alcohol content (BAC) and, 257
  fatalities and costs of, 32–33, 67, 69, 258–259
  laws on, 259–260
  protection against, 260–261
Dysphoria, 228–229

Eating behavior:
  addictive, 134–135
  early experience and, 4–5, 6
  healthful, 7–8, 139–140
  moderation concept and, 2

Eating behavior (cont.)
  stress effects on, 131
  (See also Diet; Obesity)
Eggheads (clique), 83
Elavil (amitriptyline), 161
Elderly, medications for, 181–183
Employee Assistance Program (EAP),
  145–147
Endorphins, 172
Erikson, Erik, 7
Esters, 288
Ethyl alcohol (see Alcohol consumption;
  Alcohol content; Alcoholic beverages)
Ethyl nitrite, 128–129

Family(ies):
  and alcohol consumption, 3–4
  discussion guidelines for, 33–36
  and drug use:
    discussions about, 24–26, 76–78
    limit setting on, 26–31, 44
    marijuana, 47–49
    moderation concept and, 1–3
    by parents, 50–54
    privacy vs control in, 20–23
    in problem situations, 42–47
  eating behavior in, 2, 4–5, 6–7
  pain management model in, 12–13
  parental smoking in, 54–56
Fat cells, formation of, 6
Federal Trade Commission (FTC), 192
Fetal alcohol syndrome (FAS), 50, 278
Flagyl (metronidazole), 173
Flurazepam (Dalmane), 204
Food:
  additives, 135–137
  (See also Diet; Eating behavior)
Food and Drug Administration (FDA),
  192, 193, 194
  on caffeine, 119–120
Freebasing, 226–227, 230
Freons, 288
Freud, Sigmund, 225
Functional addiction, 204, 280

Ganja, 285, 286
Gasoline, leaded, 289
Generic drugs, 158

Glycols, 289
Goldberg, Theodore, 158
Goody-Goodies (clique), 83
Gordon, Barbara, 174
Goyan, Jere, 120
Greizerstein, Hebe B., 217–218

Hallucinogens, 285–286
  in schools, 60t, 61t, 68t
Harrison Narcotic Act of 1914, 16, 207,
  225
Hashish, 68t, 285
Heads (clique), 83
Health care:
  doctor patient relations for, 151–157
  expenses on, 150
  medicine cabinet products for, 175–176
  (See also Holistic medicine)
Heart attacks:
  caffeine in, 120
  cigarette smoking in, 125
  obesity in, 133
  warning signs of, 263
Herbal cooking, 255, 256
Hitters (clique), 82
Heroin, 31–32
  abuse of, 235–236
  administration of, 234
  alcohol consumption with, 240
  cocaine with, 227
  dealer substitutions for, 221
  deaths and emergencies from, 204
  orgasmic rush with, 234–235
  Persian, 234
  price of, 234
  in schools, 60t, 61t, 64t, 65t, 68t
  sexual function and, 249
  side effects of, 282–283
Hoffman, Albert, 71
Holistic medicine:
  elements of, 150–151, 211–213
  techniques and therapies of, 213–215
Homeopathic medicine, 215
Hormone use, by athletes, 141–142
Hospice mix, 208
Hospice movement, pain management in,
  208

Hospital Corporation of America, 145
Hydrocarbons:
  aliphatic, 287
  aromatic, 287
  halogenated, 288
Hyperactivity, caffeine in, 138
Hypnosis, 214
Hypnotics, alcohol consumption with, 240

I'm Dancing as Fast as I Can (Gordon), 174
Infants:
  choking first aid for, 267
  eating behavior in, 4–5, 6–7
Inhalants:
  in schools, 60t, 61t, 64t, 68t
  volatile, 249, 286–289
Ipecac, 167, 175
International Business Machines (IBM), 145
Isobutyl nitrate, 286–287

Jews:
  alcoholism among, 33
  drug abuse among, 69–70
Jocks (clique), 83
Johnson, Lloyd, 59

Kennecott Corporation, 146
Ketamine, 282
Ketones, 288
Kimberly-Clark Corporation, 145
Koop, C. Everett, 127

Laws:
  on drinking age, 35, 69, 260
  for drug regulation, 16–19, 207
    drug dealing and, 95–96, 97–99
    of marijuana, 18, 95, 97, 299–314
  on drunk driving, 259–260
Laxatives, dependency on, 209
Leary, Timothy, 71
Leisure drugs (*see* Pleasure drugs)
Lemmon 714, 222
Life support procedures, in drug reactions, 261–270
Lithium, 9–10
Look-alike drugs, 221, 222

Lovers (clique), 83
LSD (acid):
  adverse reaction to, 261, 286
  deaths and emergencies from, 205
  in schools and colleges, 60t, 64t, 70–71
Ludes (*see* Methaqualone)
Lung cancer, cigarette smoking and, 125, 129

MAO (monoamine oxidase), 170, 171, 271, 282, 283–284
Marijuana, 284–285
  abuse of, 49–50
  alcohol consumption with, 240
  deaths and emergencies from, 205
  health effects of, 47–49, 50, 285
  laws on, 18, 95, 97
    by state, 299–314
  low-grade, 219–220
  paraquat-adulterated, 24
  PCP with, 282
  in pregnancy, 165, 285
  in schools and colleges, 59, 60t, 61t, 62, 64t, 65, 66, 68t, 71
    peer influence on, 79
  stepping stone theory of, 71–72
  super strains of, 39, 236–238
Mayer, Jean, 6, 120, 121
Medical profession (*see* Doctors)
Medications:
  activity limitations with, 171–172
  addictive, 203–211
    deaths and emergencies from, 204–205
  adverse reactions to, 162–163
  advertising and promotion of, 188, 190–191
    women in, 197
  alcohol content of, 274–277
  benefit/risk ratio for, 159–160
  for children, 176–181
  contraindications to, 168–169
  dosage instructions for, 160–161
  drug-to-drug interactions of, 172–173
  education campaign on, 192–193
  for elderly, 181–183
  expenditures on, 150–151
  with food and drink, 169–171
  for home medicine chest, 175–176

Medications (cont.)
in homeopathic medicine, 215
me-too products, 189–190
patient knowledge of, 156–158
pharmacist advice on, 184, 185–186
phenacetin in, 209–210
physician knowledge of, 188–189, 191–192
sexual function and, 245, 246–247
side effects of, 161–162
storage and dating of, 166–167
withdrawal effects of, 174
(See also Over-the counter (OTC) drugs;
Prescription drugs)
Medicine (see Holistic medicine)
Meditation, 214
Memory, stimulant drugs and, 74–75
Meprobamate (Dalmane), 280
Mescaline, 285, 286
Methaqualone, 279
adulterated, 232
alcohol consumption with, 233
as aphrodisiac, 232, 233
dealer substitutions for, 221, 222
deaths and emergencies from, 204
prescription of, 231–232
in schools, 60t
side effects of, 233, 279
Methylxanthines, 118
Miller, Sanford, 119, 120
Monoamine oxidase (see MAO)
Morgan, John, 222
Morphine, 207, 208, 240
Mothers Against Drunk Drivers (MADD),
259, 260
Murphy, Samuel, Jr., 191

Nasal septum, perforation of, 229
Nasal spray, dependency upon, 209
National Council on Alcoholism (NCA),
296
National Football League (NFL), cocaine
use in, 140–141
National Organization for the Reform of
Marijuana Laws (NORML), 18
National Organization for Women (NOW),
201
Neurotransmitters, 138

New Handbook of Prescription Drugs, The
(Burack), 189
New York Telephone Company, 145
Nicotine, 124–125, 273
(See also Cigarette smoking)
Nonprescription drugs (see Over-the
counter drugs)
Norepinephrine, 138

Obesity:
body fat and, 5
family influence on, 2, 4–5, 6–7
fat cell hypothesis of, 6
health risks of, 133
incidence of, 6
(See also Eating behavior)
Objective confrontation process, 43–44
O'Malley, Patrick, 59
Opiates, 282–283
in over-the-counter (OTC) drugs, 206–207
in schools, 60t, 61t, 68t
(See also Specific types)
Oral contraceptives, contraindications to,
168–169
Orgasm, 248, 249
Orinase, 158
Ornade, 158
Over-the-counter (OTC) drugs, 68t
addictive, 206–207, 209–210
advertising claims for, 190–191
antihistamines in, 171
caffeine content of, 117
for children, 178
cocaine in, 225
in pregnancy, 165–166
aspirin, 164
(See also Cold remedies; Medications)
Overweight (see Obesity)

Pain management:
drug use for, 8–12
by athletes, 141–142
by hospice movement, 208
of over-the counter (OTC) drugs, 206–208
family model for, 12–13
self honesty in, 11–12

Pain relief drugs, caffeine in, 117
Parents (*see* Family[ies])
Parest (*see* Methaqualone)
Party giving:
 intoxicated guests at, 258, 260
 with pleasure drugs, 253–256
 adverse reactions and, 262
Passive inhalation, 54, 126, 128
Patient package inserts (PPIs), 193, 194
PCP (phencyclidine), 281–282
 deaths and emergencies from, 205
 in schools, 60t, 68t
 side effects of, 219–220, 282
Peer group influence:
 for drug free modeling, 99–103
 and drug use, 62, 63t, 64, 78–82
 on sports teams, 142–143
Pentazocine (Talwin), 205, 208, 273
Pepsico, Inc., 145
Persian heroin, 234
Pertschuk, Michael, 190
Peterson, Robert C., 230
Pharmacists:
 ethical dilemmas of, 184–185
 relations with, 183–184, 186–187
 selection criteria for, 185–186
Phenacetin (acetophenetidim), 209–210, 273
Phencyclidine (*see* PCP)
Phenobarbital, 222
Phenothiazine, 208, 281
Physical addiction, 203
Physicians (*see* Doctors)
Physicians' Desk Reference (PDR), 188, 189–190
Pills That Don't Work (Wolfe and Coley), 192
Placebo effect, 191, 244
Pleasure drugs, 13–15, 19–20
 administration of, 217, 227, 234
 as aphrodisiacs, 228, 232, 233, 242–252
 cocaine, 224–231
 content knowledge for, 217–219
 dealer substitutions of, 220–222
 defined, 216
 dosage titration for, 222–223
 equipment sharing and, 224
 family conflict over, 14–15, 19–20

heroin, 233–236
 methaqualone, 231–233
 mixing of, 223–224, 238–242
 party giving with, 253–256
 side effects from, 219–220
 social relationships and, 85–86
 (*See also* Drug[s]; Drug taking behavior)
Poisons, in home, 166–167, 297
Polypharmacy, defined, 238
Potentiation, 239
Pregnancy:
 alcohol consumption in, 50, 164, 278
 caffeine in, 120–121
 cigarette smoking in, 121, 126, 164
 drug use in, 50, 163–166, 280, 281
 aspirin, 164
 marijuana, 285
Prescription drugs:
 abuse of, 204–206
 alcohol consumption with, 56–57
 with caffeine, 122
 dangers of sharing, 174
 dosage instructions for, 160–161
 generic substitutions in, 158
 ineffective, 192
 patient package inserts (PPIs) with, 193, 194
 patient queries about, 193–194
 for women, 196, 199–201
 (*See also* Medications)
Preston, Thomas, 154
Privacy behavior, in families, 21–23
 drug use and, 20–21
Propoxyphene (Darvon), 240, 273
Pryor, Richard, 226, 261
Psilocybin, 285, 286
Psychological addiction, 203–204
Psychotherapists:
 selection guidelines for, 201–203
 sexism among, 196
Pure Food and Drugs Act (1906), 207

Quääludes (*see* Methaqualone)

Rapoport, Judith, 138
Recreational drugs (*see* Pleasure drugs)
Reese, Don, 140

Religion, and drug use, 69–70
Rockers (clique), 83

St. Christopher's hospice, London, 208
Salt:
elimination of, 137
health problems from, 136
Sativa, 237
Schools and colleges:
alcohol consumption in, 59, 60t, 61t, 62, 64t, 66–69, 72
drug use in, 58
availability and, 64–65
clique membership and, 82–83
grade of first use, 59, 60t
of LSD, 70–71
of multiple substances, 67–68
parental action in, 73–74
peer influence on, 62, 63t, 64, 78–82
prevalence and recency of, 59, 61–62
prevention programs for, 87–94
religiosity and, 69–70
risk factors for, 69–70, 72
sports and, 84–85
as study aids, 74–78
Sedatives:
alcohol consumption with, 240, 274–277
barbiturates, 278–279
contraindications for, 277
nonbarbiturates, 279
in schools, 60t, 61t, 64t
side effects of, 277–278
(*See also* Tranquilizers)
Seizures, warning signs of, 264, 268
Selye, Hans, 129, 130
Serotonin, 138
Sexual function:
and drug enhancers, 242–252
cocaine, 228
methaqualone, 232, 233
drug interference with, 245, 246–247, 249, 283
medication effects on, 171
Sexual response cycle, drug effects on, 248
Side effects, 271–287
in drug therapy, 161–162
pharmacist advice on, 185–186
from pleasure drugs, 219–220

Sinsemilla, 236–237
Smoking (*see* Cigarette smoking; Marijuana)
Smuts, Jan Christiaan, 150
Soda, caffeine content of, 116–117
Sopor (*see* Methaqualone)
Spanish Fly, 244–245
Speed (*see* Amphetamines)
Speedball, 227
Sports, and drug use, 84–85, 140–143
Spyker, Daniel, 167
Stepping stone theory, of drug use, 71–72
Steroids, 141–142
Stimulant drugs, 271–274
alcohol consumption with, 240–241
caffeine in, 117
effects on memory, 74–75
in schools, 60t, 61t
as study aids, 74–75
in sports, 143
(*See also Specific types*)
STP (2, 5-dimethoxy-4-methyl-amphetamine), 261–262, 285, 286
Street drugs (*see* Pleasure drugs)
Stress:
defined, 129–130
eating behavior and, 131
smoking and, 130–131
Stroke, warning signs of, 264
Sugar:
effect on mood, 138, 139
elimination of, 137
health problems from, 136
Sulfur dioxide, in alcoholic beverages, 218
Supra-additive, 239
Synergism, 239

Talwin (*see* Pentazocine)
Tardive dyskinesia, 281
Tea, caffeine content of, 116
Tetracycline:
in medications, 178
side effects of, 177
Tetrahydrocannabinol (*see* THC)
THC (tetrahydrocannabinol), 8–9, 39
in marijuana, 236, 237, 240, 285
Theophylline, 273

Thorazine (chlorpromazine), 281
  for adverse reactions, 261–262
Time perception, drug alteration of, 223, 242
Titration, of drug dosage, 222–223
Tobacco:
  history of, 124
  (*See also* Cigarette smoking)
Tolerance to drugs, 203, 238
  and cross-tolerance, 238–239
Tooth development, tetracycline effect on, 177
Toughlove, 30–31, 297
Tranquilizers:
  alcohol consumption and, 240
  as antipsychotic, 280–281
  functional addiction to, 280
  in pregnancy, 165, 280
  in schools, 60t, 61t, 64t, 65, 68t
    as study aid, 76
  side effects of, 280
  for women, 196
Tricyclic antidepressants, 284
Tryptophan, 138
Tyramine, 170
Tyrosine, 138

University (*see* Schools and colleges)

Valium (diazepam), 158
  addiction to, 204, 210, 280
  for adverse reactions, 262
  alcohol consumption with, 172
  as maintenance drug, 9
  substitutions for, 221, 222
  withdrawal from, 174
Vietnam veterans, drug use by, 109–110

Vin Mariani, 225
Volatile inhalants, 286–289
  physical effects of, 287–289
  sexual function and, 249

Wegscheider, Sharon, 53
Weight loss, 134, 135
  aids to, 117, 272
Weinbaum, Barry S., 96
Withdrawal reaction:
  from alcohol, 32
  from caffeine, 115
  from medications, 174, 203
Wolfe, Sidney, 192
Women:
  doctor relations with, 194–198
  doctor selection by, 199–203
  drug taking behavior of, 196, 197
  medications for, 196, 199–201
  psychotherapy for, 201–203
  support groups for, 201
Workplace, drug use in, 106–107
  alcohol consumption, 110
  in army, 108–110
  caffeine, 114–123
  crimes related to, 112–113
  employee assistance programs for, 145–147
  nicotine, 123–133
  self-assessment of, 147–149
  in sports, 140–143
Wurtman, Judith, 138
Wurtman, Richard, 137–138

Xanthines (*see* Caffeine)

York, David and Phyllis, 30–31